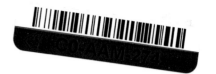

Ophthalmic Drug Delivery Systems

DRUGS AND THE PHARMACEUTICAL SCIENCES

A Series of Textbooks and Monographs

edited by

James Swarbrick
School of Pharmacy
University of North Carolina
Chapel Hill, North Carolina

58. Ophthalmic Drug Delivery Systems, *edited by Ashim K. Mitra*

ADDITIONAL VOLUMES IN PREPARATION

Pharmaceutical Skin Penetration Enhancement, *edited by Kenneth A. Walters and Jonathan Hadgraft*

Pharmaceutical Particulate Carriers: Therapeutic Applications, *edited by Alain Rolland*

Colonic Drug Absorption and Metabolism, *edited by Peter R. Bieck*

Drug Permeation Enhancement: Theory and Applications, edited by *Dean S. Hsieh*

Ophthalmic Drug Delivery Systems

edited by

Ashim K. Mitra

School of Pharmacy and Pharmacal Sciences
Purdue University
West Lafayette, Indiana

Marcel Dekker, Inc.   **New York • Basel • Hong Kong**

Library of Congress Cataloging-in-Publication Data

Ophthalmic drug delivery systems / edited by Ashim K. Mitra.
      p.   cm. -- (Drugs and the pharmaceutical sciences ; 58)
    Includes bibliographical references and index.
    ISBN 0-8247-8806-0 (alk. paper)
    1. Ophthalmic drugs. 2. Drug delivery systems. I. Mitra, Ashim
K. II. Series: Drugs and the pharmaceutical sciences ;
v. 58.
    [DNLM: 1. Eye diseases--drug therapy. 2. Ophthalmic Solutions-
-administration & dosage.   W1 DR893B v. 58 / WW 166 0603]
RE994.062 1993
617.7'061--dc20
DNLM/DLC
for Library of Congress   92-48325
                                                        CIP

This book is printed on acid-free paper.

MARCEL DEKKER, INC.
270 Madison Avenue, New York, New York 10016

Current printing (last digit):
10 9 8 7 6 5 4 3 2 1

PRINTED IN THE UNITED STATES OF AMERICA

To the memory of my mentor,
the late Professor Thomas J. Mikkelson

Foreword

Successful drug treatment of various eye pathologies depends on the intrinsic activity of the drug, the ability of the drug to cross numerous biological barriers to reach the biophase, and maintenance of the drug in the biophase for an extended period. This last factor in particular is highly dependent on the drug delivery system used, be it a frequently dosed or sustained delivery system. In an idealized case, the drug delivery system is based on the pharmaco-dynamics/pharmacokinetics of the drug. Unfortunately, the human ocular disposition characteristics of virtually every important drug are incomplete or unknown. It is therefore necessary either to employ animal models, whose relation to humans is largely unknown, or to operate empirically in designing ocular drug delivery systems. Despite these severe limitations, significant improvements in ocular drug delivery have been made over the past 10–20 years, and, although by most standards these systems are fairly primitive, they point the way to more improved drug delivery systems.

As an isolated, highly protected organ, the eye is very difficult to study from a drug delivery point of view. Because specimens of eye tissue containing drugs cannot routinely be taken from humans, one is forced to use animal models as a guide. Moreover, each of the three primary modes of drug delivery—systemic, topical application to the surface of the eye, and direct injection into the eye—carries a substantial penalty. The order of preference, in cases where a choice is possible, appears to be topical dosing, systemic delivery, and direct injection. But even the topical route has very substantial clearance mechanisms that cause removal of drugs and delivery systems, which results in typical low drug bioavailability.

An adequate description of the moving frontier of ocular drug disposition and drug delivery has not previously been brought together in a useful text. Admittedly there are several chapters, in various teaching texts, dealing with ocular drug delivery systems, but none is comprehensive enough to provide all elements in the design and evaluation of ocular drug delivery systems. From this perspective the present text is overdue. Perhaps more importantly, the present text will prove a benchmark for ocular drug delivery technology and identify those basic elements of ocular drug disposition that are pertinent to drug delivery as well as the current technical issues for improving ocular drug bioavailability and duration.

It should be clear that the primary direct beneficiary of improved ocular drug delivery is the patient. What is not as obvious—but which remains of great importance—is that drug screening for useful ocular drugs improves as our understanding and application of ocular drug delivery systems improve.

Attaching a start date to a particular field is always risky, given that earlier pioneering scientists cannot be ignored. Nevertheless, the field of ocular pharmacokinetics is about 25 years old, whereas the emerging area of ocular pharmacodynamics is much younger, perhaps 5–10 years old. Steady significant advances in ocular drug delivery have been made over the last 15 years and are growing steadily. It is hoped that this much-needed text on ocular drug delivery interfaces the past, present, and future.

Joseph R. Robinson, Ph.D.
School of Pharmacy
University of Wisconsin
Madison, Wisconsin

Preface

A major goal of pharmacotherapeutics is the attainment of an effective drug concentration at the intended site of action for a desired length of time. Efficient delivery of a drug while minimizing its systemic and/or local side effects is the key to the treatment of ocular diseases. The unique anatomy and physiology of the eye offer many challenges toward developing effective ophthalmic drug delivery systems. Currently, the body of knowledge in this field is rapidly expanding. Systems range from simple solutions to novel delivery systems such as biodegradable polymeric systems, inserts, corneal collagen shields, and iontophoresis, to name a few. An increase in the knowledge of ocular drug absorption and disposition mechanisms has led to the development of many of these new systems.

The goal of this book is to lay the foundation necessary for understanding constraints of ophthalmic drug delivery and to review the systems currently available and/or in various stages of research and development. The book begins with a brief discussion of the anatomy and physiology of the eye relevant to ocular drug delivery. Precorneal barriers as well as corneal barriers to ocular drug absorption are discussed. A review of both the conventional and novel delivery systems follows. The book attempts to stress the fact that simple instillation of drug solution in the cul-de-sac is not always acceptable and emphasizes the need for the development of newer and more efficient systems.

The introductory section (Part I) investigates the fundamental variables inherent to ocular drug delivery. The three chapters in this section review the iatrogenic pathologies incurred by topical ocular drug therapy, the relevant ocular anatomy and physiology, and the constraints imposed by the eye upon successful delivery. A quantifying model of drug permeability and ocular bioavailability is a prerequisite for the selection of an optimal drug candidate.

Part II of the book opens with a discussion of pharmacokinetics relevant to ocular drug delivery. This chapter is followed by a critique of current pharmacokinetic models. The next chapter on animal pharmacokinetic studies provides valuable practical information on the variables inherent in using rabbits as an experimental model. Cell culture and animal models for assessing the efficiency of ocular drug delivery systems are covered next. Disease state models, also presented in this section, allow the pharmaceutical scientist or ocular pharmacologist to investigate the efficacy of various treatment modalities in animals possessing disease states similar to human ocular diseases.

Parts III and IV are divided into traditional and advanced corneal delivery systems. Traditional delivery systems display typical pulsed absorption while attempts are being made to increase ocular bioavailability by minimizing the precorneal losses from topical administrations of solutions, suspensions, and semisolids. Bioadhesives, ocular inserts, corneal collagen shields, particulates, and liposomal delivery systems are discussed in the context of advanced corneal delivery systems.

Improved transcorneal permeation of topical ocular drugs through prodrug derivatization and analogue synthesis is the focus of Part V of this book.

Iontophoresis as a device for ocular antibiotic delivery and diagnostic tool is described in the section on novel drug delivery systems (Part VI). Penetration enhancers and a new ophthalmic delivery system (ocular film) are also discussed in this section. A water-soluble, drug-loaded ocular film developed to circumvent the precorneal loss of topically administered drugs is gaining increasing patient acceptance over previously introduced ocular inserts. Endophthalmous and cytomegaloviral retinitis, for example, are among a host of other ocular pathologies that are not amenable to topical drug delivery.

Part VII considers noncorneal routes of ocular drug delivery, including intracameral, intravitreal, and retinal delivery systems as well as systemic therapy for ocular disease states. The ocular delivery and therapeutics of peptides and proteins have been presented in the two chapters of Part VIII. Regulatory considerations as they pertain to ocular drug delivery constitute the final chapter (Part IX).

Considering the number of recently published papers dealing with ophthalmic drug delivery systems, it is evident that interest in the development of such systems is ever-increasing. One of the objectives of this book is to bring basic scientists, clinicians, and managerial and marketing personnel up to date in this area. I hope that it will also stimulate further research in various unexplored areas of ocular drug delivery.

It has been a pleasure for me to work with distinguished authors who contributed heavily toward the development of this book. In particular, I would like to mention Professor Joseph R. Robinson, who was involved from the inception of the idea to the finalization of the contents of the book. Without his direction and guidance, this task would not have been possible. I would like to extend my sincere appreciation and thanks to Patrick Hughes for his invaluable assistance in the preparation of this volume. Special appreciation also goes to Sandra Beberman and Carol Mayhew of Marcel Dekker, Inc., for their expert help in the preparation of this book. I am also grateful to my wife Ranjana for her encouragement.

Ashim K. Mitra

Contents

Contributors

Rajan Bawa, Ph.D. Manager, New Device Applications, Contact Lens Research & Development, Bausch & Lomb, Rochester, New York

Peter H. Bentley, B.Sc., Ph.D., C.Chem., F.R.S.C. Department of Chemical and Biological Sciences, Smith & Nephew Research Ltd., York University, Science Park, England

Nigel M. Davies, Ph.D., B.Pharm, M.R.Pharm.S. Department of Pharmaceutical Science, School of Pharmacy, University of Otago, Dunedin, New Zealand

Randall J. Erb, Ph.D. Senior Scientist, Clinical Research Foundation, Lenexa, Kansas

Jane L. Greaves, B.Sc., Ph.D. Department of Physiology and Pharmacology, Medical School, Queen's Medical Centre, Nottingham, England

James M. Hill, Ph.D. Professor, Department of Ophthalmology, Louisiana State University Medical Center School of Medicine, New Orleans, Louisiana

Kenneth J. Himmelstein, Ph.D. Professor, Department of Pharmaceutical Sciences, University of Nebraska Medical Center, Omaha, Nebraska

Jeffery A. Hobden, M.S. Graduate Student, Department of Microbiology, Louisiana State University Medical Center School of Medicine, New Orleans, Louisiana

Patrick M. Hughes, B.S. Research Assistant, Department of Industrial and Physical Pharmacy, Purdue University, West Lafayette, Indiana

Herbert E. Kaufman, M.D. Professor and Chairman, Department of Ophthalmology, Louisiana State University Medical Center School of Medicine, New Orleans, Louisiana

Ian W. Kellaway, D.Sc., F.R. Pharm.S. Professor, Welsh School of Pharmacy, University of Wales, Cardiff, Wales

Jörg Kreuter, Ph.D. Professor, Institute of Pharmaceutical Technology, Johann Wolfgang Goethe University, Frankfurt/Main, Germany

Ramesh Krishnamoorthy, M.S. Research Assistant, Department of Industrial and Physical Pharmacy, Purdue University, West Lafayette, Indiana

Vincent H. L. Lee, Ph.D. Gavin S. Herbert Professor and Chairman, Department of Pharmaceutical Sciences, University of Southern California School of Pharmacy, Los Angeles, California

Jiahorng Liaw, Ph.D.   Professor, School of Pharmacy, Taipei Medical College, Taipei, Taiwan

Philip R. Mayer, Ph.D.   Assistant Director, Department of Pharmacokinetics/Drug Metabolism, Alcon Laboratories, Fort Worth, Texas

Ashim K. Mitra, Ph.D.   Associate Professor of Physical Pharmacy, Department of Industrial and Physical Pharmacy, Purdue University, West Lafayette, Indiana

Richard J. O'Callaghan, Ph.D.   Professor, Department of Microbiology, Louisiana State University Medical Center School of Medicine, New Orleans, Louisiana

Orest Olejnik, Ph.D.   Director, Pharmaceutical Development, Allergan Pharmaceuticals, Irvine, California

Gholam A. Peyman, M.D.   Professor of Ophthalmology, Louisiana State University Medical Center School of Medicine, New Orleans, Louisiana

Mark C. Richardson, M.Sc., Ph.D.   Research Manager, Department of Pharmaceutical Sciences, Smith & Nephew Research Ltd., York University, Science Park, England

James C. Robinson, M.D.   Department of Ophthalmology, University of Wisconsin, Madison, Wisconsin

Joseph R. Robinson, Ph.D.   Professor, School of Pharmacy, University of Wisconsin, Madison, Wisconsin

Robert E. Roehrs, Ph.D.   Senior Director, Department of Regulatory Affairs, Alcon Laboratories, Fort Worth, Texas

Lotta Salminen, M.D., Ph.D.   Professor and Chairman, Department of Ophthalmology, Tampere University Hospital, Tampere, Finland

Ronald D. Schoenwald, Ph.D.   Professor, Division of Pharmaceutics, College of Pharmacy, University of Iowa, Iowa City, Iowa

Joel A. Schulman, M.D.   Associate Professor, Department of Ophthalmology, Louisiana State University School of Medicine, Shreveport, Louisiana

Arto Urtti, Ph.D.   Associate Professor, Department of Pharmaceutical Technology, University of Kuopio, Kuopio, Finland

Clive G. Wilson, B.Sc., Ph.D.   Professor, Department of Pharmaceutical Sciences, University of Strathclyde, Royal College, Glasgow, Scotland

Ophthalmic Drug Delivery Systems

1

Overview of Ocular Drug Delivery and Iatrogenic Ocular Cytopathologies

Patrick M. Hughes and Ashim K. Mitra *Purdue University, West Lafayette, Indiana*

I. OVERVIEW: OCULAR DRUG DELIVERY

A. Introduction

Ophthalmic drug delivery is one of the most interesting and challenging endeavors facing the pharmaceutical scientist. The anatomy, physiology, and biochemistry of the eye render this organ exquisitely impervious to foreign substances. The challenge to the formulator is to circumvent the protective barriers of the eye without causing permanent tissue damage. The development of newer, more sensitive diagnostic techniques and therapeutic agents renders an urgency to the development of more successful ocular delivery systems. Potent immunosuppressant therapy in transplant patients and the developing epidemic of acquired immunodeficiency syndrome have generated an entirely new population of patients suffering virulent uveitis and retinopathies. The primitive ophthalmic solution, suspension, and ointment dosage forms are clearly no longer sufficient to combat these diseases, and current research and development efforts to design better therapeutic systems are the primary focus of this text.

The goal of pharmacotherapeutics is to affect a disease state in a consistent and predictable fashion. An assumption is made that a correlation exists between the concentration of a drug at its intended site of action and the resulting pharmacological effect. The specific aim of designing a therapeutic system is to achieve the optimal concentration of a drug entity at the active site for the appropriate duration. Ocular disposition and elimination of a therapeutic agent is dependent upon its physicochemical properties as well as the relevant ocular anatomy and physiology (1). The successful design of a drug delivery system, therefore, requires an integrated knowledge of the drug entity and the constraints to delivery offered by the ocular route of administration.

The eye is subject to a milieu of assaults that can alter virtually any ocular tissues. Hence, the drug entities need to be targeted to many different sites within the globe. Receptors for the mydriatics and miotics are in the iris ciliary body. The active sites for the antibiotics, antivirals, and steroids are the infected or inflamed areas within the anterior as well as the posterior segments of the eye. A host of different tissues are involved, each of which may pose its own challenge to the formulator of ophthalmic delivery systems.

Historically, the bulk of the research has been aimed at delivery to the anterior tissues. Only recently has research been directed at delivery to the tissues of the posterior globe (the uveal tract, vitreous, choroid, and retina).

The aim of this chapter is merely to present the challenges of designing successful ophthalmic delivery systems by way of introduction. The reader is referred to specific chapters within this book for a thorough discussion of the topics introduced in this section.

B. Mechanisms of Ocular Drug Absorption

Topical delivery into the cul-de-sac is, by far, the most common route of ocular drug delivery. Absorption from this site may be corneal or noncorneal. A schematic diagram of the human eye is depicted in Figure. 1. The so-called noncorneal route of absorption

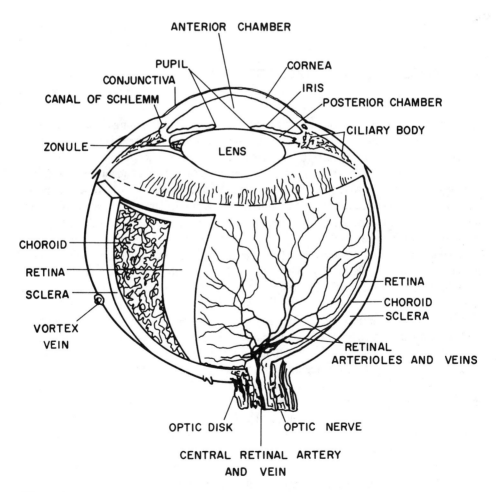

Figure 1. Anatomical structure of the human eye. (From Ref. 12.)

involves penetration across the sclera and conjunctiva into the intraocular tissues. This mechanism of absorption is usually not productive, as drug penetrating the surface of the eye beyond the corneal-scleral limbus is picked up by local capillary beds and removed to the general circulation (2). This noncorneal absorption in general precludes entry into the aqueous humor.

Recent studies, however, suggest that the noncorneal route of absorption may be significant for drug molecules with poor corneal permeability. Studies with inulin (3), timolol maleate (3), gentamicin (4), and prostaglandin PGF$_{2\alpha}$ (5) suggest that these drugs gain intraocular access by diffusion across the conjunctiva and sclera. Patton and Ahmed (3) studied the noncorneal absorption of inulin and timolol maleate. Penetration of these agents into the intraocular tissues appeared to occur from diffusion across the conjunctiva and sclera and not via reentry from the systemic circulation or via absorption into the local vasculature. Both compounds gained access to the iris-ciliary body without entry into the anterior chamber. As much as 40% of inulin absorbed into the eye was determined to be the result of noncorneal absorption.

The noncorneal route of absorption may be significant for poorly cornea-permeable drugs; however, corneal absorption represents the major mechanism of absorption for most therapeutic entities. Topical absorption of these agents, then, is considered to be rate limited by the cornea. The anatomical structures of the cornea exert unique differential solubility requirements for drug candidates. Figure 2 illustrates a cross-section of the cornea. In terms of transcorneal flux of drugs, the cornea can be viewed as a trilaminate structure consisting of three major diffusional barriers: epithelium, stroma, and endothelium. The epithelium and endothelium contain on the order of 100-fold the amount of lipid material per unit mass

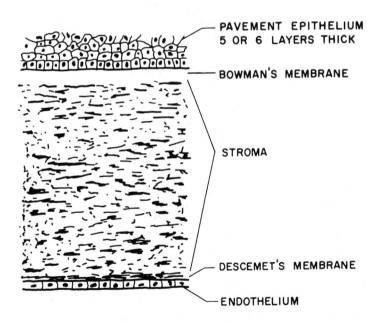

Figure 2.   Cross-sectional view of the corneal membrane depicting various barriers to drug absorption. (From Ref. 12.)

of the stroma (6). Depending on the physicochemical properties of the drug entity, the diffusional resistance offered by these tissues varies greatly (7,8).

The outermost layer, the epithelium, represents the rate-limiting barrier for trans-corneal diffusion of most hydrophilic drugs. The epithelium is composed of five to seven cell layers. The basement cells are columnar in nature, allowing for minimal paracellular transport. The epithelial cells, however, narrow distal to Bowman's membrane, forming flattened epithelial cells with zonulae occludentes interjunctional complexes. This cellular arrangement precludes paracellular transport of most ophthalmic drugs and limits lateral movement within the anterior epithelium (9). Corneal surface epithelial intracellular pore size has been estimated to be about 60 Å (10). Small ionic and hydrophilic molecules appear to gain access to the anterior chamber through these pores (11); however, for most drugs, paracellular transport is precluded by the interjunctional complexes. In a recent review, Lee (10) discusses the attempts made to transiently alter the epithelial integrity at these junctional complexes to improve ocular bioavailability. This approach has, however, only met with moderate success and has the potential to compromise the cornea severely.

Sandwiched between the corneal epithelium and endothelium is the stroma (substantia propria). The stroma comprises 85–90% of the total corneal mass and is composed mainly of hydrated collagen (12). The stroma exerts a diffusional barrier to highly lipophilic drugs owing to its hydrophilic nature. There are no tight junction complexes in the stroma and paracellular transport through this tissue is possible.

The innermost layer of the cornea, separated from the stroma by Descemet's membrane, is the endothelium. The endothelium is lipoidal in nature; however, it does not offer a significant barrier to the transcorneal diffusion of most drugs. Studies have shown that endothelial permeability depends solely on molecular weight and not the charge or hydrophilic nature of the compound (13,14).

Transcellular transport across the corneal epithelium and stroma is the major mechanism of ocular absorption of topically applied ophthalmic pharmaceuticals. This type of Fickian diffusion is dependent upon many factors; i.e., surface area, diffusivity, the concentration gradient established, and the period over which the concentration gradient can be maintained. A parabolic relationship between octanol/water partition coefficient and corneal permeability has been described for many drugs (15–19). The optimal log partition coefficient appears to be in the range of 1–3. The permeability coefficients of 11 steroids were determined by Schoenwald and Ward (15). The permeability versus log partition coefficient fit the typical parabolic relationship, with the optimum log partition coefficient being 2.9. Narurkar and Mitra studied a homologous series of 5' aliphatic esters of 5-iodo-2'-deoxyuridine (IDU) (16,17). In vitro corneal permeabilities were optimized at a log partition coefficient of 0.88, as can be seen graphically in Figure 3 and in Table 1, where CMP represents the corneal permeability values as measured by in vitro perfusion experiments on rabbit corneas (I=IDU, II=IDU-propionoate, III=IDU-butyrate, IV=IDU-isobutyrate, V=IDU-valerate, VI=IDU-pivaloate). A homologous series of n-alkyl-p-aminobenzoate esters in a study by Mosher and Mikkelson fit the parabolic relationship displaying optimal permeability at a log partition coefficient of 2.5 (18). Maximizing bioavailability of ophthalmic medications, then, requires the active compound be neither extremely hydrophilic or lipophilic. To this end, the pH of the postinstillation precorneal fluid becomes an important factor. The postinstillation pH time course will be dictated by the buffer concentration of the formulation. Most ophthalmic formulations are formulated in the pH range of 5–6; hence, depending on the pK_a of the drug to be administered, the

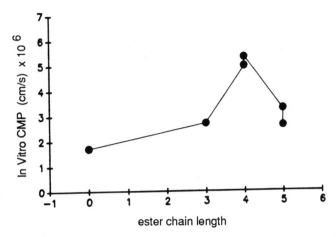

Figure 3. A plot depicting the parabolic relationship between in vitro CMP and ester chain length. (From Ref. 16.)

postinstillation buffering capacity of the formulation may greatly affect the drug's bioavailability. Mitra and Mikkelson studied the effect of varying the concentration of citrate buffer in a pH 4.5 formulation on the miosis versus time profile of a 1% pilocarpine solution (20). The area under the miosis-time profile, maximum pupillary response, and duration of miotic activity were all decreased with increasing buffer concentrations. Figure 4 displays the effect of increasing buffer concentration on the miosis-time profiles for different total molar citrate values (0.0, 0.055, 0.075, 0.110). The ratio of pilocarpinium ion to pilocarpine increases with the postinstillation buffering capacity, thus reducing the net transcorneal flux of pilocarpine.

C. Constraints to Ocular Drug Delivery

Physiological barriers to the diffusion and productive absorption of topically applied ophthalmic drugs exist in the precorneal and corneal spaces. Anterior chamber factors also

Table 1. Physicochemical Properties of IDU and Its 5′-Ester Prodrugs

Compound	m.p. (°C)	Solubility[a] in pH 7.4 phosphate buffer, 25°C (M/L ± SD [$\times 10^3$])	K^a ± SD (octanol/water)
I	168–171 (dec)	5.65 (0.5)	0.11 (0.02)
II	167–168	3.48 (0.3)	4.77 (0.1)
III	145–146	1.45 (0.1)	7.50 (0.3)
IV	144–145	1.75 (0.3)	6.92 (0.8)
V	142–143	0.40 (0.2)	27.54 (2.0)
VI	106–107	0.44 (0.1)	22.10 (1.5)

[a]N = 3.

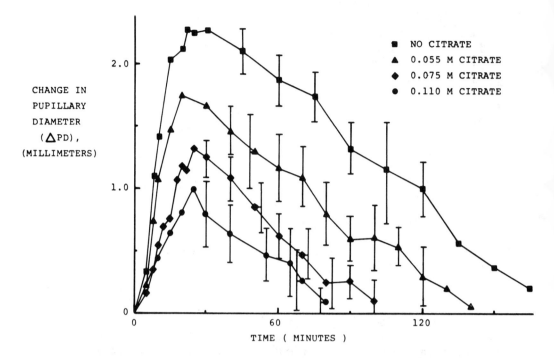

CHANGE IN
PUPILLARY
DIAMETER
(ΔPD),
(MILLIMETERS)

Figure 4. Miosis-time profiles: Plots of the average observed changes in pupillary diameter (ΔPD) as a function of time following the instillation of 25.0 µL of the isotonic 1% pilocarpine nitrate solutions, which contained the different concentrations of citrate buffer. The vertical lines through the data points are ±SD (data points with standard deviation lines omitted is for clarity of the figure). (From Ref. 20.)

greatly influence the disposition of topically applied drugs. Precorneal constraints include solution drainage, lacrimation and tear dilution, tear turnover, and conjunctival absorption. For acceptable bioavailability, a proper duration of contact with the cornea must be maintained. Drug solution drainage away from the precorneal area has been shown to be the most significant factor in reducing this contact time and ocular bioavailability of topical solution dosage forms (21,22). The instilled dose leaves the precorneal area within 5 min of instillation in humans (21,23). The natural tendency of the cul-de-sac is to reduce its fluid volume to 7–10 µL (24–26). The typical ophthalmic dropper delivers 30 µL, most of which is rapidly lost through nasolacrimal drainage immediately following dosing. The drainage may then allow the drug to be systemically absorbed across the nasal mucosa or the gastrointestinal tract (27). Systemic loss from topically applied drugs also occurs from conjunctival absorption into the local circulation. The conjunctiva possesses a relatively large surface area, making this loss significant.

Simple dilution of instilled drug solution in the tears acts to reduce the trans-corneal flux of the drug remaining in the cul-de-sac. Lacrimation can be induced by many factors, including the drug entity, the pH, and the tonicity of the dosage form (28–30). It has been shown that the formulation adjuvants can also stimulate tear production (20).

Tear turnover acts to remove drug solution from the conjunctival cul-de-sac. Normal human tear turnover is approximately 16% per minute, which can also be stimulated by many factors, as described earlier (21,31). These factors, among many others, render topical application of ophthalmic solutions to the cul-de-sac extremely inefficient. Typically, less than 1% of the instilled dose reaches the aqueous humor (27,32). The low fraction of applied dose (1%) of drug solution reaching the anterior chamber further undergoes rapid elimination from the intraocular tissues and fluids. Absorbed drug may exit the eye through the canal of Schlemm or via absorption through the ciliary body or suprachoroid into the episcleral space (27). Enzymatic metabolism of those drug entities possessing labile bonds may account for further loss. Metabolism may occur in the precorneal space or in the cornea (33,34). Age and genetics have been determined to be two important variables in ocular metabolism (35,36).

Clearly, the physiological barriers to topical corneal absorption are formidable. The result is that the clinician is forced to recommend frequent doses of drugs at extremely high concentration. This pulsed type of dosing not only results in extreme fluctuations in ocular drug concentrations but may also cause many untoward side effects. Approaches taken to circumvent this pulsed-type dosing and their ramifications to ocular therapeutics are the subject matter of this text.

II. IATROGENIC OCULAR CYTOPATHOLOGIES

Many approaches have been developed to access specific sites within the globe, including those previously discussed. These techniques are, however, not without detriment. The pulsed dosing of ophthalmic pharmaceuticals result in extremely high transient concentrations of the active drug, vehicle, preservatives, and surfactants. Such types of insults on the delicate ocular tissues, especially the corneal epithelium, can produce functional and morphological changes. The eye represents a collection of highly differentiated and specialized tissues. Morphological and functional changes to these tissues results in varying degrees of vision impairment. It is imperative that these changes be quantified and hopefully minimized or eliminated. The specialized nature of the ocular tissues allows for drug accumulation at specific sites.

The trilaminate, avascular cornea is particularly susceptible to accumulation of various compounds and their metabolites. The lens is extremely sensitive to alterations in its environment, responding by opacification. The aging lens compact lens fibers centrally rather than being sloughed off. The cataractogenic ramifications of this process are obvious.

Iatrogenic ocular cytopathologies relevant to ocular drug delivery may result from any one of the three major modalities: local toxicities resulting from the tropical delivery of ophthalmic pharmaceuticals, systemic toxicities from topical delivery, and ocular manifestations of systemic drug delivery. Numerous investigators have collected an enormous amount of data on these toxicities, a review of which is presented below with the caveat that while the clinical significance of these functional and structural changes may vary, their presence clearly necessitates caution on the part of the formulator. The first two of these modalities are of major concern to formulators of ophthalmic dosage forms. The ocular toxicities from systemic delivery of drugs, moreover can not be ignored. Particularly the synergistic ocular toxicities and cocataractogenisis from the concomitant delivery of both topical ophthalmic formulations and systemic drug administration should be considered.

A. Corneal Pathologies From Topical Delivery

1. Vehicle Effects

The ocular side effects of topically applied drugs are well documented and the corneal tissues are particularly susceptible to alteration and damage. Owing to the transient high concentrations of topically applied ophthalmic formulations, the vehicle as well as the active drug may be implicated.

Vehicles for ophthalmic medications must be adjusted to the proper tonicity, viscosity, buffering and sterility necessary for optimum therapeutics with minimum toxicities. These agents as well as many other adjuvants, however, may alter the morphology and function of the cornea. Among the most frequent adjuvants are the surfactants (i.e., benzalkonium chloride), the mercurial compounds, antioxidants, and other preservatives.

a. Benzalkonium Chloride

Benzalkonium chloride (BAK) falls into the category of surfactant preservatives which exert their bacteriocidal effect by emulsification of the bacterial cell walls. Ocular damage from these agents is most likely due to emulsification of the cell membrane lipids. Benzalkonium is a quaternary cationic surfactant primarily used in ophthalmic preparations as a preservative for its bacteriocidal effect. It is commonly used at concentrations of 0.004–0.02% w/v. Adverse reactions are not uncommon with this preservative, and the epithelial cytotoxicities with even lower concentrations of BAK are well documented (37–45). Emulsification of the cell walls is observed after instillation of a 0.01% solution of BAK (44). Most of the side effects are reversible; however, a significant number of irreversible cytopathologies are also seen. A 1:1000 BAK solution caused irreversible corneal damage with neovascularization (46). Epithelial microvilli are destroyed with 0.01% BAK, preventing adhesion of the mucoid layers of the tear film (45). The compound is known to cause edema, desquamation, punctate keratitis, and papillary conjunctivitis (46).

Morphological and ion permeability studies reveal that punctate keratitis occurs in the anterior epithelia at BAK concentrations of 0.04–0.1% (39,42). Solutions of 0.005, 0.01, and 0.02% BAK and 2 mM cetyl pyridinium chloride were all shown to increase the corneal permeability to fluorescein (43). Cetyl pyridinium chloride causes functional and morphological changes to the ocular tissues similar to those seen with BAK (43). Scanning electron microscopic studies conducted by Pfister and Burstein revealed that BAK caused the corneal epithelial cells to smooth at their edges and loose their microplicae when a 0.01% solution was topically administered to New Zealand albino rabbits (38). Loss of microvilli and elevated cell margins were seen with the application of a 0.0025% solution of BAK to the cat cornea (44). A 0.0075% solution topically applied resulted in the surface cells being peeled off.

In isolated perfused porcine corneal experiments, Camber and Edman determined the effects of various preservatives on the permeability of the corneal epithelium (47). The corneas were bathed in 0.01% BAK, 0.5% chlorobutanol (CB), 0.01% chlorohexidine digluconate (CDG), and 0.04% methylhydroxybenzoate (M) plus 0.02% propylhydroxybenzoate (P). The apparent corneal permeability coefficients for the different perfusion conditions are shown in Table 2. The transcorneal flux of pilocarpine was increased twofold for the BAK bathed corneas. The chlorobutanol-treated corneas also displayed increased pilocarpine penetration but not to the extent of the BAK-treated corneas. They reported that deepithelialization of the cornea resulted in a 2- to 15-fold increase in the transcorneal flux of pilocarpine (48). From this observation the authors postulated that the

Table 2. Effect of Various Agents on the Corneal Permeability of Pilocarpine

Substance	Perfusion condition	Permeability coefficient (cm·s^{-1}) × 10^6 mean (SD)	Mean difference (SD)[a]	Corneal uptake $\frac{\text{(DPM/g of cornea)}}{\text{(DPM/ml of solution)}}$ × 100 mean (SD)	Mean difference (SD)[a]	Number of paired corneas
Pilocarpine HCl	Normal	6.42 (0.68)	—	11.31 (0.98)	—	30[b]
	BAC	10.85 (0.91)	4.44 (1.20)***	19.77 (1.13)	8.08 (1.25)***	6
	CB	11.71 (0.72)	5.04 (1.20)***	16.70 (2.97)	6.22 (2.73)**	6
	CDG	7.15 (0.99)	1.21 (1.22)	13.40 (2.18)	2.12 (1.81)*	6
	M + P	7.89 (0.63)	1.55 (0.93)*	12.17 (1.30)	1.10 (1.32)	6
	Deepithelized cornea	16.78 (2.00)	10.07 (1.88)***	23.82 (2.79)	11.78 (2.53)***	6
Dexamethasone	Normal	0.62 (0.14)	—	10.19 (1.97)	—	30[b]
	BAC	2.07 (0.49)	1.54 (0.50)***	25.50 (5.30)	16.25 (5.66)***	6
	CB	2.91 (0.52)	2.22 (0.56)***	21.47 (5.96)	10.50 (5.68)***	6
	CDG	0.91 (0.53)	0.29 (0.40)	13.93 (3.87)	3.27 (5.59)	6
	M + P	0.93 (0.22)	0.43 (0.22)**	12.90 (1.44)	3.60 (1.40)**	6
	Deepithelized cornea	9.48 (0.63)	8.75 (0.79)***	37.33 (8.57)	26.50 (7.49)***	6

[a]Differences in corneal permeability and uptake between corneas perfused during normal and test conditions tested by Student's t-test for paired observations.
[b]The corneas used are the same as those used as controls in the paired experiments.
Significances denoted by: *$P < 0.05$, **$P < 0.01$, ***$P < 0.001$.

BAK, and to a lesser extent chlorobutanol, must have adverse effects on the functional structure of the corneal epithelium. Electrophysiological measurements revealed functional changes in the epithelium caused by 0.001% BAK, 0.004% thimerosal, and 0.05% chlorobutanol (39).

The rabbit corneal endothelial response to varying concentrations of BAK has been studied in vitro (49–52). Morphological and functional changes in the endothelium occurred even at low BAK concentrations (0.0001%) (50). Green postulated that the effect is similar to that of the corneal epithelium; i.e., swelling of the cornea and lysis and destruction of the cellular membranes (50). Unlike the corneal epithelial cells, the human adult corneal endothelial cells have no regenerative capacity. Hence, BAK should not be used to preserve formulations intended for intraocular use or for corneal preservation.

Topical administration of 0.133% BAK revealed no functional or ultrastructural alterations in the corneal endothelium (50). Caution, however, should still be taken, given the corneal permeability-enhancement effects of BAK and given the fact that direct contact with the endothelium causes the previously mentioned cytopathologies. It is also important to note that most studies are performed on healthy corneas, and it is expected that many of the disease states treated by ophthalmologists will compromise the corneal epithelial integrity. Repeated topical applications of BAK will result in accumulation in the epithelium (58), especially when used concurrently with soft contact lenses (64).

Benzalkonium chloride binds to soft contact lenses and tends to concentrate (53). Parallel use of soft contacts and vehicles contraining BAK can result in severe damage. In one case study, 14 days of concomitant use of soft contact lenses and BAK resulted in neovascularization of the cornea toward the anterior pole outside of Bowman's membrane (53). In another case study, massive superficial keratitis with corneal vascularization was seen with 3 days of parallel use (53).

Studies on most surfactants, including BAK, show a permeability enhancement of the cornea with nonionic, cationic, and anionic surfactants, suggesting at least a transient change in the functional structure of the epithelium (42,43,54–56). Experiments have revealed, however, that the pharmacokinetics and disposition of the surfactant molecules in the eye differ significantly from other hydrophilic drugs (57,58). Pilocarpine is known to leave the ocular tissues within 30 minutes of instillation (58,59). Sixty percent of the long chain detergents, however, are still present 30 min postinstillation, 12% at 6 h, and a significant amount still persists at 24 h (57,58). Age-related changes in accumulation of surfactants has been studied (59). Although elimination of the detergents from the juvenile cornea appears to parallel the adult, a much greater initial uptake is seen, possibly due to the different lipid contents of the tissues. Surfactants are known to impair corneal wound healing (40). The use of these agents as penetration enhancers demands that proper studies be undertaken to address the issue of possible cytotoxicities from their accumulation.

b.   Mercurial Compounds

Adverse ocular side effects to the organomercurials are rare but can sometimes be significant. Twenty percent of the ophthalmic preparations are preserved by one of the three organomercurials; i.e., phenylmercuric acetate, phenylmercuric nitrate, or thimerosal. Thimerosal is usually used in concentrations of 0.001 to 0.01% w/v. Seven days of treatment with 2% topical thimerosal induced no corneal epithelial defects (39). Bluish-gray mercurial deposits may develop in the corneal tissues. These are harmless deposits in the ocular and periocular tissues. They can appear in the cornea, eyelid, conjunctiva, or the lens. Conjunctival mercury deposits are seen in the blood vessels near the cornea, corneal deposits appear in the peripheral Descemet's membrane, and lens deposits occur mainly in the pupillary area (60). These deposits are harmless and rarely interfere with vision.

Hypersensitivity to the organomercurials appears to be the most dramatic side effect incurred with these agents. Hyperemia, edema, and blepharoconjunctivitis may result. Hypersensitivity to the mercurials has been estimated to occur in about 10–50% of the patients (46).

Organomercurials are also known to react with the membrane sulfhydryl groups, altering membrane permeability and transport systems (61). Even low concentrations of 0.001–0.005% w/v commonly used in ophthalmic preparations can cause functional changes (42,62). Thimerosal instilled as a 0.001% solution, however, was determined not to affect corneal wound healing in the rabbit (40). Punctate keratitis and stromal infiltrates have been noted (60). Corneal perfusion experiments with thimerosal resulted in endothelial alterations (62) but no such changes were observed from topical delivery (39).

Use of hydrophilic contact lenses preserved with thimerosal have resulted in detectable levels of mercury in the aqueous humor and cornea (63).

c. Chlorobutanol

Prolonged corneal exposure to chlorobutanol may cause diffuse epithelial damage lasting for several hours (60). This agent has also been observed to concentrate in soft contact lenses causing mild conjunctivitis (64). A concentration of 0.004% w/v in cultured epithelial cells has been known to produce granularity and small vacuole formation (65). In vivo chlorobutanol, however, for the most part is without major toxic effects. Application of a 2% solution for 7 days did not increase the corneal permeability to fluorescein (39,67). No morphological changes were noted with SEM analysis of the corneal surface (38). Chlorobutanol is known to reduce oxygen utilization in the cornea and may result in loosened epithelial adhesions (66).

d. Chlorohexidine Digluconate

Chlorohexidine digluconate at 0.1, 1.0, and 2.0% w/v revealed no gross abnormalities of the epithelial or endothelial layers (67). A mild delay in corneal healing from instillation of a 0.005% solution of chlorohexidine digluconate into rabbits was observed (40). In another study, chlorohexidine diacetate caused an increase in fluorescein permeability of the cornea in vitro but had no effect on corneal wound healing (42).

2. Active Drugs

The side effects of most drugs are known and often tolerated for therapeutic benefit. Many of the ophthalmic side effects from topical ocular delivery of active drugs are not as readily noticed and can result in considerable morbidity considering the labile nature of the ocular tissues. Most common among the side effects is contact dermatitis, usually located in the mucous membranes of local tissues. Follicular hypertrophy occurs with the prolonged use of compounds such as pilocarpine and eserine. Drug-induced keratitis may be mistaken by the clinician for worsening of the disease state, resulting in overdosing and worsening of the clinical picture. Many of the ocular side effects of drugs have been documented; however, only those with major significance will be addressed here. Among these agents are the topical anesthetics, the antiglaucoma agents, antibiotics, and the corticosteroids.

a.   Topical Anesthetics

The topical anesthetics used in ocular therapy include benoxinate, butacaine, dibucaine, dyclonine, proparacaine, and tetracaine, among others. Prolonged use of these agents may result in severe and permanent corneal damage and vision loss. Stromal keratitis and severe ulceration and opacity of the cornea results from topical anesthetic abuse (68–70). Benoxinate, cocaine, lidocaine, and tetracaine can result in the loss of microvilli and can induce plasma membrane defects (64). Morphological irregularities of the anterior epithelia, stromal infiltrates, and neovascularization associated with topical anesthetic instillation are well documented (71,72). Topical cocaine administration results in loosening of the epithelium to such a degree that cocaine is used for epithelial débridement. Topical ocular anesthetics inhibit mitosis and cellular migration (73). As one would expect, delayed epithelial wound healing is seen with these agents.

Researchers have studied the effect of topical anesthetics on the corneoconjunctival surface by measuring the amount of an antibiotic, Cefotiam (CTM), in the tear fluid after intravenous injection of 100 mg/kg CTM (75). Benoxinate 0.4%, oxybuprocaine 0.4%, benzalkonium chloride 0.005%, and NaCl 0.9% as a control were tested by this method. Benoxinate produced the highest concentration of CTM in the tear fluid at all time points, indicating that it most significantly alters the blood-tear barrier.

The stromal tissues are also affected by the topical anesthetics. Rosenwasser et al. reported that six cases of topical anesthetic abuse resulted in epithelial defects and stromal infiltrates (74). Yellowish white rings may develop in the corneal stroma. These rings occur with chronic use, appearing as early as the sixth day and as late as the sixteenth (60). It has been postulated that the stromal keratitis could be the sequelae of an antigen-antibody complex reaction (76). These dense rings resolve upon the discontinuation of therapy.

The effect of these agents on the corneal epithelial microplicae has direct bearing on the tear film layer. Obviously, erosion of the corneal surface followed with the loss of these structures will result in tear film instability.

b.   Antiglaucoma Agents

Pilocarpine.   Decreased visual function is a common side effect of the miotics. Corneal effects from topical pilocarpine therapy are relatively minimal. Instillation of a 2% pilocarpine solution in 0.5-strength Ringer's solution to rabbits caused no increase in the corneal permeability to fluorescein (43). SEM analysis suggested some loss of microvilli and wrinkling of the plasma membranes (38). A 2% solution of pilocarpine has been shown to prevent healing of punctate wounds in the rabbit cornea (77).

Direct corneal perfusion experiments of 2.5% pilocarpine solutions resulted in marked corneal swelling (78). For this reason, pilocarpine should not be used as an irrigation solution.

Epinephrine.   Dark brown or black adenochrome deposits develop in the stroma after prolonged administration of epinephrine (79). These deposits are infrequent and generally occur only after daily use for more than a year or when the corneal epithelial integrity has been compromised by disease or other influences. Administration of a single drop of a 1.25% epinephrine solution resulted in corneal endothelial swelling (55). A 1:1000 injection of a commercial preparation into the anterior chamber resulted in damage to the corneal epithelium; however, sodium bisulfite, the preservative in the formulation, was determined to be the responsible entity (80). Endothelial cell thickness was found to be much lower in nine patients receiving epinephrine as compared to nine placebo controls

(81). Iontophoresed epinephrine is also known to reactivate latent herpes simplex corneal infection (82).

Beta-Blockers. Transient epithelial irregularities are not uncommon with timolol therapy. Punctate and linear epithelial erosions have been noted (83). Timolol, betaxolol, and levobunolol all have caused slow epithelial wound healing (84). A dendritic keratopathy has been reported with topical application of 0.5% betaxolol and 0.5% levobunolol (85). Timolol produced no endothelial changes when topically applied to the cornea (59); however, application of a commercial preparation to cultured bovine endothelial cells did show endothelial toxicity resulting from the BAK preservative (86).

c. Antibiotics

A common side effect resulting from the overuse of topical antibiotics is the colonization by nonsusceptible bacteria and fungi. Gentamicin, neomycin, and tetracycline may produce ocular side effects when topically applied to the eye.

Gentamicin. Gentamicin exerts its toxic effects on cells by concentrating in lysosomes, thereby inhibiting lysosomal phospholipid metabolism (87). Topical application of gentamicin produces few cytopathologies (46). Intrastromal and intracameral injections, however, are a common component of the therapeutic regimens used in the treatment of endophthalmitis. A subconjunctival injection of 40 mg of gentamicin exhibited cellular toxicity and an induced lysosomal storage process (51). Dense bodies and a deformed nucleus were noted. A 1000 µg injection of gentamicin into the anterior chamber produced endothelial toxicity as evidenced by electron and specular microscopy (88). The effect of gentamicin on cultured rabbit corneal epithelial cells was investigated by Alfonso et al. (89). The cells were bathed in a solution of 50 µg/mL of gentamicin for 48 h. Examination of the cells revealed typical intracytoplasmic inclusions.

Neomycin. Plasma membrane injury and cell death of superficial layers is observed with chronic administration of neomycin (90). Corneal edema followed by a punctate keratitis occurs on occasion. Long-term topical use of neomycin quite often results in allergic blepharoconjunctivitis and should be avoided. It is not recommended that neomycin be administered for a period longer than 7 days.

Tetracycline. Dermal phototoxic reactions are common with systemic tetracycline administration. Although to our best knowledge, the literature does not cite any phototoxicities with respect to the inner eye structures, this compound's photoreactivity should be kept in mind in the development of new tetracycline derivatives. When tetracycline is administered in a presoaked hydrophilic matrix, it is known to cause a reversible yellow discoloration of the cornea (92).

d. Topical Corticosteroids

Interstitial keratitis often requires prolonged treatment with corticosteroids. Maudgal et al. studied the effects of various commercial preparations on the corneal epithelium. Dexamethasone resulted in the loss of microvilli, causing patches of cell degeneration and exfoliation (93). An increased tendency toward microplicae formation was observed with most of the topical corticosteroids studied. Posterior subcapsular cataracts and the precipitation of primary narrow-angle glaucoma are well documented side effects from long-term topical administration of corticosteroids and will be further examined later in this chapter.

B.   Ocular Toxicities from Systemic Administration

Reports of oculotoxicities from the systemic administration of therapeutic agents have been reported for virtually all therapeutic classes of drugs. These range from inconsequential to those that drastically threaten vision. The details of the oculotoxicities of the different pharmacological agents is not within the context of this text; however, many comprehensive reviews have been written on the subject. This section will be limited to the mechanisms involved in the ocular pathology of systemically administered drugs and a brief review of some of the classic and commonly used oculotoxic agents.

It is an unavoidable fallacy of drug therapy that therapeutic agents produce effects in organs and tissues other than those for which they are intended. Knowing the mechanisms of toxicity and the routes of access to these tissues is a prerequisite for minimizing the untoward side effects of therapeutic entities. Koneru et al. (94) addressed the roles that melanin, photosensitization, metabolism, genetics, and the environment play in ocular toxicities. Metabolism will not be addressed in this chapter; however, it is an important variable in ocular pathologies (95,96). The lens consistently responds to alterations in its metabolism by opacification. Drugs and preservatives interfering with corneal epithelial metabolism will result in cell death and desquamation. Investigators have noted that age (95) and genetic variability in metabolism (96) may have a significant impact on drug-induced ocular toxicities.

Access to the globe by systemically administered drugs is limited by two barriers: The blood-aqueous barrier and the blood-retinal barrier. The endothelium of the iridial vessels and the ciliary nonpigmented epithelium constitute the blood-aqueous barrier (97). Both cell types preclude paracellular transport via zonulae ocludentes interjunctional complexes. The blood-retinal barrier consists of the retinal vessel epithelial cells and the retinal pigmented epithelium (97,98). These cells also possess similar "tight junctions." The blood-retinal barrier is similar to the blood-brain barrier in the lipoidal nature of the cell membranes and the lack of vasoactivity to histamine (98). The rate of penetration of chemical entities into the globe, however, has been shown to be a function of the agent's octanol/water partition coefficient (99). It is important to point out that in certain disease states these barriers become compromised, allowing toxins access to the intraocular structures. Therapeutic agents possessing the proper physicochemical properties or a sufficient concentration gradient will undergo Fickian diffusion across the lipoidal cells of the above barriers, achieving significant intraocular concentrations.

More indirectly, but equally as significant, is the effect of drug accumulation in the ocular tissues. The eye is a diverse organ allowing for the accumulation of active drugs and their metabolites. Melanin of the uveal tract and retina, the cornea owing to its differential solubility characteristics, the lens, and the posterior globe all have the ability to accumulate drugs, resulting in overt or subliminal functional and morphological changes to themselves and surrounding tissues.

1.   Melanin Binding

A diverse variety of pharmacological and chemical entities possess a high affinity toward natural and synthetic melanins (100–107). These drugs become bound and are slowly released from their melanin complexes. The retina and uvea contain the highest concentration of melanin in the body. The long-term administration of entities with a high affinity for melanin has been highly correlated with ocular cytopathologies (101,102,108–111).

Ophthalmologists have for some time recognized the strong correlation between melanin binding and oculopathologies. Chloroquine, known to concentrate and then slowly clear from the pigmented tissues, when taken in high enough doses for a long duration, will result in retinal toxicities (107,110). While the literature cites an abundance of correlations between melanin binding and ocular cytopathologies, the mechanisms of binding and its causal relationship to toxicities is yet to be fully delineated.

While the exact structure of melanin is unclear, it appears to be an irregular polymer composed of indole 5–6 quinone units (113). Several carboxylic acid residues present in the melanin polymer endow it with weak cation-exchange capabilities at physiological pH. Melanin also possesses a stable free radical, and it has been postulated that this free radical may enter charge-transfer reactions with compounds donating an electron to the melanin polymer (114). The free radicals, however, appear to be sterically hindered and do not represent the major binding mechanism of melanin (105). Further work has identified other important mechanisms of melanin binding; i.e., an irreversible charge-transfer reaction and a reversible reaction involving electrostatic and dispersive van der Waals forces (115).

Larsson and Tjalve studied the binding of chlorpromazine, chloroquine, paraquat, and Ni^{+2} to pigment obtained from beef eyes (113). The drugs were incubated in a suspension of pigment granules and assayed spectrophotometrically and by liquid scintillation. The binding of these agents were highly influenced by the ionic environment, clearly suggesting an electrostatic binding mechanism. The ability of metal ions to inhibit the binding of chlorpromazine, chloroquine, and paraquat was studied and appeared to increase with the valency of the metal ion, the exception being Pb^{+2}, which is known to bind strongly to melanin. Hydrogen ions compete strongly with organic compounds for the melanin-binding sites with a marked effect seen within the pH values of 2–4. The effect of hydrogen ion concentration on the melanin binding of chlorpromazine, chloroquine, and Ni^{+2} is shown in Figure 5. The chloroquine-melanin complex was reduced from 80 to 7% as the pH of the medium was lowered to a value of 2. The binding of chlorpromazine, however, was only reduced to 29% by adjusting the pH. Studies on many other drugs showed that compounds that are cationic at physiological pH have a high affinity for melanin (114). Procaine-melanin complexes were shown to liberate procaine in 4 M NaCl washes (110). The amount of chlorpromazine un-ionized, recovered from chlorpromazine-melanin complexes after the same wash was negligible. However, chlorpromazine was released upon washing the complex with ethanol. The above studies suggest definite electrostatic and dispersive forces involved in melanin binding.

Scatchard plot analysis of melanin binding and the behavior of chlorpromazine in the Larsson and Tjalve study (113), however, lend evidence to additional binding mechanisms. In the preliminary report, Potts (115) demonstrated that dispersive forces played a major role in melanin binding. While this may not be entirely correct, it has been determined that these forces do play some role. Potts suggested that polyaromatic compounds with coplanar fused ring structures are unique in their high affinity for melanin. Atlasik et al. demonstrated, however, that compounds possessing only one aromatic ring may have significant affinity for melanin (108). In the Larsson Tjalve study (113), it was impossible to completely inhibit the binding of chlorpromazine via the adjustment of ionic strength or hydrogen ion concentration, suggesting a nonelectrostatic binding mechanism. Scatchard plot analysis of the binding of many drugs indicates that, indeed, there are many different binding sites on the melanin polymer. Chlorpromazine and chloroquine each showed three types of binding sites, whereas paraquat and Ni^{+2} exhibit only two. Differences in the

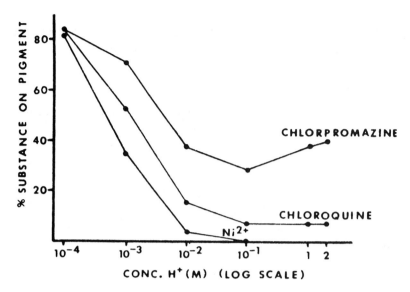

Figure 5. Effect of H⁺ on the binding of chlorpromazine, chloroquine, and Ni^{+2} to melanin. 2.5 µmol of chlorpromazine, chloroquine of $NiCl_2$ were added to pigment granule (10 mg) suspensions in distilled water containing various amounts of HCl. After 45 min incubation, the binding to the pigment was determined. (From Ref. 113.)

binding properties of blue and brown irides have been studied (100,117). Menon et al. have demonstrated different binding mechanisms for chlorpromazine to melanin in brown and blue irides (117), whereas no difference was noted in the binding of timolol to brown and blue irides (100).

Numerous studies have clearly demonstrated that although binding of a compound to melanin may be an important factor in the development of toxic retinopathy, melanin binding alone is insufficient to produce these changes. Chloroquine accumulates to a large degree in the pigmented tissues but exerts its toxic effects on many nonpigmented tissues within the globe, cornea, lens, and retina (116). Accumulation of chloroquine in the photoreceptors and neuroretina has also been noted (119). The morphological alterations attributed to chloroquine vary within the literature. Investigators have noted degeneration of the pigmented epithelium as well as the sensory retina (120). Other investigators, however, noted morphological changes in the neuroretina, but no ultrastructural changes could be observed in the retinal pigmented epithelium (RPE) (121). The effect of long-term chloroquine exposure on the phospholipid metabolism and its relationship to retinal damage was studied by Hallberg et al. (122). The appearance of cytoplasmic multilamellated bodies is pathognomic for phospholipidosis. The appearance of multilamellated bodies in the retinal cells was noted after long-term exposure with chloroquine. Examination after chloroquine treatment revealed that the ganglionic cells were the only cell type to be heavily loaded with multilamellated bodies. The phospholipid metabolism of the RPE was normal after 6 months of chloroquine treatment. These data suggest that changes in the RPE were not responsible for the chloroquine-induced toxic retinopathy. Chemical entities that accumulate in melanin-containing depots do not necessarily result in toxicities to those tissues. Beta-blockers, benzodiazepines, and topical anesthetics bind irreversibly to melanin but are not significantly correlated with damage to the RPE or uveal tract (123). Topical anesthetics have, however, been associated with posterior subcapsular lens opacities (124). Accumulation of pharmacological agents in melanin-containing tissues and resulting cytopathologies have been shown not to always correlate in studies with albino and pigmented rabbits (119).

It is possible that the retinal toxicities of melanin-bound drugs result from subliminal effects due to the accumulation of drugs in a melanin depot, resulting in pathologies to adjacent tissues over time.

2. Photosensitization

Photosensitizing agents represent another mechanism of oculotoxicity from systemically administered drugs. Photosensitizing agents absorb visible and ultraviolet (UV) radiation at specific wavelengths, forming excited singlets, triplets, or free radicals. A resonant energy transfer from these compounds to secondary molecules creates reactive toxins. These highly reactive species may in turn react with the surrounding biological tissues. Photosensitizing agents may become photobound to macromolecules in the corneal, lenticular, and retinal tissues. Allopurinol, amiodarone, phenothiazines, and psoralens are known photosensitizing agents (124–130). The cornea and lens proteins filter some of the incident UV radiation; however, a significant intraocular effect from photosensitizing agents has been well documented. Allopurinol becomes photobound to the lens. Prolonged administration of this drug, however, does not by itself result in cataracts but with a parallel history of significant UV exposure senile cataracts have appeared in very young patients (127,128). Accumulation of the drug was not found in patients not suffering from allopurinol cataract, in contrast to the cataract patients. The photobinding of allopurinol to the lens appears to be a prerequisite for cataractogenesis.

Compounds containing aromatic, conjugated systems or tricyclic ring structures may possess the ability to absorb UV energy and form triplets, ions, or free radicals. The oculotoxic potential of such drugs needs to be studied. Tetracycline, hematoporphyrin derivatives, fluorescein, and methylene blue induce photosensitized polymerization of lens proteins in vitro (130). It is, therefore, important that the possibility of a photosensitized reaction be fully investigated prior to the release of suspected photosensitizing agents.

Carotenoid retinopathies are also well known. Canthanxanthin, a skin-tanning agent, is the cause of crystalline retinopathy in humans. Delayed dark adaptation and impaired night vision have been reported by Weber et al. (131). Electroretinographic examination revealed a delay in the increase in amplitudes during the course of dark adaptation. Functional impairment was reversible after a few months; however, complete reversal of the retinopathy was not noticed even after 1 year.

The cornea, lens, and posterior portion of the globe can also act as drug depots. The corneal endothelium offers minimal resistance to diffusion of chemical agents and may not accumulate any significant amounts of drug entities. However, the corneal stroma and epithelium may accumulate different compounds depending upon their physicochemical nature. Agents entering the aqueous humor through the uveal circulation can rapidly penetrate the corneal endothelium into the stroma. The lipoidal nature of the epithelium may also result in drug accumulation. The basement cell layers of the epithelium are cuboidal and allow for diffusion into the epithelium. Lipophilic drugs reaching the aqueous humor will tend to accumulate to some extent in the corneal epithelium.

3. Oculotoxic Drugs

A milieu of drugs administered via systemic routes have been reported to cause ocular pathologies. A brief review of some of the more commonly encountered ones are presented here.

a. Corticosteroids

High-dose long-term corticosteroid therapy is recommended in a variety of conditions, including rheumatoid arthritis and renal transplant therapy. Cataracts and keratopathy have been associated with this type of therapy (131). It has long been recognized that corticosteroid therapy has been associated with cataractogenisis which correlates well with dose, both daily and total, and duration of therapy (132). Prednisolone cataracts can be observed in the majority of patients receiving more than 15 mg/day (133). Vacuole formation in the posterior subcapsular region is the first sign of cataractogenisis.

Prolonged topical and systemic administration of corticosteroids have also been implicated in decreasing aqueous humor outflow resulting in corticosteroid-induced glaucoma (134,135). Topical administration is known to result in pressure changes in the treated eye alone. The degree of pressure elevation in patients correlates with the anti-inflammatory strength of the specific corticosteroid, with dexamethasone causing the greatest elevation of intraocular pressure (136).

A host of secondary ocular pathologies have also been observed with corticosteroid therapy. Infectious invasion of the ocular tissues is a common sequelae of corticosteroids and other immunosuppressive drugs; i.e., cyclosporin. Chorioretinitis can rapidly result in peripheral and macular degeneration of the retina (137). Cytomegalovirus, a common cause of retinitis, can rapidly progress to blindness in the immunocompromised patient. Herpes simplex keratitis is potentiated by concomitant administration of corticosteroids (138). Exacerbation of fungal and bacterial corneal infections have also resulted from corticosteroid use (139).

b. Phenothiazines

Phenothiazines also display ocular pathologies related to dose and duration of treatment. Multiple punctate deposits develop in the posterior corneal surface (133). Stromal clouding and visual impairment can result. The typical purple syndrome associated with phenothiazine therapy will have concurrent corneal and lenticular deposits (140). Diffuse cataractous lesions in the anterior lens develop and retinal pigmentation can also occur.

c. Amiodarone

Amiodarone has long been known to induce corneal deposits located in the basal epithelium (141–143,145). The keratopathy does not normally affect vision but is related to both dose and duration (142). Miller has defined three stages of amiodarone keratopathy (141,142):

1. Coalescence of punctate grayish golden brown opacities into a horizonal linear pattern in the inferior cornea
2. Additional arborizing and horizontal lines
3. A verticillate whorl-like pattern extending into the visual axis.

Flach has shown the keratopathy to be related to both dose and duration of therapy (144). Patients receiving 100–200 mg/day generally did not progress past stage 1 keratopathy. The threshold for stages 2 and 3 keratopathies appears to be 400 mg/day. The pathology is a drug-induced lipidosis with supranuclear intracytoplasmic inclusions in the epithelial basal cells (143). Flach et al. were the first to notice lipid deposits in the anterior lens associated with amiodarone therapy (144). These anterior white-yellow opacities appeared in the pupillary axis, possibly suggesting a photosensitizing mechanism.

d. Chloroquine

Chloroquine retinopathy is seen more significantly in patients receiving more than 100 g total dose or a duration of therapy of greater than 1 year (146). Macular degeneration occurs with optic atrophy and diffuse retinal pigmentation. Defects in color vision is an early sign of the retinopathy. Corneal punctate opacities and papilledema have also been noticed (147).

C. Systemic Absorption from Topical Delivery

The precorneal loss of topical ophthalmic medications has implications beyond that of low ocular bioavailability. As little as 1% or less of the instilled topical dose reaches the anterior chamber. More importantly, nonproductive conjunctival absorption coupled with nasolacrimal drainage and absorption of the topical dose can result in significant systemic availability of the topically administered drug avoiding the hepatic first-pass metabolism. The low ocular bioavailability of topically instilled drugs requires the clinician to recommend a pulse dosing method, utilizing frequent dosing of very high concentrations. It is known that administration of topical timolol in the treatment of open-angle glaucoma has resulted in therapeutic concentrations of timolol in the systemic circulation (148,149). The side effects incurred with this type of absorption into the systemic circulation is consistent with direct systemic administration of the drug agent. Depending upon the physicochemical nature of the drug agent and formulation factors (e.g., contact time, drainage rate, surfactants), the plasma levels of a therapeutic agent and hence its systemic side effects may be significant.

A brief literature review of the systemic side effects from topical ocular delivery of therapeutic agents used in the treatment of glaucoma illustrates this point. While therapeutic agents such as carbonic anhydrase inhibitors and hyperosmotic agents are useful in the treatment of glaucoma and not without side effects, they will not be addressed here as they are administered systemically.

Two general classes of drugs are utilized in the treatment of glaucoma. Those that increase outflow of the aqueous humor and those that decrease its input (formation). Parasympathetic agents are known to relieve obstructive egress pathways, increasing outflow (150). The sympathetic agents appear to act via decreasing the formation of aqueous humor (151). Carbonic anhydrase inhibitors exert effects both by increasing outflow and decreasing aqueous humor formation (151).

1. Cholinergic Agents

The miotics increase the outflow of aqueous humor by their action in the iris–ciliary body and via dilation of the veins peripheral to the canal of Schlemm. Pilocarpine is the most common of these agents and is used in the treatment of primary open-angle glaucoma. It is administered in concentrations of 0.5–1.0% and given two to three times per day up to every 2 h. Carbachol is also used topically in the treatment of open-angle glaucoma.

Miotics may cause conjunctival irritation, blepharitis, headache, and periorbital pain. Indirect or long-acting agents may induce salivation, gastrointestinal disturbances (nausea, vomiting, and diarrhea), muscle spasms, bradycardia, hypotension, bronchial spasm, and other typical cholinergic effects. These agents as such would be contraindicated in disease states such as parkinsonism, bronchial asthma, and gastrointestinal ulcerations.

2. Beta-Blockers

Beta-blockers are commonly administered topically to the eye in the treatment of open-angle glaucoma. In a 1987 review of the systemic toxicities of timolol since its introduction in 1978, Fraunfelder and Meyer have indicated that over 2000 cases of systemic toxicities from topical ocular administration of timolol have been reported to the National Registry of Drug Induced Ocular Side Effects (150). It must be noted, however that such incidental reports are without experimental design or controls and by themselves do not offer proof of a causal relationship. Timolol maleate and levobunolol are nonselective $beta_1$ and $beta_2$ antagonists used topically in the treatment of glaucoma. Betaxolol is a $beta_1$ cardioselective agent that has recently been approved for topical application in primary open-angle glaucoma. Side effects from these agents include bradycardia and hypotension. Headache and depression are known central nervous system (CNS) disturbances. The use of timolol may precipitate bronchospasms (153). Bronchospasms are by far the most serious side effect of topical ocular timolol therapy in the asthmatic or emphysema patient and as such its use is contraindicated in this patient population. Hypothetically, bronchospasms would not be expected to be manifested as a side effect of betaxolol therapy, as it possesses $beta_1$ selectivity. Caution should be exercised in the diabetic patient when using these agents, as systemic absorption has been infrequently reported to mask the symptoms of hypoglycemia in insulin-dependent diabetics (152).

3. Sympathomimetics

Epinephrine is used in the treatment of open-angle glaucoma, administered as a 1–2% w/v solution and given every 6–8 h. Hypertension and cardiac irregularities such as palpitations and tachycardia have been reported after topical ocular epinephrine administration. The dipivaloyl HCl diester (DPV) of epinephrine has been approved for use and its penetration through the cornea into the aqueous humor is 17-fold greater than epinephrine (154). A 0.1% w/v solution of the dipivaloyl diester was found to be equipotent to a 2% w/v solution of epinephrine in reducing intraocular pressure (155). Despite the higher ocular bioavailability of the dipivaloyl ester than epinephrine, its systemic absorption is similar to epinephrine and topical ocular administration of DPV results in fewer side effects than topical epinephrine (156). Topical ocular application of 1% epinephrine has been reported to cause toxic coma (157). There have been many reports of systemic toxicity associated with topical administration of 10% phenylephrine eye drops (158).

III. CONCLUSIONS: FUTURE DIRECTIONS

Clearly, in an effort to achieve better ophthalmic delivery systems, the pharmaceutical scientist must weigh the benefits of improved ocular bioavailability against the possible detriments of the delivery system. As previously described, many of the reported oculotoxicities of various agents are without statistical evaluations. This may be a result of retroactive studies without a baseline or poor experimental controls and design. Even well-designed studies suffer from lack of quantifying models of low-level cytopathologies. Recent work has progressed far beyond the initial models of Draize and Kelly and enable the researcher to detect low-level cytotoxicities and subliminal influences on the ocular tissues.

An inordinately high number of ocular conditions are aggravated by overtreatment with topical ocular drugs. Repeated applications can cause biochemical or mechanical injury as well as sensitivity reactions resulting in blepharoconjunctivitis. The local and systemic toxicities can be significantly minimized by interventions with newer ophthalmic delivery systems.

As has been repeatedly emphasized, frequent local instillations of antiglaucoma agents, antibiotics, antivirals, and sulfonamides provide an unusually high drug and preservative concentration at the epithelial surface. Improvements in dosing by controlled and enhanced delivery, prolonged contact time, and targeting within the globe will go a long way toward achieving safe and reliable ophthalmic dosage forms.

REFERENCES

1. Gibaldi, M., and Perrier, D. (1982). *Pharmacokinetics*, Vol. 15, 2nd ed., Marcel Dekker, New York, p. 145.
2. Maurice, D. M. (1969). In: *The Eye*, Vol. 1, *Vegetative Physiology and Biochemistry* (H. Davsoned, ed.), Academic Press, New York, p. 541.
3. Patton, T. F., and Ahmed, I. (1985). Importance of the noncorneal absorption route in topical ophthalmic drug deliver, *Invest. Ophthalmol. Vis. Sci., 26*:585.
4. Bloomfield, S. E., Miyata, T., Dunn, M. W., Byeser, N., Stenzclik, H., and Pubin, A. L. (1978). Soluble gentamicin ophthalmic inserts as a drug delivery system, *Arch. Ophthalmol., 96*:885.
5. Bito, L. Z., and Baroody, R. A. (1982). The penetration of exogenous prostaglandin and arachidonic acid into, and their distribution within, the mammalian eye, *Curr. Eye Res., 1*:659.
6. Cogan, D. G., and Hirch, E. D. (1944). Cornea: Permeability to weak electrolytes, *Arch. Ophthalmol., 32*:276.
7. Kinsey, V. E. (1965), 43th ed. In: *Physiology of the Eye* (F. H. Adler, ed.), Mosby, St. Louis.
8. Huang, H. S., Schoenwald, R. D., and Lach, J. L. (1983). Corneal penetration of b-blocking agents II. Assessment of barrier contributions, *J. Pharm. Sci., 72*:1272.
9. Grass, G. M., and Robinson, J. R. (1988). Mechanisms of corneal drug penetration II. Ultrastructural analysis of potential pathways for drug movement, *J. Pharm. Sci., 77*:15.
10. Lee, V. H. L. (1990). Mechanisms and facilitation of corneal drug penetration, *J. Controlled Rel., 11*:79.
11. Klyce, S. D., and Crosson, C. E. (1985). Transport processes across the rabbit corneal epithelium: A review. *Curr. Eye Res., 4*:323.
12. Mitra, A. K. (1988). Ophthalmic drug delivery, *Drug Delivery Devices* (P. Tyle, ed.), Marcel Dekker, New York, p. 455.
13. Tonjum, A. M. (1975). Permeability of horseradish peroxidase in the rabbit corneal epithelium, *Acta Ophthalmol., 52*:650.
14. Mishima, S. (1981). Clinical pharmacokinetics of the eye, *Invest. Ophthalmol. Vis. Sci. 21*:504.
15. Schoenwald, R. D., and Ward, R. L. (1978). Relationship between steroid permeability across excised rabbit cornea and octanol-water partition coefficients, *J. Pharm. Sci., 67*:786.
16. Narurkar, M. M., and Mitra, A. K. (1989). Prodrugs of 5-iodo-2′-deoxyuridine for enhanced ocular transport, *Pharm. Res., 6*:887.
17. Narurkar, M. M., and Mitra, A. K. (1988). Synthesis physicochemical properties, and cytotoxicity of a series of 5′-ester prodrugs of 5-Iodo-2′-deoxyuridine, *Pharm. Res., 5*:734.
18. Mosher, G. L., and Mikkelson, T. J. (1979). Permeability of the n-alkyl p-ammino benzoate esters across the isolated corneal membrane of the rabbit, *Int. J. Pharm., 2*:239.

19. Schoenwald, R. D., and Huang, H. (1983). Corneal penetration behavior of beta-blocking agents I: Physicochemical factors, *J. Pharm. Sci., 72*:1266.
20. Mitra, A. K., and Mikkelson, T. J. (1982). Ophthalmic solution buffer systems I. The effect of buffer concentration on the ocular absorption of pilocarpine, *Int. J. Pharm., 10*:219.
21. Chrai, S. S., Patton, T. F., Mehta, A., and Robinson, J. R. (1973). Lacrimal and instilled fluid dynamics in rabbit eyes, *J. Pharm. Sci., 62*:1112.
22. Chrai, S. S., Makoid, M. C., Eriksen, S. P., and Robinson, J. R. (1974). Drop size and initial dosing frequency problems of topically applied ophthalmic drugs, *J. Pharm. Sci., 63*:333.
23. Sieg, J. W., and Robinson, J. R. (1976). Mechanistic studies on transcorneal permeation of pilocarpine, *J. Pharm. Sci., 65*:1816.
24. Maurice, D. M. (1973). The dynamics and drainage of tears, *Int. Ophthalmol. Clin., 13*:73.
25. Mishima, S., Gasset, A., Klyce, Jr., S. D., and Baum, J. L. (1966). Determination of tear volume and tear flows, *Invest. Ophthalmol. Vis. Sci., 5*:264.
26. Ehlers, N. (1965). The precorneal film, biomicroscopical, histological, and chemical investigations, *Acta Ophthalmol., 81*(Suppl.):1.
27. Lee, V. H. L., and Robinson, J. R. (1986). Review: Topical Ocular drug delivery: Recent developments and future challenges, *J. Ocul. Pharmacol., 2*:67.
28. Kupferman, A., Prah, M. V., Syckewer, K., and Leibowitz, H. M. (1974). Topically applied steroids in corneal disease III. The role of drug derivative in stromal absorption of dexamethasone, *Arch. Ophthalmol., 91*:373.
29. Sieg, J. W., and Robinson, J. R. (1977). Vehicle effects on ocular drug bioavailability II: Evaluation of pilocarpine, *J. Pharm. Sci., 66*:1222.
30. Conrad, J. M., Reay, W. A., Polcyn, R. E., and Robinson, J. R. Influence of tonicity and pH on lacrimation and ocular drug bioavailability (1978), *J. Parent. Drug Assoc., 32*:149.
31. Mishima, S., Gasset, A., Klyce, S. D., and Baum, J. L. (1966). Determination of tear volume and tear flow, *Invest. Ophthalmol. Vis. Sci., 5*:264.
32. Mikkelson, T. J., Chrai, S. S., and Robinson, J. R. (1973). Competitive inhibition of drug-protein interaction in eye fluids and tissues, *J. Pharm. Sci., 62*:1942.
33. Lee, V. H. L., Morimoto, K. W., and Stratford, Jr., R. E. (1982). Esterase distribution in the rabbit cornea and its implications in ocular drug bioavailability, *Biopharm. Drug Dispos., 3*:291.
34. Lee, V. H. L., Hui, H. W., and Robinson, J. R. (1980). Corneal metabolism of pilocarpine in pigmented rabbits, *Invest. Ophthalmol. Vis. Sci., 9*:210.
35. Lee, V. H. L., Stratford, Jr., R. E., and Morimoto, K. W. (1983). Age-rebated changes in esterase activity in rabbit eyes, *Int. J. Pharm., 13*:183.
36. Shichi, H., and Nebert, D. W. (1982). Genetic differences in drug metabolism associated with ocular toxicity, *Environ. Health Perspect., 44*:107.
37. Swan, K. C. (1944). Reactivity of the ocular tissues to wetting agents, *Am. J. Ophthalmol., 27*:1118.
38. Pfister, R. R., and Burstein, N. (1976). The effects of ophthalmic drugs, vehicles, and preservatives on corneal epithelium: a scanning electron microscope study, *Invest. Ophthalmol. Vis. Sci., 15*:246.
39. Gasset, A. R., Ishii, Kaufman, H. E., and Miller, T. (1974). Cytotoxicity of ophthalmic preservatives, *Am. J. Ophthalmol., 78*:98.
40. Green, K., Johnson, R. E., Chapman, J. M., Nelson, E., and Cheeks, L. (1989). Surfactant effects on the rate of corneal epithelial healing, *J. Toxicol. Cutan. Ocul. Toxicol., 8*:253.
41. Tonjum, A. M. (1975). Effects of benzalkonium chloride upon the corneal epithelium studies with scanning electron microscopy, *Acta Ophthalmol., 53*:358.
42. Burstein, N. L., and Klyce, S. D. (1977). Electrophysiologic and morphologic effects of ophthalmic preparations on rabbit corneal epithelium, *Invest. Ophthalmol. Vis. Sci., 16*:899.
43. Green, K., and Tonjum, A. M. (1971). Influence of various agents on corneal permeability, *Am. J. Ophthalmol., 72*:897.

44. Burstein, N. L. (1980). Preservative cytotoxic threshold for benzalkonium chloride and chlohexidine digluconate in cat and rabbit corneas, *Invest. Ophthalmol., 19*:308.
45. Holly, F. J. (1978). Surface chemical evaluation of artificial tears and their ingredients II. Interaction with a superficial lipid layer, *Contact Intraocul. Lens Med. J., 4*:52.
46. Fraunfelder, F. T. (1976). *Drug-Induced Ocular Side Effects and Drug Interactions*, Lee & Febiger, Philadelphia.
47. Camber, O., and Edman, P. (1987). Influence of some preservatives on the corneal permeability of pilocarpine and dexamethasone, in vitro, *Int. J. Pharm., 39*:229.
48. Camber, O., and Edman, P. (1987). Factors influencing the corneal permeability of prostaglandin F_2 and its isopropyl ester in vitro, *Int. J. Pharm., 37*:27.
49. Lavine, J. B., Binder, P. S., and Wickham, M. G. (1979). Antimicrobials and the corneal endothelium, *Ann. Ophthalmol., 11*:1517.
50. Green, K., Hull, D. S., Vaughn, E. D., Malizia, Jr., A. A., and Bowman, K. (1977). Rabbit endothelial response to ophthalmic preservatives, *Arch. Ophthalmol., 95*:2218.
51. Sasamoto, K., Akagi, Y., Kodama, Y., and Ittoi, M. (1984). Corneal endothelial changes caused by ophthalmic drugs, *Cornea, 3*:37.
52. Britton, B., Hervey, R., and Kasten, K. (1976). Intraocular irrigation evaluation of benzalkonium chloride in rabbits, *Ophthalmol. Surg., 7*:46.
53. Kilp, H., Heisig-Salentin, B., Poss, W., Thode, C., and Rogalla, K. (1987). Acute and chronic influence of benzalkonium chloride as a preservative, *Concepts Toxicol., 4*:59.
54. Marsh, R. J., and Maurice, D. M. (1971). Influence of nonionic detergents and other surfactants on human corneal permeability, *Exp. Eye Res., 11*:43.
55. Green, K., and Tonjum, A. M. (1971). Influence of various agents on corneal permeability, *Am. J. Ophthalmol., 72*:897.
56. Green, K. (1976). Electrophysiological and anatomical effects of cetylpyridinium chloride on the rabbit cornea, *Acta Ophthalmol., 54*:145.
57. Green, K., Chapman, J., Cheeks, L., and Clayton, R. M. (1987). Surfactant penetration into the eye, *Concept Toxicol., 4*:126.
58. Clayton, R. M., Green, K., Wilson, M., Zehir, A., Jack, J., and Searle, L. (1985). The penetration of detergents into adult and infant eyes, possible hazards of additives to ophthalmic preparations, *Fed. Chem. Toxicol., 23*:239.
59. Green, K., and Chapman, J. M. (1986). Benzalkonium chloride kinetics in young and adult albino and pigmented rabbit eyes, *J. Toxicol Cutan. Ocular Toxicol., 5*:132.
60. Fraunfelder, F. T., and Meyer, S. M. (1986). Corneal complications of ocular medications, *Cornea, 5*:55.
61. Van Horn, D. L., Edelhauser, H. F., Prodanovich, G., et al. (1977). Effect of the ophthalmic preservative thimerosal on rabbit and human corneal endothelium, *Invest. Ophthalmol. Vis Sci., 16*:273.
62. Van Horn, D. L., Edelhauser, H. F., Prodanovic, G., Eiterman, R., and Pederson, H. J. (1977). Effect of the ophthalmic preservative thimerosal on rabbit and human corneal endothelium, *Invest. Ophthalmol. Vis. Sci., 16*:273.
63. Winder, A. F., Sheraidah, G. A. K., Astbury, N. J., and Ruben, M. (1980). Penetration of mercury from ophthalmic preservatives into the human eye, *Lancet, 2*:237.
64. Burstein, N. (1980). Corneal cytotoxicity of topically applied drugs, vehicles and preservatives, *Surv. Ophthalmol., 25*:15.
65. Krejci, L., and Harrison, R. (1970). Antiglaucoma effects on corneal epithelium: A comparative study in tissue culture, *Arch. Ophthalmol., 84*:766.
66. Grant, W. M. (1974). *Toxicology of the Eye*, 2nd ed., Springfield, Illinois, Thomas.
67. Gasset, A. R., and Ishii, Y. (1975). Cytotoxicity of chlorohexidine, *Can. J. Ophthalmol., 10*:98.
68. Michaels, P. H., Wilson, F. M., and Grayson, M. (1979). Infiltrative keratitis from abuse of anesthetic eyedrops, *J. Indiana St. Med. Assoc., 72*:51.

69. Burns, R. P., Forster, R. K., Laibson, P., and Gipson, K. (1977). Chronic toxicity of local anesthetics on the cornea. *In: Symposium on Ocular Therapy*, Vol. 10 (I. H. Leopold and R. P. Burns, eds.). Wiley, New York, p. 31.

70. Epstein, D. L., and Paton, D. (1968). Keratitis from misuse of corneal anesthetics, *N. Engl. J. Med., 279*:396.

71. Marr, W. G., Wood, R., Senterfit, L., and Singleman, S. (1957). Effects of topical anesthetics, *Am. J. Ophthalmol., 43*:606.

72. Behrendt, T. (1957). Experimental secondary effects of topical anesthetics of the cornea, *Am. J. Ophthalmol., 44*:74.

73. Gundersen, T., and Liebman, S. D. (1944). Effects of local anesthetics on regeneration of corneal epithelium, *Arch. Ophthalmol., 31*:29.

74. Rosenwasser, G., et al. (1990). Topical anesthetic abuse, *Ophthalmology, 97*:967.

75. Ishida, T., Shigeyoshi, H., and Nakamura, Y. (1987). Topical anesthetic and its effect on the corneoconjunctival surface, *In: Concepts in Toxicology*, Vol. 4 (O. Hockwin, ed.), New York, Karger, p. 121.

76. Harnisch, J. P., Hoffman, F., and Dumitrescu, L. (1975). Side effects of local anesthetics on the corneal epithelium of the rabbit eye, *Albrecht von Graefes Klin. Arch. Ophthalmol., 197*:71.

77. Marr, W. G., Wood, R., and Starck, M. (1951). Effect of some agents on regeneration of corneal epithelium, *Am. J. Ophthalmol., 34*:609.

78. Augsburger, A. R., and Hill, R. M. (1972). Corneal anesthetics and epithelial oxygen flux, *Arch. Ophthalmol., 88*:305.

79. Reinecke, R. D., and Kuwabara, T. (1963). Corneal deposits secondary to topical epinephrine, *Arch. Ophthalmol., 70*:170.

80. Hull, D. S., Chemotti, M. T., Edelhauser, H. F., Van Dorn, D. L., and Hyndick, R. A. (1975). Effect of epinephrine on the corneal epithelium, *Am. J. Ophthalmol., 79*:245.

81. Waltman, S. R., Yarian, D., Hart, W., and Becker, B. (1977). Corneal endothelium changes with long term topical epinephrine therapy, *Arch. Ophthalmol., 95*:1357.

82. Laibson, P. R., and Kibrick, S. (1966). Reactivation of herpetic keratitis by epinephrine in rabbit, *Arch. Ophthalmol,, 75*:254.

83. Van Buskirk, E. M. (1980). Adverse reactions from timolol administration, *Ophthalmology, 87*:447.

84. Trope, G. E., Lia, G. S., and Basu, T. K. (1988). Toxic effects of topically administered betagan, betoptic and timoptic on regenerating corneal epithelium, *J. Ocul. Pharmacol., 4*:359.

85. Wilhelmus, K. R., McCulloch, R. R., and Gross, R. L. (1990). Dendritic keratopathy associated with beta-blocker eye drops, *Cornea, 9*:335.

86. Staats, W. D., Radius, R. L., Van Horn, D. L., and Schultz, R. O. (1981). Effects of timolol on bovine corneal endothelial cultures, *Arch. Ophthalmol., 99*:660.

87. Bleckmann, H., and Wollensak, J. (1975). Inhibition of corneal metabolism by glucocorticosteroids, *Albrecht von Graefes Arch. Klin. Ophthalmol., 193*:57.

88. Petroutsos, G., Savaldelli, M., and Pouliquen, Y. (1990). The effect of gentamicin on the corneal endothelium: An experimental study, *Cornea, 9*:62.

89. Alfonso, E. C., Albert, D. M., Kenyon, K. R., and Robinson, N. L. (1990). In vitro toxicity of gentamicin to corneal epithelial cells, *Cornea, 9*:55.

90. Belfort, Jr. R., Smolin, G., Olumoto, M., and Kim, H. B. (1975). Nebicin in the treatment of experimental pseudomonas keratitis, *Br. J. Ophthalmol., 59*:725.

91. David, D. S., and Berkowitz, J. S. (1969). Ocular side effects of topical and systemic corticosteroids, *Lancet, 2*:149.

92. Krejci, L., and Brettschneider, I. (1978). Yellow-brown cornea: A complication of topical use of tetracycline, *Ophthalmic Res., 10*:131.

93. Maudgal, P. C., Cornelis, H., and Missollen, L. (1989). Effects of commercial ophthalmic drugs on the rabbit corneal epithelium, *Graefes Arch. Ophthalmol., 216*:191.

94. Koneru, B. P., Lien, E. J., and Koda, R. T. (1986). Review: Oculotoxicities of systemically administered drugs, *J. Ocul. Pharmacol., 2*:385.

95. Lee, V. H., Stratford, Jr., R. E., and Morimoto, K. W. (1983). Age related changes in esterase activity in rabbit eyes, *Int. J. Pharm., 13*:183.

96. Hitoshi, S., and Nebert, W. (1982). Genetic differences in drug metabolism associated with ocular toxicity, *Environ. Health Perspect., 44*:107.

97. Chuna-Vaz, J. G. (1979). The blood-ocular barriers, *Surv. Ophthalmol., 23*:279.

98. Chuna-Vaz, J. G. (1976). The blood-retinal barriers, *Doc. Ophthalmol., 41*:287.

99. Blekker, G. M., and Maas, E. H. (1958). Penetration of penethamate penicillin ester into the tissue of the eye, *Arch. Ophthalmol., 60*:1013.

100. Persad, S. D., Menon, I. A., Basu, P. K., and Haberman, H. F. (1986). Binding of imipramine, 8-methoxypsoralen, and epinephrine to human blue and brown eye melanins, *J. Toxicol. Cutan. Ocul. Toxicol., 5*:125.

101. Menon, I. A., Trope, G. E., Basu, P. K., Walkham, D. L., and Persad, S. D. (1989). Binding of timolol to iris-ciliary body and melanin: An in-vitro model for assessing the kinetics and efficacy of long-acting antiglaucoma drugs, *J. Ocul. Pharmacol., 5*:313.

102. Calissendor, B. (1976). Melanotropic drugs and retinal function I: Effects of quinine and chloroquine on the sheep ERG, *Acta Ophthalmol., 54*:109.

103. Calissendor, B. (1976). Melanotropic drugs and retinal function II: Effects of phenothiazine and rifampicin on the sheep ERG, *Acta Ophthalmol., 54*:118.

104. Lindquist, N. G. (1973). Accumulation of drugs on melanin, *Acta Radiol. 325*(Suppl.):1.

105. Potts, A. M. (1964). Further studies concerning accumulation of polycylic compounds on uveal melanin, *Invest. Ophthalmol., 3*:399.

106. Salminen, L., Urtti, A., and Periviita, L. (1984). Effect of ocular pigmentation in the rabbit eye. I. Drug distribution and metabolism, *Int. J. Pharm., 18*:17.

107. Ings, R. M. J. (1984). The melanin binding of drugs and its implications, *Drug Metab. Rev., 15*:1183.

108. Atlasik, B., Stepien, K., and Wilcox, T. (1980). Interaction of drugs with ocular melanin in vitro, *Exp. Eye Res., 30*:325.

109. Henkind, P., Carr, R. E., and Siegel, I. M. (1964). Early chloroquine retinopathy: Clinical and functional findings, *Arch. Ophthalmol., 71*:157.

110. Bernstein, H. N., and Ginsberg, J. (1964). The pathology of chloroquine retinopathy, *Arch. Ophthalmol., 71*:238.

111. Weiter, J. J., Delori, F. C., Wing, G. L., and Fitch, K. A. (1985). Relationship of senile macular degeneration to ocular pigmentation, *Ann. of Ophthalmol., 99*:185.

112. Meier-Ruge (1965). Experimental investigations of the morphogenesis of chloroquine retinopathy, *Arch. Ophthalmol., 73*:540.

113. Larsson, B., and Tjalve, H. (1979). Studies on the mechanism of drug binding to melanin, *Biochem. Pharmacol., 28*:1181.

114. Mason, H. S., Ingram, D. J., and Allen, B. (1960). The free radical property of melanin, *Arch. Biochem. Biophys., 86*:225.

115. Potts, A. M. (1964). The reaction of uveal pigment in-vitro with polycyclic compounds, *Invest. Ophthalmol. Vis Sci., 3*:405.

116. Hobbs, H. E., Sorsby, A., and Freedman, A. (1959). Retinopathy following chloroquine therapy, *Lancet, 2*:478.

117. Menon, I. A., Persad, S., Haberman, H. F., Kurian, C. J., and Basu, P. K. (1982). A qualitative study of the melanins from blue and brown human eyes, *Exp. Eye Res., 34*:531.

118. Rosenthal, A. R., Kolb, H., Bergsma, P., Huxsoll, D., and Hopkins, J. (1978). Chloroquine retinopathy in the rhesus monkey, *Invest. Ophthalmol. Vis. Sci., 17*:1158.

119. Abraham, R., and Hendy, R. J. (1970). Irreversible lysosomal damage induced by chloroquine in the retinae of pigmented and albino rabbits, *Exp. Mol. Pathol., 12*:185.

120. Hodgkinson, B. J., and Kolb, H. (1970). A preliminary study of the effect of chloroquine on the rat retina, *Arch. Ophthalmol., 84*:509.

121. Ramsey, M. S., and Fine, B. S. (1972). Chloroquine toxicity in the human eye: Histopathologic observations by electron microscopy, *Am. J. Ophthalmol., 73*:229.

122. Hallberg, A., Naeser, P., and Andersson, A. (1990). Effects of long-term exposure on the phospholipid metabolism in retina and pigment epithelium, *Acta Ophthalmol., 68*:125.

123. Howard, R. O., McDonald, C. J., Dunn, B., and Creasey, W. A. (1969). Experimental chlorpromazine cataracts, *Invest. Ophthalmol. Vis. Sci., 8*:413.

124. Koch, H. R., Beitzen, R., Kremer, F., Chioralia, G., Baurmann, H., Megaw, J., Gardner, K., and Lerman, S. (1982). 8-Methoxypsoralen and long ultraviolet effects on the rat lens: Experiments with high dosage, *Graefes Archiv. Klin. Exp. Ophthalmol., 218*:193.

125. Wulf, H. C., and Andreasen, M. P. (1982). Concentration of ^{3}H-8-Methoxypsoralen and its metabolites in eye after a single oral administration, *Invest. Ophthalmol. Vis. Sci., 22*:32.

126. Jose, J. J., and Yielding, K. L. (1978). Photosensitive cataractogens, chlorpromazine and methoxypsoralen, cause DNA synthesis in lens and epithelial cells, *Invest. Ophthalmol. Vis. Sci., 17*:687.

127. Lerman, S., Megaw, J. M., and Gardner, K. (1982). Allopurinol therapy and cataractogenesis, *Am. J. Ophthalmol., 94*:141.

128. Lerman, S., Megaw, J. M., and Gardner, K. (1984). Further studies on allopurinol and human cataractogenesis, *Am. J. Ophthalmol., 97*:205.

129. Flach, A. J., Dolan, B. J., Sudduth, B., and Weddell, J. (1983). Amiodarone-induced lens opacities, *Arch. Ophthalmol., 101*:1554.

130. Roberts, J. E., and Dillon, D. J. (1984). A comparison of the photodynamic effect of photosensitizing drugs on lens protein, *Lens Res., 2*:133.

131. Weber, U., Goerz, G., Kern, W., and Michaelis, L. (1987). Clinical and experimental findings in carotenoid retinopathy, *Concepts in Toxicology*, Vol. 4 (O. Hockwin, ed.), Karger, Basel, p. 105.

132. Black, R. L., Oglesby, R. B., von Sallmann, L., and Bunim, I. J. (1960). Posterior subcapsular cataracts induced by corticosteroids in patients with rheumatoid arthritis, *J.A.M.A., 174*:166.

133. Oglesby, R. B., Black, R. L., von Sallmann, L., and Bunim, I. J. (1961). Cataracts in patients with rheumatic diseases treated with corticosteroids, *Arch. Ophthamol., 66*:625.

134. Bernstein, H. N., and Schwartz, Z. B. (1962). Effects of long term systemic steroids on ocular pressure and tonographic values, *Arch. Ophthalmol., 68*:742.

135. Bernstein, H. N., Mills, D. W., and Becker, B. (1963). Steroid induced elevation of intraocular pressure, *Arch. Ophthalmol., 70*:15.

136. Mindel, J. S., Tavitian, H. O., Smith, H., and Walker, E. C. (1980). Comparative ocular pressure elevation by medrysone, fluoromethalone and dexamethasone phosphate, *Arch. Ophthalmol., 98*:1577.

137. Berger, B. B., Weinberg, R. S., Tessler, H. H., Whyhinny, G. J., and Vygantas, C. M. (1979). Bilateral cytomegalovirus panuveitis after high dose corticosteroid therapy, *Am. J. Ophthalmol., 88*:1020.

138. Aronson, S. B., and Moore, T. E. (1969). Corticosteroid therapy in central stromal keratitis, *Am. J. Ophthalmol., 67*:843.

139. Mitsui, T. (1955). Corneal infections after cortisone therapy, *Br. J. Ophthalmol., 39*:244.

140. Greiner, A. C., and Berry, K. (1964). Therapy of chlorpromazine melanosis: A preliminary report, *Can. Med. Assoc. J., 90*:663.

141. Chew, E., Gosh, M., and McCulloch, C. (1982). Amiodarone induced cornea verticillata, *Can. J. Ophthalmol., 17*:96.

142. Kaplan, L., and Cappaert, W. (1982). Amiodarone keratopathy correlation to dosage and duration, *Arch. Ophthalmol., 100*:601.

143. D'Amico, D. L., Kenyon, K. R., and Ruskin, J. N. (1981). Amiodarone Keratopathy: Drug-induced lipid storage disease, *Arch. Ophthalmol., 99*:257.
144. Flach, A. J., Dolan, B. J., Sudduth, B., and Weddell, J. (1983). Amiodarone induced lens opacities, *Arch. Ophthalmol., 101*:1554.
145. Wilson, F. M., II, Schmitt, T. E., and Grayson, M. (1980). Amiodarone induced cornea verticillata, *Ann. Ophthalmol., 12*:657.
146. Carr, R. E., Gouras, P., and Gunkel, R. D. (1966). Chloroquine retinopathy: Early detection by retinal threshold test, *Arch. Ophthalmol., 75*:171.
147. Vopio, H. (1966). Incidence of chloroquine retinopathy, *Acta Ophthalmol., 44*:349.
148. Kaila, T., Salminen, L., and Huupponen, R. (1985). Systemic absorption of topically applied ocular timolol, *J. Ocul. Pharmacol., 1*:79.
149. Passo, M., Palmer, E., and Van Buskirk, E. (1984). Plasma timolol in glaucoma patients, *Ophthalmology, 91*:1361.
150. Fraunfelder, F. T., and Meyer, S. M. (1987). Systemic side effects from ophthalmic timolol and their prevention, *J. Ocul. Pharmacol., 3*:177.
151. Havener, W. H. (1983). *Autonomic Drugs in Ocular Pharmacology* (W. H. Havener, ed.), Mosby, St. Louis, p. 311.
152. Kohn, A. N., Moss, A. P., Hargett, N. A., Ritch, R., Smith, H., and Podos, S. M. (1979). Clinical comparisons of dipivalyl epinephrine and epinephrine in the treatment of glaucoma, *Am. J. Ophthalmol., 87*:196.
153. Mandell, A. I., Stentz, F., and Kitabchi, A. E. (1978). Dipivalyl epinephrine: A new prodrug in the treatment of glaucoma, *Trans. Am. Acad. Ophthalmol. Otolaryngal., 85*:268.
154. Kaas, M. A., Mandell, A. I., Goldberg, T., Paine, J. M., and Becker, B. (1979). Dipivefrin and epinephrine treatment of elevated intraocular pressure, *Arch. Ophthalmol., 97*:1865.
155. Nadal, J., De La Fuente, V., Abadias, M., Torrent, J., and Jané, F. (1987). Toxic coma induced by anticholinergic eyedrops, *Br. Med. J., 295*:1352.
156. Kumar, V., Schoenwald, R. D., Chien, D. S., Packer, A. J., and Choi, W. W. (1985). Systemic absorption and cardiovascular effects of phenylephrine eyedrops, *Am. J. Ophthalmol., 99*:180.
157. Willetts, G. S. (1969). Ocular side effects of drugs, *Br. J. Ophthalmol., 53*:252.
158. Ellis, P. P. (1969). Carbonic anhydrase inhibitors: Pharmacologic effects and problems of long term therapy, *Symposium on Ocular Therapy*, Vol. 4 (I. H. Leopold, ed.), Mosby, St. Louis, p. 32.

2
Ocular Anatomy and Physiology Relevant to Ocular Drug Delivery

James C. Robinson *University of Wisconsin, Madison, Wisconsin*

I. INTRODUCTION

The eye is an isolated organ that maintains connection to the rest of the body through its vascular network as well as nerve fibers and selected muscular attachments. As an isolated and highly protected organ, access to specific tissues is seriously constrained by the numerous physiological and protective defense mechanisms that shield the vision pathway from exogenous substances. To design effective drug delivery approaches, it is first necessary to understand the relevant anatomical and physiological constraints that impede or modify ocular drug and vehicle disposition.

The eye is referred to as a globe; however, it is not a true sphere. Indeed, the eye is actually two spheres, one set in the other, as shown in Figure 1. The front sphere is the smaller of the two and is bordered anteriorly by the cornea, whereas the larger posterior sphere is an opaque fibrous shell encased by the sclera (1). The combined weight of both spheres has been given as 6.77–7.5 g, with a volume of approximately 6.5 mL (2). The circumference of the eye is about 75 mm. Along with the rest of the orbital contents, the eye is located within the boney orbital cavity of the head. The eye is approximately 80% of its adult size at birth.

This chapter is intended to provide a description of selective ocular anatomy and physiology that is relevant to ocular drug delivery. Because of space limitations, it is expected that the depth of certain subjects will be insufficient for some readers and they are encouraged to consult cited references.

II. STRUCTURAL SUPPORT

A. The Orbit

The eyes rest in two boney cavities; i.e., the orbits, located on either side of the nose, as shown in Figure 2. The anterior two-thirds of the orbit is roughly the shape of a

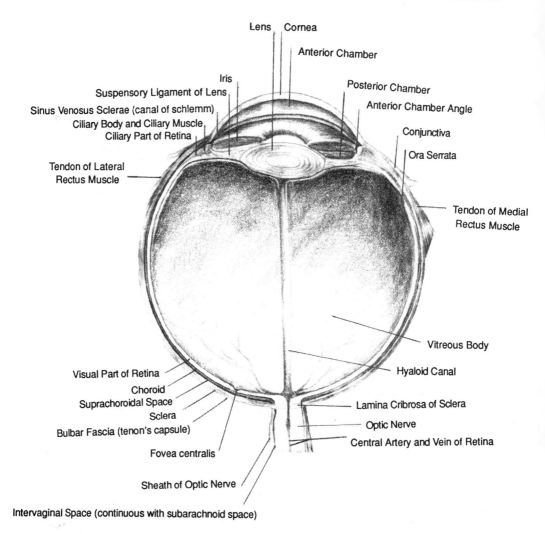

Figure 1. Cross-sectional view of the eye.

quadrilateral pyramid, whereas the posterior one-third of the orbit narrows to the shape of a triangular pyramid (3). The globe occupies approximately 20% of the cavity, lying slightly nearer the upper and lateral sides but never in contact with the orbital bones (4).

    Seven bones make up the orbit: the maxilla, the palatine, the frontal, the sphenoidal, the zygoma, the ethmoid, and the lacrimal bones.

    The optic foramen, located at the apex of the orbit in the body of the sphenoid bone, is the conduit for the optic nerve. In addition, the ophthalmic artery and sympathetic nerves pass through the optic foramen.

    Orbital contents are bound together and supported by connective tissue, the orbital fascia. Although these tissues are connected, they divide the orbit into spaces of clinical importance in limiting the spread of hemorrhage and inflammation, whereas at the same time providing barriers to the external world and the remainder of the head.

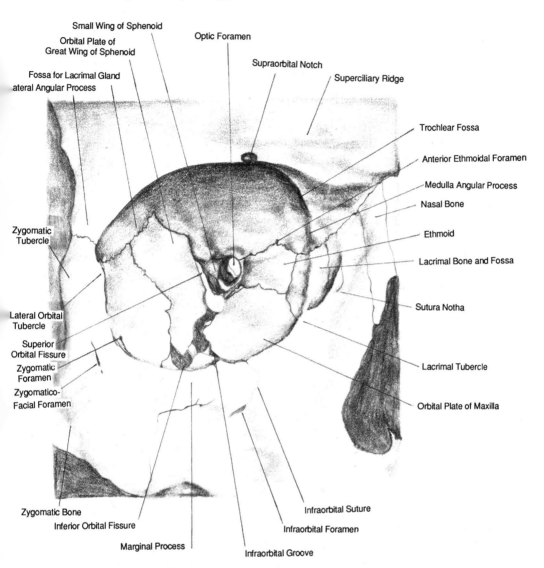

Small Wing of Sphenoid

Orbital Plate of
Great Wing of Sphenoid

Optic Foramen

Supraorbital Notch

Superciliary Ridge

Fossa for Lacrimal Gland
Lateral Angular Process

Trochlear Fossa

Anterior Ethmoidal Foramen

Medulla Angular Process

Nasal Bone

Zygomatic
Tubercle

Ethmoid

Lacrimal Bone and Fossa

Sutura Notha

Lateral Orbital
Tubercle

Superior
Orbital Fissure

Zygomatic
Foramen

Zygomatico-
Facial Foramen

Lacrimal Tubercle

Orbital Plate of Maxilla

Zygomatic Bone

Inferior Orbital Fissure

Marginal Process

Infraorbital Suture

Infraorbital Foramen

Infraorbital Groove

Figure 2. Major landmarks for the orbit of the eye.

III. EXTERNAL OCULAR TISSUES

A. Eyebrows and Eyelids

The eyebrows separate the upper eyelids from the forehead and may move as part of changing facial expressions or in concert with changes in the direction of the visual axis and position of the eyelids.

The eyebrows perform a variety of specialized functions. They have a major influence on nonverbal communication by way of facial expression. In addition, owing to their position and curvature, the eyebrows help shield the eyes from bright sunlight coming from directly above and are efficient barriers to keep liquids, such as perspiration on the forehead, from running into the eyes. Moreover, their sensory innervation is quite extensive, so that they are extremely sensitive to tactile stimulation and thus aid in the protection of the eye by providing an early warning system. Finally, they also participate directly in certain ocular movements and can be important indicators in certain disease processes (5).

The external part of the eye is covered by the eyelids. These mobile folds protect the eye from mechanical or chemical injury by sweeping the external surface of the eye at periodic intervals and, when closed, as a first line of defense. In addition, the lids also keep out excessive light and assist in spreading the secreted tear film over the cornea as well as retarding evaporation from the surface of the eye.

The upper lid is the more mobile of the two. When the lid is open, it covers about 1 mm of the cornea in caucasians and even more in Orientals. This is an important issue in the relative comfort of ocular products. Thus, the cornea is one of the most higher innervated tissues of the body, and movement of an uncomfortable dosage form across this area can lead to patient discomfort. The lower lid lies at the lower edge of the cornea and rises only slightly when the lids shut. Opening and closing movements of the lids are controlled primarily by the levator palpebrae superioris and orbicularis muscles, respectively.

The coordinated opening and closing movements of the eyelids make up the act of blinking. High-speed photography shows that a blink has a zipperlike action beginning in the temporal region and concluding in the nasal region. This zipperlike action helps propel tears toward the drainage apparatus. A single blink averages from 290–750 ms in length (5). Additionally, the average pressure exerted on the globe by the apposition of the lids during blinking is 10 mmHg (6). When a foreign body sensation is present, lid pressure rises dramatically in an attempt to squeeze the intruding material away from the eye. On average, humans blinks 15–20 times per minute, although this can vary widely, depending on the subject and external conditions.

When the eye is open, the angles created by the junctions of the upper and lower lids are called the canthi. The junction closest to the nose is called the medial canthus and on the other side of the cornea it is called the lateral canthus. These landmarks are shown in Figure 3.

The borders of the eyelids are about 2 mm thick and contains the eyelashes and a number of secretory glands. These eyelashes are long hairs arranged in two or three rows with the lashes of the upper lid being longer and more numerous. Eyelashes help sweep foreign substances away from the eye and assist in diverting perspiration away from direct contact with the eye surface. An efficient "window wiper" action of the lids is maintained, since the posterior border of the lid margin is sharp and fits tightly against the front surface of the eye.

By depressing the lower lid you can see a thin, gray line that separates the two borders of the lid. This anatomical landmark is used in many surgical procedures to split the eyelids into two portions.

The lid margins also contain tiny openings which lead to the sweat and oil glands. The largest oil-secreting glands are embedded in the posterior tissue of the lids and are called the meibomian glands (Figure 4). Secretions from these glands provide lubrication, help retard evaporation of tears, and probably play an antimicrobial role similar to that of the sebaceous glands of the skin.

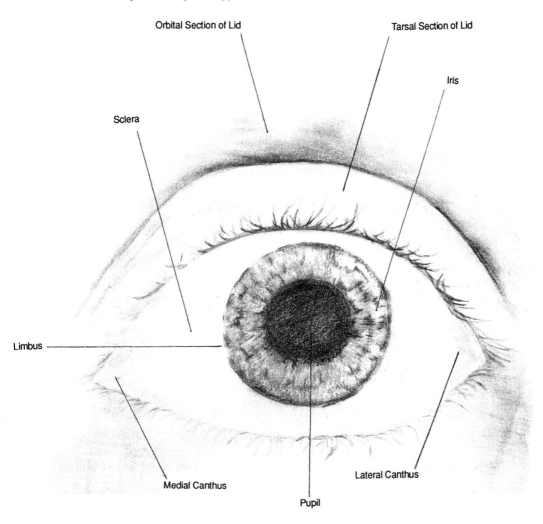

Figure 3. Front view of the eye with associated landmarks.

B. Conjunctiva

The conjunctiva is a vascularized mucous membrane that covers the anterior surface of the globe with the exception of the cornea, as shown in Figure 5. Conjunctival epithelium is continuous with that of the cornea and with the epidermis of the lids and has a surface area that is about five times that of the cornea. Mucus-producing goblet cells which are important for wetting and tear film stability are located in the conjunctiva (7). In addition to physical protection of the globe, the conjunctiva has great potential for combating infection for four reasons:

1. It is a highly vascular tissue, thus able to mobilize and deliver defense cells and antimicrobial agents.
2. It contains many immunocompetent cells.

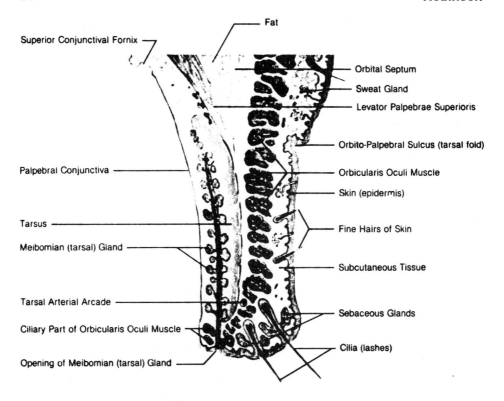

Figure 4. Cross-sectional view of the eyelid showing various glands.

3. The different cells types located within the conjunctiva can initiate and participate in inflammatory reactions.
4. The anatomy and biochemistry of conjunctival cells enable it to phagocytize and neutralize foreign particles (8,9).

Anatomically the conjunctiva is divided into three areas:

1. The palpebral (lid) conjunctiva
2. The conjunctival fornix
3. The bulbar (globe) conjunctiva

The palpebral conjunctiva may be further subdivided into the marginal, tarsal, and orbital portions. The conjunctiva of the lid margin is actually a transition zone between the skin and conjunctiva and the tear drainage puncta open on the marginal portion of the conjunctiva. In contrast, the tarsal conjunctiva is thin, transparent, very vascular, and tightly adherent to the tarsal plate. The orbital zone of the conjunctiva lies between the tarsal plate and the fornix. Its surface is cast into horizontal folds, which are folds of movement that are deepest when the eyes are open and almost disappear when the eyes are shut.

The conjunctival fornix is subdivided into superior, inferior, lateral, and medial regions. Located within the conjunctival fornix are the glands of Krause and the nonstriated muscle of Mueller. The fornix has a rich vascular supply.

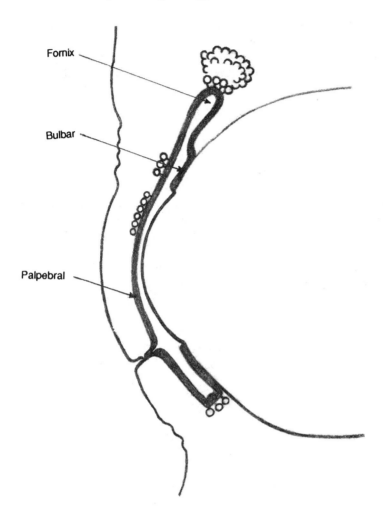

Fornix

Bulbar

Palpebral

Figure 5. The conjunctival membrane.

Finally, the bulbar conjunctiva is thin and transparent, so that the underlying sclera appears white. It lies loosely on the underlying tissues and thus may be easily moved. Owing to its exposed position, degenerative and traumatic conditions are common in the bulbar conjunctiva.

The arterial supply of the conjunctiva comes from the peripheral arterial and marginal arterial arcades as well as the anterior ciliary arteries (10). This arterial plexus is arranged in two layers, a superficial conjunctival and a deep episcleral. The superficial portion is engorged in superficial infections of the cornea, whereas the deeper portion is engorged in conditions affecting the iris, ciliary body, or deep portions of the cornea.

As a protective tissue, the conjunctiva is richly endowed with sensory nerve endings. This sensory nerve supply is derived from the ophthalmic branch of the trigeminal nerve (11). The conjunctival sensory system is closely associated with those of the eyelids, eyebrows, and cornea. Pain associated with the conjunctiva may be caused by almost any stimulus if it is of sufficient intensity, but some of the more common causes of pain in and about the eye include inflammation, hypoxia, denudation, and deformation or compression of receptors. The last two causes are especially difficult to deal with when designing a drug delivery system that is intended to remain in contact with the eye for extended periods of time.

C. Muscles

The extraocular muscles include the four rectus muscles and two oblique muscles (Fig. 6). The various combinations of their simultaneous contractions and relaxations allow a multitude of different rotation axes about which the eye may move. The specific muscles and associated innervation and function are shown in Table 1.

All of the rectus muscles originate in the orbital apex from the annulus of Zinn. The superior oblique muscle originates in the apex of the orbit from the annulus of Zinn, whereas the inferior oblique muscle originates on the anterior nasal floor.

In humans, the two eyes work as though they were one; i.e., binocular. Both eyes project to the same point in space and fuse their images so that a single mental impression is obtained by this collaboration. Without this delicate balance, we would see double because two images would be formed by the independent action of each eye. The ability of the eyes to fuse two images into a single picture is called binocular vision.

Fixation involves the simple task of looking straight ahead toward an object in space. To operate effectively, fixation requires stability of the eyes and good eye function. If the eyes are constantly moving, such as occurs with nystagmus, the eyes can only make

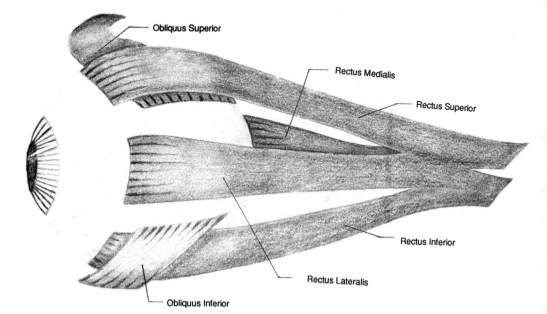

Figure 6. The extraocular muscles.

Table 1. Extraocular Muscles: Innervation and Function

Muscle	Innervation	Function
Medial rectus	3rd cranial nerve	Adduction[a]
Lateral rectus	6th cranial nerve	Abduction[a]
Superior rectus	3rd cranial nerve	Supraduction[b] Intorsion[c]
Inferior rectus	3rd cranial nerve	Infraduction[b] Extorsion[c]
Superior oblique	4th cranial nerve	Infraduction[b] Intorsion[c]
Inferior oblique	3rd cranial nerve	Supraduction[b] Extorsion[c]

[a]Adduction is a horizontal movement directed medially and abduction is a horizontal movement directed laterally from the vertical axis.
[b]Supraduction is a vertical movement directed superiorly and infraduction is a vertical movement directed inferiorly from the horizontal axis.
[c]Incycloduction (intorsion) is a torsional movement of the eye about the anteroposterior axis that displaces the superior pole of the eye medially. Excycloduction (extorsion) is a torsional movement of the eye about the anteroposterior axis that displaces the superior pole of the eye laterally.

scanning motions about an object and never adequately see it in detail. If the ability to fixate becomes compromised by constant eye movements, then the visual acuity of the affected eye is reduced.

Fusion is the power exerted by both eyes to keep the position of the eyes aligned so that both foveas project to the same point in space. Since movement of the entire eyeball is controlled by a small number of attached muscles, it is possible to shorten one or more of these muscles to correct a poorly directed eye or crossed eye (esotropia).

Depth perception is a higher quality of binocular vision. Each eye views an object at a slightly different angle, so that fusion of images occurs by combining slightly dissimilar images. It is the combination of these angular views that yields depth perception.

IV. LACRIMAL SYSTEM

A. Tears

1. Physiology

The tear film is a highly specialized moist film that covers the bulbar and palpebral conjunctiva and the cornea. Abnormalities of the tear film can result in dysfunction of the eyelids and conjunctiva as well as a loss of corneal transparency.

The cul-de-sac normally holds 7–9 µL of tears but can retain up to approximately 20–30 µL without overflowing if care is taken not to blink. Under baseline conditions, the normal tear flow rate and tear film thickness are 1 µL/min; i.e., approximately 16%/min and 4–9 µm, respectively (12). Additionally, the normal pH of tears is ~6.5–7.6. An oft-repeated statement in the literature is that tears are a well-buffered system, in part, because instilled solutions of lower pH are quickly returned to physiological conditions. The rapid return of pH is likely due to high tear turnover rather than a well-buffered tear. The turnover of tears is heavily dependent on environmental conditions, such as temperature, relative humidity, and wind as well as age and the physiological state of the patient.

Eyelid movement is of paramount importance in the continual renewal and reformation of the preocular tear film. Tears from the lacrimal gland do not flow across all external eye tissues but rather flow down to the lid margins and from there to the drainage ducts. Thus, adequate wetting of external eye tissues is accomplished by the sweeping action of the lids which moves the secreted tears across the cornea and conjunctiva. Movement of the lids is thus responsible for moving tears into the collection portion of the lacrimal apparatus as well as the distribution of new tears over the ocular surface (13,14). Drainage of tears and instilled solutions away from the front of the eye is an extremely efficient process; i.e., removal of a 25–50 μL volume of instilled solution in the human is essentially completed at around 90 s.

2. Biochemistry

The tear film is a trilaminar structure with each layer distinctive in its own composition (Fig. 7). Beginning with the corneal surface, there is a layer of mucin. Just anterior to this layer is an aqueous phase that makes up the bulk of the tear film, and the outermost layer of the tears is a monolayer of lipid.

The anterior layer of the tear film is made up predominantly of a lipid fraction as well as small amounts of mucin and proteins. Mucus and proteins, although they may be surface active, do not retard evaporation. Lipids do, however, reduce evaporation to about 10% of that found in other fluid systems without such a surface layer. The lipids secreted by the tarsal glands along the eyelid margins are neutral oils (4%), phospholipids (16%), sterol ester fractions (32%), mixed waxes (35%), and other lipids (13%) (15,16). The surface-active compounds present in conjunctival mucus facilitate the spreading of tears across precorneal tissues as well as movement of tarsal gland lipids over the surface of the tear film.

The middle layer of the tear film constitutes about 98% of this trilaminar film. This layer is composed mainly of water, electrolytes, and various proteins. The osmotic pressure of the tear film is ~311–350 mOsm in normal eyes and is regulated by the principal inorganic ions Na^+, K^+, Cl^-, HCO_3^-, and proteins (17). The osmotic pressure of tears is slightly higher than blood owing to constant evaporation of the tear film. Under basal conditions, the oxygen tension in the precorneal tear film varies from 140 to 160 mmHg. A minimal precorneal oxygen tension, which is needed to avoid corneal edema, is ~74 mmHg (18).

The posterior layer of the tear film is a mucin layer, i.e., a glycoprotein, which chemically consists of about one-quarter protein and three-fourths carbohydrate. Conjunctival mucus is a mixture of neutral and acidic mucopolysaccharides which are secreted by the approximately 1.5 million goblet cells located on the conjunctival surface. This secreted mucous contributes stability to the tear film as well as furnishing an attachment for the tear film to the underlying cornea and conjunctiva.

Lysozyme (muramidase), an antimicrobial enzyme, is an important protein component of the tear film (19,20). Lysozyme helps to prevent infectious agents from reaching the blood stream via the conjunctival surface and helps maintain sterile conditions in the front of the eye.

ATMOSPHERIC AIR

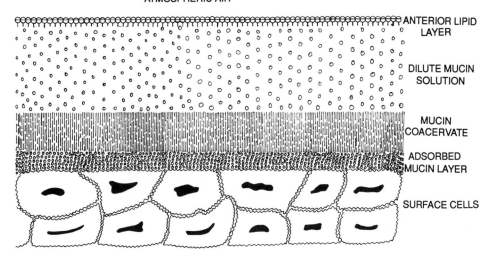

Figure 7.   Proposed structure of the tear film in the human eye.

B.   Secretory and Drainage Apparatus

The lacrimal system consists of a secretory and a collection portion. The collection aspect has been discussed previously. Tears are a complex mixture of salts, proteins, lipids, phospholipids, and enzymes in a water base. The secretory portion of the lacrimal system consists of the main and accessory lacrimal glands. The main lacrimal gland lies in the lacrimal fossa of the frontal bone and occupies the lateral one-third of the orbital roof; i.e., in the temporal region on both sides of the head. In an adult, the main lacrimal gland measures approximately $20 \times 12 \times 15$ mm and weighs about 0.78 g (21) and constitutes the bulk of tear fluid (Fig. 8). The main excretory ducts from this gland empty into the superior fornix just above the lid margin.

Secreted tears do not normally flow across the cornea but must be assisted by the wiperlike action of the lids. It is assumed that secreted tears mix relatively rapidly and thoroughly with tears held in the lower cul-de-sac; an assumption that has not been experimentally verified and which is very important in drug delivery.

There are approximately 60 accessory lacrimal glands located within the conjunctival stroma which empty onto the epithelial surface of the conjunctiva via small ducts. Approximately two-thirds of these are the glands of Krause and are located in the lateral part of the upper fornix near the main lacrimal gland. Along the orbital margin of each lid are a group of slightly larger glands known as the glands of Wolfring (Fig. 9). These accessory lacrimal glands help produce the aqueous phase of the tear film.

The openings into which tears drain are the four puncta; one for each eyelid of each eye. Each punctum is round or slightly oblong and measures approximately 0.3 mm. They are located on the medial portion of each eyelid directly in line with the openings of the tarsal glands. Fluid is directed into the puncta by the blinking action of the lids. From the puncta fluid enters the lacrimal canaliculi which transport the fluid to the lacrimal sac. The removal of tears by the zipperlike closure of the lids is assisted by a negative pressure in the

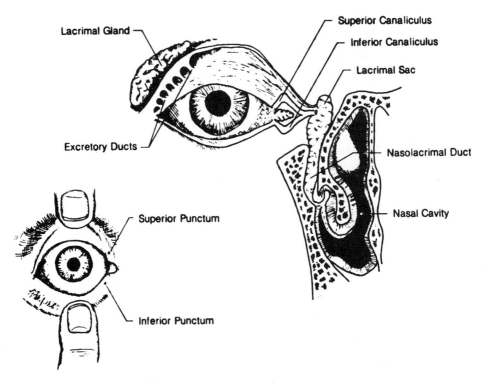

Figure 8. The tear drainage apparatus of the eye.

lacrimal sac. These two events help propel tears away from the eye and into the drainage apparatus. Fluid from the lacrimal sac drains into the nasolacrimal duct which leads to the nose, where it empties into the inferior nasal meatus (see Fig. 8).

The nasal meatus is a highly vascular area, and hence normal tears and drugs contained in tears are absorbed into the systemic circulation from this area. One has to tear copiously to exceed the capacity of this area to absorb tears and have the tears leak out of the nose.

C. Issues in Drug Delivery

There are a substantial number of issues relating to the precorneal area of the eye that can have a major impact on ocular drug delivery. Some of these issues appear intractable to study at present owing to analytical limitation, whereas others are being considered by investigators in the field. The purpose of this tabulation of statements and questions is to attempt to identify important areas for consideration in developing ocular drug delivery systems.

1. Since both lacrimation and blinking profoundly influence residence time of liquid ocular drug delivery systems, comfort of the drug delivery system seems essential. Comfort of specific drugs, buffer components, and drug delivery systems is not well understood.
2. Placement of the drop, solid, or semisolid system as deep as possible into the lower cul-de-sac will assist in patient comfort as well as residence time.

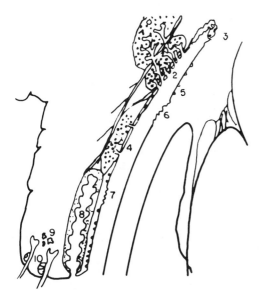

MAIN LACRIMAL GLAND
1 orbital lobe
2 palpebral lobe
ACCESSORY LACRIMAL GLANDS

3 glands of Krause
4 glands of Wolfring
MUCIN SECRETORS
5 goblet cells
6 glands of Manz
7 crypts of Henle

OIL SECRETORS
8 meibomian gland
9 glands of Moll
10 glands of Zeis

Figure 9. Cross-sectional view showing lacrimal glands.

3. How well do liquid delivery systems coat and/or adhere to the cornea and conjunctival surface?
4. The smallest instilled drop (5 μL) will minimize systemic load through drainage loss.
5. Because of eyeball shape and movement, as well as lid pressure during blinking, soluble and insoluble ocular drug inserts must be small, thin, and carefully shaped to avoid movement and perhaps expulsion from the eye.
6. For local treatment, good mixing of the drug delivery system with all areas of the front of the eye is necessary. There is no literature evidence that present ocular drug delivery systems adequately cover all precorneal tissues in a short period of time postdosing, but considering the power and frequency of the blinking process, it is probably a good assumption.

Table 2. Comparison of Some Precorneal Characteristics in the Human and Rabbit

	Rabbit	Human
Tear volume	7–8 µL	7–8 µL
Tear turnover	8%/min	16%/min
Blink rate	2–5/min	15–20/min
Drainage rate constant 50 µL solutions	0.545 min^{-1}	1.40 min^{-1}
Protein content of tears	0.5%	0.7%

7. Very little work has been reported on the precorneal metabolism of drugs in large measure because of severe analytical limitation. Given the usual short contact time of drug, even with a reasonably sensitive drug, it is not likely that extensive precorneal drug metabolism occurs. As contact time of drug increases, with certain prolonged-release systems, the issue of local metabolism increases accordingly.
8. Given the frequent use of the rabbit as an experimental animal in ocular drug delivery research, it may be helpful to compare some precorneal characteristics in the rabbit and human. Table 2 compares the rabbit and human.

V. ANTERIOR SEGMENT

A. Anterior Chamber

The anterior chamber is bounded in front by the cornea and a small portion of the sclera. Posteriorly the anterior chamber is bounded by the front surface of the iris, a variable area of the anterior surface of the lens, and a part of the ciliary body (see Fig. 1). At the periphery of the anterior chamber is the so-called drainage angle. It is here that the trabecular meshwork is located and conventional outflow of aqueous humor occurs. The anterior chamber is deepest centrally and shallowest at the periphery, holding a volume of aqueous humor that has been shown to be ~250 µL in the human, with a turnover rate of ~1%/min (22). The discussion of certain tissues in either the anterior or posterior segment sections were done in an attempt to move from the front to the back of the eye. Naturally, there is some overlap of tissues between the anterior and posterior segments.

1. Cornea

The cornea, or window of the eye, is an optically transparent tissue that conveys images to the back of the eye. Any change in the cornea, such as curvature, the presence of blood vessels, excessive thickness, or edema, will interfere with the visual pathway.

The cornea, being an avascular tissue, receives nutrients and oxygen from the bathing solutions, i.e., the tears and aqueous humor as well as from the blood vessels that line the junction between the cornea and sclera, i.e., the limbal blood vessels. Depriving the cornea of any of its nutrient or oxygen supply can create a physiological disaster. Thus, hard contact lenses with low oxygen permeability can only be worn for a limited period of time and then must be removed to allow the cornea to become resupplied with oxygen.

Corneal diameter is about 11.5 mm with a radius of curvature of the anterior corneal surface of 7.8 mm. The cornea measures approximately 0.5 mm thick centrally and increases to approximately 0.7 mm at the limbus (23,24). The surface area of the cornea and conjunctiva in a normal adult human is approximately 16 cm^2.

The cornea is composed of the following five layers (Fig. 10).

1. Epithelium
2. Bowman's membrane
3. Substantia propria (stroma)
4. Descemet's membrane
5. Endothelium

a. Epithelium

The corneal epithelium is ~50 μm thick and represents the most important barrier to invasion by foreign substances, including drugs. It is composed of five or six layers of epithelial cells, which are continuous with those of the conjunctiva, and which replace themselves at a rate of approximately a cell layer per day. There is a basal layer of columnar cells, two to three layers of wing-shaped cells and one to two layers of nonkeratinized flattened superficial cells. The basement membrane of the basal epithelial cells is a continuous well-defined osmophilic layer about 400 Å in thickness (25). There are zonulae occludentes between the lateral surfaces of the superficial cells, and it is these zonulae occludentes that determines the degree of impermeability of the corneal epithelium to water-soluble drugs. In general, the intercellular space in the lower superficial space of the epithelium allows passage of horseradish peroxidase, a 40-kd material. However, the uppermost layers have an upper limit of about 1 kd, or perhaps smaller size, for permeation of the intercellular spaces. The anterior surface of the superficial cells display microvilli and microplicae which help in holding the tear film to the anterior surface of the eye.

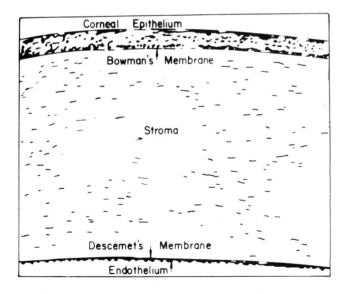

Figure 10. The cornea.

The corneal epithelium is a reasonably hydrophobic tissue and, indeed, ophthalmic literature commonly states that useful ocular drugs intended to cross the cornea should have an oil/water partition coefficient of greater than one and preferably 10–100.

b. Bowman's Membrane

Bowman's membrane is an 8–14 μm thick, homogeneous sheet between the basement membrane and substantia propria. It is separated from the epithelium by a sharply defined border and is acellular except under pathological conditions.

c. Substantia Propria (Stroma)

The stroma forms about 90% of the cornea and is composed of a modified connective tissue. Water constitutes ~70% of the volume of the stroma. There are approximately 200–250 alternating lamellae of collagenous tissue in the stroma. Each lamellae is ~2 μm thick and 10–25 μm wide. In each lamellae, the fibers lie in parallel to each other, whereas in alternating layers they lie at right angles to each other. This arrangement provides physical strength while permitting optical transparency.

d. Descemet's Membrane

Descemet's membrane is 10–15 μm thick and lies between the stroma and the endothelium. It is very elastic and remarkably resistant to proteolytic enzymes, often remaining intact when the epithelium and stroma have been destroyed.

e. Endothelium

The endothelium is the most posterior layer of the cornea and consists of a single layer of flattened epithelial-like cells. The cells are separated from each other via a substantial intercellular space. Indeed, few drugs will be impeded in their transcorneal movement by the endothelial layer. With age, lost endothelial cells are replaced by thinning and spreading out of the surrounding cells rather than by cell proliferation. This layer houses the water pump responsible for maintaining corneal thickness (26).

2. Limbus

The corneoscleral limbus is a transitional zone 1–2 mm wide between the cornea proper and the sclera and conjunctiva. Externally, the limbus is covered by peripheral corneal epithelium and anterior conjunctival epithelium. Internally, the limbus includes aqueous veins, the canal of Schlemm, and the trabecular meshwork (Fig. 11) (4). Since the cornea is an avascular tissue, the limbal blood supply is an important source of nutrients and defense mechanisms. Indeed, activation of this defense can present problems with vision. After trauma, infection, or an inflammatory process to the cornea, blood vessels can penetrate the cornea from the limbal region, presumably in an attempt to bring defense cells to the area. This neovascularization of the cornea can lead to visual impairment. Additionally, the limbus is an important anatomical landmark because of surgical procedures employing a limbal incision.

3. Trabecular Meshwork and Schlemm's Canal

The trabecular meshwork and canal of Schlemm form the conventional pathway of aqueous humor outflow from the anterior segment of the eye. The trabecular meshwork is divided into uveal and corneoscleral portions, each with their own distinct anatomy. Aqueous humor leaves the eye at the anterior chamber angle, where it enters the trabecular meshwork. Once aqueous percolates through the trabecular meshwork, it enters into Schlemm's canal, and once in the lumen of Schlemm's canal, it flows into the 25 to 35 endothelial

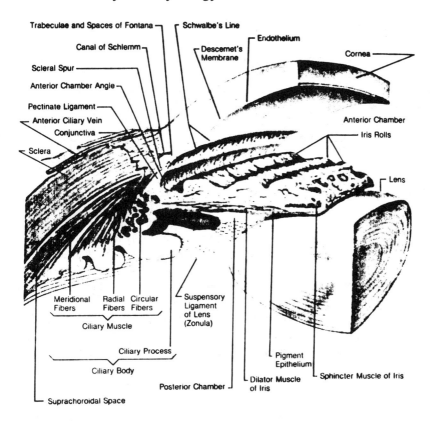

Figure 11. Illustration of the anterior segment of the eye showing the aqueous humor drainage apparatus.

tubules that exit from the circumference of the outer wall of Schlemm's canal. Some of these external collector channels connect directly to the deep scleral venous plexus; however, most penetrate through the sclera and join the episcleral venous plexus, where aqueous humor is drained into the venous system (27). Although the majority of aqueous humor leaves the eye via the trabecular meshwork, a portion of it is drained by the uveoscleral or unconventional pathway (28,29). In the uveoscleral pathway, aqueous humor courses through the ciliary muscle, between muscle bundles, to the suprachoroidal space to be carried away by the choroidal vessels. In addition, some aqueous humor actually drains through the sclera to orbital lymph and blood vessels. In addition, a portion of aqueous humor leaves the anterior and posterior chambers through the iris and through the vitreous to the optic nerve and retinal vessels.

Inasmuch as the eye is a hollow sphere, its interior pressure must exceed that of the surrounding atmosphere to prevent collapse. Thus, normal intraocular pressure is between 13 and 19 mmHg (30). Two factors are primarily concerned with the maintenance of intraocular pressure: the rate of aqueous humor secretion and the rate of outflow of aqueous humor. Glaucoma is an increase in intraocular pressure, the cause of which has many etiologies.

B. Posterior Chamber

The posterior chamber is somewhat triangular in appearance. The apex of the triangle is located where the edge of the iris rests on the lens. The base is formed by the ciliary processes, the posterior wall is formed by the lens and zonule, and the anterior wall is the posterior surface of the iris. The posterior chamber is filled with about 50 μl of aqueous humor. Aqueous produced by the ciliary processes, at a rate of 2.0–2.5 μl/min, flows into the posterior chamber through the pupil and from there into the anterior chamber (31,32).

1. Iris and Pupil

The pupil is a circular opening located near the center of the iris (see Figs. 1, 3, and 11). There are two sets of smooth muscle in the iris that regulate pupillary diameter: the sphincter and the dilator muscles. The pupillary sphincter is primarily parasympathetically innervated, whereas the dilator is primarily sympathetically innervated. The diameter of the normal pupil varies from 2 to 9 mm depending upon illumination, emotional state, fatigue, and amount of accommodation. In the normal eye, both the sphincter and dilator muscles are continuously working and the pupillary diameter is a function of the relative activity of these two muscles (33). Pupillary dilation increases the amount of light entering the eye and enhances the ability of the rods to function. In contrast, pupillary constriction increases the depth of focus of the eye and decreases optical aberrations from the lens periphery.

The iris separates the anterior and posterior chambers. It is bathed by aqueous humor on its anterior and posterior surfaces and permits the free flow of aqueous from the posterior to the anterior chamber.

Arterial blood supply to the iris is provided by the long posterior ciliary arteries and the anterior ciliary arteries.

Color of the iris depends upon the amount of melanin in its stroma. If there is only a small amount of melanin, reflection from the pigment located in the posterior layer of the iris causes scattering of light with a blue appearance. Conversely, a heavily pigmented iris will cause minimal light scattering and thus a brown appearance. There is often a considerable quantitative difference in drug response between light and heavily pigmented eyes. Some of this difference can be ascribed to simple drug binding to melanin granules, whereas a portion is attributable to metabolic differences.

Perhaps not surprisingly, the majority of drug in the aqueous humor from a topical dose will leave the eye via bulk flow. In addition, it is expected that a portion will enter the iris and leave via the vascular bed in this tissue.

2. Ciliary Body

The ciliary body is responsible for many functions in the eye. It secretes aqueous humor, nourishes the lens, provides the muscle power for accommodation, and may secrete the unique zonular fibers. In cross-section, the shape of the ciliary body is triangular with its shortest side anterior. The anterior ciliary is known as the pars plicata (Fig. 12) and contains 70 to 80 folds known as the ciliary processes where aqueous humor is secreted. The posterior portion of the ciliary body is known as the pars plana. The ciliary body is attached posteriorly to the retina at the ora serrata. Ciliary epithelium consists of two layers: an inner nonpigmented layer (NPE) and an outer pigmented layer (PE) (34). The NPE of the ciliary body stretches from the root of the iris to the ora serrata in a continuous layer. Aqueous

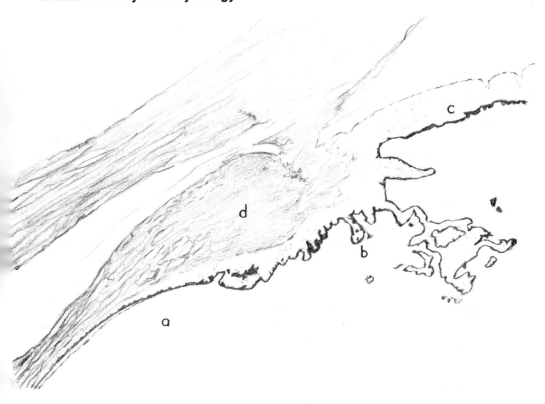

Figure 12. The ciliary body, a = pars plana ciliaris, b = plicata ciliaris, c = iris, d = ciliary muscle.

humor is secreted by the ciliary epithelium and it is hypothesized that the NPE is actually responsible for its production.

The ciliary muscle, which expands and contracts the lens to accommodate the visual process, is traditionally divided into three portions: an outer longitudinal, a middle radial, and an inner circular portion. These regions are felt to be interconnected, so that upon contraction the muscle undergoes a three-dimensional anterior and inward movement. The greatest bulk of the ciliary muscle lies in the anterior two-thirds of the ciliary body. The action of ciliary muscle contraction is to decrease tension on the zonules, resulting in a decreased tension on the lens capsule, which therefore becomes more convex. This process is known as accommodation and is used to look at near objects.

The blood supply to the ciliary body is derived from the two long posterior ciliary arteries and from the anterior ciliary arteries. Innervation of the ciliary body is parasympathetic, sympathetic, and sensory. It has been estimated that 1–2% of ciliary muscle innervation is sympathetic in origin with the rest being parasympathetic (35,36).

3. Aqueous Humor

The aqueous humor is produced both by active and passive secretion from the ciliary processes. Under normal conditions, it has been estimated that active secretion accounts for

~80–90% of total aqueous humor formation. There are two enzymes located in the nonpigmented epithelium of the ciliary processes that are intimately involved in the active secretion of aqueous (37,38). These are the sodium-potassium activated adenosine triphosphate enzyme (Na^+-K^+-ATPase) and carbonic anhydrase.

The composition of aqueous humor differs from that of plasma as a result of two distinct physiological processes. One process is the active transport of organic and inorganic substances by the ciliary epithelium, and the other is diffusion across the blood-aqueous barrier. The physiological manifestation of these two processes is the low protein and high ascorbate concentration in the aqueous relative to the plasma. Additionally, the aqueous concentration of lactate is higher than that in plasma (39).

C. Issues in Drug Delivery

1. Coverage of the cornea by the lids is an important consideration in patient comfort with certain types of delivery systems. As will be discussed later, the cornea is one of the most highly innervated tissues of the body. Physically immobile dosage forms such as inserts and gels when swept across the cornea cause a certain discomfort to the patient. Moreover, it appears that differences in tightness of the lid to the globe, as well as extent of corneal coverage, can account for why certain ocular delivery systems show racial differences. Thus, systems designed for North American Caucasians can be uncomfortable when placed in Oriental eyes.

2. From a drug permeability point of view, it appears that the cornea consists of a lipophilic epithelial layer, a thick layer of water beneath this, i.e., the stroma, and finally a porous endothelial layer. As a result, the corneal epithelium represents the primary barrier for water-soluble drugs and drugs with small oil/water partition coefficients, whereas the stroma is the primary barrier for very lipophilic drugs. In light of the unfavorable oil/water partition coefficient for many drugs, i.e., if it has a high partition into the corneal epithelium it will have low partition into the stroma, low bioavailability will result unless there is prolonged residence time.

3. It is physically difficult to maintain a drug delivery system on the cornea unless it is a contact lens. Thus, all drug delivery systems will typically be housed elsewhere in the front of the eye with appreciable drug loss to those tissues. As an illustration, the conjunctiva is about five times the surface area of the cornea and is commonly more permeable to drugs. It is likely, therefore, that an upper limit to corneal absorption of an externally applied drug is 10–15%. A desirable solution would be to have a drug that shows good corneal but poor conjunctival absorption. This is, to a large extent, wishful thinking.

VI. POSTERIOR SEGMENT

A. Lens

The lens is a transparent bioconvex structure located behind the iris and in front of the vitreous. Like all lenses, that of the eye has two surfaces, anterior and posterior, and a border where these surfaces meet; i.e., the equator. At its equator, the lens has a diameter of ~10 mm. The average radius of curvature of the anterior surface is ~10 mm, whereas that of the posterior surface is ~6 mm (40).

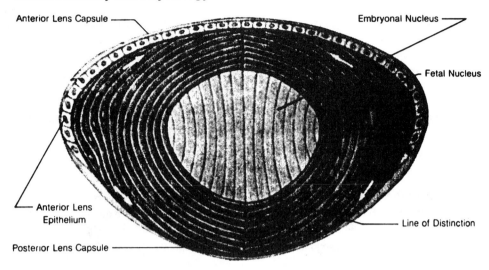

Figure 13. Cross-sectional view of the lens.

The lens is composed of components (Fig. 13) (41):

1. Lenticular capsule
2. Lenticular epithelium
3. Lens cells or fibers

1. Lenticular Capsule

The lens capsule is a hypertrophied basement membrane. Its thickness varies with age and position. It is thickest both preequatorially and postequatorially and thinnest posteriorly. One of the most important functions of the lens capsule is that it serves as a point of attachment for the zonules.

2. Lenticular Epithelium

The lens grows throughout life, although at decreasing rates with increasing age. All lens growth is dependent upon mitotic activity of the lens epithelium. The lens epithelium is a monolayer of cells that occupy the anterior surface of the lens but does not extend to the posterior side of the lens.

3. Lens Fibers

Lens fibers are located internally to the epithelium with newer fibers being laid down externally to the older deeper ones, so that the lens acquires a laminated structure. The superficial youngest fibers are nucleated while the older fibers lose their nuclei. New lens fibers are produced throughout life; however, since the older fibers cannot be shed, the lens keeps on growing. This growth is not proportional to the number of new fibers, since the older fibers shrink, thus by age 65 the lens is approximately one-third larger than at age 25. Additionally, the consistency of the lens varies with the superficial portion of cortex being softer than the central part, the nucleus. As a result of this density difference between the outer and inner portion of the lens, it is likely that drug distribution from a topically applied drug, especially as a function of time, would be different. There are numerous references that describe the content of drug in the lens as if it were a homogeneous tissue. Unless a differential in drug concentration as a function of lens section is reported, this homogeneous view of lens-drug distribution does not give a true profile of drug levels.

4. Lens Color

The color of the lens also changes with age. In the very young, it is usually colorless but with age it acquires a yellowish tinge, so that often in the elderly, the lens has an amber color.

5. Zonules

The zonules are a system of fibers that emanate from the ciliary body and attach to the equator of the lens, both anteriorly and posteriorly. These suspensory ligaments support the lens in the visual axis. The zonular fibers are dense bundles up to 60 μm in diameter and are made up of 0.35- to 1.0-μm fibers, which are in turn composed of microfibrils 8–12 nm in diameter.

6. Accommodation

Accommodation is the adjustment by the eye for vision at different distances (42). This adjustment is accomplished by changing the shape of the lens. As an object is moved closer to the eye, the rays of light entering the eye must be continuously converged so as to prevent a blurred image. This change in focusing power is achieved by contraction of the ciliary muscle, which in turn relaxes the tension of the zonules. Once the zonular tension has relaxed, the lens is able to achieve a more spherical shape. This change in shape increases the thickness of the lens and thus increases its refractive power. The ability to accommodate decreases with age and is called presbyopia.

B. Sclera

The outer coat of the eye is fibrous and serves a protective function. The white opaque sclera constitutes the posterior five-sixths of the globe, whereas the transparent cornea comprises the anterior one-sixth of the globe (see Fig. 1).

The scleral shell has a diameter of 22 mm and a radius of curvature of 12 mm (43). It is 1 mm thick posteriorly and at the equator it thins to 0.6 mm. Immediately posterior to the insertions of the rectus muscles, the sclera is only 0.3 mm thick. The scleral coat does thicken to 0.6 mm where the tendons of the rectus muscles attach. Adjacent to the limbus, the sclera is 0.8 mm thick.

The anterior surface of the sclera is covered by the episclera and the inner surface is covered by the lamina fusca. The episclera is a thin fibrovascular layer that covers the outer surface of the sclera and contains many arteriolar branches from the anterior ciliary vessels. These vessels form a distinct layer from the conjunctival vessels. Sandwiched between these two vascular layers, the subconjunctival vessels and the episcleral plexus, is Tenon's capsule. Tenon's capsule is an avascular layer of collagen that surrounds the globe. Clinically, ophthalmologists have used injection into Tenon's capsule for prolonged release of drug. Anteriorly Tenon's is inseparable from the conjunctiva and posteriorly it blends with the dura of the optic nerve. The inner surface of the sclera is light brown in color and is called the lamina fusca. The brown color is due to a thin irregular coating of melanocytes.

The sclera consists of dense bundles of collagen fibers, which vary in width, with the outer fibers being thicker than the inner fibers (44). These bundles do not lie in an orderly pattern but are interlaced in an irregular fashion.

There are two major openings in the scleral sphere. Anteriorly, the anterior scleral foramen, approximately 12 mm in diameter, surrounds the cornea; and posteriorly, approximately 3.8 mm nasal to the posterior pole, the posterior scleral foramen, the optic nerve canal pierces the sclera. There are approximately 20 small openings known as emissaria present in the posterior sclera. These carry the posterior long and short ciliary nerves and arteries. Between the equator and the posterior pole there are four to eight larger channels through which the vortex veins exit. Anteriorly, the anterior ciliary arteries pierce the sclera delivering blood to the ciliary body and other anterior segment tissues. Additionally, small veins pass outwards carrying drainage from the anterior uvea and aqueous humor from Schlemm's canal.

C. Choroid

The choroid (Fig. 14) is the vascular coat of the eye and is divided into four layers:

1. Suprachoroid
2. Layer of vessels
3. Choriocapillaris
4. Bruch's membrane

The suprachoroid is a transition zone between the choroid and the sclera. It is ~30 μm thick and consists of flattened lamellae of collagen fibers (45). The vascular layer of the choroid receives its blood supply from three sources, all of which are orbital branches of the ophthalmic artery (46). These three sources are the short and long posterior ciliary arteries and the anterior ciliary arteries. There are 15 to 20 short posterior ciliary arteries that perforate the sclera near the optic nerve. Two branches of the ophthalmic artery become the long nasal and temporal posterior ciliary arteries. These vessels pierce the sclera along with the long posterior ciliary nerves 3–4 mm from the optic nerve. The arteries of the four rectus muscles follow their tendons to their scleral insertions, where they perforate the sclera as the anterior ciliary arteries. The anterior ciliary arteries pass through the sclera, traverse the suprachoroidal space, enter the ciliary muscle, and join with the major arterial circle of the iris. Venous drainage of the choroid is by the four vortex veins.

The choriocapillaris is a single layer of capillaries lying in a plane internal to the vessels and external to Bruch's membrane, and these capillaries supply the outer part of the retina. Bruch's membrane is the inner layer of the choroid. It is about 2 μm in thickness and lies next to the pigmented layer of the retina (47).

D. Vitreous

The vitreous humor comprises 80% of the internal volume of the eye. Human vitreous weighs ~4 g and occupies a volume of almost 4 mL. The vitreous cavity is surrounded by the retina and optic nerve posteriorly. Anteriorly, it is bounded by the ciliary body, zonules, and the posterior surface of the lens. In its normal state, the vitreous is a clear gel composed almost entirely of water (99%) (48). The vitreous is important as a supporting structure and a metabolic pathway for nutrients for the lens and retina. However, of equal importance is its clarity and ability to transmit light to the retina.

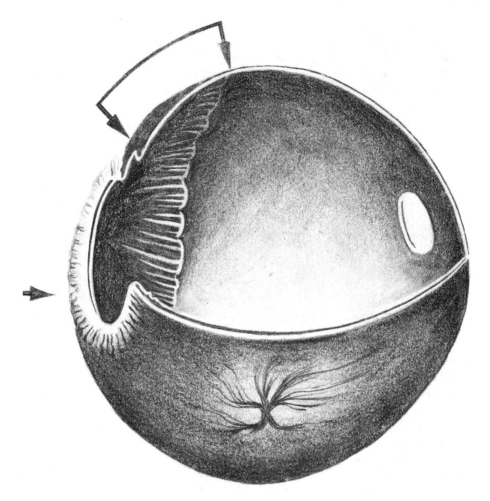

Figure 14. The uveal sphere with the ciliary body (bracketed), iris (arrow), and the choroid on right.

E. Retina

The retina is the innermost coat of the eye. It is a transparent tissue that lines the posterior two-thirds of the eyeball (49). The only firm attachments of the retina are at its anterior termination, the ora serrata, and at the margins of the optic nerve.

Histology of the retina shows it to have nine layers (Fig. 15). From internally (vitreal side) these are:

1. Internal limiting membrane
2. Nerve fiber layer
3. Ganglion cell layer
4. Inner plexiform layer
5. Inner nuclear layer

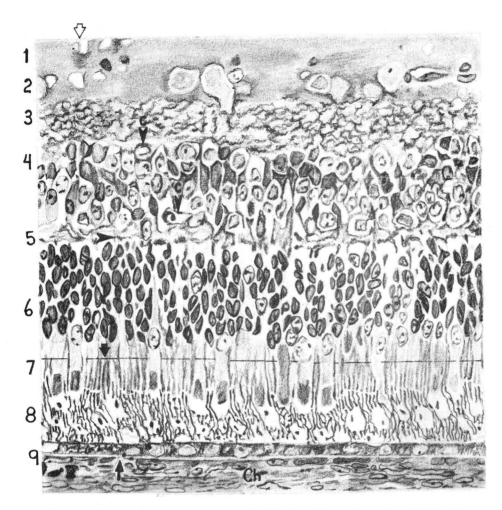

Figure 15. Illustration of light micrograph of retina. Bruch's membrane (arrow): 9 = pigment epithelium, 8 = rod and cone outer segments, 7 = rod and cone inner segments. External limiting membrane (solid thick arrow): 6 = nuclei of photoreceptors (outer nuclear layer), 5 = outer plexiform layer. Middle limiting membrane (arrow head): 4 = inner nuclear layer, 3 = inner plexiform layer, 2 = ganglion cell layer, 1 = nerve fiber layer. Inner limiting membrane (clear arrow): c = capillary; Ch = choroid.

6. Outer plexiform layer
7. Outer nuclear layer
8. External limiting membrane
9. Rod and cone inner and outer segments

The retina is approximately 0.18 mm thick at the equator and thins peripherally to about 0.11 mm at the ora serrata. This thinning is due to decreased density of all the neuronal elements.

The central posterior retina is known as the area centralis (Fig. 16), which is 5–6 mm in diameter and lies between the superior and inferior temporal arteries. Within the center

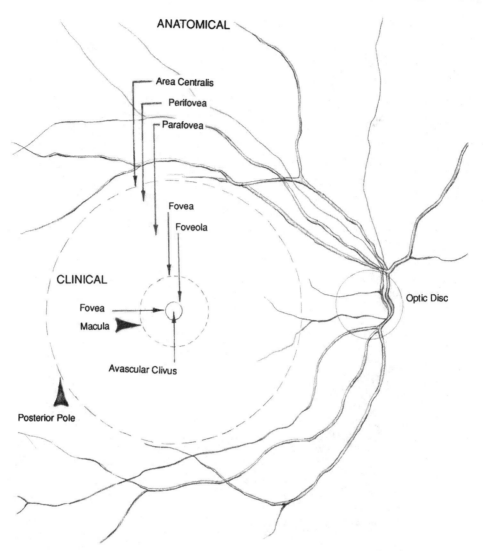

Figure 16. The posterior retina.

of this region is a 0.35-mm depression that consists of cones only. This pit is called the foveola by anatomists and the fovea by clinicians. The fovea is located ~3.4 mm from the temporal margin of the optic disc. The macula lutea, named for its yellowish coloration, is the 1.5-mm diameter central retina that surrounds the foveola.

Photoreceptor cells of the retina consists of rods and cones. The cones are concerned with visual acuity and color discrimination, whereas the rods are concerned with peripheral vision under decreased illumination. In the entire retina the rods far outnumber the cones with a ratio of 125 million rods to 6.5 million cones. The cones are present primarily in the foveal region.

The retina has the highest oxygen consumption per unit weight of any tissue in the body and has two circulatory systems to meet these high metabolic demands. The outer one-third of the retina is supplied by the choroidal circulation, whereas the inner two-thirds receives nutrition from the retinal circulation. Retinal circulation is driven by the central retinal artery. The central retinal artery and vein emerge on the surface of the optic disc.

F. Optic Nerve

The optic nerve is a bundle of myelinated nerve fibers through which the entire output of the retina travels (see Fig. 1). It travels from the retina to the optic chiasm (50) and is divided into four portions:

1. Intraocular portion
2. Intraorbital portion
3. Intracanalicular portion
4. Intracranial portion

The optic nerve is sheathed by the meninges, which are continuous with those of the brain, and it is the ophthalmic artery that is the primary source of all arterial branches to the optic nerve (51). In contrast, venous drainage of the intraocular and intraorbital portions of the nerve is primarily by the central retinal veins.

G. Issues in Drug Delivery

Placement of drug into the posterior part of the eye by other than direct injection is difficult. Reliance on systemic delivery of drug to supply adequate levels of drug to the back of the eye is on a case by case basis but is commonly difficult. Nevertheless, there are a number of ocular pathologies in the posterior part of the eye requiring drug treatment. Some issues in posterior drug delivery are:

1. Injection of liposomes, microcapsules, and nanoparticles must not interfere with the visual pathway and their component parts and physical properties must be compatible with ocular tissues.
2. Drug disposition in the back of the eye has not been thoroughly studied. It is known that vitreous humor presents a low diffusional barrier to drug movement and the periphery of the posterior segment is quite vascular, leading to an expected rapid and extensive drug loss unless the availability of drug is rate limited by release of drug from the delivery system.

VII. CONCLUSIONS

This chapter has attempted to provide a topical overview of anatomy and physiology of the eye relevant to drug delivery. Recognizing that drug delivery strategies should be based on mechanism(s) of drug absorption, distribution, metabolism, and elimination, it is essential that a thorough understanding of how the eye acts on a drug be available. For many reasons, not the least of which is severe analytical limitations, the fields of ocular pharmacokinetics and pharmacodynamics are not as mature as these fields perhaps elsewhere in the body. This lack of detailed understanding, in many cases, leads to an empirical or semiempirical approach to drug delivery, especially optimized drug delivery. The reader of this chapter may be struck by what we do not know as much as by what we do know. Thus, to a large extent, ocular drug delivery, while continuously improving, needs considerable effort to effectively utilize drugs that are protecting the visual pathway.

REFERENCES

1. Warwick, R. (1976). The eyeball, *Eugene Wolff's Anatomy of the Eye and Orbit*, 7th ed., Saunders, Philadelphia, p. 30.
2. Duke-Elder, S., and Wybar, K. C. (1961). The anatomy of the visual system, *System of Ophthalmology*, Vol. 2 (S. Duke-Elder, ed.), Mosby, St. Louis, p. 81.
3. Warwick, R. (1976). The boney orbit and paranasal sinuses, *Eugene Wolff's Anatomy of the Eye and Orbit*, 7th ed., Saunders, Philadelphia, p. 1.
4. Jakobiec, F. A., and Ozanics, V. (1989). General topographic anatomy of the eye, *Foundations of Clinical Ophthalmology*, Vol. 1, (M. M. Rodrigues, ed.), Lippincott, Philadelphia, Chap. 1.
5. Records, R. E. (1989). Eyebrows and eyelids, *Foundations of Clinical Ophthalmology*, Vol. 2 (W. Tasman and E. A. Jaeger, eds.), Lippincott, Philadelphia, Chap. 1.
6. Miller, D. (1967). Pressure of the lid on the eye, *Arch. Ophthalmol., 78*:328.
7. Holly, F. J. (1973). Formation and stability of the tear film, *Int. Ophthalmol. Clin., 13*(1):73.
8. Pfister, R. R. (1975). The normal surface of conjunctiva epithelium: A scanning electron microscopic study, *Invest. Ophthalmol., 14*:267.
9. Allansmith, M. R., and O'Connor, G. R. (1970). Immunoglobulins: Structure, function and relation to the eye, *Surv. Ophthalmol., 14*:367.
10. Duke-Elder, S. (1961). The anatomy of the visual system, *System of Ophthalmology*, Vol. 2 (S. Duke-Elder, ed.), Mosby, St. Louis, p. 543.
11. Warwick, R. (1976). The ocular appendages, *Eugene Wolff's Anatomy of the Eye and Orbit*, 7th ed., Saunders, Philadelphia, p. 218.
12. Maurice, D. N. (1967). The use of fluorescein in ophthalmological research, *Invest. Ophthalmol., 6*:464.
13. Brieman, J. A., and Snell, C. (1969). The mechanisms of lacrimal flow, *Ophthalmologica, 159*:223.
14. Brown, S. I., and Dervichian, D. G. (1969). Hydrodynamics of blinking, *Arch. Ophthalmol., 82*:541.
15. Andrews, J. S. (1970). Human tear film lipids, *Exp. Eye Res., 10*:223.
16. Nicolaides, N., Kaitaranta, J., and Rawdah, T. (1981). Meibomian gland studies: Comparison of sheep and human lipids, *Invest. Ophthalmol., 20*:522.
17. Mastman, G. L., Blades, E. J., and Henderson, J. W. (1961). The total osmotic pressure of tears in normal and various pathological conditions, *Arch. Ophthalmol., 65*:509.
18. Holden, B., Sweeney, D., and Sanderson, G. (1984). The minimal precorneal oxygen tension to avoid corneal edema, *Invest. Ophthalmol., 25*:476.
19. Janssen, E., and van Bijsterreld, O. (1983). Origin and biosynthesis of human tear fluid proteins, *Invest. Ophthalmol., 24*:623.
20. Sen, D. K., and Sarin, G. S. (1980). Immunoassay of human tear lysozyme, *Am. J. Ophthalmol., 90*:715.
21. Records, R. E. (1989). The conjunctiva and lacrimal system, *Foundations of Clinical Ophthalmology*, Vol. 2 (W. Tasman, and E. A. Jaeger, eds.), Lippincott, Philadelphia, Chap. 2.
22. Brubaker, R. F. (1989). Clinical evaluation of the circulation of aqueous humor, *Clinical Ophthalmology*, Vol. 3 (R. K. Parrish, ed.), Lippincott, Philadelphia, Chap. 46.
23. von Bahr, G. (1948). Measurement of the thickness of the cornea, *Acta Ophthalmol., 26*:247.
24. Martola, E. L., and Baum, J. L. (1968). Central and peripheral corneal thickness: A clinical study, *Arch. Ophthalmol., 79*:28.
25. Edelhauser, H. F., Van Horn, D. L., and Records, R. E. (1989). Cornea and Sclera, *Foundations of Clinical Ophthalmology*, Vol. 2 (P. L. Kaufman, ed.), Lippincott, Philadelphia, Chap. 4.

26. Harris, J. E., and Nordquist, L. T. (1955). The hydration of the cornea: I. Transport of water from the cornea, *Am. J. Ophthalmol., 40*:100.
27. Kaufman, P. L. (1984). Aqueous humor outflow, *Current Topics in Eye Research*, Vol. 4 (J. A. Zadunaisky and H. Davson, eds.), Academic Press, New York, p. 97.
28. Bill, A., and Phillips, C. I. (1971). Uveoscleral drainage of aqueous humor in human eyes, *Exp. Eye Res., 12*:275.
29. Bill, A. (1965). The aqueous humor drainage mechanism in the cynomolgus monkey (Macaca irus) with evidence for unconventional routes, *Invest. Ophthalmol., 4*:911.
30. Moses, R. A. (1981). Intraocular pressure, *Adler's Physiology of the Eye: Clinical Application*, 7th ed. (R. A. Moses, ed.), Mosby, St. Louis, Chap. 8.
31. Yablonski, M. E., Zimmerman, T. J., and Wattman, S. R. (1978). A fluorophotometric study of the effect of topical timolol on aqueous humor dynamics, *Exp. Eye Res., 27*:135.
32. Townsend, D. J., and Brubakes, R. F. (1980). Immediate effect of epinephrine on aqueous formation in the normal human eye as measured by fluorophotometry, *Invest. Ophthalmol. Vis. Sci., 19*:256.
33. Thompson, H. S. (1981). The pupil, *Adler's Physiology of the Eye: Clinical Application*, 7th ed. (R. A. Moses, ed.), Mosby, St. Louis, Chap. 12.
34. Streeten, B. W. (1989). Ciliary body, *Foundations of Clinical Ophthalmology*, Vol. 1 (M. M. Rodrigues, ed.), Lippincott, Philadelphia, Chap. 13.
35. Warwick, R. (1954). The ocular parasympathetic nerve supply and its mesencephalic sources, *J. Anat., 88*:71.
36. Ruskell, G. L. (1973). Sympathetic innervation of the ciliary muscle in monkey, *Exp. Eye Res., 16*:183.
37. Shiose, Y., and Sears, M. L. (1966). Fine structural localization of nucleoside phosphatase activity in the ciliary epithelium of albino rabbits, *Invest. Ophthalmol., 5*:152.
38. Maren, T. H. (1967). Carbonic anhydrase: Chemistry, physiology, and inhibition, *Physiol. Rev., 47*:595.
39. Sears, M. L. (1981). The aqueous, *Adler's Physiology of the Eye: Clinical Application*, 7th ed. (R. A. Moses, ed.), Mosby, St. Louis, Chap. 7.
40. Charles, M. W., and Brown, N. (1975). Dimensions of the human eye relevant to radiation protection, *Phys. Med. Biol., 20*:202.
41. Paterson, C. A. (1989). Crystalline lens, *Foundations of Clinical Ophthalmology*, Vol. 1 (P. L. Kaufman, eds.), Lippincott, Philadelphia, Chap. 10.
42. Moses, R. A. (1981). Accommodation, *Adler's Physiology of the Eye: Clinical Application*, 7th ed. (R. A. Moses, ed.), Mosby, St. Louis, Chap. 11.
43. Hogan, M. J., Alvarado, J. A., and Weddell, J. E. (1971). The sclera, *Histology of the Human Eye*, Saunders, Philadelphia, Chap. 5.
44. Spitznas, M. (1971). The fine structure of human scleral collagen, *Am. J. Ophthalmol., 71*:68.
45. Hogan, M. J., Alvarado, J. A., and Weddell, J. E. (1971). Choroid, *Histology of the Human Eye*, Saunders, Philadelphia, Chap. 8.
46. Duke-Elder, S., and Wybar, K. C. (1961). The anatomy of the visual system, *System of Ophthalmology*, Vol. 2 (S. Duke-Elder, ed.), Mosby, St. Louis, pp. 131, 339.
47. Hollenberg, M., and Burt, W. (1969). The fine structure of Bruch's membrane in the human eye, *Can. J. Ophthalmol., 4*:296.
48. Schepens, C. L. (1954). Clinical aspects of pathological changes in the vitreous body, *Am. J. Ophthalmol., 38*:8.
49. Sigelman, J., and Ozanics, V. (1989). Retina, *Foundations of Clinical Ophthalmology*, Vol. 1 (M. M. Rodrigues, ed.), Lippincott, Philadelphia, Chap. 19.
50. Anderson, D. R., and Hoyt, W. F. (1969). Ultrastructure of intraorbital portion of human and monkey optic nerve, *Arch. Ophthalmol., 82*:506.
51. Anderson, D. R. (1970). Vascular supply to the optic nerve in primates, *Am. J. Ophthalmol., 70*:341.

3
Precorneal, Corneal, and Postcorneal Factors

Vincent H. L. Lee *University of Southern California School of Pharmacy, Los Angeles, California*

I. INTRODUCTION

Designing formulations and delivery systems for topically applied ophthalmic drugs is challenging. It requires a thorough understanding of the physiological basis of the protective mechanisms designed by the eye to allow only 1–10% of the topically applied dose to be absorbed ocularly. These protective mechanisms include solution drainage, lacrimation, diversion of exogenous chemicals into the systemic circulation via the conjunctiva, and a highly selective corneal barrier to exclude exogenous compounds from the internal eye. Improvement of ocular drug delivery then amounts to determining the outer boundaries as well as the maximum duration over which these protective mechanisms can be compromised without causing harm to this vital organ. According to Grass and Robinson (1), to significantly alter the fraction of drug absorbed into the eye, it will be necessary to either increase the corneal drug absorption rate constant by one to two orders of magnitude or to reduce the precorneal loss rate constant by a similar extent—a formidable task.

This chapter discusses the role of key precorneal, corneal, and postcorneal factors in determining the ocular bioavailability of topically applied drugs. These factors include 1) precorneal fluid dynamics, 2) drug binding to tear proteins, 3) conjunctival drug absorption, 4) systemic drug absorption, 5) resistance to corneal drug penetration, 6) drug binding to melanin, and 7) drug metabolism. Although drug uptake by the lens is gaining attention owing to a growing interest in aldose reductase inhibitors as drugs for retarding the progress of sugar-induced cataracts (2,3), it will not be discussed here, since relatively little information exists on this topic.

II. PRECORNEAL FACTORS

A. Precorneal Fluid Dynamics

All liquid dosage forms, including aqueous solutions, oil solutions, suspensions, and liposomes, are rapidly drained from the conjunctival sac to the nasolacrimal duct. The residence time of an instilled dose ranges from 4–23 min (Table 1). Such a rapid drainage

Table 1. Residence Time of Liquid Aqueous Ophthalmic Dosage Forms in the Conjunctival Sac Following Topical Instillation in Rabbit Eyes[a]

Dosage form	Drug	Residence time (min.)	Ref.
Aqueous solution	Cromolyn Na	6.8 ± 0.46	173
Aqueous solution	Epinephrine	5.9 ± 0.35	60
Aqueous solution	Inulin	7.3 ± 0.71	60
Aqueous solution	Pilocarpine	4.8 ± 0.18	53
Oil solution	Vitamin A	9.7 ± 0.62	174
Microspheres	None	23.0	19
Liposomes (neutral)[b]	None	6.5 ± 0.57	60
Liposomes (positive)[c]	None	4.3 ± 0.37	6

[a]Residence time is defined as the time required for loss of 95% of the instilled dose.
[b]Phospholipid composition—Dipalmitoyl phosphatidylcholine
[c]Phospholipid composition—Stearylamine:L-α-phosphatidylcholine:cholesterol:α-tocopherol (1:4:4.95:0.05)

rate results from the tendency of the eye to maintain the residence volume at 7–10 µL at all times (4). This rate becomes even higher when the formulation is perceived to be irritating. The irritancy of positively charged liposomes to the eye (5) is probably the main reason for its relatively rapid rate of clearance from the precorneal area when compared with solutions (6). Indeed, it is the desire to minimize the irritation potential of suspended particles to the eye that underlies the many attempts to render the particle size in suspensions as small as possible. While the irritating potential versus size relationship has never been documented, reduction in particle size does affect drug dissolution rate and bioavailability. A significant rank-order correlation was observed by Schoenwald and Stewart (7) between increasing dexamethasone concentrations in the aqueous humor and decreasing particle size over the range of 5.75–22.0 µm in a 1% suspension of the drug. A similar relationship was reported by Hui and Robinson (8) for a 0.1% suspension of fluorometholone over the size range of 2.0–10.4 µm; there was no further gain in ocular drug bioavailability upon further reducing the particle size from 2 to 1 µm. Not surprisingly, varying the particle size has no effect on the corneal permeability coefficient (9).

Several factors influence the drainage rate: instilled volume, viscosity, pH, tonicity, and drugs.

1. Instilled Volume

The human eye can hold about 30 µL without overflow or spillage at the outer angle, provided that great care is exercised and that the subject does not blink (4). This volume reduces to 10 µL if blinking is allowed (10). The seminal work of Robinson and his colleagues (11,12) based on gamma scintigraphy has established that the rate of solution drainage from the conjunctival sac is directly proportional to the instilled volume. In the rabbit, 90% of the dose is cleared within 2 min for an instilled volume of 50 µL (the volume delivered by most commercial ophthalmic preparations), 4 min for an instilled volume of 25 µL, 6 min for an instilled volume of 10 µL, and 7.5 min for an instilled volume of 5 µL (11). This volume dependency of solution drainage rate has been found to exert its expected effect on the percent of dose absorbed into the eye and on the pharmacological effect that ensues (13–16). Using a model that predicts ocular drug bioavailability from tear drug concentration-time data, Keister et al. (17) proposed that reducing the instilled drop would increase only the ocular bioavailability of drugs with low permeability four times and would not affect the ocular bioavailability of drugs with high corneal permeability. Since high corneal permeability is the exception rather than the rule, the clinical implication is that appropriate reduction of instilled volume and the simultaneous increase in instilled drug concentration should permit substantial dosage reductions without sacrifice of drug concentration in the eye (18).

The above volume dependency of the drainage rate has also been observed for suspensions (3 μm in size) (19), but it has not been observed in liposomes (20). Lee et al. (20) reported that multilamellar, neutral liposomes prepared from phosphatidylcholine and cholesterol were cleared from the conjunctival sac of the albino rabbit, with approximately the same first-order rate constant, 0.45 min^{-1}, over the instilled volume range of 10–50 μL. As a result, the ocular absorption of inulin from these liposomes was not affected by changes in instilled dose volume over the above range. The size and number of liposomes were believed to be more important factors than instilled volume influencing the extent of ocular drug absorption from liposomes.

The volume dependency of the drainage rate for solutions has implications in multiple drop therapy in terms of 1) minimum time interval in between drops and 2) order of addition of drops. Using radioactive technetium (^{99m}Tc) as the test substance in rabbits, Chrai et al. (21) showed that a 5-min interval between drops minimized drainage loss of drug, and that the first drug administered suffered a greater loss than the second drug. These findings constitute a very strong argument for combination drug products whenever multiple drug therapy is indicated.

2. Viscosity

Compared with reducing instilled solution volume, increasing solution viscosity is a more popular method of prolonging the residence time of an instilled dose in the conjunctival sac. Various polymers have been used to increase solution viscosity, including poly(vinyl alcohol), poly(pyrrolidone), hydroxypropylcellulose, and other cellulose derivatives. Based upon a comparison of the reduction in solution drainage rate by methylcellulose and poly(vinyl alcohol) and the resulting increase in aqueous humor pilocarpine concentrations in the albino rabbit (22,23), Patton and Robinson (23) concluded that it is the flow properties of the vehicle in question and its viscosity, not the concentration, that determines the effect of polymers on solution drainage and ocular drug absorption. It appears that the optimum viscosity to use is in the range of 12–15 cps, beyond which the gain in ocular absorption would be minimal, while the risks of inaccuracy of instillation and blurring of vision would increase. Even with a 100-fold increase in viscosity, the gain in ocular drug absorption is modest, being less for oil-soluble than for water-soluble drugs (1).

The hypothesis that all polymers affect ocular drug absorption similarly so long as they yield the same viscosity assumes that these polymers do not interact with the corneal surface. Work by Saettone et al. (24,25) indicates that this may not be the case in human subjects. These investigators demonstrated that equiviscous solutions of carboxymethylcellulose, hydroxypropylcellulose, poly(vinyl alcohol), poly(vinylpyrrolidone), while equally effective in rabbits, enhanced the ocular absorption of pilocarpine as well as tropicamide to different extents. The most effective polymers were poly(vinyl alcohol) and poly(vinylpyrrolidone). The different activity of these polymers was attributed to their influence on the spreading characteristics and the thickness of the medication layer over the precorneal area in humans. Saettone et al. (26) showed that soluble, mucoadhesive polyanionic polymers, such as hyaluronic acid, poly(galacturonic acid), mesoglycan (a complex mixture of mucopolysaccharides), carboxymethylchitin, and polyacrylic acid, enhanced the ocular absorption of pilocarpine more so than poly(vinyl alcohol) of equivalent viscosity. Similar favorable effects with hyaluronic acid over hydroxypropylmethylcellulose and polyacrylic acid (Carbopol 934P) over poly(vinyl alcohol) have been reported by Camber et al. (27) and Davies et al. (28). Cyanoacrylate block copolymer, another mucoadhesive polymer, has also been found to improve the ocular absorption of pilocarpine by 53% (29).

3. pH and Tonicity

For stability reasons, most eye drops are formulated at pHs other than pH 7.4. They are, therefore, potentially irritating to the eye, stimulating tear production. Lacrimal gland fluid secretion can be stimulated by reflexes from afferent pathways arising in the cornea, conjunctiva, and optic nerve. In rabbits, lacrimal gland fluid stimulated by ocular surface reflexes was 3.0 ± 0.5 μL/10 min as compared with a baseline level of 1.0 ± 0.2 mL/10 min. There was a concomitant rise in the protein concentration in tears (30), which could affect the amount of free drug available for corneal absorption. Conrad et al. (31) reported that alkaline pHs induced greater lacrimation than acidic pHs in the albino rabbit. This is consistent with the lower buffer capacity of tears in the basic than in the acidic range (32,33). Since tears are poorly buffered (32), a strategy to minimize the impact of induced lacrimation is to use the most dilute buffer possible; i.e., to keep the tonicity low. By progressively reducing the buffer concentration of a pH 4.5 citrate buffer from 0.11 M to zero, Mitra and Mikkelson (34) observed a fivefold increase in the ocular bioavailability of pilocarpine. In addition to buffer concentration, the buffer type used also affects the absorption efficiency of pilocarpine owing to its effect on the rate at which pH reequilibration will occur (33). Thus, a phosphate buffer (pH 4) which is resistant to pH reequilibration near the pK_a of pilocarpine owing to its high residual buffer capacity, yields a lower bioavailability of pilocarpine than does an acetate buffer, even though its buffer capacity is lower (Fig. 1) (33). Nevertheless, the phosphate buffer is still preferred because the acetate buffer causes excessive lacrimation and may be inherently irritating to the eye.

4. Drugs

Drugs that act on the lacrimal gland can affect precorneal fluid dynamics. Examples include epinephrine (35), pilocarpine (36), the local anesthetics tetracaine and proparacaine (37), certain beta-blockers (35), and the tear stimulants currently in development (38). Thus, epinephrine has been shown to accelerate the removal of topically applied liposomes from the conjunctival sac by inducing tear production (39). Induced lacrimation by epinephrine and pilocarpine (and possibly their prodrugs) has also been suggested as a reason for the reduction in ocular absorption of topically applied timolol when used in the same drop with either of the above two drugs (40,41). On the other hand, suppression of tear turnover by the topical instillation of five drops of 0.5% tetracaine has been shown to double the amount of pilocarpine absorbed in the aqueous humor of the albino rabbit eye (37).

B. Drug Binding to Tear Proteins

Although the protein content of tears is much less than that of blood, it is still appreciable and ranges from 0.5% total protein in rabbits to about 0.7% total protein in humans (42). Of

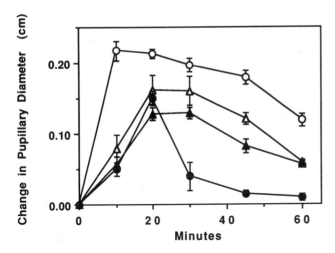

Figure 1. Time course of changes in pupillary diameter following topical instillation of 25 μL of various formulations containing 1% pilocarpine (pH 4) to the albino rabbit eye. Key: O, unbuffered; Δ, acetate-buffered; ▲, phosphate-buffered; ●, citrate-buffered. (From Ref. 33.)

the several proteins in tears (43,44), at least three (albumin, globulins, and lysozyme) are necessary to quantitate the binding of some drugs in the tears (45). There exists, therefore, the possibility of drug binding to tear proteins, resulting in a reduction in the free drug concentrations for absorption. Such a possibility was first pointed out by Mikkelson et al. (42) for pilocarpine. These investigators showed that the miotic response to topically applied pilocarpine in the albino rabbit was reduced about two times as the albumin concentration in the precorneal fluid was increased from 0 to 3%. This problem of reduced drug bioavailability due to binding of drugs to tear proteins could be exacerbated when there is an elevation of tear proteins in certain extraocular disease states, such as corneal inflammation (13,46), herpes simplex infection (47), and allergic conjunctivitis (47). Increased loss of timolol to protein binding due to an increase in tear protein concentration caused by reduction in tear turnover rate by tetracaine and propracaine has been proposed as a reason for the reduced ocular absorption of timolol when coadministered with the two local anesthetics (40).

C. Conjunctival Drug Absorption

The conjunctiva is a vascularized, thin mucous membrane lining the inside of the eyelids and the anterior sclera. The conjunctiva is known to differ from the cornea in several aspects: metabolic activity (48), length and density of microvilli (49), and permeability to water-soluble compounds such as mannitol, inulin, and FITC-dextran (MW 20,000) (50). The conjunctiva possesses two important features that render it more effective in competing with the cornea for drug absorption: 1) a 9 times larger surface area in the rabbit and a 17 times larger surface area in the human (51), and 2) a 2 to 30 times greater permeability to drugs (52). It is, therefore, not surprising that drug uptake by the conjunctiva is as important as solution drainage loss in reducing the fraction of pilocarpine available for corneal absorption (53). The early hint that conjunctival drug uptake is a significant precorneal drug loss factor lies in the many observations that in spite of a 10-fold reduction in drainage rate by a 100-fold increase in solution viscosity, the maximum improvement in drug activity, be it miosis, inhibition of infection, or aqueous humor levels, is about twice that of an aqueous solution (23). To date, no attempts to reduce conjunctival drug absorption have been reported, even though this is a desirable goal from the standpoint of increasing the fraction of drug available for corneal absorption.

There is now evidence that it may be possible to reduce conjunctival drug absorption in two ways: varying drug lipophilicity or changing the drug formulation. Wang et al. (52) reported that although lipophilicity affected the conjunctival and corneal permeability to beta-blockers in a qualitatively same but quantitatively different way, the conjunctival permeability coefficient was less sensitive to changes in lipophilicity (log PC) compared with the corneal permeability coefficient. Within the log PC range of –0.62 (sotalol) and 3.44 (betaxolol), there was only an eightfold difference in the conjunctival permeability coefficient as compared with a 48-fold difference in the corneal permeability coefficient. Therefore, provided that the drug candidates are sufficiently lipophilic, it should be possible to improve corneal drug penetration without markedly affecting conjunctival drug absorption.

In addition to its lesser sensitivity to changes in drug lipophilicity, the conjunctival permeability coefficient is also less sensitive to a given formulation change than is the corneal permeability coefficient (54). Formulation changes that are most effective in minimizing the ratio of conjunctival to corneal drug absorption are increasing solution pH, lowering solution tonicity, and lowering the percentage of ethylenediaminetetraacetic acid (EDTA) and benzalkonium chloride in the formulation. The first hint that the conjunctiva and cornea are different from the standpoint of drug penetration is the different magnitude by which a given pH change alters the corneal and conjunctival permeability to the four beta-blockers studied: atenolol, timolol, levobunolol, and betaxolol. For instance, whereas raising the pH from 7.4 to 8.4 increased the corneal permeability to timolol 2.4 times, it only increased the conjunctival permeability by 28%. The magnitude of increase in both instances was much less than the factor of 8 increase in the fraction of timolol (pK$_a$ 9.21) in the nonionized, preferentially absorbed form.

Besides maximizing the fraction of topically applied drug for corneal absorption, minimizing drug uptake by the conjunctiva is also desirable from the standpoint of minimizing drug absorption into systemic circulation, at least in theory. Nevertheless, the resulting reduction in systemic absorption is expected to be minimal, since the conjunctiva plays only a minor role, compared with the nasal mucosa, in contributing to systemic drug absorption (15,55).

The vascularized nature of the conjunctiva has generated the perception that drugs absorbed by the conjunctiva would all be swept into systemic circulation and would not be available for distribution to the uveal tract underneath. This assumption has now been proven to be incorrect, first by Doane et al. (56) and then by Ahmed and Patton (57,58). Thus, an unknown fraction of the drug absorbed by the conjunctiva could lead to direct drug entry into the uveal tract, bypassing the cornea. This route of drug entry into the eye following topical dosing is called the noncorneal route, as depicted in Scheme 1. There is indirect evidence that the ratio of noncorneal to corneal drug absorption is increased whenever inefficient mixing of the instilled dose with tears occurs, as when very viscous solutions or when dispersed systems such as nanoparticles and liposomes are instilled (39,59–63). Noncorneal drug absorption is also facilitated by drug administration in an

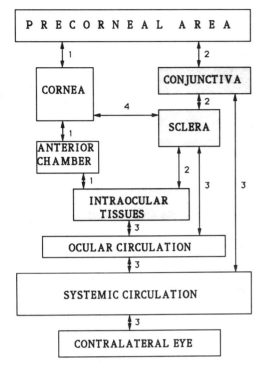

Scheme 1. Ocular penetration routes for topically applied drugs. Key: 1 = transcorneal pathway; 2 = noncorneal pathway; 3 = systemic return pathway; 4 = lateral diffusion. (From Ref. 58.)

insert. This is indicated by the unequal concentrations of timolol in the superior and inferior parts of the pigmented rabbit eye and very low timolol concentrations in the aqueous humor when a silicone cylindrical device containing timolol (1.46 × 1.94 × 0.24 mm, ID × OD × wall thickness) was placed in the inferior cul-de-sac (64). A smaller difference between timolol concentrations in the superior and inferior portions of the anterior segment tissues was found when the device was placed in the superior cul-de-sac.

D. Systemic Drug Absorption

An often-neglected aspect of ocular drug therapy is systemic absorption of the topically applied dose that has reached the nasal mucosa following solution drainage. This is partly due to the fact that the drugs involved then had wide therapeutic indices or that the patient population who had suffered from systemic side effects elicited by topically applied ophthalmic drugs was small. This situation changed dramatically when timolol, a potent mixed beta$_1$ and beta$_2$ antagonist, was introduced into glaucoma therapy in 1978. Systemic risk associated with topical timolol was emphasized by Van Buskirk then (65). Six years later, Nelson et al. (66) reported 450 cases of serious systemic side effects attributed to timolol, of which 32 resulted in patient deaths. As many as 23% of the patients experienced their adverse event on the first day of timolol therapy and 33% did so within the first week (66).

Table 2. Percent of Topically Applied Dose Absorbed into the
Systemic Circulation

Drug	% Applied dose	Ref.
Cortisol	30–35	175
Dipivalylepinephrine	65	176
Epinephrine	55	176
Flurbiprofen	74	179
Imirestat	50–75	177
Inulin	3	55
Insulin, with 1% Na glycocholate	5	178
Levobunolol	46	180
[D-Ala^2]Metenkephalinamide	36	55
Tetrahydrocannabinol	23	150
Timolol	80	181

Restricting entry of a topically applied ophthalmic dose into the nasal cavity is an obvious approach to reducing the extent of systemic absorption of topically applied ophthalmic drugs. This objective can be achieved by nasolacrimal occlusion for 5 min, with or without eyelid closure (67,68), or by changes in vehicle composition such as incorporation of polymers (16,69), changes in vehicle type (41,70), alteration in solution pH and tonicity (16), and adjustment of preservative concentration (16). Other means to reducing systemic drug absorption include 1) coadministration with low doses of vasoconstrictors such as phenylephrine and epinephrine (40,41,69); 2) designing ophthalmic drugs that are poorly absorbed into the bloodstream (71) or are rapidly inactivated in the systemic circulation (72,73)—so-called prodrug and soft drug approaches, respectively; and 3) selecting a dosing time that minimizes systemic absorption while maximizing ocular drug absorption (74–77). The effectiveness of the above approaches has been reviewed (78). Because the majority of the above approaches aim primarily at the nasal mucosa (the main site of systemic drug absorption) rather than at the conjunctival sac, reduction in systemic drug absorption may not necessarily lead to enhanced corneal drug absorption. This has been found to be the case when epinephrine was coadministered with timolol to reduce the systemic absorption of timolol (41). Table 2 summarizes the percent of topically applied dose that has been found to be absorbed into the bloodstream of rabbits.

III. CORNEAL FACTORS: RESISTANCE TO CORNEAL DRUG PENETRATION

The majority of topically applied drugs enter the eye by passage across the cornea (79). This is an extremely inefficient process owing largely to the resistance exerted by the corneal epithelium to drug penetration. Generally, resistance due to metabolism is low, except for pilocarpine (80), fluorometholone (81), and peptides such as methionine enkephalin (82) and triglycine (83). The corneal epithelium contributes to over 90% of the corneal resistance to penetration for hydrophilic beta-blockers, decreasing to about 50% for the moderately lipophilic and to less than 10% for the lipophilic. This is accompanied by a rise in the contribution due to the corneal endothelium from less than 5% for hydrophilic compounds through 30% for the moderately lipophilic and to 50% for the lipophilic. A similar trend is seen in the contribution from the corneal stroma (84).

A measure of the corneal penetration efficiency of drugs is the permeability coefficient. This is generally on the order of $0.1–4.0 \times 10^{-5}$ cm/s (52). Unless the drug is very lipophilic, e.g., prednisolone acetate (85), fluorometholone (85), betaxolol (86), and timolol ester prodrugs (87), at least a twofold increase in the extent of corneal penetration occurs when the corneal epithelial barrier is absent. The degree of penetration enhancement can be as high as 10- to 30-fold, as is the case for 5-fluorouracil, which penetrates the cornea poorly because of its hydrophilicity (log PC = –0.96) (52); 14-fold, as is the case for methionine enkephalin (82), which penetrates the cornea poorly mainly because of susceptibility to aminopeptidase-mediated hydrolysis (88); and 60-fold, as is the case for inulin, which penetrates the cornea poorly because of its size (MW 5000) and hydrophilicity (log PC = –2.90) (89).

Changes in corneal epithelial permeability during ocular inflammation have also caused an increase in the permeability to such drugs as cyclosporine (90) and dexamethasone phosphate (91). Kupferman et al. (91) and Cox et al. (92) demonstrated that dexamethasone alcohol and phosphate were absorbed across the corneal epithelium of the inflamed but not the noninflamed eye, even though no macroscopic changes were obvious in the structural integrity of the corneal epithelium in the inflamed eye. Similarly, Pavan-Langston and Nelson (93) reported that trifluridine, an antiviral agent, was well absorbed across the corneas of patients with herpetic iritis but not in the corneas of healthy subjects. Baum et al. (94) found that the type of injury to the cornea affected the extent of improvement in corneal drug absorption. Six times more gentamicin penetrated lye-burned ulcers than corneal ulcers caused by *Pseudomonas*. However, for unknown reasons, a corneal ulcer induced by the vaccinia virus, manifested as a frank erosion of the corneal epithelium and Bowman's membrane, did not affect the ocular uptake of cortisol.

Corneal integrity can be compromised by sufficiently high concentrations of certain formulation excipients, such as preservatives (e.g., benzalkonium chloride and other cationic surfactants) and chelating agents (e.g., EDTA). Thus, benzalkonium chloride and other cationic surfactants have been shown to enhance the ocular absorption of drugs varying in molecular size and lipophilicity, including pilocarpine (95), carbachol (96), prednisolone (97), homatropine (98), inulin (99), and horseradish peroxidase (100). Grass et al. (101) demonstrated that EDTA at 0.5% altered the permeability of the corneal epithelium, probably at the intercellular junction level, to enhance the corneal permeability of water-soluble but not oil-soluble drugs. Moreover, EDTA reached the iris–ciliary body at concentrations high enough to alter the permeability of the uveal vessels, thereby indirectly accelerating drug removal from the aqueous humor.

Interpretation of corneal penetration data usually assumes homogeneity in lipophilic characteristics in the corneal epithelium. In actuality, the corneal epithelium is five to six cell layers thick and consists of three groups of cells with unique biochemical characteristics: 1) two to three layers of flattened platelike superficial cells, 2) two to three layers of wing or polygonal cells comprising the intermediate zone, and 3) a single row of columnar basal cells. In 1979, Godbey et al. (102) made the interesting observation that disrupting the top two epithelial layers by treatment with 0.02% cetylpyridinium chloride, an ophthalmic preservative, was as effective as removing all layers of the corneal epithelium in allowing penicillin G to pass through the cornea. The implication of this finding is that the top two layers of the corneal epithelium bear all the resistance to the corneal penetration of this drug.

The above finding also raises the interesting possibility that a lipophilicity gradient exists across five to six cell layers within the corneal epithelium, with the most lipophilic layer on the tear side. This hypothesis has been confirmed by Shih and Lee (86) using a technique developed by Wolosin et al. (103,104) to strip off selective layers of the corneal epithelium. This was achieved by pretreating the cornea with 20–100 µM of digitonin for 15 min. Such pretreatment did not affect the corneal penetration of betaxolol, a very lipophilic drug (log PC = 3.65). Pretreatment with 40 µM digitonin to cause exfoliation of the top two corneal epithelial cell layers enhanced the corneal penetration of timolol (log PC = 2.64) and levobunolol (log PC = 3.22) to the same extent as deepithelizing the corneal epithelium. Unlike timolol and levobunolol, atenolol (log PC = 0.15) encounters resistance beyond the superficial cell layers in its penetration across the corneal epithelium. Even when the intermediate zone of wing cells was removed by treating the cornea with 60–100 µM digitonin, the corneal permeability coefficient was only 68% of that seen in the deepithelized cornea. This finding is somewhat surprising, since atenolol, given its hydrophilic characteristics, is anticipated to cross the corneal epithelium via the paracellular pathway, the permeability of which is presumably controlled by the tight junctions in the superficial cells. Although direct confirmation is required, the above findings are consistent with the hypothesis that a lipophilicity gradient exists across the five to six cell layers within the corneal epithelium; i.e., the number of corneal epithelial cell layers limiting the corneal penetration of ocularly administered drugs is inversely related to drug lipophilicity. From the standpoint of maximally improving the corneal penetration of a hydrophilic drug such as atenolol, it will therefore be necessary 1) to modify the drug properties to match those exhibited by all the five to six cell layers in the corneal epithelium, or 2) to design a penetration enhancer capable of disrupting the integrity of all those cell layers.

The existence of a lipophilicity gradient within the corneal epithelium has implications on how the parabolic relationships between corneal penetration and lipophilicity reported for steroids (105), n-alkyl p-aminobenzoate esters (106), substituted anilines (107), timolol ester prodrugs (108), and beta-blockers (84) should be interpreted. The usual interpretation is a shift in the rate-limiting layer from the corneal epithelium to the corneal stroma as drug lipophilicity is increased. In light of the new finding noted above, such a shift in the rate-limiting layer could have occurred within the corneal epithelium, far removed from the corneal stroma. Nevertheless, deciding on where in the cornea such a shift actually occurs must await resolution of the controversy on whether a parabolic relationship best describes the influence of drug lipophilicity on corneal drug penetration. As shown by Wang et al. (52), a sigmoidal relationship (Fig. 2) statistically described the influence of lipophilicity on the corneal penetration of beta-blockers better than the parabolic relationship reported by Schoenwald and Huang (84), which weighted heavily on one lipophilic compound (penbutolol) beyond the purported maximum in their parabola. The same argument probably holds for steroids (84). Deviation from the parabolic relationship has also been reported by Grass and Robinson (1) when compounds of diverse chemical structure and molecular size are considered. Such deviations are to be expected because not all the compounds selected for study utilize the usual transcellular pathway for penetration. Compounds that penetrate via the less common paracellular pathway include low molecular weight alcohols and the ionized form of such drugs as pilocarpine (109,110), sulfonamides (111), and cromolyn Na (101). It is important to resolve the controversy on

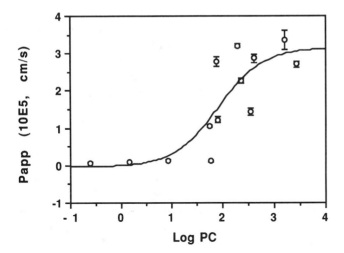

Figure 2. Influence of drug lipophilicity (log PC) on the permeability coefficients (Papp) of beta-blockers across the cornea of the pigmented rabbit. Error bars represent standard error of the mean for n = 5–12. Where not shown, the error bar is smaller than the size of the symbol. (From Ref. 52.)

the influence of lipophilicity on corneal drug penetration, since parabolic relationships have been guiding the design of prodrugs or analogs for improved corneal penetration (112).

IV. POSTCORNEAL FACTORS

A. Drug Binding to Melanin

Drug binding to melanin pigments in the iris and ciliary body can affect the bioavailability of topically applied drugs both positively and negatively. The impact is usually a negative one, however, owing to 1) the high binding capacity of the pigments relative to the amount of drug typically reaching the eye and 2) the slow rate and small fraction of bound drug that is subsequently released (113–118). For instance, the mydriatic response to topically applied ephedrine diminished progressively with increasing pigmentation of the iris (113). Moreover, the hypotensive effect of timolol in individuals with pigmented irides was much reduced relative to those with light irides (119), even though the amount of drug accumulating in the pigmented irides was considerably higher (120).

Theoretically, the amount of drug within the eye can be increased to saturate all the binding sites in the pigments so that the bound drug would be released at a pharmacologically active concentration. Urtti et al. (121) confirmed the feasibility of this approach using pilocarpine in pigmented rabbits. Specifically, whereas the miotic response at doses of 0.11 and 0.43 mg of pilocarpine was reduced in the pigmented relative to the albino rabbit, the response at higher doses of the drug, 0.85 and 2.30 mg, was two to three times higher and more sustained in the pigmented than in the albino rabbit. Based upon an evaluation of 27 acidic and basic compounds, Zane et al. (122) concluded that compounds containing strongly basic functionalities, such as piperidine or piperazine moieties and other amines, were most likely to be retained at high concentrations in the melanin-containing tissues, and that binding was further enhanced by increased lipophilicity. Since drug binding to melanin is saturable, the rate at which the drug is released and absorbed from its delivery system can markedly affect the consistency of the pharmacological response from patient to patient. Conceivably, a larger fraction of the released drug would be bound at low than at high release rates.

B. Drug Metabolism

Drug metabolism in ocular tissues (123) is an important area that has yet to be fully explored in ocular drug pharmacokinetics. This is partly because of the limitations in the sensitivity required to detect metabolites and partly because of the expectation that the eye, as a whole, is not a primary drug-metabolizing organ. For instance, Cheng-Bennett et al. (124) reported that neither human nor rabbit cornea, iris–ciliary body, and sclera possessed the enzymes that typically deactivate prostaglandins, such as $PGF_{2\alpha}$, by 15-OH dehydrogenation, ω-oxidation, and β-oxidation. This finding is consistent with the observation that drugs that are degraded by oxidation or reduction are less likely to be metabolized than those that are degraded by hydrolysis. Thus, pilocarpine, a cyclic ester, is hydrolyzed to the extent of 30% in the cornea of pigmented rabbits at 10 min postinstillation (80), whereas cyclophosphamide (125) and timolol (126), which degrade chemically by oxidation, remain intact in isolated pigmented rabbit corneas and iris–ciliary bodies.

Nonetheless, a number of enzymes that may participate in ocular drug metabolism have been identified or proposed. Several of these, such as esterases (127), monoamine oxidase (128), and catecholamine O-methyl transferase (128), play an important role in the metabolism of classic neurotransmitters. Others, such as NADPH cytochrome P-450(c) reductase (129,130), N-demethylase (131), deethylase (132), 11-β-oxidoreductase (133–135), N-acetyltransferase (136,137), sulfatase (138), and glucuronidase (138), have been implicated to exist in the eye based on the in vitro or in vivo biotransformation of dexamethasone, fluorometholone, cortisol, cortisone, progesterone, testosterone, N-methylacetazolamide, aminozolamide, and 7-ethoxycoumarin. Except for levobunolol (139) and aminozolamide (136), the concentration of metabolites is usually very low when compared to the parent drug.

Of the anterior segment tissues, the corneal epithelium and the iris–ciliary body are metabolically most active. This has been shown to be the case for esterases (140–142), aminopeptidases (88,143), ketone reductase (139), and N-acetyltransferase (137). The enrichment of drug-metabolizing enzymes in these tissues indicates that drugs which are good substrates for these enzymes may suffer substantial degradation both during transport across the corneal epithelium and after reaching their sites of action in the iris–ciliary body. A good case in point is the massive destruction of topically applied methionine enkephalin by aminopeptidases, in spite of pretreatment with six sequential 25-μL doses, at 5 min apart, of 25 μM bestatin (82) (a potent aminopeptidase inhibitor (144)). Although one may modify the structure of the drug molecule or potentially alter the pathway of drug penetration to minimize drug metabolism in these tissues, neither approach has been thoroughly investigated. A possible exception is methionine enkephalin (82).

Except for the glutathione-conjugating enzymes (145,146), the drug-metabolizing enzymes that have been identified in the eye typically exist in levels that are a fraction of their counterparts in the liver, the leading drug-metabolizing organ in the body. In one extreme, the activity of 7-ethoxycoumarin deethylase in the iris–ciliary body of rabbits is less than 0.06% of hepatic activity (132). In the other extreme, N-acetyltransferase (137) and ketone reductase activities (139) in the iris–ciliary body are higher, about 13 and 18% of hepatic activity, respectively. Given the low dose of most topically applied drugs, those which are labile could be extensively metabolized nonetheless. This is precisely the case with chloramphenicol, about 45% of which that was recovered in the aqueous humor of the albino rabbit 2 h after solution instillation was in metabolite form (147).

Of the ocular drug-metabolizing enzymes, the esterases and ketone reductase are perhaps the most important owing mainly to their potential role in the activation of prodrugs or soft drugs which are designed to improve the ocular delivery characteristics of their parent drugs. Prodrugs are bioreversible derivatives of drugs with the potential to alter absorption, decrease side effects, or prolong duration of action (148). Soft drugs are biologically active drugs which are predictably metabolized to nontoxic moieties after achieving their therapeutic role (149).

1. Ketone Reductase

Ketone reductase is a cytosolic enzyme which is strongly dependent on NADPH but which is inhibited by quercetin and p-chloromercuribenzoate and, to a lesser extent, by pyrazole or barbital. This enzyme has been shown to mediate the conversion of topically applied levobunolol to dihydrolevobunolol (139) and, in concert with esterases, the activation of diisovaleryl adrenalone via the diisovaleryl epinephrine intermediate to epinephrine, preferentially in the iris–ciliary body of the albino rabbit (150). Naturally, this enzyme is believed to play a key role in the activation of the ketoxime analogs of propranolol and timolol (151) following their hydrolysis to ketones. Activation is assumed to be stereospecific, since only the S-(-) form of propranolol was obtained from a racemic mixture of the soft drug (152). Provided that the same activation process does not take place systemically, this approach is viable in reducing the systemic toxicities of topically applied beta-blockers.

Ocular ketone reductase differs from other ocular drug-metabolizing enzymes such as esterases (140,153) and aminopeptidases (154) in two ways. First, its activity relative to the liver is rather high—as high as 18%. Second, it is not ubiquitous, being confined to the conjunctiva, corneal epithelium, iris–ciliary body and the lens and being conspicuously absent in the tears, corneal stroma, sclera, and aqueous humor. Recent work by Ashton et al. (155) has revealed a nonuniform distribution of ketone reductase in the corneal epithelium of the pigmented rabbit, with maximal activity possibly residing in the zone of wing cells.

2. Esterases

Esterases play a very important role in the activation of ester prodrugs; the only type of prodrugs that have been considered in ophthalmology to date (112). Susceptibility of these prodrugs to esterase-mediated hydrolysis is an important factor that affects not only the onset of drug action but also the extent of corneal penetration. Chien et al. (108) demonstrated that the enzymatically more labile straight-chain alkyl ester prodrugs of timolol penetrated the cornea more readily than the more stable branched-chain esters of comparable lipophilicity.

Esterases are widely distributed in anterior segment tissues (140). Their activities are twice as high in the iris–ciliary body as in the cornea, where about 70% of the activity resides in the epithelium (141). The esterase activity in the bovine eye is predominantly microsomal (156), amounting to about 80% in the corneal epithelium and the iris–ciliary body. By contrast, almost all of the esterase activity in the corneal stroma is cytosolic or extracellular.

Two types of esterases exist in the ocular tissues of the rabbit: acetyl- and butyryl-cholinesterase (157). Except in the corneal epithelium, butyrylcholinesterase contributes to over 75% of the esterase activity in the anterior segment tissues (157). The different proportion of these esterases rather than the existence of specific esterases contributes to the tissue differences in esterase activity.

Ocular butyrylcholinesterase appears to prefer lipophilic to hydrophilic esters. A means to increase the lipophilicity of an ester prodrug is to extend the number of carbon atoms in the ester side chain. Chang et al. (158) reported that in a homologous series of 1- and 2-naphthyl esters, there existed a chain length which optimized hydrolysis and that this optimal chain length was influenced by the orientation of the ester side chain with respect to the basic naphthalene nucleus. The peak hydrolytic rate was reached at the caproate and the valerate esters for the 1- and 2-naphthyl ester series, respectively. The same is true of timolol (87,159–162) and pilocarpine ester prodrugs (163–165).

V. CONCLUSION

Delivery of drugs to their target tissues in the eye is difficult because of the multiple protective barriers imposed by the eye against the entry of xenobiotics. For more than a decade, attempts to improve ocular drug bioavailability have been focused on overcoming precorneal solution drainage through manipulation of solution viscosity with polymers that may or may not undergo a phase transition driven by changes in tear pH (166), electrolyte composition (167), or temperature (168). The desire to further prolong the corneal contact time over that which can be achieved by manipulation of solution viscosity has led to new approaches based on mucoadhesive polymers (28,169) and collagen shields (170–172). Thus far, improvement in ocular drug bioavailability using the above approaches has been modest, since none of them affords the requisite one to two orders of reduction in the magnitude of precorneal drug loss (1). Consequently, it seems logical to also consider improving corneal drug permeability using the grossly underutilized but potentially very useful approach of prodrug derivatization as an adjunct to improve ocular drug bioavailability. Given the distinct possibility of absorption of topically applied drugs into the blood stream, the success of such a hybrid system will be measured not only by how much it will improve ocular drug bioavailability but also by how much it will reduce systemic drug load.

ACKNOWLEDGMENTS

This work was supported in part by grant EY7389 from the National Institutes of Health, Bethesda, Maryland, and by the Gavin S. Herbert Professorship. The author thanks Esther Ashby, Yilson Tang, and Udaya Bhaskar Kompella for editorial assistance.

REFERENCES

1. Grass, G. M., and Robinson, J. R. (1984). Relationship of chemical structure to corneal penetration and influence of low-viscosity solution on ocular bioavailability, *J. Pharm. Sci.*, 73:1021.

2. Brazzell, R. K., Woolridge, C. B., Hackett, R. B., and McCue, B. A. (1990). Pharmacokinetics of the aldose reductase inhibitor imirestat following topical ocular administration, *Pharm. Res.*, 7:192.

3. Ohtori, A., Yamamoto, Y., and Tojo, K. J. (1991). Penetration and binding of aldose-reductase inhibitors in the lens, *Invest. Ophthalmol. Vis. Sci.*, 32:189.

4. Mishima, S., Gasset, A., Klyce, S. D., and Baum, J. L. (1966). Determination of tear volume and tear flow, *Invest. Ophthalmol.*, 5:264.

5. Taniguchi, K., Yamamoto, Y., Itakura, K., Miichi, H., and Hayashi, S. (1988). Assessment of ocular irritability of liposome preparations, *J. Pharmacokinet. Biopharm.*, 11:607.

6. Lee, V. H. L., and Carson, L. W. (1986). Ocular disposition of inulin from single and multiple doses of positively charged multilamellar liposomes: Evidence for alterations in tear dynamics and ocular surface characteristics, *J. Ocul. Pharmacol.*, 2:353.

7. Schoenwald, R. D., and Stewart, P. (1980). Effects of particle size on ophthalmic bioavailability of dexamethasone suspensions in rabbits, *J. Pharm. Sci.*, 69:391.

8. Hui, H. W., and Robinson, J. R. (1985). Effect of particle dissolution rate on ocular drug bioavailability, *J. Pharm. Sci.*, 75:280.

9. Bisrat, M., Nyström, C., and Edman, P. (1990). Influence of dissolution rate of sparingly soluble drugs on corneal permeability in vitro, *Int. J. Pharm.*, 63:49.

10. Wright, J. C., and Meger, G. E. (1962). A review of the Schirmer test for tear production, *Arch. Ophthalmol.*, 67:564.

11. Chrai, S. S., Patton, T. F., Mehta, A., and Robinson, J. R. (1973). Lacrimal and instilled fluid dynamics in rabbit eyes, *J. Pharm. Sci.*, 62:1112.

12. Chrai, S. S., Makoid, M., Eriksen, S. P., and Robinson, J. R. (1974). Drop size and initial dosing frequency problems of topically applied ophthalmic drugs, *J. Pharm. Sci.*, 63:333.

13. Berman, M. B., Barber, J. C., Talamo, R. C., and Langley, C. E. (1973). Corneal ulceration and the serum antiproteases. I. α-Antitrypsin, *Invest. Ophthalmol.*, 12:759.

14. File, R. R., and Patton, T. F. (1980). Topically applied pilocarpine. Human pupillary response as a function of drop size, *Arch. Ophthalmol.*, 98:112.

15. Chang, S. C., Chien, D. S., Bundgaard, H., and Lee, V. H. L. (1988). Relative effectiveness of prodrug and viscous solution approaches in maximizing the ratio of ocular to systemic absorption of topically applied timolol, *Exp. Eye Res.*, 46:59.

16. Podder, K., Moy, K. C., and Lee, V. H. L. (1992). Improving the safety of topically applied timolol in the pigmented rabbit through manipulation of formulation composition, *Exp. Eye Res.*, 54:747.

17. Keister, J. C., Cooper, E. R., Missel, P. J., Lang, J. C., and Hager, D. F. (1991). Limits on optimizing ocular drug delivery, *J. Pharm. Sci.*, 80:50.

18. Patton, T. F. (1977). Pharmacokinetic evidence for improved ophthalmic drug delivery by reduction of instilled volume, *J. Pharm. Sci.*, 66:1058.

19. Sieg, J. W., and Triplett, J. W. (1980). Precorneal retention of topically instilled micronized particles, *J. Pharm. Sci.*, 69:863.

20. Lee, V. H. L., Takemoto, K. A., and Iimoto, D. S. (1984). Precorneal factors influencing the ocular distribution of topically applied liposomal inulin, *Curr. Eye Res.*, 3:585.

21. Chrai, S. S., Makoid, M. C., Eriksen, S. P., and Robinson, J. R. (1974). Drop size and initial dosing frequency problems of topically applied ophthalmic drugs, *J. Pharm. Sci.*, 63:333.

22. Chrai, S. S., and Robinson, J. R. (1974). Ocular evaluation of methylcellulose vehicle in albino rabbits, *J. Pharm. Sci.*, 63:1218.

23. Patton, T. F., and Robinson, J. R. (1975). Ocular evaluation of polyvinyl alcohol vehicle in rabbits, *J. Pharm. Sci.*, 64:1312.

24. Saettone, M. F., Giannaccini, B., Teneggi, A., Savigni, P., and Tellini, N. (1982). Vehicle effects on ophthalmic bioavailability: The influence of different polymers on the activity of pilocarpine in rabbit and man, *J. Pharm. Pharmacol., 34*:464.

25. Saettone, M. F., Giannaccini, B., Ravecca, S., La Marca, F., and Tota, G. (1984). Polymer effects on ocular bioavailability—the influence of different liquid vehicles on the mydriatic response of tropicamide in humans and in rabbits, *Int. J. Pharm., 20*:187.

26. Saettone, M. F., Monti, D., Torracca, M. T., Chetoni, P., and Giannaccini, B. (1989). Muco-adhesive liquid ophthalmic vehicles—evaluation of macromolecular ionic complexes of pilocar-pine, *Drug Dev. Indust. Pharm., 15*:2475.

27. Camber, O., Edman, P., and Gurny, R. (1987). Influence of sodium hyaluronate on the meiotic effect of pilocarpine in rabbits, *Curr. Eye Res., 6*:779.

28. Davies, N. M., Farr, S. J., Hadgraft, J., and Kellaway, I. W. (1991). Evaluation of mucoadhesive polymers in ocular drug delivery. I. Viscous solutions, *Pharm. Res., 8*:1039.

29. Cheeks, L., Green, K., Stone, R. P., and Riedhammer, T. (1989). Comparative effects of pilocarpine in different vehicles on pupil diameter in albino rabbits and squirrel monkeys, *Curr. Eye Res., 8*:1251.

30. Dartt, D. A., Markin, C., and Gray, K. (1988). Comparison of proteins in lacrimal gland fluid secreted in response to different stimuli, *Invest. Ophthalmol. Vis. Sci., 29*:991.

31. Conrad, J. M., Reay, W. A., Polcyn, E., and Robinson, J. R. (1978). Influence of tonicity and pH on lacrimation and ocular drug bioavailability, *J. Parent. Drug Assoc., 32*:149.

32. Carney, L. G., Mauger, T. F., and Hill, R. M. (1989). Buffering in human tears: pH responses to acid and base challenge, *Invest. Ophthalmol. Vis. Sci., 30*:747.

33. Ahmed, I., and Chaudhuri, B. (1988). Evaluation of buffer systems in ophthalmic product development, *Int. J. Pharm., 44*:97.

34. Mitra, A. K., and Mikkelson, T. J. (1982). Ophthalmic solution buffer systems I. The effect of buffer concentration on the ocular absorption of pilocarpine, *Int. J. Pharm., 10*:219.

35. Åberg, G., Adler, G., and Wikberg, J. (1978). Inhibition and facilitation of lacrimal flow by β-adrenergic drugs, *Ophthalmol. Acta, 57*:225.

36. de Haas, E. B. H. (1960). Lacrimal gland response to parasympathomimetics after parasym-pathomimetics denervation, *Arch. Ophthalmol., 64*:34.

37. Patton, T. F., and Robinson, J. R. (1975). Influence of topical anesthesia on tear dynamics and ocular bioavailability in albino rabbits, *J. Pharm. Sci., 64*:267.

38. Schoenwald, R. D., Barfknecht, C. F., Ignace, C., Wei, T., Spawn, C., Jensen, V., and Cheng, B. (1991). Evaluation of tear stimulants related to bromhexine [BH], *Invest. Ophthalmol. Vis. Sci., 32(Suppl.)*:1294.

39. Stratford, R. E., Yang, D. C., Redell, M. A., and Lee, V. H. L. (1983). Ocular distribution of liposome-encapsulated epinephrine and inulin in the albino rabbit, *Curr. Eye Res., 2*:377.

40. Luo, A. M., Sasaki, H., and Lee, V. H. L. (1991). Ocular drug interactions involving topically applied timolol in the pigmented rabbit, *Curr. Eye Res., 10*:231.

41. Lee, V. H. L., Luo, A. M., Li, S., Podder, S. K., Chang, S. C., Ohdo, S., and Grass, G. M. (1991). Pharmacokinetic basis for nonadditivity of IOP lowering in timolol combinations, *Invest. Ophthalmol. Vis. Sci., 32*:2948.

42. Mikkelson, T. J., Chrai, S. S., and Robinson, J. R. (1973). Altered bioavailability of drugs in the eye due to drug-protein interaction, *J. Pharm. Sci., 62*:1648.

43. Coyle, P. K., Sibony, P. A., and Johnson, C. (1989). Electrophoresis combined with immunologic identification of human tear proteins, *Invest. Ophthalmol. Vis. Sci., 30*:1872.

44. Kuizenga, A., van Haeringen, N. J., and Kijlstra, A. (1991). SDS-minigel electrophoresis of human tears, *Invest. Ophthalmol. Vis. Sci., 32*:381.

45. Chrai, S. S., and Robinson, J. R. (1976). Binding of sulfisoxazole to protein fractions of tears, *J. Pharm. Sci., 65*:437.

46. Woodward, D. F., and Ledgard, S. E. (1985). Effect of LTD_4 on conjunctival vasopermeability and blood-aqueous barrier integrity, *Invest. Ophthalmol. Vis. Sci., 26*:481.

47. Anderson, J. A., and Leopold, I. H. (1981). Antiproteolytic activities found in human tears, *Ophthalmology, 88*:82.
48. Nichols, B., Dawson, C. R., and Togni, B. (1983). Surface features of the conjunctiva and cornea, *Invest. Ophthalmol. Vis. Sci., 24*:570.
49. Nichols, B. A., Chiappino, M. L., and Dawson, C. R. (1985). Demonstration of the mucus layer of the tear film by electron microscopy, *Invest. Ophthalmol. Vis. Sci., 26*:464.
50. Huang, A. J. W., Tseng, S. C. G., and Kenyon, K. R. (1989). Paracellular permeability of corneal and conjunctival epithelia, *Invest. Ophthalmol. Vis. Sci., 30*:684.
51. Walsky, M. A., Jablonski, M. M., and Edelhauser, H. F. (1988). Comparison of conjunctival and corneal surface areas in rabbit and human, *Curr. Eye Res., 7*:483.
52. Wang, W., Sasaki, H., Chien, D. S., and Lee, V. H. L. (1991). Lipophilicity influence on conjunctival drug penetration in the pigmented rabbit: A comparison with corneal penetration, *Curr. Eye Res., 10*:571.
53. Lee, V. H. L., and Robinson, J. R. (1979). Mechanistic and quantitative evaluation of precorneal pilocarpine disposition in albino rabbits, *J. Pharm. Sci., 68*:673.
54. Ashton, P., Podder, S. K., and Lee, V. H. L. (1991). Formulation influence on the conjunctival penetration of four beta blockers in the pigmented rabbits: Comparison with corneal penetration, *Pharm. Res., 8*:1166.
55. Stratford, R. E., Carson, L. W., Dodda-Kashi, S., and Lee, V. H. L. (1988). Systemic absorption of ocularly administered enkephalinamide and inulin in the albino rabbit: Extent, pathways, and vehicle effects, *J. Pharm. Sci., 77*:838.
56. Doane, M. G., Jense, A. D., and Dohlman, C. H. (1978). Penetration routes of topically applied eye medications, *Am. J. Ophthalmol., 85*:383.
57. Ahmed, I., and Patton, T. F. (1985). Importance of the noncorneal absorption route in topical ophthalmic drug delivery, *Invest. Ophthalmol. Vis. Sci., 26*:584.
58. Ahmed, I., and Patton, T. F. (1987). Disposition of timolol and inulin in the rabbit eye following corneal versus non-corneal absorption, *Int. J. Pharm., 38*:9.
59. Ahmed, I., and Patton, T. F. (1986). Selective intraocular delivery of liposome encapsulated inulin via the non-corneal absorption route, *Int. J. Pharm., 34*:163.
60. Stratford, R. E., Redell, M. A., Yang, D. C., and Lee, V. H. L. (1983). Ocular distribution of liposome-encapsulated epinephrine and inulin in the albino rabbit, *Curr. Eye Res., 2*:377.
61. Lee, V. H. L., Swarbrick, J., Redell, M. A., and Yang, D. C. (1983). Vehicle influence on ocular disposition of sodium cromoglycate in the albino rabbit, *Int. J. Pharm., 16*:163.
62. Li, V. H.-K., and Robinson, J. R. (1989). Solution viscosity effects on the ocular disposition of cromolyn sodium in the albino rabbit, *Int. J. Pharm., 53*:219.
63. Diepold, R., Kreuter, J., Himber, J., Gurny, R., Lee, V. H. L., Robinson, J. R., Saettone, M. F., and Schnaudigel, O. E. (1989). Comparison of different models for the testing of pilocarpine eyedrops using conventional eyedrops and a novel depot formulation (nanoparticles), *Graefes Arch. Clin. Exp. Ophthalmol., 227*:188.
64. Attia, M. A., Kassem, M. A., and Safwat, S. M. (1988). In vivo performance of [^{3}H]dexamethasone ophthalmic film delivery systems in the rabbit eye, *Int. J. Pharm., 47*:21.
65. Van Buskirk, E. M. (1980). Adverse reactions from timolol administration, *Ophthalmology, 87*:447.
66. Nelson, W. L., Fraunfelder, F. T., Sills, J. M., Arrowsmith, J. B., and Kruitdky, J. N. (1986). Adverse respiratory and cardiovascular events attributed to timolol ophthalmic solution, *Am. J. Ophthalmol., 102*:606.
67. Zimmerman, T. J., Kooner, K. S., Kandarakis, A. S., and Ziegler, L. P. (1984). Improving the therapeutic index of topically applied ocular drugs, *Arch. Ophthalmol., 102*:551.
68. Kaila, T., Huupponen, R., and Salminen, L. (1986). Effects of eyelid closure and nasolacrimal duct occlusion on the systemic absorption of ocular timolol in human subjects, *J. Ocul. Pharmacol., 2*:365.

69. Kyyrönen, K., and Arto, U. (1990). Improved ocular:systemic absorption ratio of timolol by viscous vehicle and phenylephrine, *Invest. Ophthalmol. Vis. Sci., 31*:1827.
70. Urtti, A., Pipkin, J. D., Rork, G., Sendo, T., Finne, U., and Repta, A. J. (1990). Controlled drug delivery devices for experimental ocular studies with timolol: 2. Ocular and systemic absorption in rabbits, *Int. J. Pharm., 61*:241.
71. Sasaki, H., Bundgaard, H., and Lee, V. H. L. (1989). Design of prodrugs to selectively reduce systemic timolol absorption on the basis of the differential lipophilic characteristics of the cornea and the conjunctiva, *Invest. Ophthalmol. Vis. Sci., 30(Suppl.)*:25.
72. Sugrue, M. F., Gautheron, P., Grove, J., Mallorga, P., Viader, M. P., Baldwin, J. P., Ponticello, G. S., and Varga, S. L. (1988). L-653,328: An ocular hypotensive agent with modest beta receptor blocking activity, *Invest. Ophthalmol. Vis. Sci., 29*:776.
73. Bodor, N., Ohiro, Y., Loftsson, Y., Katovich, M., and Cladwell, W. (1984). Soft drugs IV. The application of the inactive metabolite approach for design of soft β-blockers, *Pharm. Res., 1*:120.
74. Ohdo, S., Grass, G. M., and Lee, V. H. L. (1991). Improving the ocular:systemic ratio of topical timolol by varying the dosing time, *Invest. Ophthalmol. Vis. Sci., 32*:2790.
75. Kompella, U., Ohdo, S., Gurny, R., Martenet, M., Bundgaard, H., and Lee, V. H. L. (1991). Varying the dosing time to further improve the ocular:systemic ratio of 0-1'-methyl-cyclopropanoyl timolol in the pigmented rabbit, *Invest. Ophthalmol. Vis. Sci., 32(Suppl.)*:733.
76. Ohdo, S., Podder, S. P., and Lee, V. H. L. (1990). Ocular chronopharmacology in the pigmented rabbit: Ocular timolol concentrations are dependent on the time of drop instillation, *Invest. Ophthalmol. Vis. Sci., 31(Suppl.)*:232.
77. Lee, V. H. L., Zhu, J., Kompella, U., and Huang, C.-L. (1991). Diurnal changes in ocular and systemic absorption of topically applied betaxolol in the pigmented rabbit, *Invest. Ophthalmol. Vis. Sci., 32(Suppl.)*:1296.
78. Lee, V. H. L. (1992). Minimizing the systemic absorption of topically applied ophthalmic drugs, *STP Pharma, 2*:5.
79. Benson, H. (1974). Permeability of the cornea to topically applied drugs, *Arch. Ophthamol., 91*:313.
80. Lee, V. H. L., Hui, H. W., and Robinson, J. R. (1980). Corneal metabolism of pilocarpine in pigmented rabbits, *Invest. Ophthalmol. Vis. Sci., 9*:210.
81. Richman, J. B., and Tang-Lui, D. D.-S. (1990). A corneal perfusion device for estimating ocular bioavailability in vitro, *J. Pharm. Sci., 79*:153.
82. Lee, V. H. L., Carson, L. W., Dodda Kashi, S., and Stratford, R. E. (1986). Metabolic and permeation barriers to the ocular absorption of topically applied enkephalins in albino rabbits, *J. Ocul. Pharmacol., 2*:345.
83. Dodda Kashi, S., Wang, W., and Lee, V. H. L. (1989). Corneal penetration of angiotensin converting enzyme inhibitors and related peptides in the albino rabbit, *Invest. Ophthalmol. Vis. Sci., 30(Suppl.)*:21.
84. Schoenwald, R. D., and Huang, H. S. (1983). Corneal penetration behavior of β-blocking agents I: Physicochemical factors, *J. Pharm. Sci., 72*:1266.
85. Hull, D. S., Hine, J. E., Edelhauser, H. F., and Hyndiuk, B. A. (1974). Permeability of the isolated rabbit cornea to corticosteroids, *Invest. Ophthalmol., 13*:457.
86. Shih, R. L., and Lee, V. H. L. (1990). Rate limiting barrier to the penetration of ocular hypotensive beta blockers across the corneal epithelium in the pigmented rabbit, *J. Ocul. Pharmacol., 6*:329.
87. Chien, D. S., Bundgaard, H., and Lee, V. H. L. (1988). The influence of corneal integrity in the ocular absorption of timolol prodrugs, *J. Ocul. Pharmacol., 4*:137.
88. Dodda Kashi, S., and Lee, V. H. L. (1986). Hydrolysis of enkephalins in anterior segment tissue homogenates of the albino rabbit eye, *Invest. Ophthalmol. Vis. Sci., 27*:1300.
89. Lee, V. H. L., Carson, L. W., and Takemoto, K. A. (1983). Macromolecular drug absorption in the albino rabbit eye, *Int. J. Pharm., 72*:1272.
90. BenErza, D., and Maftzir, G. (1990). Ocular penetration of cyclosporin A, *Invest. Ophthalmol. Vis. Sci., 31*:1362.

91. Kupferman, A., Pratt, M. V., Suckewar, K., and Leibowitz, H. M. (1974). Topically applied steroids in corneal disease. III. The role of drug derivative in stromal absorption of dexamethasone, *Arch. Ophthalmol., 91*:373.

92. Cox, W. V., Kupferman, A., and Leibowitz, H. W. (1972). Topically applied steroids in corneal disease. I. The role of inflammation in stromal absorption of dexamethasone, *Arch. Ophthalmol., 88*:308.

93. Pavan-Langston, D., and Nelson, D. J. (1979). Intraocular penetration of trifluridine, *Am. J. Ophthalmol., 87*:814.

94. Baum, J. L., Barza, M., Shushan, D., and Weinstein, L. (1974). Concentration of gentamicin in experimental corneal ulcers. Topical vs. subconjunctival therapy, *Arch. Ophthalmol., 92*:315.

95. Mikkelson, T. J., Chrai, S. S., and Robinson, J. R. (1973). Competitive inhibition of drug-protein interaction in the eye fluids and tissues, *J. Pharm. Sci., 62*:1942.

96. Smolen, V. F., Clevenger, J. M., Williams, E. J., and Bergdolt, H. W. (1973). Biophasic availability of ophthalmic carbachol. I: Mechanism of cationic polymers- and surfactant-promoted miotic activity, *J. Pharm. Sci., 62*:958.

97. Green, K., and Downs, S. J. (1974). Prednisolone phosphate penetration into and through the cornea, *Invest. Ophthalmol., 13*:316.

98. Kassem, R. M., El-Nimr, A. E. M., Salama, H. A., and Khalil, R. M. (1983). "Effect of Quarternary Ammonium Compounds on the Mydriatic Activity of Homatropine in Man," Proceedings of the 3rd International Conference of Pharmaceutical Technology., A.P.G.I., Paris, p. 275.

99. Keller, N., Moore, D., Carper, D., and Longwell, A. (1980). Increased corneal permeability induced by the dual effect of transient tear film acidification and exposure to benzalkonium chloride, *Exp. Eye Res., 30*:203.

100. Tonjum, A. M. (1974). Permeability of horseradish peroxidase in the rabbit corneal epithelium, *Ophthalmol. Acta, 52*:650.

101. Grass, G. M., Wood, R. W., and Robinson, J. R. (1985). Effects of calcium chelating agents on corneal permeability, *Invest. Ophthalmol. Vis. Sci., 26*:110.

102. Godbey, R. E. W., Green, K., and Hull, D. S. (1979). Influence of cetylpyridinium chloride on corneal permeability to penicillin, *J. Pharm. Sci., 68*:1176.

103. Wolosin, J. M. (1988). Regeneration of resistance and ion transport in rabbit corneal epithelium after induced surface cell exfoliation, *J. Membr. Biol., 104*:45.

104. Sokol, J. L., Masur, S. D., Asbell, P. A., and Wolosin, J. M. (1990). Layer-by-layer desquamation of corneal epithelium and maturation of tear-facing membranes, *Invest. Ophthalmol. Vis. Sci., 31*:294.

105. Schoenwald, R. D., and Ward, R. L. (1981). Relationship between steroid permeability across excised rabbit cornea and octanol-water partition coefficients, *J. Pharm. Sci., 67*:786.

106. Mosher, G. L., and Mikkelson, T. J. (1979). Permeability of the n-alkyl p-aminobenzoate esters across the isolated corneal membranes of the rabbit, *Int. J. Pharm., 2*:239.

107. Kishida, K., and Otori, T. (1980). A quantitative study on the relationship between transcorneal permeability of drugs and their hydrophobicity, *Jpn. J. Ophthalmol., 24*:251.

108. Chien, D. S., Sasaki, H., Bundgaard, H., Buur, A., and Lee, V. H. L. (1991). Role of enzymatic lability in the corneal and conjunctival penetration of timolol ester prodrugs in the pigmented rabbit, *Pharm. Res., 8*:728.

109. Francoeur, M. L., Sitek, S. J., Costello, B., and Patton, T. F. (1985). Kinetic disposition and distribution of timolol in the rabbit physiologically based ocular model, *Int. J. Pharm., 25*:275.

110. Mitra, A. K., and Mikkelson, T. J. (1988). Mechanism of transcorneal permeation of pilocarpine, *J. Pharm. Sci., 77*:771.

111. Jankowska, L. M., Bar-Ilan, A., and Maren, T. H. (1986). The relations between ionic and non-ionic diffusion of sulfonamides across the rabbit cornea, Invest. *Ophthalmol. Vis. Sci., 27*:29.

112. Lee, V. H. L., and Li, V. H. K. (1989). Prodrugs for improved ocular drug delivery, *Adv. Drug Deliv. Rev., 3*:1.

113. Patil, P. N., and Jacobowitz, D. (1974). Unequal accumulation of adrenergic drugs by pigmented and nonpigmented iris, *Am. J. Ophthalmol.*, *78*:470.

114. Shimada, K., Baweja, R., Sokoloski, T., and Patil, P. N. (1976). Binding characteristics of drugs to synthetic levodopa melanin, *J. Pharm. Sci.*, *65*:1057.

115. Larsson, B., and Tjalve, H. (1979). Studies on the mechanism of drug-binding to melanin, *Biochem. Pharmacol.*, *28*:1181.

116. Atlasik, B., Stepien, K., and Wilczok, T. (1980). Interaction of drugs with ocular melanin *in vitro*, *Exp. Eye Res.*, *30*:325.

117. Araie, M., Takase, M., Sakai, Y., Ishii, Y., Yokoyama, Y., and Kitagawa, M. (1982). Beta-adrenergic blockers: Ocular penetration and binding to the uveal pigment, *Jpn. J. Ophthalmol.*, *26*:248.

118. Lee, V. H. L., and Robinson, J. R. (1982). Disposition of topically applied pilocarpine in the pigmented rabbit eye, *Int. J. Pharm.*, *11*:155.

119. Katz, I. M., and Berger, E. T. (1979). Effects of iris pigmentation on response of ocular pressure to timolol, *Surv. Ophthalmol.*, *23*:395.

120. Urtti, A., and Salminen, L. (1985). A comparison between iris-ciliary body concentration and receptor affinity of timolol, *Ophthalmol. Acta*, *63*:16.

121. Urtti, A., Salminen, L., and Miinalainen, O. (1985). Systemic absorption of ocular pilocarpine is modified by polymer matrices, *Int. J. Pharm.*, *23*:147.

122. Zane, P. A., Brindle, S. D., Gause, D. O., O'Buck, A. J., Raghavan, P. R., and Tripp, S. L. (1990). Physicochemical factors associated with binding and retention of compounds in ocular melanin of rats: Correlations using data from whole-body autoradiography and molecular modeling for multiple linear regression analyses, *Pharm. Res.*, *7*:935.

123. Shichi, H., and Nebert, D. W. (1980). Drug metabolism in ocular tissues, *Extrahepatic Metabolism of Drugs and Other Foreign Compounds* (T. E. Gram, ed.), Spectrum, New York, p. 333.

124. Cheng-Bennett, A., Poyer, J., Weinkam, R. J., and Woodward, D. F. (1990). Lack of prostaglandin $F_{2\alpha}$ metabolism by human ocular tissues, *Invest. Ophthalmol. Vis. Sci.*, *31*:1389.

125. Schoenwald, R. D., and Houseman, J. A. (1982). Disposition of cyclophosphamide in the rabbit and human cornea, *Biopharm. Drug Dispos.*, *3*:231.

126. Putterman, G. J., Davidson, J., and Albert, J. (1985). Lack of metabolism of timolol by ocular tissues, *J. Ocul. Pharmacol.*, *1*:287.

127. Petersen, R. A., Lee, K.-J., and Donn, A. (1965). Acetylcholinesterase in the rabbit cornea, *Arch. Ophthalmol.*, *73*:370.

128. Waltman, S., and Sears, M. (1964). Catechol-O-methyl transferase and monoamine oxidase activity in the ocular tissues of albino rabbits, *Invest. Ophthalmol.*, *3*:601.

129. Abraham, N. G., Lin, J. H. C., Dunn, M. W., and Schwartzman, M. L. (1987). Presence of heme oxygenase and NADPH cytochrome P-450 (c) reductase in human corneal epithelium, *Invest. Ophthalmol. Vis. Sci.*, *2*:1464.

130. Matsumoto, K., Kishida, K., Manabe, R., and Sugiyama, T. (1987). Induction of cytochrome P-450 in the rabbit eye by phenobarbital, as detected immunohistochemically, *Curr. Eye Res.*, *6*:847.

131. Duffel, M. W., Ing, I. S., Segarra, T. M., Dixson, T. M., Barfknecht, C. F., and Schoenwald, R. D. (1986). N-Substituted sulfonamide carbonic anhydrase inhibitors with topical effects on intraocular pressure, *J. Med. Chem.*, *29*:1488.

132. Aimoto, T., and Chiou, G. C. Y. (1985). 7-Ethoxycoumarin deethylase activity as indicator of oxidative metabolism in rabbit eyes, *J. Ocul. Pharmacol.*, *1*:279.

133. Southren, A. L., Altman, K., Vittek, J., Boniuk, V., and Gordon, G. G. (1976). Steroid metabolism in ocular tissues of the rabbit, *Invest. Ophthalmol.*, *15*:222.

134. Yamauchi, H., Kito, H., and Uda, K. (1975). Studies on intraocular penetration and metabolism of fluorometholone in rabbit: A comparison between dexamethasone and prednisolone acetate, *Jpn. J. Ophthalmol.*, *19*:339.

135. Weinstein, B. I., Kandalaft, N., Ritch, R., Camras, C. B., Morris, D. J., Latif, S. A., Vecsei, P., Vittek, J., Gordon, G. G., and Southren, A. L. (1991). 5α-Dihydrocortisol in human aqueous humor and metabolism of cortisol by human lenses in vitro, *Invest. Ophthalmol. Vis. Sci.,* 32:2130.

136. Putnam, M. L., Schoenwald, R. D., Duffel, M. W., Barfknecht, C. F., Segarra, T. M., and Campbell, D. A. (1987). Ocular disposition of aminozolamide in the rabbit eye, *Invest. Ophthalmol. Vis. Sci.,* 28:1373.

137. Campbell, D. A., Schoenwald, R. D., Duffel, M. W., and Barfknecht, C. F. (1991). Characterization of arylamine acetyltransferase in the rabbit eye, *Invest. Ophthalmol. Vis. Sci.,* 32:2190.

138. Ono, S., Hirano, H., and Obara, K. (1972). Study on the conjugation of cortisol in the lens, *Ophthal. Res.,* 3:307.

139. Lee, V. H. L., Chien, D. S., and Sasaki, H. (1988). Ocular ketone reductase distribution and its role in the metabolism of ocularly applied levobunolol in the pigmented rabbit, *J. Pharmacol. Exp. Ther.,* 246:871.

140. Lee, V. H. L. (1983). Esterase activities in adult rabbit eyes, *J. Pharm. Sci.,* 72:239.

141. Lee, V. H. L., Morimito, K. W., and Stratford, R. E. (1982). Esterase distribution in the rabbit cornea and its implications in ocular drug bioavailability, *Biopharm. Drug Dispos.,* 3:291.

142. Lee, V. H. L., Stratford, R. E., and Morimoto, K. W. (1983). Age-related changes in esterase activity in rabbit eyes, *Int. J. Pharm.,* 13:183.

143. Stratford, R. E., and Lee, V. H. L. (1985). Aminopeptidase activity in the albino rabbit extraocular tissues relative to the small intestine, *J. Pharm. Sci.,* 74:731.

144. Sharma, K. K., and Ortwerth, B. J. (1987). Purification and characterization of an aminopeptidase from bovine cornea, *Exp. Eye Res.,* 45:117.

145. Saneto, R. P., Awasthi, Y. C., and Srivastava, S. K. (1982). Mercapturic acid pathway enzymes in bovine ocular lens, cornea, retina and retinal pigmented epithelium, *Exp. Eye Res.,* 34:107.

146. Kishida, K., Akaki, Y., Sasabe, T., and Yamamoto, C. (1990). Glutathione conjugation of methazolamide and subsequent reactions in the ciliary body in vitro, *J. Pharm. Sci.,* 79:638.

147. Green, K., and MacKeen, D. L. (1976). Chloramphenicol retention on, and penetration into, the rabbit eye, *Invest. Ophthalmol. Vis. Sci.,* 15:220.

148. Sinkula, A. A., and Yalkowsky, S. H. (1975). Rationale for design of biologically reversible drug derivatives: Prodrugs, *J. Pharm. Sci.,* 64:181.

149. Bodor, N. (1984). Soft drugs: Principles and methods for the design of safe drugs, *Med. Res. Rev.,* 4:449.

150. Chiang, C. W. N., Barnett, G., and Brine, D. (1983). Systemic absorption of Δ1-tetrahydrocannabinol after ophthalmic administration to the rabbit, *J. Pharm. Sci.,* 72:136.

151. Bodor, N., ElKoussi, A., Kano, M., and Nakamura, T. (1988). Improved delivery through biological membranes. 26. Design, synthesis, and pharmacological activity of a novel chemical delivery system for β-adrenergic blocking agents, *J. Med. Chem.,* 31:100.

152. Bodor, N., and Prokai, L. (1990). Site- and stereospecific ocular drug delivery by sequential enzymatic bioactivation, *Pharm. Res.,* 7:723.

153. Lee, V. H. L., and Smith, R. E. (1985). Effect of substrate concentration, product concentration, and peptides on the *in vitro* hydrolysis of model ester prodrugs by corneal esterases, *J. Ocular Pharmacol.,* 1:269.

154. Stratford, R. E., and Lee, V. H. L. (1985). Ocular aminopeptidase activity and distribution in the albino rabbit, *Curr. Eye Res.,* 4:995.

155. Ashton, P., Wang, W., and Lee, V. H. L. (1991). Location of penetration and metabolic barriers to levobunolol in the pigmented rabbit, *J. Pharmacol. Exp. Ther.,* 259:719.

156. Lee, V. H. L., Iimoto, D. S., and Takemoto, K. A. (1983). Subcellular distribution of esterases in the bovine eye, *Curr. Eye Res.,* 2:869.

157. Lee, V. H. L., Chang, S. C., Oshiro, C. M., and Smith, R. E. (1985). Ocular esterase composition in albino and pigmented rabbits: Possible implications in ocular prodrug design and evaluation, *Curr. Eye Res., 4*:1117.

158. Chang, S. C., and Lee, V. H. L. (1983). Influence of chain length on the *in vitro* hydrolysis of model ester prodrugs by ocular esterases, *Curr. Eye Res., 2*:651.

159. Chang, S. C., Bundgaard, H., Buur, A., and Lee, V. H. L. (1987). Improved corneal penetration of timolol by prodrugs as a means to reduce systemic drug load, *Invest. Ophthalmol. Vis. Sci., 28*:487.

160. Chang, S. C., Bundgaard, H., Buur, A., and Lee, V. H . L. (1988). Low dose O-butyryl timolol improves the therapeutic index of timolol in the pigmented rabbit, *Invest. Ophthalmol. Vis. Sci., 29*:626.

161. Bundgaard, H., Buur, A., Chang, S. C., and Lee, V. H. L. (1986). Prodrugs of timolol for improved ocular delivery: Synthesis, hydrolysis kinetics and lipophilicity of various timolol esters, *Int. J. Pharm., 33*:15.

162. Bundgaard, H., Buur, A., Chang, S. C., and Lee, V. H. L. (1988). Timolol prodrugs: Synthesis, stability and lipophilicity of various alkyl, cycloalkyl and aromatic esters of timolol, *Int. J. Pharm., 46*:77.

163. Bundgaard, H., Falch, E., Larsen, C., and Mikkelson, T. J. (1986). Pilocarpine prodrugs I. Synthesis, physicochemical properties and kinetics of lactonization of pilocarpic acid esters, *J. Pharm. Sci., 75*:36.

164. Bundgaard, H., Falch, E., Larsen, C., Mosher, G., and Mikkelson, T. J. (1986). Pilocarpine prodrugs II. Synthesis, stability, bioconversion, and physicochemical properties of sequentially labile pilocarpic acid diesters, *J. Pharm. Sci., 75*:775.

165. Mosher, G. L., Bundgaard, H., Falch, E., Larsen, C., and Mikkelson, T. J. (1987). Ocular bioavailability in pilocarpic acid mono- and diester prodrugs as assessed by miotic activity in the rabbit, *Int. J. Pharm., 39*:113.

166. Gurny, R., Ibrahim, H., Aebi, A., Buri, P., Wilson, C. G., Wahington, N., Edman, P., and Camber, O. (1987). Design and evaluation of controlled release systems for the eye, *J. Contr. Rel., 6*:367.

167. Rozier, A., Mazuel, C., Grove, J., and Plazonnet, B. (1989). Gelrite: A novel, ion-activated, in-situ gelling polymer for ophthalmic vehicles. Effect on bioavailability of timolol, *Int. J. Pharm., 57*:163.

168. Miller, S. C., and Donovan, M. D. (1982). Effect of poloxamer 407 gel on the miotic activity of pilocarpine nitrate in rabbits, *Int. J. Pharm., 12*:147.

169. Hui, H. W., and Robinson, J. R. (1985). Ocular drug delivery of progesterone using a bio-adhesive polymer, *Int. J. Pharm., 26*:203.

170. Sawusch, M. R., O'Brien, T. P., Dick, J. D., and Gottsch, J. D. (1988). Use of collagen corneal shields in the treatment of bacterial keratitis, *Am. J. Ophthalmol., 106*:279.

171. Hobden, J. A., Reidy, J. J., O'Callaghan, R. J., Insler, M. S., and Hill, J. M. (1990). Quinolones in collagen shields to treat aminoglycoside-resistant pseudomonal keratitis, *Invest. Ophthalmol. Vis. Sci., 31*:2241.

172. Hobden, J. A., Reidy, J. J., O'Callaghan, R. J., Insler, M. S., and Hill, J. M. (1990). Cipro-floxacin iontophoresis for aminoglycoside-resistant pseudomonal keratitis, *Invest. Ophthalmol. Vis. Sci., 31*:1940.

173. Lee, V. H. L., Swarbrick, J., Stratford, R. E., and Morimoto, K. W. (1983). Disposition of topically applied sodium cromoglycate in the albino rabbit eye, *J. Pharm. Pharmacol., 35*:445.

174. Lee, V. H. L., and Carson, L. W. (1985). Possible mechanisms for the retention of topically applied vitamin A (retinol) in the albino rabbit eye, *J. Ocul. Pharmacol., 1*:297.

175. Janes, R. B., and Stiles, J. F. (1964). The penetration of cortisol into normal and pathologic rabbit eyes, *Am. J. Ophthalmol., 56*:84.

176. Anderson, J. A. (1980). Systemic absorption of topical ocularly applied epinephrine and dipivefrin, *Arch. Ophthalmol., 98*:350.

177. Vaidyanathan, G., Jay, M., Bera, R. K., Mayer, P. R., and Brazzell, R. K. (1990). Scintigraphic evaluation of the ocular disposition of ^{18}F-imirestat in rabbits, *Pharm. Res., 7*:1198.
178. Yamamoto, A., Luo, A. M., Dodda Kashi, S., and Lee, V. H. L. (1989). The ocular route for systemic insulin delivery in the albino rabbit, *J. Pharmacol. Exp. Ther., 249*:249.
179. Tang-Liu, D. D.-S., Liu, S. S., and Weinkam, R. J. (1984). Ocular and systemic bioavailability of ophthalmic flurbiprofen, *J. Pharmacokinet. Biopharm., 12*:611.
180. Tang-Liu, D. D.-S., Lui, S., Neff, J., and Sandri, R. (1987). Disposition of levobunolol after an ophthalmic dose to rabbits, *J. Pharm. Sci., 76*:780.
181. Chang, S. C., and Lee, V. H. L. (1987). Nasal and conjunctival contributions to the systemic absorption of topical timolol in the pigmented rabbit: Implications in the design of strategies to maximize the ratio of ocular to systemic absorption, *J. Ocul. Pharmacol., 3*:159.

4

Ocular Pharmacokinetics/ Pharmacodynamics

Ronald D. Schoenwald *College of Pharmacy, University of Iowa,
Iowa City, Iowa*

I. INTRODUCTION

The study of pharmacokinetic processes—called absorption, distribution and elimination—is fundamental to determining the appropriate dosing regimen for an individual patient administered a drug by systemic routes. Pharmacokinetics has also been indispensable in designing an improved therapeutic agent or the means by which it is delivered. Quite often, pharmacokinetic analysis of systemically useful drugs is approached by dividing the body into a series of compartments which mathematically represent tissue levels of drug over time as a summation of exponentials. The number of compartments that are chosen are equal to and limited by the number of exponentials that can be assigned to the concentration of drug found in a particular body tissue and/or fluid over time.

The compartments are often interpreted physiologically or anatomically to contain tissues and/or organs which are "kinetically homogeneous." The term *kinetically homogeneous compartments* refers to tissues and/or organs which show similar if not identical kinetics for certain drugs even though the tissues and/or organs within the compartment may be dissimilar physiologically or anatomically. Although the rates within these groups of tissues and/or organs are similar for a particular drug, the extent of drug distribution to each is usually not equal.

The ophthalmic literature contains many reports of drug concentrations measured in eye tissues over time. However, when classic pharmacokinetic approaches have been applied to ophthalmic drugs, a number of limitations have been found to restrict the usefulness of pharmacokinetics in the practice of ophthalmology. Although quantitative interpretations of reported literature values often do not consider the limitations imposed by the eye on the classic pharmacokinetic equations, qualitative explanations of these data do serve as a guide. Noncompartmental approaches, such as moment analysis, circumvent the difficulty in choosing an appropriate compartmental model; however, the assumption of linearity remains as well as various intractable experimental difficulties.

Limitations in the use of classic pharmacokinetic approaches and difficulties in designing and implementing animal studies for the eye as well as interpretation of the results obtained from animal models are discussed in the following sections.

II. LIMITATIONS TO THE PRACTICAL USE OF CLASSIC MODELING

At the present time, it is not possible to predict optimal dosing regimens in the human eye for different drugs or for the same drug in different dosage forms. The most significant reason for not conducting ocular pharmacokinetic studies in the human eye is the inability to sample tissues or fluids from the intact eye without risking pain and/or injury. Although the rabbit eye is useful in predicting human ocular toxicities (1), the eyes of each species are dissimilar in anatomy and physiology (see Table 1) such that predicting human ocular pharmacokinetics from rabbit data may not be very precise for certain drugs. As a further complication in predicting human ocular pharmacokinetics based upon animal data, samples from eye tissues cannot be continuously sampled over time. Although a number of tissues can be removed quickly and precisely from the rabbit eye, one animal must be used to determine drug concentration at a single time point. Therefore, in order to construct a kinetic profile of drug concentration over time, a number of rabbits must be sacrificed at each time point. As many as 150 to 250 rabbit eyes may be required to complete a bioequivalence test between two ophthalmic drugs. It is often assumed that a representative pharmacokinetic profile can be constructed from "noncontinuous sampling" if enough time intervals and sufficient eyes per time interval are chosen; however, this number is not always chosen by a sound statistical approach.

III. ADEQUATE CHOICE OF TIME INTERVALS

Studies often use as few as 4 or 6 rabbit eyes per time interval or as many as 22, depending on the objective of the study (2–6). A statistical basis for choosing an appropriate number of rabbit eyes in ophthalmic bioavailability studies has been established using areas under the concentration-time curve (AUC) (7,8). The AUC is related to the extent of absorption

Table 1. Anatomical and Physiological Differences in the New Zealand Rabbit and Human Eye Pertinent to Ophthalmic Pharmacokinetics

Pharmacokinetic factor	Rabbit eye	Human eye
Tear volume	7.5 μL	7.0–30.0 μL[a]
Tear turnover rate	0.6–0.8 μL/min	0.5–2.2 μL/min
Spontaneous blinking rate[b]	4–5 times/min	15 times/min
Nictitating membrane[c]	Present	Absent
pH of tears	[d]	7.14–7.82
Milliosmolarity of tears	[d]	305 mOsm/L
Corneal thickness	0.40 mm	0.52 mm
Corneal diameter	15 mm	12 mm
Aqueous humor volume	[d]	310 μL
Aqueous humor turnover rate	[d]	1.53 μL/min

[a]Range depending on blinking rate and conjunctival sac volume.
[b]Occurs during normal waking hours without apparent external stimuli.
[c]Significance of nictitating membrane is small relative to overall loss rate from precornea area.
[d]Approximately same measurement as human.

which, similar to systemically administered drugs, is most important in determining therapy for chronic medication. The rate of absorption into the eye is less precise a measurement and also less pertinent to chronic therapy.

How many intervals and the length of time between each interval has not always been decided upon using a rational approach. Some general guidelines can be applied based upon the importance of absorption, distribution, and elimination to the kinetic profile. Each kinetic process is practically complete after 5 half-lives (96.875%); therefore, if the half-life for each kinetic process is known or can be easily arrived at, the theoretical length of time that should be used to generate a concentration x time profile can be estimated (Fig. 1).

A. Elimination Phase

Elimination of drug from the eye is the least complicated process and can be discussed first. It occurs over the entire concentration-time profile, and as long as it is the slowest of pharmacokinetic processes, the latter log-linear phase of the drug concentration-time profile represents the elimination phase and its slope allows for the calculation of elimination half-life and the time necessary for completion of the process. For example, the half-life for elimination of phenylephrine from rabbit aqueous humor is 83.5 min (9); therefore, the process is complete in 5 x 83.5 min or 6.96 h. Ideally, at least four or five time intervals should be equally spaced over 7 h following the completion of distribution within the eye. Obviously, a practical limitation to measuring phenylephrine for 7 h in the postdistributive phase is the sensitivity of the assay. Phenylephrine can be measured to a

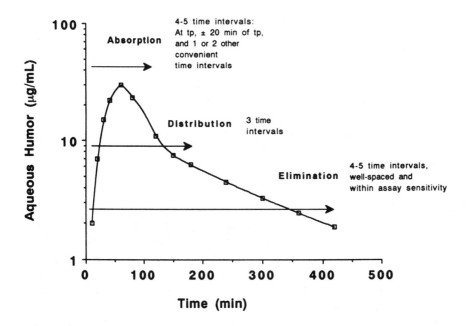

Figure 1. Ideal choice of sampling times for measurement of ocular absorption, distribution, and elimination of a topically administered drug.

sensitivity of 5–10 ng/mL using fluorescent detection methods (9,10) and providing tissues concentrations of at least 200 ng/mL can be attained from drug instillation, it would be possible to measure the decline over 5 elimination half-lives.

B. Absorption Phase

Absorption is somewhat more complex to estimate in the eye, since lag time and drainage lengthen and shorten, respectively, the length of time that the absorption process is operative. For example, the first-order absorption rate constant for phenylephrine is 4.5×10^{-5} min^{-1}, which gives a half-life of 128.3 h; however, drainage permits drug to remain at the corneal absorption site for approximately 3–6 min only, depending on the volume and viscosity of the instilled solution (3,11–14). Consequently, the absorption process is abruptly terminated from theoretical expectations. The short residence time of drug at the absorption site results in exceptionally poor bioavailability.

Phenylephrine is atypical, since it is very hydrophilic and transverses the cornea at a very slow rate. On the other hand, pilocarpine is moderately lipophilic and therefore more rapidly absorbed. Nevertheless, the difference between the theoretically expected time and the actual time during which absorption occurs remains large. For example, Makoid and Robinson reported an accurate K_a of 6.2×10^{-3} min for pilocarpine (15), which gives an absorption half-life of 111.8 min and predicts that the process is complete in about 10 h. However, the drainage rate constant is approximately 100 times larger with an estimated completion of the process in about 6 min (15). As a result of the very short residence time of drug at the absorption site, the extent of absorption of ophthalmic drugs is about 1–10% (2,3,6,9,16,17). The competing processes, referred to as nonabsorptive processes, have been specifically defined as drainage, conjunctival absorption, nictitating membrane absorption, tear turnover, drug protein binding and drug metabolism (3).

The initial time for drug to transverse the cornea, referred to as the lag time, is sufficiently long that most often the time to peak occurs over a much longer time period than the time that a drug solution resides on the cornea (i.e., 3–6 min). The majority of ophthalmic drugs requires between 20 and 60 min after instillation to reach the time to peak. Therefore, a reasonable time period exists so that up to three to four time intervals can be chosen to characterize the absorption phase. Because of the very low extent of absorption for ophthalmic drugs as well as the large correction needed for the drainage rate, the classic deconvolution technics (Wagner-Nelson and Loo-Riegelman) (18) cannot be used without severely overestimating the first-order absorption rate constant, K_a.

C. Distribution Phase

The distribution phase can be identified visually as the concave portion of the log concentration-time curve immediately following the time to peak. The latter log linear phase is the elimination or postdistributive phase (see Fig. 1). The distribution phase, which is expected to be shorter than the elimination phase, cannot be visually identified as easily as absorption and elimination. Depending on the numerical relationship between the micro-transfer constants associated with drug disposition, it is possible that the profile representing drug concentration over time cannot be characterized by the proper number of exponentials. Often one less exponential occurs than actually exists, particularly when $k_{21} > K_a$ and $\alpha > K_a$ (19). In addition, the concave portion of the log concentration-time curve may not be apparent because distribution is rapid. On the other hand, when drug concentrations from just after the time to peak to the beginning of the postdistributive phases are concave to the time axis, then the distributive phase is discernable and the concave portion of the profile should be represented by an additional two to four time intervals.

As shown in Figure 1, 10 to 12 time intervals will suffice if they are properly chosen to represent absorption, distribution, and elimination. However, if variability is too great, a larger number of eyes could be chosen at each interval to characterize adequately the drug's ocular pharmacokinetics. It is assumed that a smooth representative profile will result if a large enough sample size is chosen. For bioequivalence, the time to peak (tp) is a critical concentration to obtain, since it represents a maximum concentration. Because of the relatively large and constant nature of the drainage rate for topically administered solutions and suspensions, the tp only varies from about 20 to 60 min for ophthalmic drugs regardless of a drug's physicochemical behavior. As discussed previously, in practice, the distribution phase is usually not apparent either because of inherent variability or because the magnitude of the microconstants representing distribution to peripheral tissues prevents observation of the characteristic concavity shown in Figure 1.

D. Other Factors Influencing Choice of Sampling Times

Unfortunately, more subtle factors may be operating to complicate the choice of sampling times and obscure the expected shape of the profile shown in Figure 1. For example, for some drugs, most notably pilocarpine (20), rapid equilibration with aqueous humor does not occur. As a result, the terminal log-linear elimination phase of the concentration of drug in aqueous humor versus time curve is difficult to identify unless time intervals are extended well beyond what is usually considered adequate for ocular studies (i.e, 2–5 h). For pilocarpine, when drug concentration was measured for 11 h, a biexponential decline was evident and an elimination half-life of 2.75 h was observed (15) compared to earlier studies which estimated the half-life to be about 40–60 min. However, the latter log-linear decline of pilocarpine may be due to residual drug slowly redistributing from the lens. Since these levels are low and released slowly, the use of 40–60 min is probably more useful in practical situations.

Another limiting factor is the sensitivity of the assay. Significant advances have been made over the last 10 years, so that it is not necessary to prepare a radioactive tracer for adequate detection of drug in eye tissues. High-pressure liquid chromatography (HPLC) with ultraviolet, radioactive, or fluorescence detectors or gas chromatography using nitrogen or electron capture can measure drug concentrations in ocular tissues at levels as low as 2–5 ng per milliliter or gram of tissue (21–24).

IV. OCULAR PHARMACOKINETIC MODELING

The classic pharmacokinetic approach of expressing the concentration-time curve into a sum of exponentials has been applied to the eye (2,3,17,25–29) but much less extensively than other routes of administration. At the present time, limited application has resulted from these studies in developing new ophthalmic drugs with optimal pharmacokinetic behavior or more specifically in estimating dosing regimens. Although the reasons given above are a contributing factor, it is also true that ophthalmic drugs are a relatively small commercial market compared to systemically administered drugs, and there are intractable difficulties in clearly and unambiguously defining pharmacokinetic parameters exclusively for the eye, such as clearance and volume of distribution, as well as rate and extent of absorption.

Although the classic pharmacokinetic approach has limitations when applied to the eye, in situ or in vitro experiments have been developed which directly measure a kinetic phenomena, and are more accurate when compared to results obtained from classic compartmental approaches. Very specific technics have been developed to measure precorneal drug disposition, permeability of various corneal layers, and the measurement of fluorescein kinetics, which have led to the understanding of tear, aqueous, and vitreous dynamics (5,30–33), and have been responsible for the development of very useful clinical applications (5,34). These latter approaches are discussed in another chapter.

A. Classic Modeling Approaches

Initially, a classic pharmacokinetic approach is applied to concentration-time curves derived from topical instillation to the eye in much the same manner as data derived from systemically administered drugs. The curve is first expressed by a computer-determined sum of exponentials which closely fit the experimental data and likewise show no systemic deviation. In the eye, aqueous humor is most often assigned to the central compartment, which is reversibly connected to one or more peripheral compartments and/or a reservoir compartment, in the various models (or schemes) that have been derived. This choice is compatible with physiological reality, since aqueous humor, which fills the anterior and posterior chambers, is the circulating fluid bathing the peripheral tissues. Drugs instilled topically on the eye primarily reach the first third of the eye which encompasses these regions. Topically applied ophthalmic drugs do not reach the retina in significant concentrations.

In the eye, the cornea, conjunctiva, lens, iris–ciliary body, choroid, and vitreous are specific tissues that are often lumped together into one or more peripheral compartments. A peripheral compartment can be reversibly connected to a central compartment, but if redistribution into aqueous humor is negligible or nonexistent, peripheral tissues can act as a sink or reservoir compartment. The exit out of the eye is into the blood or circulating fluid of the body.

Figure 2 lists the compartmental schemes that are most commonly applied to ophthalmic drugs following topical application. In particular, pilocarpine has received the most attention. The most appropriate scheme seems to depend heavily on the design of the study (i.e., number and length of sampling periods and number of tissues measured for drug content over time), the specificity and sensitivity of the assay, and the sophistication of the curve-fitting routine used to analyze the data. When aqueous humor concentrations of drug are measured over time, either mono- or biexponential equations adequately describe the disposition of drug (2,3,5,35). Since it is relatively easy to remove cornea, conjunctiva, lens, iris–ciliary body, and/or choroid tissues along with aqueous humor, the assignment of barriers and peripheral and/or reservoir compartments is not particularly difficult with the exception of the cornea.

Although the cornea is clearly a physical barrier to drug entry into the anterior chamber, it is actually divided into three significant kinetic barriers—the multilayered lipophilic epithelium, the aqueouslike stroma, and the single-celled lipophilic endothelium. The specific corneal permeability rate for each drug depends on the drug's partitioning properties and molecular weight relative to the individual properties of each barrier

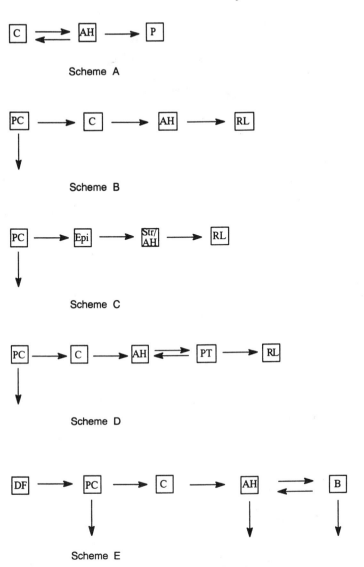

Figure 2. Classic pharmacokinetic schemes used to express compartmentalization for topically applied ophthalmic drugs. Key: C = cornea, AH = aqueous humor, P (or PT) = peripheral tissues, PC = precorneal area, RL = reservoir loss, Epi = corneal epithelium, str/AH = stroma, endothelium and aqueous humor (i.e., kinetic homogeneity), DF = dosage form, and B = biophase.

(36–42). The sum of the resistances of each layer represents the apparent corneal permeability rate. However, for pilocarpine, a closer study of its kinetics in each barrier by Lee and Robinson (25) indicated that the stroma and endothelium could be more correctly associated with the aqueous humor compartment and only the corneal epithelium was a barrier for entry of drug into the anterior chamber. Although the endothelium is lipophilic, it is only one cell thick and is apparently not as significant a barrier as the much thicker, more torturous epithelium with 9 or 10 layers.

This latter division of corneal layers into a single epithelial barrier and the assignment of stroma and endothelium into a compartment along with aqueous humor may be correct not only for pilocarpine but also other hydrophilic drugs for which the epithelium is the major significant barrier. These drugs likely penetrate the epithelium predominately by intercellular pathways. Consequently, as long as the drug is soluble, a high topical concentration can be applied to the cornea to promote a high penetration rate and overcome poor penetrability.

B. Pharmacometric Measurements

Today, computer curve-fitting routines are designed for microcomputers to easily accommodate mathematical treatment of tissue concentrations of drug over time (43). Regardless of the statistical approach employed to arrive at the best representation of the data, it is desirable to characterize and express absorption, distribution, and elimination of drugs. Over the years, the most appropriate parameters to express pharmacokinetic drug behavior has been the fraction absorbed (F), the first-order rate absorption rate constant (K_a), or the time to peak (tp), the volume of distribution (V_d) and clearance. Clearance is expressed as either excretory (Cl_e), metabolic (Cl_m), or their total, which represents elimination out of the "body" (Cl_t). In the eye, Cl_t becomes ocular clearance, Cl_o. Difficulties in measuring ocular pharmacokinetic behavior is summarized in Figure 3 and discussed in more detail in the following sections.

1. Absorption

As discussed more fully in another chapter, the rate and extent of ophthalmic drug absorption is restricted largely by noncorneal absorption in the precorneal area and the drainage

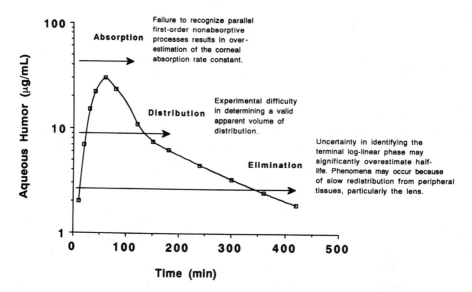

Figure 3. Critical problems associated with clearly identifying and quantitating absorption, distribution, and elimination phases associated with ophthalmic pharmacokinetic behavior.

rate. The latter process, because of its rapidity, limits the ocular contact time for drugs residing at the absorption site to about 3–6 min, whereas the rate and extent of penetration across the cornea is restricted by the physicochemical properties of the drug and/or its formulation (2–6,44–53).

a. Fraction Absorbed

For drugs administered systemically, the fraction absorbed is determined by taking the ratio of the area under the plasma concentration-time curve or the total amount excreted in the urine for a bolus intravenous dose and an oral dose, respectively. On occasion, a drug cannot be given by a bolus intravenous dose and, therefore, equations have been developed so that a slow intravenous infusion could be used instead (54,55).

When applied in an analogous manner to the eye, a small volume of drug is injected intracamerally using a small-bore needle followed by sampling of aqueous humor and measuring drug concentration over time (16,56). Using this approach, the fraction absorbed for 75 µg and 150 µg ocular doses of flurbiprofen was 10 and 7%, respectively.

Patton and Robinson (27) estimated the fraction absorbed using a different approach. Topical dosing studies were conducted in both anesthetized and awake rabbits and with the drainage ducts plugged and unobstructed. Pilocarpine nitrate was measured as the disappearance of drug from the tears of rabbit eyes whose ducts had been plugged and also as appearance of drug in aqueous humor in both experiments. After correcting for dilution due to tear production, and determining the areas under the tear concentration-time curve (AUC), the fraction absorbed in anesthetized rabbits whose ducts had been plugged was calculated as 0.0187. Equation 1 was used to calculate F:

$$AUC = \frac{FD}{k_{10}V} \qquad (1)$$

In equation 1, D is the instilled dose (25 µL), k_{10} is the loss of drug from the precorneal area $(1 \times 10^{-2} \text{ min}^{-1})$, and V is estimated as 0.3 mL. Extrapolating the results to normal rabbits, assuming a volume of distribution approximately equal to the aqueous humor volume and assuming that negligible drug distributes out of the aqueous humor were approximations required in order to estimate F.

Since drug absorption across the cornea and loss of drug from the precorneal area are parallel loss processes, it was possible to confirm the results of Patton and Robinson (27) by the use of equation 2:

$$F = \frac{k_{10}}{k_{10} + K_a} \qquad (2)$$

The fraction absorbed for a 25 µL instilled dose of pilocarpine nitrate in the rabbit eye was estimated to be 1–2% (27,28). Using equation 2, Chiang and Schoenwald calculated that for a 30-µL dose of 0.4% clonidine, an F of 1.6% was calculated for the rabbit eye (17).

Ling and Combs (24) compared the areas under the concentration-time curves for ketorolac tromethamine 0.5% administered topically (50 µL) and intracamerally, respectively. The ratio of the areas indicated a fraction absorbed of 3.7%. An identical approach was used by Tang-liu et al. (56) in determining that 2.5% of the instilled dose of levobunolol was absorbed after a topical dose (50 µL of 0.5%), similar in range to other drugs administered topically.

b. Rate of Absorption

The loss of drug from the precorneal area is a net effect of tear secretion, drainage, noncorneal, and corneal absorption rate processes. When drug concentration in aqueous humor is described biexponentially, the latter, shallower log-linear slope represents elimination out of the eye, whereas the steeper slope is the net effect of the precorneal processes. Because the drainage rate is approximately 100 times more rapid than K_a (25), it is correct to assign the more shallow log-linear slope from aqueous humor concentration-time curves as elimination from aqueous humor. Consequently, estimation of the steepest slope and subsequent calculation of K_a can be obtained from nonlinear curve-fitting techniques if the other precorneal processes are known.

Table 2 lists drugs for which a K_a has been estimated. These values, when interpreted as half-lives, show how slowly drug is actually absorbed across the cornea. Because of the very rapid loss of drug from the precorneal area, and in particular the drainage rate, it is not surprising to find only a small fraction of the instilled dose is actually absorbed across the cornea. In addition, the cornea is relatively thick, variable in hydrophilic/lipophilic properties for each layer, and small in surface area. These factors, along with the rapid precorneal loss rate, combine to have a significant effect on the time to peak following topical instillation of drugs to the eye regardless of the drug's physicochemical properties or its elimination rate from internal eye tissues. In general, the time to peak is 20–60 min for nearly all ophthalmic drugs when instilled topically to the eye. This has been shown by Makoid and Robinson (15), who determined the ophthalmic pharmacokinetics of pilocarpine following topical application to the rabbit eye. From their work an equation was developed for tp:

$$tp = \frac{\ln (K_{na}/K_a)}{K_{na} - K_a} \qquad (3)$$

In equation 3, K_{na} and K_a are the nonabsorptive loss rate constant and the transcorneal absorption rate constant, respectively. Equation 3 assumes that K_{na} is much larger than uptake into the epithelium of the cornea from the precorneal area. This assumption can be

Table 2. Transcorneal First-Order Absorption Rate Constant and Accompanying Half-Life for Corneal Absorption

Drug	K_a (min^{-1})	t $_{1/2}$ (h)	Ref.
Pilocarpine	0.004	2.88	25
Clonidine	0.0014	8.25	17
Phenylephrine	0.00001	1155	9
Ibuprofen	0.000964	12	105
Ibufenac	0.000603	18.3	105
Ethoxzolamide	0.0015	7.7	57
Aminozolamide	0.0014	8.25	22
2-Benzothiazolesulfonamide	0.0013	8.88	57
6-Hydroxyethoxy-2-benzothiazolesulfonamide	0.0042	5.37	57
N-Methylacetazolamide	0.00126	9.17	103
Acetazolamide	0.000153	75.5	103

applied to most, if not all, ophthalmic drugs, since K_{na} is approximately twofold larger than K_a.

Eller et al. (44,57) developed a topical infusion technique for estimating the ophthalmic pharmacokinetics of drugs which was based upon noncompartmental methods. The procedure consisted of maintaining a constant concentration of drug on the cornea through the use of a plastic cylinder secured over the sclera which allowed only the cornea to be exposed to drug solution (Table 3). A volume of 0.7 mL is maintained over the cornea of an anesthetized rabbit until steady-state ocular concentrations are reached. Rabbits are sacrificed at various time intervals, ocular tissues are excised, and then assayed for drug content. This topical infusion approach permits an estimate of K_a, the apparent volume of distribution at steady state (V_{ss}) and ocular clearance (Q_e). Figure 4 shows a semilogarithmic plot of the corneal concentration of phenylephrine HCl following topical infusion of 1% maintained on the cornea for 180 min. Table 3 lists the equations and pharmacokinetic parameter values for drugs for which this procedure has been used.

2. Distribution

The volume of distribution serves primarily as a proportionality constant to relate concentration to amount or dose and also as a relative measure of tissue accumulation. In the eye, distribution is the most difficult pharmacokinetic process to measure because the amount of drug in ocular tissue at any time is not known. Aqueous humor is the circulating fluid of the eye and in order to measure V_{ss} accurately, an instantaneous input (i.e., intracameral injection) or an infusion delivered at a known rate must be introduced.

Table 3. Topical Infusion Method Depicting Well[a] and Equations[b]

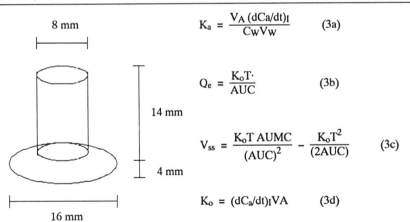

$$K_a = \frac{V_A (dC_a/dt)_I}{C_W V_W} \quad (3a)$$

$$Q_e = \frac{K_o T \cdot}{AUC} \quad (3b)$$

$$V_{ss} = \frac{K_o T\ AUMC}{(AUC)^2} - \frac{K_o T^2}{(2AUC)} \quad (3c)$$

$$K_o = (dC_a/dt)_I V A \quad (3d)$$

Ocular Well Used for Topical Infusion   Equations Used for Topical Infusion Method

[a]Well is affixed over cornea of anesthetized rabbit; drug solution is maintained at a constant concentration for 90–160 min until steady-state concentrations of drug are reached in the aqueous humor.
[b]K_a = First/order transcorneal rate constant; V_a = volume of the anterior chamber; $(dC_a/dt)_I$ = initial rate of appearance of drug in aqueous humor minus lag time; Q_e = ocular clearance ($\mu L/min$); K_o = constant rate of input into anterior chamber; AUC and AUMC = areas (to infinity) under the aqueous humor concentration × time curve and concentration × time-time curve, respectively; C_W = constant concentration maintained on the cornea over time (90–160 min); V_W = volume of drug solution maintained in well.

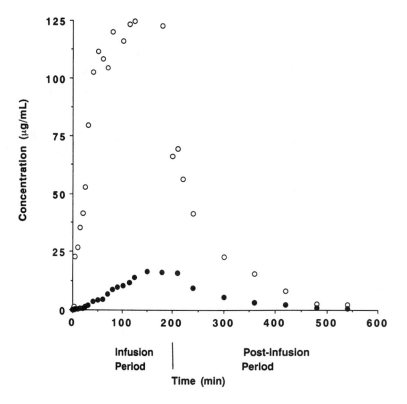

Figure 4. Corneal (o) and aqueous humor (●) concentrations of phenylephrine (HCl) measured over time following the maintenance of a constant concentration (1% of 0.7 mL buffered to pH 7.6) on the rabbit cornea (topical infusion technique) for 180 min with the use of a well affixed to the sclera. Infusion and postinfusion periods are identified.

Estimates of precise apparent volumes of distribution are lacking for ocular drugs. Table 4 lists values estimated either from an intracameral injection (Fig. 5) or from topical infusion. These values are relatively small when compared to the total aqueous humor volume of 0.31 mL for the rabbit eye (3,35). The volume of distribution for ketorolac tromethamine and for levobunolol are 1.65 and 1.93 mL, respectively, which are about five- to sixfold larger than aqueous humor volume. However, with so few drugs for comparison, it is difficult to establish if these values are extraordinary.

Nevertheless, tissues in the anterior and posterior chamber are adjacent to circulating aqueous humor and, therefore, readily available for transfer of drug. Also, protein concentration in aqueous humor measures about 10% of protein concentration in plasma, so that it is not likely that tissue distribution is greatly restricted because of preferential binding to components in aqueous humor. Consequently, it is surprising that V_{ss} is so small. Although accurate determinations of V_{ss} are necessary for estimates of optimal multiple dosing regimens, few are available mainly because of the pharmacokinetic difficulties in obtaining such measurements.

The pharmacokinetic parameter, V_{ss}, provides a general assessment of distribution. However, it does not allow for differentiation between reservoir sites which are active and

Table 4.   Volumes of Distribution (V_d) for Drugs of Ophthalmic Interest

Drug	V_d (mL)	Method	Reference
Pilocarpine	0.58	EXT [a]	28
Clonidine	0.53	SS [b]	17
Phenylephrine	0.42	SS	9
Flubiprofen	0.62	EXT	16
Levobunolol	1.65	EXT	56
Dihydrolevobunolol	1.68	EXT	56
Phenylephrine	0.42	SS	9
Ketorolac tromethamine	1.93	EXT	24
Ethoxzolamide	0.28	SS	57
Aminozolamide	0.53	SS	22
2-Benzothiazolesulfonamide	0.24	SS	57
6-Hydroxyethoxy-2-benzothiazolesulfonamide	0.33	SS	57
N-methylacetazolamide	0.42	SS	103
Acetazolamide	0.47	SS	103

[a] EXT = extrapolated method; determined by extrapolating log-linear elimination phase to C at t_0 and dividing into the intracameral dose.

[b] SS = steady state method; determined by maintaining a constant concentration of drug on the cornea of an anesthetized rabbit and measuring aqueous humor concentrations of drug over time during infusion and post-infusion. See Table 3 for equation for V_{ss}.

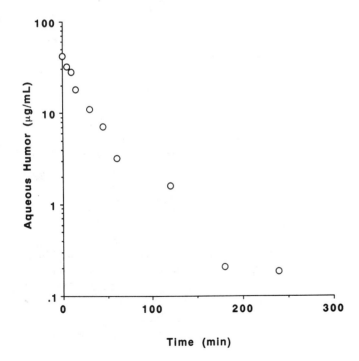

Figure 5.   Concentration of levobunolol (o) in aqueous humor following a 5 μL intracameral injection. The concentration vs time profile is a representation of the data necessary for determination of V_d for an ophthalmic drug by the "extended" method.

those which are either devoid of activity or potentially responsible for side effects. In lieu of making V_{ss} measurements, it is not difficult to measure tissue concentrations over time. Steady state tissue concentrations provide a direct indication of whether or not drug distributes to the presumed anatomical location of the active site. In contrast to the paucity of pharmacokinetic measurements for ophthalmic drugs, tissue concentrations of drug have been widely reported for many years even when radioactive methodology was the only technology available to conduct such measurements. With recent improvements in assay methodology, tissue profiles over time are routinely measured for aqueous humor and cornea but less frequently for lens, iris–ciliary body, conjunctiva, choroid, lacrimal gland, and/or retina.

It is reasonable to expect that if drug is instilled topically to the eye, and no unusual tissue affinity occurs for a particular drug, the order of decreasing tissue concentrations are: cornea > conjunctiva > aqueous humor > iris–ciliary body > lens, vitreous, and/or choroid-retina. However, for certain drugs, such as, clonidine, timolol, dapiprazole, oxymetazoline, and ketorolac tromethamine, iris–ciliary body concentrations are higher than aqueous humor concentrations even though the dose was instilled topically to the cornea. A number of reasons have been suggested to account for this phenomena. For example, the drug may distribute extensively to the iris–ciliary body but may likewise equilibrate rapidly with aqueous humor, so that the elimination rate is equally rapid from the iris–ciliary body as from aqueous humor. If this explanation is correct, the iris–ciliary body might have a large capacity for drug but not exhibit an unusually high binding affinity, and, therefore, not retain or accumulate drug over time. It is also conceivable that the binding affinity as well as its capacity is very high, so that the elimination rate from the iris–ciliary body and aqueous are not the same but drug remains in the former tissue much longer. This latter observation was observed by Putnam et al. (22) for aminozolamide, a topically active carbonic anhydrase inhibitor (CAI). Aminozolamide showed a relatively slow elimination for drug and its metabolite, 6-acetamido-2-benzothiazolesulfonamide, from the iris–ciliary body compared to aqueous humor following topical administration to the rabbit eye.

Certain studies (58,59), however, support the possibility of scleral absorption for explaining high concentrations of drug in the iris–ciliary body following topical administration of CAIs. Certain drugs, when applied topically to the eye, may be preferentially absorbed across the sclera, as opposed to the cornea, and enter the iris–ciliary body without first entering the aqueous humor. As an alternative, drug entering aqueous humor prior to entering the iris–ciliary body would be diluted and also required to diffuse against the flow of aqueous. Consequently, drug reaching the iris–ciliary body via corneal absorption may not reach high concentrations at the active site (as opposed to reaching the same site via scleral absorption) which, in effect, may be insufficient for the lowering IOP.

In a study by Ahmed et al. (47) to confirm the possibility of scleral absorption and to determine what properties are optimal, both corneal and scleral penetration were evaluated for propranolol, timolol, nadalol, penbutolol, sucrose, and inulin. The results of the study showed that the outer layer of the sclera provides much less resistance to penetrability for hydrophilic drugs than the corneal epithelium. For lipophilic drugs, such as propranolol, timolol, and penbutolol, the difference in penetrability between the tissues was not appreciably different.

In another study by Chien et al. (48), various anterior chamber tissue levels were measured over time for clonidine, p-aminoclonidine, and a 6-quinoxalinyl derivative of clonidine (AGN 190342). Drug was administered with the aid of a plastic cylinder (0.7 mL volume) affixed to the corneoscleral junction using cyanoacrylate adhesive. Drug solution could be placed within the well in direct contact with the cornea or outside the well which would exclude contact with the cornea but allow drug to bath the conjunctiva. Whenever drug was maintained on the conjunctiva or cornea for a period of 60 min, tissue concentration followed a clear trend. The order of highest to lowest concentration of drug following conjunctival contact was conjunctiva > cornea > ciliary body > aqueous humor. When drug solution was in contact with the cornea only, the order was corneal > aqueous humor > ciliary body > conjunctiva. From the results of the study, various pathways of ocular absorption were proposed and are summarized in Figure 6.

Although many anterior and, to a lesser extent, posterior tissues have been measured for drug concentration over time following topical or systemic administration, little definitive information exists regarding the ability of tissues to accumulate drug either through partitioning and/or binding of drug. Of critical importance is the iris–ciliary body, which is the biophasic and anatomical location for many pharmacological responses acting on the eye. Also of interest is the lens, since drug accumulation may be responsible for inducing cataract formation. Both of these tissues are easily removed and often treated as kinetically

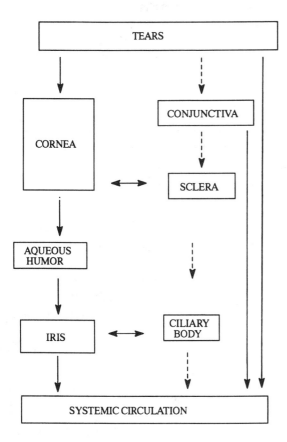

Figure 6. Possible absorption pathways of an ophthalmic drug following topical application to the eye. Solid line represents corneal route, whereas the dashed line represents conjunctival/scleral route. (Data from Ref. 48.)

homogeneous tissues; however, drug concentrations within these tissues are likely to be quite variable in concentration, since these tissues are not anatomically homogeneous.

For example, iris tissue in the rabbit eye is porous and highly vascular with a large surface area in direct contact with aqueous humor; consequently, distribution equilibrium between iris and aqueous humor should occur rapidly. Also, as the iris becomes darker, the capacity for pigmented iris to bind to catecholamines, and perhaps other drugs, increases (60). Dark-eyed individuals have a delayed onset and a reduced response but a prolonged effect to catecholamines, presumably due to the reservoir effect that the pigmented iris has on ocular disposition of catecholamines. In contrast to iris tissue, the ciliary body epithelial layer of the pars plicata, in which resides a high concentration of carbonic anhydrase and shown to be the active site for CAIs, is not easily reached via topical instillation (61,62), requiring a lipophilic drug substance to readily penetrate cellular membranes. Although the separation of these tissues from one another would provide useful information, it is usually not done because of the difficulty in separating one tissue entirely from the other.

The entire lens is also easy to remove during kinetic studies; nevertheless, the lens should not be treated as a kinetically homogeneous tissue. Maurice and Mishma (5) reported that fluorescein, a water-soluble dye, spreads laterally and rapidly in the outer layers of the lens but does not diffuse readily into the lens nucleus. In addition, Maurice (63) observed that fluorescein and also rhodamine B, which is a lipophilic dye, redistribute very slowly into aqueous humor. The slow redistribution observed by Maurice may explain why aqueous humor concentrations of some drugs measured over time do not show distribution equilibrium within a few hours after reaching the time to peak.

3. Elimination

Drug is eliminated from the anterior chamber, at least in part, by aqueous humor turnover, which in the rabbit eye is 1.5% of the volume of the anterior chamber per minute or expressed as a half-life, 46.2 min (64). Half-life representing loss from aqueous humor is the most common pharmacokinetic parameter measured following topical administration to the eye. Table 5 lists half-lives for drugs of ophthalmic interest. Surprisingly, nearly all the drugs fall within a range from 0.6 to 3.0 h, which is less than when these same drugs are studied systemically. Either there are few tissue-binding sites in the eye to lower clearance or the pathways by which drugs are eliminated are very efficient. The latter may be the most likely explanation, since aqueous humor volume is relatively large compared to ocular tissue volume.

Elimination can be expressed as a clearance, and if the anterior chamber of the rabbit contains about 0.311 mL, an average aqueous humor clearance due to bulk flow becomes 4.67 µL/min based upon equation 4 below. Ocular clearances can be calculated from the following equations:

$$Q_e = K_e V_d \qquad (4)$$

$$Q_e = \frac{K_o T}{AUC_{INF}} \qquad (5)$$

$$Q_e = \frac{D_{IC}}{AUC_{INF}} \qquad (6)$$

where K_e represents the first-order elimination rate constant out of aqueous humor, V_d is the apparent volume of distribution for the eye, K_o is the constant rate input into the anterior

Table 5. Aqueous Humor Half-Lives[a] of Drugs Administered to the Rabbit Eye Either Topically, Intracamerally, or Subconjunctivally

Drug	Half-life (h)	Ref.
Dapiprazole	5.8	99
Imirestat	4.75	88
6-Mercaptopurine	4.6	96
Falintolol	3.0	88
Fusidic acid	2.8	101
Suprofen	2.6	111
Histamine	2.2	108
Cimetidine	2.2	108
Ketorolac tromethamine	2.1	24
Benzolamide	2.0	91
Ceftazidime	2.0	93
Gentamicin	1.9	107
L-Alphamethyldopa[b]	1.8	23
I-643,799[c]	1.8	90
Diclofenac	1.7	97
Flurbiprofen	1.7	102
Fluorometholone acetate	1.5	7
Cefamandole	1.5	107
Phenylephrine	1.4	9
D-Alphamethyldopa[b]	1.4	23
Timolol	1.2	100
	0.84	89
Lincomycin	1.2	110
6-Amino-2-benzothiazolesulfonamide	1.15	22
L-662,583[d]	1.11	92
Acetbutolol	1.1	89
Cefsulodin	1.0	112
Fluorouracil	1.0	94
Dihydrolevobunolol	0.98	56
N-Methylacetazolamide	0.98	103
6-Hydroxyethoxy-2-benzothiazolesulfonamide	0.97	57
6-Acetamido-2-benzothiazolesulfonamide	0.93	22
L-650,719[e]	0.81	90
Tobramycin	0.75	7
Trifluoromethazolamide	0.78	91
Pilocarpine	0.72	113
Methazolamide	0.58	91
Cefotaxime	0.57	29
Bufuralol	0.50	89
Levobunolol	0.67	56
Ethoxzolamide	0.63	57
	0.23	91
Pyrilamine	0.61	108
Clonidine	0.49	17
Acetazolamide	0.35	103
1,3-Bis(2-chloroethyl)-1,1-nitrosurea (BCNU)	0.34	25
2-Benzothiazolesulfonamide	0.29	57

[a]Concentrations from the last two to four time intervals were used in calculating $t_{1/2}$ values.
[b]A small dose dependency was observed (statistically NS); IV dose = 10 mg/kg.
[c]6-Hydroxybenzo[b]thiophene-2-sulfonamide.
[d]6-Hydroxybenzo[b]thiophene-2-sulfonamide.
[e]6-Hydroxy-2-benzothiazidesulfonamide.

chamber, T_o is time for the constant rate input, D_{IC} is an intracameral dose, and AUC_{INF} is the area (to infinity) under the aqueous humor concentration-time curve.

Each equation above depends on assumptions that require experimentation to be carefully planned. In equation 4, K_e can be obtained from the latter linear slope of the logarithm of drug concentration in aqueous humor measured over time or obtained from any other tissue concentration in distribution equilibrium with aqueous humor. The V_d term in equation 3 has been correctly determined for the eye by either of two methods. One method, the topical infusion technique (9,17,57), has been discussed previously and is the basis for equation 5, also shown in Figure 4. The other method for determining V_d is based upon measuring drug concentration in aqueous humor over time following an intracameral injection of a very small volume (5 μL) of drug solution. Whenever an intracameral injection is made, there is concern that drug elimination can be altered because of a breakdown of the blood-aqueous barrier. However, Tang-Liu and coworkers (16,56) have established that for intracameral injections of 5 μL solutions containing flurbiprofen and levobunolol, no significant breakdown of the blood-aqueous barrier had occurred, since protein concentration was <1 mg/mL. Equation 6, sometimes referred to as a "dose-area" determination, was used by Tang-liu et al. (16,56) to calculate V_d for flurbiprofen and levobunolol.

Table 6 contains Q_e values for those drugs for which accurate determinations have been made. Values range from 13.0 to 28.7 mL/min, which are 2.8 to 6.1 times higher than aqueous humor clearance, suggesting additional pathways of elimination other than aqueous turnover. The two most likely alternate routes of elimination are metabolism and systemic uptake by the vascular tissues of the anterior uvea. However, accumulation and retention by the lens (over the time course of the experiment) as well as back diffusion into the cornea and tears followed by subsequent drainage are all minor routes that may contribute to apparent ocular clearance values.

Table 6. Ocular Clearances (Q_e)[a] for Drugs of Ophthalmic Interest

Drug	Q_e (μL/min)	Ref.
Pilocarpine	13.0	20
Clonidine	14.9	17
Phenylephrine	14.6	9
Flurbiprofen	14.4	16
Levobunolol	28.7	56
Dihydrolevobunolol	19.7	56
Phenylephrine	14.6	9
Ketorolac tromethamine	11.0	24
Ethoxzolamide	9.0	57
2-Benzothiazolesulfonamide	1.15	57
6-Hydroxyethoxy-2-benzothiazolesulfonamide	3.0	57
N-Methylacetazolamide	1.56	103
Acetazolamide	5.27	103

[a]Q_e calculated from equations 4–6 in text.

C. Metabolic Models

Although the eye is not a primary drug-metabolizing organ, a knowledge of metabolic pathways in the eye has become increasingly important in order to optimize drug action and therapeutic effect. Esterases have been studied most extensively (65–68); no doubt because of their importance in the development of prodrugs for use in the eye. Prodrugs which have shown a significant improvement in corneal penetrability are phenylephrine (10,21), timolol (69), pilocarpine (70,71), idoxuridine (72), and the tromethamine salt of prostaglandin $F_{(2\alpha)}$ (73,74). Acetyl-, butyrl-, and carboxylesterases have been identified in the pigmented rabbit eye (65) and are responsible for rapid conversion of ester prodrugs to the active drug species.

Other enzyme systems have been identified within ocular tissues. As summarized by Plazonnet et al. (4), these are catechol-O-methyltransferase, monoamine oxidase, steroid 6-betahydroxylase, oxidoreductase, lysosomal enzymes, peptidases, glucuronide and sulfate transferase, and glutathione-conjugating enzymes. Arylamine acetyltransferase activity was demonstrated by Campbell et al. (75) in anterior chamber tissues using p-aminobenzoate, aminozolamide, and sulfamethazine as substrates. The rank order of arylamine acetyltransferase activity regardless of substrate was liver > iris–ciliary process > corneal epithelium > stroma-endothelium. Although fast- and slow-acetylating rabbits, classified with respect to their rate of hepatic acetylation (76), metabolized aminozolamide at different rates in liver tissue, no differences between phenotypes was observed for aminozolamide either in ocular disposition or in decline of IOP following topical instillation.

The distribution of ketone reductase activity in anterior chamber tissues was determined by Lee et al. (83) in order to explain the metabolism of levobunolol to dihydrolevobunolol. The rank order of activity was corneal epithelium > iris–ciliary body > conjunctiva > lens. No activity was detected in the tears, corneal stroma, sclera, or aqueous humor. Bovine ciliary body apparently contains aldehyde oxidase, which is responsible for the reduction of a number of compounds: N-oxide, hydroxamic acid, sulfoxide, and nitro compounds (84).

Metabolic models have been devised for levobunolol (56) and aminozolamide (22) and reproduced in Figure 7. In general, the iris–ciliary body and the epithelium of the cornea appear to be anterior chamber tissues with the greatest capacity for metabolism; however, additional research is necessary.

V. PHARMACODYNAMICS

Because ophthalmic drugs are relatively potent and because of the difficulty in routinely measuring ophthalmic pharmacokinetics, the measurement of pharmacological responses in the animal or human eye has become a convenient aid in anticipating clinical experience of an ophthalmic drug. The principal shortcoming to the use of pharmacological measurements to either optimize therapy or for use as an aid in the development of new ophthalmic drugs is that the same dose often produces a different intensity of effect in different individuals. This variability occurs because of differences in dose-response relationships as well as differences in ocular pharmacokinetic behavior between individuals. Factors which contribute to variability are eye pigmentation, whether or not an individual wears contact lenses, allergies to the drugs or preservatives, and a number of physiological factors that

A. Metabolic Scheme for Aminozolamide

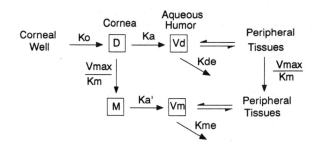

B. Metabolic Scheme for Levobunolol

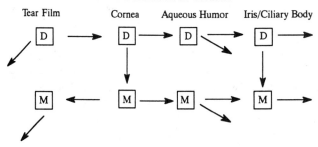

Figure 7. Metabolic schemes devised for aminozolamide and levobunolol following absorption into the eye. (Data from Refs. 22, 51, and 56.)

also determine intrasubject variation, such as eye discomfort leading to induced tearing, changes in blood pressure, hormonal concentrations, and/or changes in autonomic tone.

Although many ophthalmic pharmacological responses, such as miosis, mydriasis, IOP, flicker fusion, tear secretion, and aqueous turnover, can be measured over time, variability has been a major reason why mathematical model development has been elusive. Pilocarpine and carbachol, muscarinic agonists which constrict the pupil, have been studied extensively with respect to their miotic response. The response of an isolated strip of human sphincter muscle to carbachol and pilocarpine follows a typical sigmoid-shaped dose-response relationships (77). Figure 8 is a log-log plot of a reproduction of the classic responses of carbachol and pilocarpine to the human sphincter muscle (87). Mishima (78) showed that this response, which represents one molecule binding competitively to a single muscarinic receptor, can be described by equation 7:

$$\frac{R}{R_{max} - R} = qC \tag{7}$$

In equation 7, R_{max} is the largest response that can be achieved by drug when all receptors are occupied, C is the drug concentration present in the incubation media, and q is a proportionality constant which is equal to 1 if a single molecule binds to a single receptor. Mishima (78) further reported that equation 7 also correctly characterized the miosis of

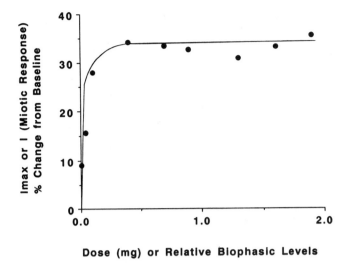

Figure 8. Dose-response (miotic) curve for pilocarpine following the topical instillation of 50 μL of various concentrations to the rabbit eye (N=5). Curve is used in the conversion of miotic response intensities into biophasic drug levels over time.

carbachol on the sphincter muscle of the cat, mydriasis of isoproterenol on bovine and rabbit sphincter muscle, mydriasis of l-epinephrine and atropine on guinea pig iris, and mydriasis of epinephrine and acetylcholine on cat iris.

Smolen and coworkers (79–85) developed a mathematical model for which pharmacological response intensities were transformed into biophasic drug levels for tropicamide (80–82), tridihexethylchloride (83,84), carbachol (85), and pilocarpine (79). The transformation was accomplished with the use of a precisely determined dose-response curve. The method requires a graded response that can be measured over time. Figure 9 is an example of dose-response curve constructed from miosis measurements made over time for nine separately administered topical doses (D) of pilocarpine HCl to the rabbit eye (79). The ordinate, plotted as a percent of baseline values, was obtained from the averages of the computer-fitted maximum response intensities (I_{max}) of the miotic versus time profiles following administration of each dose. Equation 8 was used to construct the line of best fit shown in Figure 8.

$$I_{max} = \frac{719.4\,D}{I + 20.4D} + 0.5\,D \qquad (8)$$

The numbered values in equation 7 were obtained from the weighted least-squares regression curves (79) applied to the data shown in Figure 9. Use of equation 8 requires that the following assumptions are valid: 1) the same biophasic concentration of drug produces the same intensity of response (i.e., nonhysteresis), 2) binding to the receptor site is rapid and reversible, and 3) the pharmacokinetic processes are first order and, therefore, do not differ with dose. Once the assumptions have been verified, equation 8 becomes equation 9:

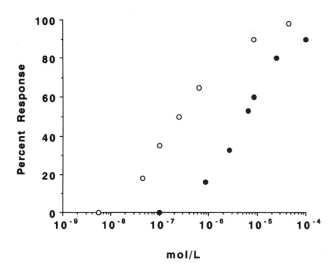

Figure 9. Dose-response relationships for carbachol (o) and pilocarpine (●) following incubation with an isolated human sphincter muscle strip. (Data from Ref. 78.)

$$I = \frac{K_1\, Q'_B}{I + K_2\, Q'_B} + P\, Q'_B \tag{9}$$

where I is the intensity of response at any time and Q'_B is the concentration of drug in the biophase at the same time of measurement (normalized for dose: $Q'_B = Q_B/D$) and K_1, K_2, and P are constants derived from the fitting procedure. Application of this approach permits the optimization of a delivery system for an ophthalmic drug, insight into a drug's kinetics of response, and determination of a product's "biophasic bioavailability." The latter term refers to the drug's absorption into the eye as well as uptake into the site of action (79).

A mydriatic tolerance of the pupil response has been interpreted for phenylephrine from the application of the classic pharmacodynamic E_{max} model (86):

$$K_m' = \left(\frac{\Delta E_{max}}{\Delta E(t)} - 1\right) C_a(t) \tag{10}$$

In equation 10, $K_m'(t)$ is the drug concentration in aqueous humor required to produce one-half of the maximal mydriatic response of phenylephrine (1/2 E_{max}), E(t) is the change in the mydriatic response from baseline at any time, and $C_a(t)$ is the concentration of drug in aqueous humor at the same time of measurement of E. In equation 10, $K_m'(t)$ is linearly related to $C_a(t)$ for a drug that does not develop tolerance; however, if mydriatic tolerance is developed following topical instillation, the value of K_m' will vary with time. Chien and Schoenwald (86) measured the aqueous humor concentration of phenylephrine and its corresponding mydriatic response over time in the rabbit eye following a 10-μL topical instillation of phenylephrine HCl viscous solution (10%). A clockwise hysteresis effect of mydriasis versus $C_a(t)$ was interpreted as a consequence of the development of tolerance over time. A plot of K_m' versus time agreed with that conclusion. K_m' was linear up to 90 min but steadily increased beyond 90 min through 240 min postinstillation.

Nonlinear pharmacokinetic behavior may be more common than has been observed, since many ophthalmic drugs are known to alter physiological processes. Drugs that affect aqueous humor turnover or blood flow within the iris–ciliary body would be expected to show some degree of nonlinear pharmacokinetic behavior. Nevertheless, the inability to routinely measure concentrations of drug in the human eye provides a strong incentive to continue exploring the use of pharmacological response intensities to either optimize therapy or provide a screening tool for use in developing new ophthalmic agents.

VI. CONCLUSIONS

It is important that the ocular pharmacokinetic behavior for drugs of ophthalmic interest be determined. Without a detailed knowledge of these processes, we must rely on the screening of new ophthalmic drugs intended for systemic use. In the past, drugs originally intended for systemic use and screened for use in the eye have provided good leads but rarely have they been optimized for ophthalmic potency or structurally altered to be devoid of systemic side effects when instilled topically to the eye. A knowledge of ocular pharmacokinetic behavior is also critical for optimizing therapeutic regimens following single, and particularly, multiple doses. It is not for lack of interest that prevents study of the ocular pharmacokinetic behavior of drugs but because of the problems that have yet to be solved.

First of all, an animal model is needed that is readily available and can accurately predict human ocular pharmacokinetics and, in particular, apply to patients. It would be more desirable if measurements could be made directly from the human eye without injury, pain, or risk of infection. At the present time, pharmacokinetic determinations in the human eye can only be made in subjects undergoing eye surgery. The patient is given the ophthalmic drug prior to entering surgery and a sample of aqueous humor (or other tissue) is removed when it does not interfere with the surgery. In these experiments, the time interval may not be measured accurately and each patient's sample represents only one time interval. Consequently, a number of patient determinations at different time intervals must be averaged.

The ideal animal model, whether a rabbit or monkey eye, should allow for accurate predictions in the human eye. The pharmacokinetic measurements should be capable of assessing absorption (rate and extent), distribution, and elimination in volunteers, and, in particular, patients. The model may be mathematically based but capable of use without extensive training and/or require specialized computer programs for its use. It should also allow for accurate predictions even though the drug itself may alter its own pharmacokinetic or pharmacodynamic processes over time. No doubt as these limitations are solved, the application of pharmacokinetics will become as extensively studied and applied to the human eye as it is now for drugs administered systemically.

REFERENCES

1. McDonald, T. O., and Shadduck, J. A. (1977). Eye irritation, *Dermatatoxicology and Pharmacology* (H. Maibach and F. N. Marzulli, eds.), Wiley, New York, pp. 139–191.
2. Schoenwald, R. D. (1990). Ocular drug delivery. Pharmacokinetic considerations, *Clin. Pharmacokinet., 18*:255.
3. Lee, V. H. L., and Robinson, J. R. (1986). Review: Topical ocular drug delivery: Recent developments and future challenges, *J. Ocul. Pharmacol., 2*:67.

4. Plazonnet, B., Grove, J., Durr, M., Mazuel, C., Quint, M., and Rozier, A. (1977). Pharmacokinetics and biopharmaceutical aspects of some anti-glaucoma drugs, *Ophthalmic Drug Delivery Biopharmaceutical Technological and Clinical Aspects*, Vol. 11 (M. F. Saettone, M. Bucci, and P. Speiser, eds.), Liviana Press, Springer-Verlag, Berlin, pp. 118–139.

5. Maurice, D. M., and Mishima, S. (1984). Ocular pharmacokinetics, *Pharmacology of the Eye* (M. L. Sears, ed.), Springer-Verlag, Berlin, pp. 19–116.

6. Schoenwald, R. D. (1985). The control of drug bioavailability from ophthalmic dosage forms, *Controlled Drug Bioavailability*, Vol. 3 (V. F. Smolen and L. A. Ball, eds.), Wiley, New York, pp. 257–306.

7. Schoenwald, R. D., Harris, R. G., Turner, D., Knowles, W., and Chien, D. S. (1987). Ophthalmic bioequivalence of steroid/antibiotic combination formulations, *Biopharm. Drug Dispos., 8*:527.

8. Tang-Liu, D. D. S., and Burke, S. S. (1988). The effect of Azone on ocular levobunolol absorption: Calculating the area under the curve and its standard error using tissue sampling compartments, *Pharm. Res., 5*:238.

9. Schoenwald, R. D., and Chien, D. S. (1988). Ocular absorption and disposition of phenylephrine and phenylephrine oxazolidine, *Biopharm. Drug Dispos., 9*:527.

10. Chien, D. S., and Schoenwald, R. D. (1986). Improving the ocular absorption of phenylephrine, *Biopharm. Drug Dispos., 7*:453.

11. Chrai, S. S., Makoid, M. C., Eriksen, S. P., and Robinson, J. R. (1974). Drop size and initial dosing frequency problems of topically applied ophthalmic drugs, *J. Pharm. Sci., 63*:333.

12. Chrai, S. S., and Robinson, J. R. (1974). Ocular evaluation of methylcellulose vehicle in albino rabbits, *J. Pharm. Sci., 63*:1218.

13. Chrai, S. S., Patton, T. F., Mehta, A., and Robinson, J. R. (1973). Lacrimal and instilled fluid dynamics in rabbit eyes, *J. Pharm. Sci., 62*:1112.

14. Burstein, N. L., and Anderson, J. A. (1985). Corneal penetration and ocular bioavailability of drugs, *J. Ocul. Pharmacol., 1*:309.

15. Makoid, M. C., and Robinson, J. R. (1979). Pharmacokinetics of topically applied pilocarpine in the albino rabbit eye, *J. Pharm. Sci., 68*:435.

16. Tang-Liu, D. D. S., Liu, S. S., and Weinkam, R. J. (1984). Ocular and systemic bioavailability of ophthalmic flurbiprofen, *J. Pharmacokinet. Biopharm., 12*:611.

17. Chiang, C. H., and Schoenwald, R. D. (1986). Ocular pharmacokinetic models of clonidine-^{3}H hydrochloride, *J. Pharmacokinet. Biopharm., 14*:175.

18. Gibaldi, M., and Perrier, D. (1982). *Pharmacokinetics*, 2nd ed., Marcel Dekker, New York, pp. 145–166.

19. Wagner, J. G. (1975). *Fundamentals of Clinical Pharmacokinetics*, Drug Intelligence Publications, Hamilton, Illinois, pp. 102–106.

20. Miller, S. C., Himmelstein, K. J., and Patton, T. F. (1981). A physiologically based pharmacokinetic model for the intraocular distribution of pilocarpine in rabbits, *J. Pharmacokinet. Biopharm., 9*:653.

21. Schoenwald, R. D., Folk, J. C., Kumar, V., and Piper, J. G. (1987). In vivo comparison of phenylephrine and phenylephrine oxazolidine instilled in the monkey eye, *J. Ocul. Pharmacol., 3*:333.

22. Putnam, M. L., Schoenwald, R. D., Duffel, M. W., Barfknecht, C. F., Segarra, T. M., and Campbell, D. A. (1987). Ocular disposition of aminozolamide in the rabbit eye, *Invest. Ophthalmol. Vis. Sci., 28*:1373.

23. Auclair, E., Laude, D., Wainer, I. W., Chaouloff, F., and Elghozi, J. L. (1988). Comparative pharmacokinetics of D- and L-alphamethyldopa in plasma, aqueous humor, and cerebrospinal fluid in rabbits, *Fundam. Clin. Pharmacol., 2*:283.

24. Ling, T. L., and Combs, D. L. (1987). Ocular bioavailability and tissue distribution of [^{14}C] ketorolac tromethamine in rabbits, *J. Pharm. Sci., 76*:289.

25. Lee, V. H. L., and Robinson, J. R. (1979). Mechanistic and quantitative evaluation of precorneal pilocarpine disposition in albino rabbits, *J. Pharm. Sci., 68*:673.

26. Himmelstein, K. J., Guvenir, I., and Patton, T. P. (1978). Preliminary pharmacokinetic model of pilocarpine uptake and distribution in the eye, *J. Pharm. Sci., 67*:603.
27. Patton, T. F., and Robinson, J. R. (1976). Quantitative precorneal disposition of topically applied pilocarpine nitrate in rabbit eyes, *J. Pharm. Sci., 65*:1295.
28. Conrad, J. M., and Robinson, J. R. (1977). Aqueous chamber drug distribution volume measurements in rabbits, *J. Pharm. Sci., 66*:219.
29. Vigo, J. F., Rafart, J., Concheiro, A., Martinez, R., and Cordido, M. (1988). Ocular penetration and pharmacokinetics of cefotaxmine: An experimental study, *Curr. Eye Res., 7*:1149.
30. Bourne, W. M., Nagataki, S., and Brubaker, R. F. (1984). The permeability of the corneal endothelium to fluorescein in the normal human eye, *Curr. Eye Res., 3*:509.
31. Nagataki, S., and Mishima, S. (1980). Pharmacokinetics of instilled drugs in the human eye, *Clinical Pharmacology of the Anterior Segment* (F. Holly, ed.), Little, Brown, Boston, p. 33.
32. Occhipinti, J. R., Mosier, M. A., LaMotte, J., and Monji, G. T. (1988). Fluorophotometric measurement of human tear turnover rate, *Curr. Eye Res., 7*:995.
33. Palestine, A. G., and Brubaker, R. F. (1981). Pharmacokinetics of fluorescein in the vitreous, *Invest. Ophthalmol. Vis. Sci., 21*:542.
34. Lee, D. A., and Brubaker, R. F. (1982). Effect of phenylephrine on aqueous humor flow, *Curr. Eye Res., 2*:89.
35. Patton, T. (1980). Ocular drug disposition, *Ophthalmic Drug Delivery Systems* (J. R. Robinson, ed.), American Pharm. Association, Washington, D.C., pp. 28–54.
36. Igarashi, H., Sato, Y., Hamada, S., and Kawasaki, T. (1984). Studies on rabbit corneal permeability of local anesthetics, *Jpn. J. Pharmacol., 34*:429.
37. Schoenwald, R. D., and Huang, H. S. (1983). Corneal penetration behavior of beta-blocking agents I: Physicochemical factors, *J. Pharm. Sci., 72*:1266.
38. Huang, H. S., Schoenwald, R. D., and Lach, J. L. (1983). Corneal penetration behavior of beta-blocking agents II: assessment of barrier contributions, *J. Pharm. Sci., 72*:1272.
39. Chiang, C. H., Huang, H. S., and Schoenwald, R. D. (1986). Corneal permeability of adrenergic agents potentially useful in glaucoma, *J. Taiwan Pharm. Assoc., 38*:67.
40. Grass, G. M., and Robinson, J. R. (1988). Mechanisms of corneal drug penetration II: Ultrastructural analysis of potential pathways for drug movement, *J. Pharm. Sci., 77*:15.
41. Camber, O., Edman, P., and Olsson, L. I. (1986). Permeability of prostaglandin F_{2alpha} and prostaglandin F_{2alpha} esters across cornea in vitro, *Int. J. Pharm., 29*:259.
42. Corbo, D. C., Liu, J. C., and Chien, Y. W. (1990). Characterization of the barrier properties of mucosal membranes, *J. Pharm. Sci., 79*:202.
43. Gibaldi, M., and Perrier, D. (1982). *Pharmacokinetics*, 2nd ed., Marcel Dekker, New York, pp. 475–477.
44. Eller, M. G., Schoenwald, R. D., Dixson, J. A., Segarra, T., and Barfknecht, C. F. (1985). Topical carbonic anhydrase inhibitors III: Optimization model for corneal penetration of ethoxzolamide analogues, *J. Pharm. Sci., 74*:155.
45. Mosher, G. L., and Mikkelson, T. J. (1979). Permeability of the n-alkyl p-aminobenzoate esters across the isolated corneal membrane of the rabbit, *Int. J. Pharm., 2*:239.
46. Shell, J. W. (1985). Ophthalmic drug delivery systems, *Drug Dev. Res., 6*:245.
47. Ahmed, I., Gokhale, R. D., Shah, M. V., and Patton, T. F. (1987). Physicochemical determinants of drug diffusion across the conjunctiva, sclera, and cornea, *J. Pharm. Sci., 76*:583.
48. Chien, D. S., Homsy, J. J., Gluchowski, C., and Tang-liu, D. D. S. (1990). Corneal and conjunctival/scleral penetration of p-aminoclonidine, AGN 190342, and clonidine, *Curr. Eye Res., 9*:1051.
49. Ahmed, I., and Patton, T. F. (1985). Importance of the noncorneal absorption route in topical ophthalmic drug delivery, *Invest. Ophthalmol. Vis. Sci., 26*:584.
50. Maurice, D. M. (1980). Factors influencing the penetration of topically applied drugs, *Clinical Pharmacology of the Anterior Segment* (F. Holly, ed.), Little, Brown, Boston, pp. 21–32.

51. Lewis, R. A., Schoenwald, R. D., Barfknecht, C. F., and Phelps, C. D. (1986). Aminozolamide gel. A trial of a topical carbonic anhydrase inhibitor in ocular hypertension, *Arch. Ophthalmol., 104*:842.

52. Lewis, R. A., Schoenwald, R. D., and Barfknecht, C. F. (1988). Aminozolamide suspension: The role of the vehicle in a topical carbonic anhydrase inhibitor, *J. Ocul. Pharm., 4*:215.

53. Lee, V. H. L., Urrea, P. T., Smith, R. E., Schanzlin, D. J., and Kreuter, J. (1985). Ocular drug bioavailability from topically applied liposomes, *Surv. Ophthalmol., 29*:335.

54. Wagner, J. G. (1975). *Fundamentals of Clinical Pharmacokinetics*, Drug Intelligence Publications, Hamilton, Illinois, pp. 91–102.

55. Gibaldi, M., and Perrier, D. (1982). *Pharmacokinetics*, 2nd ed., Marcel Dekker, New York, pp. 409–417.

56. Tang-Lui, D. D. S., Liu, S., Neff, J., and Sandri, R. (1987). Disposition of levobunolol after an ophthalmic dose to rabbits, *J. Pharm. Sci., 76*:780.

57. Eller, M. G., Schoenwald, R. D., Dixson, J. A., Segarra, T., and Barfknecht, C. F. (1985). Topical carbonic anhydrase inhibitors IV: Relationship between excised corneal permeability and pharmacokinetic factors, *J. Pharm. Sci., 74*:525.

58. Hitoshi, S., Bundgaard, H., and Lee, V. H. L., (1989). Design of prodrugs to selectively reduce timolol absorption on the basis of the differential lipophilic characteristics on the cornea and the conjunctiva. *Invest. Ophthalmol. Vis. Sci., 30*(Suppl.): 25.

59. Edelhauser, H. F., and Maren, T. H. (1988). Permeability of human cornea and sclera to sulfonamide carbonic anhydrase inhibitors, *Arch. Ophthalmol., 106*:110.

60. Havener, W. H. (1983). Ocular pharmacology, *Autonomic Drugs*, 5th ed., Mosby, St. Louis, pp. 264–269.

61. Friedland, B. R., and Muther, T. F. (1978). Autoradiographic localization of carbonic anhydrase in the ciliary body, *Invest. Ophthalmol. Vis. Sci. 18*(Suppl.):162.

62. Lutjen-Drecoll, E., Lonnerholm, G., and Ober, M. (1978). Carbonic anhydrase activity in the monkey anterior ocular segment. *Invest. Ophthalmol. Vis. Sci., 18*(Suppl.):162.

63. Maurice, D. (1987). Kinetics of topically applied ophthalmic drugs, *Ophthalmic Drug Delivery: Biopharmaceutical, Technological and Clinical Aspects*, Vol. 11 (M. F. Saettone, M. Bucci, and P. Speiser, eds.), Fidia Research Series, Liviana Press, Springer-Verlag, Berlin, pp. 19–26.

64. Maurice, D. M. (1980). Structures and fluids involved in the penetration of topically applied drugs, *Clinical Pharmacology of the Anterior Segment* (F. Holly, ed.), Little, Brown, Boston, pp. 7–20.

65. Lee, V. H. L., Chang, S. C., Oshiro, C. M., and Smith, R. E. (1985). Ocular esterase composition in albino and pigmented rabbits: Possible implications in ocular prodrug design and evaluation. *Curr. Eye Res., 4*:1117.

66. Chien, D. S., Bundgaard, H., and Lee, V. H. L. (1988). Influence of corneal epithelial integrity on the penetration of timolol prodrugs, *J. Ocul. Pharmacol., 4*:137.

67. Lee, V. H. L., Morimoto, K. M., and Stratford, Jr., R. E. (1982). Esterase distribution in the rabbit cornea and its implications in ocular drug bioavailability, *Biopharm. Drug Dispos., 3*:291.

68. Lee, V. H. (1983). Esterase activities in adult rabbit eyes, *J. Pharm. Sci., 72*:239.

69. Chang, S. C., Bundgaard, H., Buur, A., and Lee, V. H. L. (1987). Improved corneal penetration of timolol by prodrugs as a means to reduce systemic drug load, *Invest. Ophthalmol. Vis. Sci., 28*:487.

70. Bundgaard, H., Falch, E., Larsen, C., and Mikkelson, T. (1986). Pilocarpine prodrugs I. Synthesis, physicochemical properties and kinetics of lactonization of pilocarpic acid esters, *J. Pharm. Sci., 75*:36.

71. Bundgaard, H., Falch, E., Larsen, C., Mosher, G. L., and Mikkelson, T. (1996). Pilocarpine prodrugs II. Synthesis, stability, bioconversion, and physicochemical properties of sequentially labile pilocarpine acid diesters, *J. Pharm. Sci., 75*:775.

72. Narukar, M. M., and Mitra, A. K. (1989). Prodrugs of 5-Iodo-2'-deoxyuridine for enhanced ocular transport, *Pharm. Res., 6*:887.

73. Bito, L. Z., and Baroody, R. A. (1987). The ocular pharmacokinetics of eicosanoids and their derivatives. 1. Comparison of ocular eicosanoid penetration and distribution following the topical application of PGF 2alpha, PGF 2alpha-1-methyl ester, and PGF 2alpha-1-isopropyl ester, *Exp. Eye Res., 44*:217.
74. Bito, L. Z. (1986). Prostaglandins and other eicosanoids: Their ocular transport, pharmacokinetics, and therapeutic effects, *Trans. Ophthalmol. Soc. U.K., 105*:162.
75. Campbell, D. A., Schoenwald, R. D., Duffel, M. W., and Barfknecht, C. F. (1991). Characterization of arylamine acetyltransferase in the rabbit eye, *Invest. Ophthalmol. Vis. Sci., 32*:2190.
76. Hearse, D. J., and Weber, W. W. (1973). Multiple N-acetyltransferases and drug metabolism, *Biochem. J., 132*:519.
77. OHara, K. (1977). Effects of cholinergic agonists on isolated iris sphincter muscles: A pharmacodynamic study, *Jpn. J. Ophthalmol., 21*:516.
78. Mishima, S. (1981). Clinical pharmacokinetics of the eye, *Invest. Ophthalmol. Vis. Sci., 21*:504.
79. Smolen, V. F. (1981). Noninvasive pharmacodynamic and bioelectrometric methods for elucidating the bioavailability mechanisms of ophthalmic drug preparations, *Prog. Drug Res., 25*:421.
80. Smolen, V. F., and Schoenwald, R. D. (1971). Drug absorption analysis from pharmacological data. I. The method and its confirmation exemplified for a mydriatic drug, tropicamide, *J. Pharm. Sci., 60*:96.
81. Schoenwald, R. D., and Smolen, V. F. (1971). Drug absorption analysis from pharmacological data. II. Transcorneal biophasic availability of tropicamide, *J. Pharm. Sci., 60*:1039.
82. Smolen, V. F., and Schoenwald, R. D. (1974). Drug absorption analysis from pharmacological data. III. Influence of polymers and pH on transcorneal biophasic availability and mydriatic response of tropicamide, *J. Pharm. Sci., 63*:1582.
83. Smolen, V. F. (1972). Applications of a pharmacological method of drug absorption analysis to the study of the bioavailability characteristics of mydriatic drugs, *Can. J. Pharm. Sci., 7*:7.
84. Smolen, V. F. (1971). Quantitative determination of drug bioavailability and biokinetic behavior from pharmacological data for ophthalmic and oral administration of a mydriatic drug, *J. Pharm. Sci., 60*:354.
85. Smolen, V. F. (1975). Drug bioelectrometric study of the mechanisms of carbachol interactions with the cornea and its relation to miotic activity, *J. Pharm. Sci., 64*:526.
86. Chien, D. S., and Schoenwald, R. D. (1990). Ocular pharmacokinetics and pharmacodynamics of phenylephrine and phenylephrine oxazolidine in rabbit eyes, *Pharm. Res., 7*:476.
87. Anderman, G., Guggenbuhl, P., de Burlet, G., and Himber, J. (1989). Pharmacokinetics of falintolol II. Absorption, distribution and elimination from tissues and organs following ocular administration and intravenous injection of falintolol in albino rabbits, *Methods and Find Exp. Clin. Pharmacol., 11*:747.
88. Brazzell, R. K., Woolridge, C. B., Hackett, R. B., and McCue, B. A. (1990). Pharmacokinetics of the aldose reductase inhibitor imirestat following topical ocular administration, *Pharm. Res., 7*:192.
89. Huang, H. S., Schoenwald, R. D., and Lach, J. L. (1983). Corneal penetration behavior of beta-blocking agents III: In vitro-in vivo correlations, *J. Pharm. Sci., 72*:1279.
90. Grove, J., Gautheron, P., Plazonnet, B., and Sugrue, M. F. (1988). Ocular distribution studies of the topical carbonic anhydrase inhibitors L-643,799 and L-650,719 and related alkyl prodrugs, *J. Ocul. Pharmacol., 4*:279.
91. Maren, T. H., and Jankowska, L. (1985). Ocular pharmacology of sulfonamides: The cornea as barrier and depot, *Curr. Eye Res., 4*:399.
92. Sugrue, M. F., Gautheron, P., Mallorga, T. E., Nolan, S. L., Graham, H., Schwam, H., Shepard, K. L., and Smith, R. L. (1990). L-662,583 is topically effective ocular hypotensive carbonic anhydrase inhibitor in experimental animals, *Br. J. Pharmacol., 99*:59.
93. Walstad, R. A., Hellum, K. B., Blika, S., Dale, L. G., Fredriksen, T., Myhre, K. I., and Spencer, G. R. (1983). Pharmacokinetics and tissue penetration of ceftazidime: Studies on lymph, aqueous humor, skin blister, cerebrospinal and pleural fluid, *J. Antimicrob. Chemother., 12*(Suppl. A): 275.

94. Rootman, J., Ostry, A., and Gudauskas, G. (1984). Pharmacokinetics and metabolism of 5-fluorouracil following subconjunctival versus intravenous administration, *Can. J. Ophthalmol., 19*:187.

95. Ueno, N., Refojo, M. F., and Liu, L. H. S. (1982). Pharmacokinetics of the antineoplastic agent 1,3-bis(2-chloroethyl)-1-nitrosurea (BCNU) in the aqueous and vitreous of rabbit, *Invest. Ophthalmol. Vis. Sci., 23*:199.

96. Gudauskas, G., Kumi, C., Dedhar, C., Bussanich, N., and Rootman, J. (1985). Ocular pharmacokinetics of subconjunctivally versus intravenously administered 6-mercaptopurine, *Can. J. Ophthalmol., 20*:110.

97. Agata, M., Tanaka, M., Nakajima, A., Fujii, A., Kuboyama, N., Tamura, T., and Araie, M. (1984). Ocular penetration of topical diclofenac sodium, a non-steroidal anti-inflammatory drug, in rabbit eye, *Nippon Ganka Gakkai Zashi, 88*:991.

98. Fantes, F., Heuer, D. K., Parrish, R. K., Sossi, N., and Gressel, M. G. (1985). Topical fluorouracil: Pharmacokinetics in normal rabbit eyes, *Arch. Ophthalmol., 103*:953.

99. Valeri, P., Palmery, M., Severini, G., Piccinelli, D., and Catanese, B. (1986). Ocular pharmacokinetics of dapiprazole, *Pharmacol. Res. Commun., 18*:1093.

100. Huupponen, R., Kaila, T., Salminen, L., and Urtti, A. (1987). The pharmacokinetics of ocularly applied timolol in rabbits, *Acta Ophthalmol., 65*:63.

101. Taylor, P. B., Burd, E. M., and Tabbara, K. (1987). Corneal and intraocular penetration of topical and subconjunctival fusidic acid, *Br. J. Ophthalmol., 71*:598.

102. Anderson, J. A., Chen, C. C., Vita, J. B., and Shackleton, M. (1982). Disposition of topical flurbiprofen in normal and aphakic rabbit eyes, *Arch. Ophthalmol., 100*:642.

103. Eng, I. S. (1986). N-Methylacetazolamide ocular disposition and enzyme kinetics. Ph.D. Thesis, University of Iowa College of Pharmacy, Iowa City, Iowa.

104. Hussain, A., Hirai, S., and Sieg, J. (1980). Ocular absorption of propranolol in rabbits, *J. Pharm. Sci., 69*:736.

105. Rao, C. S. (1991). Ph.D. Thesis, University of Iowa College of Pharmacy, Iowa City, Iowa.

106. Barza, M., Kane, A., and Baum, J. L. (1979). Intraocular levels of cefamandole compared with cefazolin after subconjunctival injection in rabbits, *Invest. Ophthalmol. Vis. Sci., 18*:250.

107. Barza, M., and McCue, M. (1983). Pharmacokinetics of aztreonam in rabbit eyes, *Invest. Ophthalmol. Vis. Sci., 24*:468.

108. Hui, H. W., Zeleznick, L., and Robinson, J. R. (1984). Ocular disposition of topically applied histamine, cimetidine and pyrilamine in the albino rabbit, *Curr. Eye Res., 3*:321.

109. Huupponen, R., Kaila, T., and Salminen, L. (1987). The pharmacokinetics of oculary applied timolol in rabbits, *Acta Ophthalmol., 65*:63.

110. Leibowitz, H. M., Ryan, W. J., Kupferman, A., and DeSantis, L. (1986). Bioavailability and corneal anti-inflammatory effect of topical suprofen, *Invest. Ophthalmol. Vis. Sci., 27*:628.

111. Kleinberg, J., Dea, F. J., Anderson, J. A., and Leopold, I. H. Intraocular penetration of topically applied lincomycin hydrochloride in rabbits, *Arch. Ophthalmol., 97*:933.

112. Mester, U., Krasemann, C., and Werner, H. (1982). Cefsulodine concentrations in rabbit eyes after intravenous and subconjunctival administration, *Ophthalmol. Res., 14*:129.

113. Lee, V. H . L., and Robinson, J. R. (1982). Disposition of pilocarpine in the pigmented rabbit eye, *Int. J. Pharm., 11*:155.

5
Cell Cultures to Assess Corneal Permeability

Jiahorng Liaw *School of Pharmacy, Taipei Medical College, Taipei, Taiwan*

Joseph R. Robinson *School of Pharmacy, University of Wisconsin, Madison, Wisconsin*

I. INTRODUCTION

Multicellular organisms exchange material, mostly solutes and water, with their environment. This is achieved by transport through their outer and inner body surfaces; e.g., in humans, through the skin, intestine, and urinary tract. All these organs are covered by epithelia; i.e., a sheet of cells, which are held together by a junction of some sort (Fig. 1). The key questions of research in the field of epithelial transport are as follows: 1) What is transported along which pathways and across which barriers? 2) How does the transport work and where is it located? Logically, all analyses start with intact epithelial cell layers. The usual approach is black box; i.e., variation of the outer compartments, mucosal-serosal or epithelial-endothelial, and measurement of the respective transport rates. This approach has not yet provided complete answers to the above questions.

Because of analytical sensitivity problems, identification of transport routes or transport mechanisms requires sophisticated and sensitive techniques. For example, by using a voltage scanning microelectrode probe, it is possible to identify transport across individual cells or to separate transcellular and paracellular pathways (1,2). The transcellular pathway proceeds through the cell and membranal transport processes are required to understand their interaction with the surface of the membrane in achieving net transepithelial transport. In other words, the physiological function of transepithelial transport can be understood only if the molecular events at each cell side are elucidated by biochemical and biophysical methods. Once these molecular events (i.e., transporter and their location within the cell) are known, it may be useful for the design of drugs and drug delivery systems for tissues.

Because of the complexity of multicellular or whole tissue specimens, it is advantageous to use cell cultures where individual cells or a monolayer of cells can be studied. Such "simple" biological specimens are indeed still very complex and numerous assumptions are made to permit extrapolation of transport data from this level to the tissue, organ, or whole animal. An organ of the body wherein cell culture studies have been particularly

111

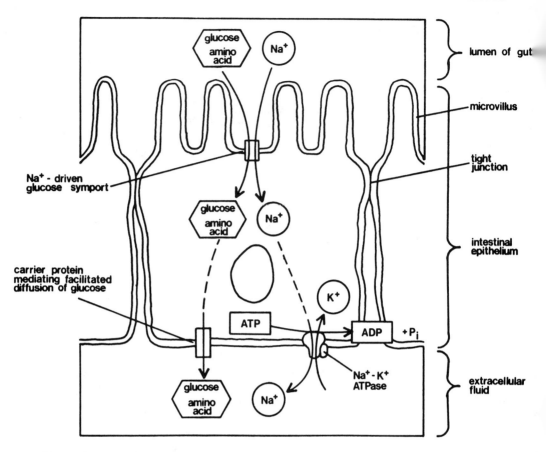

Figure 1. Diagramatic representation of epithelial transport processes.

helpful is the eye. As a small isolated organ, it is quite difficult analytically to study the physiological processes of the eye. However, ocular human cell lines are available for virtually every important tissue of the eye (J. Polanasky, personal communication) and have found increasing use in identifying and using receptors, expression of important proteins, drug metabolism studies, and so forth. Such cells, however, have not been used in drug permeability studies of ocular tissues, as judged by the available literature. In part, this reflects the relatively recent availability of certain tissue lines, e.g., the corneal epithelium and endothelium and, in part, the lack of effort to learn the detailed mechanism of movement of permeant molecules across corneal tissues.

In an effort to develop strategies for delivery of drug candidates arising from drug design, some pharmaceutical scientists have begun to employ the technique of epithelial cell culture to study drug transport and metabolism in specific biological barriers (3). In vitro cultures of the cells have many advantages over conventional techniques, including 1) rapid assessment of the potential permeability and metabolism of a drug; 2) the opportunity to elucidate the molecular mechanisms of drug transport or the pathway(s) of drug degradation (or activation); 3) rapid evaluation of strategies for achieving drug targeting, enhancing drug transport, and minimizing drug metabolism; 4) the opportunity to use human rather than animal tissues; and 5) the opportunity to minimize time-consuming expensive and sometimes controversial animal studies (4).

The objective of this chapter is to describe some of the general factors that should be considered in developing a cell culture model for transport studies. In addition, we review corneal epithelial properties and the potential use of cell cultures of the corneal epithelium, which is known as the major barrier for drug transport (5).

II. GENERAL FACTORS TO CONSIDER IN DEVELOPING A CELL CULTURE MODEL SYSTEM FOR DRUG TRANSPORT AND METABOLISM STUDIES

In order to successfully mimic a biological barrier with an in vitro cell culture system, selection of the appropriate cell line is essential (4). The transport and metabolic properties of cultured cells can vary depending on 1) whether the cells are primary cultures, passaged lines, or transformed lines; 2) the number of times the cells have been passaged; 3) the phenotypic stability of the cell line; 4) the heterogeneity of the cell line; and 5) the inherent ability of the cell line to undergo differentiation. Once the cell line has been selected, the properties may vary depending on 1) cell seeding density; 2) whether the cells have reached confluency; 3) the stage of cellular differentiation; and 4) the presence or absence of essential nutrients, growth factors, or associated cells that produce topic factors. During transport experiments the properties may change depending on 1) the composition of the transport media (e.g., concentration of the solute, temperature, pH, presence or absence of a metabolic source of energy or ions, presence or absence of proteins that might bind the solute, presence or absence of competing solutes); and 2) whether the solute is added to the apical or basolateral side of the monolayer. All of these factors need to be carefully optimized and regulated so as to best mimic the biological barrier.

The development of a cell culture system that will mimic a specific biological barrier requires not only an appropriate cell line but also a microporous support membrane, which by itself or after treatment with an appropriate matrix (i.e., collagen) will support cell attachment and cell growth. Ideally, the microporous membrane should also be 1) sufficiently translucent so that development of the cell monolayer can be verified by microscopic techniques; 2) readily permeable to hydrophilic and hydrophobic solutes; and 3) readily permeable to both low and high molecular weight solutes.

Another critical factor, particularly in the study of the transport of lipophilic molecules, is selection of the diffusion apparatus. Whether the diffusion apparatus is stagnant or stirred can influence the thickness of the aqueous boundary layer on the surface of the cell monolayer and thus permeability of lipophilic solutes. The types of diffusion apparatus currently employed for studying transport across cell monolayers include 1) the unstirred cell-insert system; 2) the side-by-side diffusion system stirred mechanically (5); and 3) the side-by-side diffusion system stirred by gas lift (4). Stirring should produce minimal damage to the cell monolayer and minimize the thickness of the aqueous boundary layer.

Since it is possible to readily manipulate the experimental conditions in a cell culture system, these in vitro models have tremendous potential to help in elucidation of the various pathways by which a drug can penetrate a biological barrier. Experiments can be designed to determine whether the permeability of a small solute is via passive diffusion or active or facilitated diffusion and/or paracellular diffusion. The extracellular milieu, including nutrients, growth factors, and substrate, is easily manipulated. For macro-molecules, experiments can be designed to determine whether the molecule penetrates the barrier by a paracellular or a transcellular mechanism. Most importantly, these systems may provide basic information about transport mechanisms in biological barriers to allow development of novel strategies for targeting drugs to a specific tissue compartment or enhancing drug permeability through an impermeable biological barrier.

III. CORNEAL STRUCTURE AND FUNCTION

The cornea is composed of three major layers: two boundary cellular layers, the epithelium and the endothelium, and a thick connective tissue, the stroma, between these two layers (Figs. 2 and 3). The total thickness of the cornea is around 500–600 µm, of which some 90% is the stroma. The corneal epithelium is a nonkeratinized stratified squamous epithelium, five to six cell layers in thickness. Junctional complexes are more numerous, and particularly important are the zonulae occludentes of tight junctions between the adjacent superficial cells, which form an important permeability barrier for the cornea. The apical surface of the epithelium alone contributes more than half of the total electrical resistance of the entire cornea when intact (6). This indicates that it is the major barrier of transport of ionic or polar molecules. The function of the tight junction is to exclude all solute movement except that which occurs by partitioning process. Thus, compounds which are lipophilic can easily be absorbed across the epithelium. While molecular size appears not to be the decisive factor in determining the rate of corneal penetration for lipophilic compounds (7), it is crucial for penetration of hydrophilic molecules, with the exception of very small molecular weight polar compounds such as water, methanol, and butanol (5). In fact, it was found that the molecular size of the aqueous diffusional pathway of the cornea wherein considerable resistance is noted is approximately the size of a glycerol molecule (MW 92) or molecular weight 400–500 of polyethylene glycol molecule. The intercellular spaces underlying the apical layer have larger dimension and are perme-able to molecules as large as horseradish peroxidase (MW 40,000), and this permeability continues through the entire thickness of the corneal stroma and endothelium (8).

The stroma is composed mainly of regularly arranged optically transparent collagen fibrils, with smaller amounts of proteoglycan and some migrant cells. All molecular weights over 500,000 D are impeded from movement through the stroma unless it is edematous (7). Unlike the lipophilic epithelium, and because of its high water content, the aqueous stroma presents less retardation to movement of hydrophilic compounds as com-pared to that for lipophilic substances. The endothelium comprises a single layer of regularly spaced hexagonal cells of uniform thickness. The endothelial cells are joined to each other by zonulae occludentes, maculae occludentes, and maculae adherences but no desmosomes. All these junctions at the lateral cell membranes have an oblique and tortuous course with complex interdigitations. The intercellular spaces are approximately 50 µm and are open to the entry of molecules as large as colloidal gold, lanthanum, and ferritin (9). Since it constitutes less than 1% of the total mass of the cornea, it is usually ignored as a reservoir for solutes or as a barrier.

The primary role of transport phenomena across the cornea is related to the preserva-tion of hydration and transparency of this tissue. The basic process consists of an ionic pump located in the boundary cell layer that limit the amount of water in the stroma. At a low degree of hydration, the cornea is transparent, but becomes opaque when water is

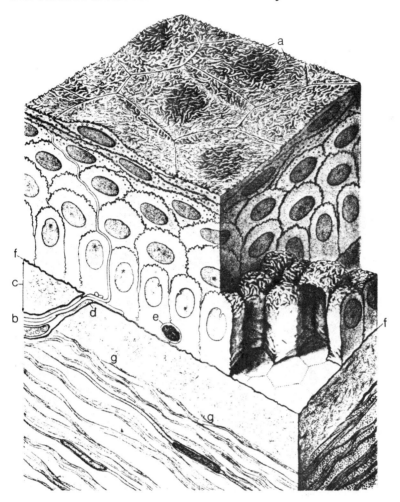

Figure 2. Diagrammatical representation of the corneal epithelium. The cell surface shows an extensive net of microplicae (a) and microvilli. A corneal nerve (b) passes through Bowman's layer (c); it has lost its Schwann sheath (d) near the basement membrane (f) of the basal epithelium. A lymphocyte (e) is seen between two basal epithelium cells. Some of the most superficial corneal stroma lamellae (g) are seen curving forward to merge with Bowman's layer. (From Ref. 37.)

accumulated in the tissue. Through membrane-activated transport systems, the cornea generates a transepithelial potential which is negative on the epithelial side and positive on the endothelial side (10). This corneal potential originates from asymmetries in specific ionic conductances in the apical and basal membranes.

In the rabbit cornea, active sodium transport accounts for about half of the total transport current with the remaining being balanced by an outward chloride transport (11). Transepithelial sodium transport is dependent on its ability to cross the apical and basolateral membranes. The movement of sodium from the tears into the epithelium can be accounted for simply in terms of passive diffusion along its electrochemical gradient. This passive movement is the rate-limiting step in the active absorption of sodium into the

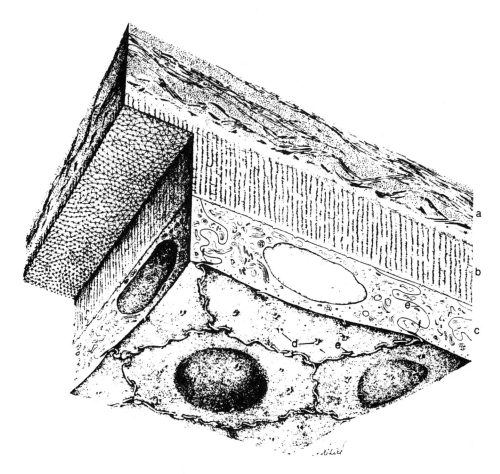

Figure 3. Three-dimensional representational of the deep cornea showing the deepest corneal lamellae (a), Descemet's membrane (b), and the endothelium (c). The endothelial cells are polygonial in shape, measuring approximately 3.5 μm in thickness and 7–10 μm in length. Microvilli (d) protrude into the anterior chamber from the posterior cell, and the marginal folds (e) at intercellular junctions project into the anterior chamber. The intercellular space near the anterior chamber is closed by a zonula occludens (f). (From Ref. 37.)

stroma, as demonstrated by a direct correlation between apical membrane cation conductance and short circuit current (6). Unlike sodium entry, the extrusion of sodium from the cells into the stroma occurs in opposition to an electrochemical gradient, a process that requires an active transport mechanism in the basolateral membrane.

The addition of ouabain, a sodium pump inhibitor, to the bathing solutions has been shown to reduce transepithelial potential and the spontaneous short-circuit current (12). This indicates that Na/K ATPase and the associated "pump" are involved in ion transport at the basolateral membrane. Klyce (13) have similarly shown the presence of an active Cl^- transport, which operates synergistically with the sodium pump, against the electrochemical potential gradient from the stroma to the tears. In fact, the epithelium alone is capable of deswelling a previously edematous cornea, when its Cl^- transport is stimulated

(14). Although the fluid-transporting capability of the epithelium in terms of maintenance of corneal hydration is small in comparison with that of the endothelium, its function can be modulated by activation of specific receptors under neural control, whereas no such regulation has been demonstrated for the endothelium.

A. Corneal Epithelial Cells

Recently, a number of cell culture models for drug absorption studies have been developed (15), such as using an intestinal epithelial (Caco-2) cell line to determine cellular permeability coefficients and aqueous boundary layer thickness (16), using pulmonary epithelium to study the effect of beta-adrenergic agonist on ion absorption (17), and using MDCK kidney cell line to characterize the enzyme on the surface membrane (18). Drug delivery by the ophthalmic route is generally concerned with delivering a therapeutic substance across the corneal barrier to intraocular tissue target sites. Consequently, approaches to meet the continuing needs of clinical activity have been directed at improving intraocular bioavailability by extending topical ocular contact time, modifying corneal permeability properties, and the design of prodrugs. In part, the success of these approaches will depend on further characterization of the biochemical and molecular level properties of the corneal barrier. Although the ophthalmic route can also be considered for systemic delivery of drugs with poor oral bioavailability, for our purpose, only those tissue culture models relevant to the corneal epithelial barrier to intraocular drug delivery will be mentioned.

In recent years, several investigators have reported success in culturing corneal epithelial cells of several species, including humans (19), rabbit (20,21), and rats (22). Many investigators have used the technique of cell cultures reported by Stocker et al. (23). This technique, although relatively simple in concept, may lead to cell cultures that are often contaminated with corneal stromal keratocytes, which rapidly reproduce and overgrow the slow-growing epithelial and endothelial cells. Most investigators resort to physical and enzymatic dissociation of the corneal epithelial surface as a means of obtaining a starting cell population. Numerous cell culture systems, originating primarily from the rabbit and human cornea, by enzymatic methods are the most popular methods for establishing a homogeneous tissue culture system (24,25). However, cells grown in these systems retain biochemical and morphological features that are similar but, again, not identical to the parent cell types (4).

One of the cell lines, derived from normal rabbit corneal epithelial cells (SIRCs), has been recently characterized as to biochemistry and morphology (26,27). By using the pH-sensitive absorbance of intracellularly trapped 5(and 6)-carboxy-4',5-dimethylfluorescein, they showed that a Na^+/H^+ exchange and lactate-H^+ cotransport are present in SIRC rabbit corneal epithelial cells to maintain the intracellular pH of epithelial cells. This is of importance in drug transport. In other words, extracellular pH may affect the cytoplasmic pH of viable cells when drug transport through the transcellular pathway is sensitive to the pH medium.

Corneal epithelial cell cultures have been employed in studies that are directly relevant to drug delivery problems. To test beta-adrenergic and serotonergic responsiveness of rabbit corneal epithelial cells culture, Jumblatt et al. (28) showed that the cell is able to synthesize cyclic adenosine monophosphate (cAMP) in response to beta-adrenergic stimulation but lack the ability to respond to serotonergic stimulation. This may be important in the regulation of ionic transport and as well as corneal transparency. The normal corneal epithelium responds to catecholamine stimulation via beta-adrenergic receptor–mediated activation of cAMP, which can produce a sustained increase in the chloride current and the chloride net flux (29).

In addition, Reinach and Holmberg (30) showed that the increase in cAMP content responded to either adrenergic agonists or adenylate cyclase stimulation. However, they found that this enzymatic dissociation procedure does not affect the cAMP response to adrenergic agonist. Thus, the relationship was considered between an increase in calcium concentration and the effects of isoproterenol on cAMP accumulation. There were no changes in any of the cAMP responses at bathing solution calcium concentrations between 0.1 and 1.0 μM. However, in cells permeabilized to Ca^{2+} with 10 μM ionomycin, increases within this concentration range depressed the baseline level of cAMP content. Furthermore, the stimulatory effects of isoproterenol on cAMP accumulation were significantly blunted in this concentration range and these blunting effects by Ca^{2+} were not the result of any measurable decrease in adenosine triphosphate (ATP) content. This negative relationship between increases in calcium concentration and increases in cAMP content indicates that changes in intracellular calcium concentration modulate the second-messenger function of cAMP linked to these agents. This would be an important factor in terms of permeability of the cornea; i.e., the calcium environment can modify the cytoskeletal protein structure, which is known as the major controlling factor of the tight junction (31).

Furthermore, Soong et al. (32) used cytochalasin D, an inhibitor of actin polymerization, in corneal epithelial cell cultures to determine cell-cell attachment. The results have indicated that this cytochalasin-induced cytoskeletal changes were associated with cellular detachment from the substratum. Also examined have been the effect of polymer substrate irritants on cell growth (33). In addition, chemical induction of plasminogen activator secretion (34) has included the use of corneal epithelial cell cultures. The success in quantitating the sensitivity of corneal epithelial cell cultures to chemical and polymer substrate irritants suggests that these in vitro systems eventually replace the Draize test (4,35).

Another popular use of corneal epithelial cell culture systems is to study wound repair (25,36,37). By testing cholera toxin and chickenpox/shingles virus (varicella-zoster viruses, VZV) effects on corneal epithelial wound closure (38), cultured corneal epithelial cells may be used as an assay which is a useful alternative to in vivo toxicity testing. Also, Simmons et al. (39), using 13 test agents (e.g., DMSO, Tween 80, benzalkonium chloride, ethanol, and ethylene glycol), showed that the ocular tissue culture model is conceptually simple, quantitative, and an alternative to the corneal component of whole animal drug screen testing for ocular irritancy. However, details of the metabolic activity and transcellular permeability properties have not apparently been addressed in these corneal epithelial cell culture systems.

IV. CONCLUSIONS

Cultured corneal epithelial cells provide a useful model system for investigating the events governing drug irritation tests, closure of superficial epithelial defects, and assaying the actions of exogenous agents on these events. However, the use of cell culture techniques to study the transport and metabolic characteristics of specific biological barriers to drug delivery is in its infancy. It will be very important to fully characterize the cell culture at the biochemical level before its widespread use as a tool in drug delivery.

REFERENCES

1. Ullrich, K. J. (1990). Epithelial transport: An introduction, *Methods Enzymol., 192*:1–4.
2. Nagel, W. (1981). In: *Epithelial Ion and Water Transport: Microelectrode Demonstration of Rheogenic Sodium Transport in Tight Epithelia*, (Macknight et al., eds.), Raven Press, New York, pp. 63–83.
3. Wilson, G., Davis, S. S., and Illum, L. (1990). *Pharmaceutical Applications of Cell and Tissue Culture*, Plenum Press, New York.
4. Audus, K. L., Borchardt, R. T., et al. (1990). The use of cultured epithelial and endothelial cells for drug transport and metabolism studies, *Pharm. Res., 7*:435–451.
5. Grass, G. M., and Robinson, J. R. (1988). Mechanisms of corneal drug penetration. II: Ultra-structural analysis of potential pathways for drug movement, *J. Pharm. Sci., 77*:15–23.
6. Klyce, S. D. (1972). Electrical profiles in the corneal epithelium, *J. Physiol. (Lond.), 226*:407–429.
7. Maurice, D. M. (1984). In: *The Eye*, 3rd ed. (Davson, ed.), Academic Press, New York, pp. 1–158.
8. Tonjum, A. M. (1974). Permeability of horseradish peroxidase in rabbit corneal epithelium, *Acta Ophthalmol., 52*:650–658.
9. Burstein, N. L. (1979). Corneal epithelium permeability to electron opaque tracers demonstrated by modified proprane jet cryofixation, *J. Cell Biol., 83*:300a.
10. Donn, A., Maurice, D. M., et al. (1959). The active transport of sodium across the epithelium, *Arch. Ophthalmol., 62*:748–757.
11. Klyce, S. D., Neufeld, A. H., et al. (1973). The activation of chloride transport by epinephrine and DB c-AMP in the cornea of the rabbit, *Invest. Ophthalmol., 12*:127–139.
12. Green, K. (1970). Stromal cation binding alters inhibition of epithelial transport in the cornea, *Am. J. Physiol., 218*:1642–1648.
13. Klyce, S. D., and Marshall, W. S. (1982). Effect of Ag^+ on ion transport by the corneal epithelium of the rabbit, *J. Membr. Biol., 66*:133–144.
14. Klyce, S. D. (1977). Enhancing fluid secretion by the corneal epithelium, *Invest. Ophthalmol. Vis. Sci., 16*:968–978.
15. Borchardt, R. T., Hidalgo, I. J., Hillgren, K. M., and Hu, M. (1991). Pharmaceutical applications of cell culture: An overview. In: *Pharmaceutical Applications of Cell and Tissue Culture*, NATO ASI series (G. Wilson, L. Ilum, and S. S. Davies, eds.), Plenum Press, New York.
16. Karlsson, J., and Artursson, P. (1991). A method for the determination of cellular permeability coefficients and aqueous boundary layer thickness in monolayers of intestinal epithelial (Caco-2) cells grown in permeable filter chambers, *Int. J. Pharm., 71*:55–64.
17. Gatzy, J. T., Krochmal, E. M., and Ballard, S. T. (1990). In: *The Epithelia Advances in Cell Physiology and Cell Culture: Solution Transport Across Alveolar Epithelia of Foetal and Adult Lungs* (C. J. Jones, ed.), Kluwer, London, pp. 233–254.
18. Montrose, M. H. (1990). In: *The Epithelia Advances in Cell Physiology and Cell Culture: Transport Physiology of Renal and Intestinal Cell Culture Models* (C. J. Jones, ed.), Kluwer, London, pp. 145–172.
19. Sun, T. T., and Green, H. (1977). Cultured epithelial cells of cornea, conjunctiva, and skin: Absence of marked intrinsic divergence of their differentiated states, 269:489–492.
20. Chan, K. Y., and Haschke, R. H. (1983). Epithelial-stromal interactions: Specific stimulation of corneal epithelial cell growth in vitro by a factor from cultured stromal fibroblasts, *Exp. Eye Res., 36*:231–246.
21. Jumblatt, M. M., and Neufeld, A. H. (1983). β-Adrenergic and serotonergic responsiveness of rabbit corneal epithelial cells in culture, *Invest. Ophthalmol. Vis. Sci., 24*:1139–1143.

22. Forbes, D. J., Pozos, R. S., Nelson, D., et al. (1984). Characterization of rat corneal epithelium maintained in tissue cultures, *Curr. Eye Res., 3*:1471–1479.
23. Stocker, F. W., Eiring, A., et al. (1958). Tissue culture technique for growing corneal epithelial, stromal, and endothelial tissues, separately, *Am. J. Ophthalmol., 46*:294–298.
24. Xie, L., and Gebhardt, B. (1989). A simplified technique for the short-term tissue culture of rabbit corneal cells, *In Vitro Cell. Devel. Biol., 25*:20–22.
25. Jumblatt et al. (1984). See ms. pp. 212 & 214.
26. Korbmacher, C., and Helbig, H., et al. (1988). Characterization of Na^+/H^+ exchange in a rabbit corneal epithelial cell line (SIRC), *Biochim. Biophys. Acta, 943*:405–410.
27. Bonanno, J. A. (1990). Lactate-proton cotransport in rabbit corneal epithelium, *Curr. Eye Res., 9*:707–712.
28. Jumblatt et al. (1983). β-adrenergic and serotonergic responsiveness of rabbit corneal epithelial cells in culture, *Invest. Ophthalmol. Vis. Sci., 24*:1139–1143.
29. Zadunaisky, J. A., and Spinowitz, B. (1976). In: *Drugs and Ocular Tissues: Drugs Affecting the Transport and permeability of the Corneal Epithelium* (S. J. Dicksten, ed.), Karger, pp. 57–78.
30. Reinach, P., and Holmberg, N. (1989). Inhibition of calcium of beta adrenoceptor mediated c-AMP responses in isolated bovine corneal epithelial cells, *Curr. Eye Res., 8*:85–90.
31. Rojanasakul et al. (1990). See ms. p. 213.
32. Soong, H. K., Dass, B., and Lee, B. (1990). Effect of cytochalasin D on actin and vinculin in cultured corneal epithelial cells, *J. Ocul. Pharmacol., 6*:113–121.
33. Pettit, D. K., Horbett, T. A., et al. (1990). Quantitation of rabbit corneal epithelial cell outgrowth on polymeric substrates in vitro, *Invest. Ophthalmol. Vis. Sci., 31*:2269–2277.
34. Chan, K. Y. (1986). Chemical injury to an in vitro ocular system: differential release of plasminogen activator, *Curr. Eye Res., 5*:357–362.
35. Neville, R., Dennis, P., et al. (1986). Preservative cytotoxicity to cultured corneal epithelial cells, *Curr. Eye Res., 5*:367–372.
36. Nelson, J. D., Silverman, V., et al. (1990). Corneal epithelial wound healing: A tissue culture assay on the effect of antibiotics, *Curr. Eye Res., 9*:277–285.
37. Jumblatt, M. M., and Neufeld, A. H. (1986). A tissue culture assay of corneal epithelial wound closure, *Invest. Ophthalmol. Vis. Sci., 27*:8–13.
38. Dunkel, E. C., Geary, P. A., et al. (1988). Varicella zoster virus infection in vitro: A corneal epithelial cell culture model, *Mol. Biol. Eye*, 355–364.
39. Simmons, S. J., Jumblatt, M. M., et al. (1987). Corneal epithelial wound closure in tissue culture: an in vitro model of ocular irritancy, *Toxicol. Appl. Pharmacol., 88*:13–23.

6
Animal Pharmacokinetic Studies

Arto Urtti   *University of Kuopio, Kuopio, Finland*

Lotta Salminen   *Tampere University Hospital, Tampere, Finland*

I. INTRODUCTION

Animal experimentation is an essential part in the research and development of ocular drug delivery systems. The interplay between the properties of a delivery system (either chemical or physical) and the ocular pharmacokinetics determine the final system performance. In order to obtain systematic and mechanistic views of the ocular pharmacokinetics, determinations of drug concentrations from the ocular fluids and tissues have to be made. It is obvious that such experiments can not be made in humans and the picture of human ocular pharmacokinetics is far from complete.

Human ocular pharmacokinetic experimentation is limited to the noninvasive observation of fluorescent (1,2) or gamma-scintigraphic (3) probes and to the determination of drug concentrations from the aqueous humor during cataract surgery (4). In addition, pharmacodynamic bioassays of drugs acting on the autonomous nervous system, especially miotics and mydriatics, are used to interpret ocular pharmacokinetics in humans (5).

The rabbit is by far the most commonly used animal model in the ocular pharmacokinetic studies. Larger mammals are rarely used, because a considerable number of experimental animals must be sacrificed in invasive ocular pharmacokinetic studies. For example, in order to generate mean drug concentration vs time curve of seven animals with eight time points, 28 or 56 animals are required depending on whether one or both eyes are used. The figures must be multiplied by the number of different delivery systems that are compared. It is obvious that so many dogs or primates cannot be sacrificed and the ocular drug testing with these animals is limited to the noninvasive kinetic measurements and pharmacodynamics. The small ocular size of mice and rats limits their value in ocular drug delivery studies.

Owing to its dominant position as an animal model this chapter emphasizes the rabbit as an animal model in ocular pharmacokinetic studies.

II. CONSCIOUS RABBIT AS AN ANIMAL MODEL

A. General Methods

In invasive ocular pharmacokinetic studies with rabbits, an adequate number of eyes must be used per each time point, because variation in the data is greater than in noninvasive studies. This is due to the extensive interindividual variability. In interpretation of the results, an assumption is made that a similar concentration vs time profile would result from a noninvasive study. Consequently, special statistical data treatment is recommended when bioavailabilities are calculated from the invasive ocular pharmacokinetic results (6).

In animal pharmacokinetic studies, tear fluid sampling can be carried out noninvasively (7). Usually, disposable glass capillaries of 1 µL are used for sampling. The samples are collected from the marginal tear strip of the rabbits. The capillary force fills the capillary tube rapidly and the small volume collected does not interfere with the ocular pharmacokinetics. Extreme care must be undertaken to avoid any corneal contact and possible induced lacrimation.

After sacrificing the animal, aqueous humor is withdrawn with a tuberculin syringe and a small needle. The needle is pushed carefully through the limbus into the anterior chamber. During this procedure the researcher should be careful in avoiding contamination of the needle from the corneal epithelium or pigmented iris. In some cases, these tissues may have much higher drug concentrations than the aqueous humor. Also, touching the iris may cause dispersion of pigmentation to the aqueous humor and elevated drug concentrations in the aqueous humor.

Ocular tissues may be dissected directly after the collection of the aqueous humor or the remaining eye may be frozen in liquid nitrogen and dissected later. These procedures have been shown to produce similar results (8). The samples are analyzed with a method that is appropriate for a given drug.

B. Preocular Pharmacokinetics

After instillation of any eye drop to the human or rabbit eye, the drug is subject to several preocular elimination processes. These include drainage of the extra solution, conjunctival systemic drug absorption, normal tear turnover, and induced lacrimation (9). Drugs may also bind to proteins in the lacrimal fluid (10). Corneal permeability and these parallel nonproductive loss processes determine the ocular bioavailability of the drug (9).

1. Preocular Fluid Dynamics

a. Tear Turnover

The normal rate of tear turnover is 1.2 µL/min (16%/min) in humans (11) and 0.5 µl/min (7%/min) in rabbits (12). From the rabbit eye, lacrimal fluid flows via one punctum, whereas in humans, there are two puncta (13). Because the instilled eye drops are mostly removed from the precorneal area by the drainage of the extra solution volume and by the conjunctival systemic drug absorption, the normal rate of tear turnover has only a minor role in the removal of the instilled solutions from the ocular surface (9). Thus, the different rates of the basal tear turnover do not limit usefulness of rabbit as an experimental animal.

The pH of the lacrimal fluid is close to 7.4 both in rabbits (14) and humans (15). Buffering capacity is poor in the lacrimal fluid of both species (14,16,17).

b. Instilled Solution Drainage

Movement of ocularly instilled solutions on the ocular surface and lacrimal drainage system has been followed using ^{99m}Tc-labeled tracers (18) and different eye solutions (19). The initial drainage rate of instilled eye drops from the ocular surface is 1.6 min^{-1} in humans and 0.55 min^{-1} in rabbits when eye drop volume is 25 μL (12,20,21). In both species, the fractional rate of solution drainage from the ocular surface is increased with larger instilled volumes (22,23). The fast initial solution drainage continues until the solution volume on the ocular surface plateaus to the normal lacrimal volume, which is 7 μL in rabbits and humans (11,12).

The faster precorneal loss of instilled solutions in humans is due to the higher blinking frequency compared to rabbits (21). Different blinking frequencies, 6–7 min^{-1} in humans and only 4 h^{-1} in rabbits, is a major limitation of the rabbit as an animal model (24,25). Lid closure retards the precorneal drainage of solutions in humans (18,26). Since eyelid closure, blinking frequency, and position affect precorneal pharmacokinetics (18,26), these factors should be properly controlled in human studies. These factors cause variability in the ocular drug absorption in patients.

c. Induced Blinking

The problem of infrequent blinking in rabbits was overcome by inducing blinking electrically (16,27). Blinking was induced every 5 s by exposing the orbicularis muscle of the upper eyelid to electrical pulses of 5–7 V for 20 ms. The limitation of this procedure is that anesthetized rabbits have to be used. General anesthesia in rabbits decreases induced lacrimation and solution drainage from the precorneal area and, thus, increases ocular drug absorption (28,29). In addition, many intraocular factors may be affected (e.g., intraocular pressure) (30).

Another way to induce blinking is air puffing. Recently, air puffing was used to induce blinking in conscious rabbits at a frequency of 1 min^{-1} (31). It is not known, however, whether this method would work at frequencies that correspond better to the human blinking; i.e., 6–7 min^{-1}. Blinking once per minute was insufficient in causing homogeneous mixing of timolol in the precorneal area in rabbits. This was evidenced by vastly different drug concentrations in the inferior and superior parts of the ocular tissues after administration of a silicone insert in the lower conjunctival sac (31).

In contrast to air puffing, flashing light turned out to be an inefficient way of inducing blinking, because the rabbits get accustomed to the flashing light and close their eyelids permanently (31).

d. Induced Lacrimation

Lacrimation may be induced by irritation or a foreign body sensation in the eye. This is an important factor in the removal of instilled solutions from the eye (7). The extent of the induced lacrimation is difficult to predict. In humans, even major induced increases in the tear turnover rates may remain unobserved by the person (11). Quantitative similarity or difference in terms of induced lacrimation of the two species is not known.

2. Nonproductive Absorption Processes

Nonproductive preocular absorption processes include drug absorption from the lacrimal fluid to the nictitating membrane and the conjunctiva (7). Nonproductive absorption routes compete with the transcorneal absorption and in this way they limit ocular bioavailability (7,9).

Nictitating membrane is a clearly visible difference between the human and rabbit eyes. In rabbits, the nictitating membrane is large, whereas in humans, only a negligible reminiscent of the membrane is present (13). The role of the nictitating membrane in drug absorption to the rabbit eyes has been studied by DeSantis and Schoenwald (32). They found no difference in miotic responses to pilocarpine in rabbits with intact and removed nictitating membranes. This result suggests that the nictitating membrane is not an important factor in preocular pharmacokinetics.

In rabbits, owing to the large surface area and increased permeability in the conjunctiva, the clearance of timolol from the lacrimal fluid to the systemic circulation via conjunctiva is about 10 μL/min, whereas the clearance due to the corneal ocular absorption is less than 1 μL/min (33). The conjunctival surface area is 17 times larger than the corneal surface in humans but the difference in rabbits is only ninefold (34). In addition, the corneal surface area in rabbits varies from 1.5 to 2.0 cm^2 depending on the rabbit size. In humans, the mean corneal surface area is only 1.04 cm^2 (34). Assuming that the conjunctival drug permeabilities in rabbits and humans are in the same range, the nonproductive absorption is expected to impair ocular absorption more in humans than in rabbits.

3. Protein Binding

Protein binding may decrease drug absorption from the tear fluid to the eye (10). In uninflamed eyes, this factor is not expected to contribute significantly, because the protein concentrations in the tear fluid are only 0.5 and 0.7% for rabbit and human eyes, respectively (9). In addition, the concentration is further diluted after instillation of an eye drop. This factor does not impair the clinical predictability of rabbit experiments.

4. Formulation Effects

a. Rheological Effects

Ocular drug absorption to the human eye is more sensitive to changes in eye drop viscosity than absorption to rabbit eyes (25). Consequently, the rabbit studies may underestimate the benefit obtained from viscous vehicles. The reasons of this are not known in detail.

Several other factors in addition to viscosity are involved in the vehicle-blink interaction. In theory, the shear caused by frequent blinking in human eyes could cause thinning of pseudoplastic vehicles and subsequently more rapid precorneal solution drainage. Experimental results, however, are conflicting. Pseudoplasticity of hydroxypropyl methyl cellulose did not lead to more rapid precorneal solution drainage compared to isoviscous polyvinyl alcohol (21), whereas ocular bioavailability of pilocarpine given in pseudoplastic hydroxypropyl cellulose solution was less than the bioavailability after administration in polyvinyl alcohol (35). Since the shear caused by blinking is absent in rabbit eyes, this effect is not seen nor expected in rabbits (35). In theory, shear induced by blinking could also cause shear thickening of dilatant materials but this has not been shown experimentally.

Spreading properties of the polymers on the ocular surface are different from each other and this factor contributes to the ocular drug absorption. Isoviscous polymer solutions resulted in similar mydriatic responses to tropicamide in rabbits, but in humans the ocular bioavailability of tropicamide was increased with the increased ability of the solution to spread on the corneal surface (36). This suggests that blinking not only accelerates the bulk solution removal from the ocular surface but it may also spread a thin film of solution from the lower conjunctival sac to the corneal surface (36,37), the main route of ocular drug absorption from eye drops (9). In most cases, the rank-order in the performance of the eye drops (25,35,36) or gels (38) is similar both in humans and in rabbits but the extent of the pharmacokinetic modification induced by the vehicles is greater in humans.

b. Inserts

In the case of polymeric drug inserts, drainage of the extra volume from the eye is not an important factor in the precorneal kinetics, because no solution is instilled in the eye. The drug released from the insert is removed from the ocular surface mainly by the conjunctival absorption and the normal tear turnover (33). Thus, differences in blinking-induced solution removal do not limit the predictive value of rabbit experiments. However, in this case, poor mixing of the lacrimal fluid of rabbits may cause problems (31,39). This was previously shown when timolol distribution in the rabbit eyes was compared between silicone inserts placed either in the superior or inferior conjunctival sac (31). From the superior conjunctival sac the amount of timolol absorbed to the eye was greater and the absorption took place predominantly via the corneal route, whereas from the inferior cul-de-sac timolol was absorbed mostly via the noncorneal route and very small drug concentrations were observed in the upper conjunctiva and sclera compared to their lower counterparts (31). In humans, mixing on the ocular surface is probably better owing to the frequent blinking. For example, pilocarpine Ocusert™ (Alza Corp., Palo Alto, CA) is advised to be placed either in the lower or upper conjunctival sac. Thus, in some cases, the rabbit experiments may underestimate drug absorption from the ocular inserts to the eye.

B. Corneal and Scleral Permeability

1. Cornea

The detailed descriptions of the corneal and scleral barriers can be found elsewhere in this book. In this chapter, only comparison between the rabbit and human corneas in terms of drug permeability has been provided.

Mean thicknesses of the human and rabbit corneas are 0.52 and 0.35–0.45 mm, respectively (40). The surface area of the rabbit cornea is 1.5–2.0 times greater than the surface of the human cornea (34). Permeabilities of cyclophosphamide (41) and four different carbonic anhydrase inhibitors (42) in isolated human and rabbit corneas have been studied. For most compounds, permeabilities in the rabbit and human corneas were similar (41,42). Edelhauser and Maren (42), however, concluded that for most hydrophilic compounds permeability, presumably via aqueous channels, was less in the rabbit cornea than in the human cornea. It is not known whether the conclusions drawn from these two comparative permeability studies (41,42) are applicable to other compounds with different molecular weights and lipophilicities. The anatomical similarities (13,43) and similarities in the experimental permeabilities, however, suggest that the rabbit cornea is a fairly good model of the human cornea.

It must be also remembered that both human and rabbit corneas change with age (24). Permeability of pilocarpine has been shown to change with the age of the rabbit cornea (44).

2. Sclera

Although the cornea is the main route of drug penetration to the eye (9), the scleral penetration route is important, especially for hydrophilic compounds with large molecular weights (8).

In general, the rabbit sclera is more permeable than the cornea for most compounds (45). Interestingly, the permeabilities of isolated scleras from rabbits and humans had similar permeabilities for carbonic anhydrase inhibitors (42). In both species, scleral permeability of carbonic anhydrase inhibitors was substantially higher than the corneal permeability (42).

Scleral drug permeability is expected to play an important role in ocular drug penetration after subconjunctival injections (24). This is not, however, always the case, because regurgitation of the solution from the injection site to the preocular tear fluid may take place (24,46). Consequently, substantial transcorneal drug penetration may also occur (46). Regurgitation is generally less severe in humans than in rabbit eyes (24).

The passage of subconjunctivally injected fluorescein was an order of magnitude greater in humans than it was in rabbits (47). The reason for this observation is not known. In contrast, gentamicin, tobramycin, and lincomycin penetrated similarly to the human and rabbit aqueous humor after they were injected subconjunctivally (24). It is, however, difficult to compare different studies, because the experimental procedures (e.g., injected volumes and injection sites) vary. These factors may give rise to changes in the proportions of the absorption routes and results. In both species, subconjunctivally injected drug is absorbed mostly and rapidly to the systemic circulation even though the injection bleb may remain visible long after injection (24,46).

Comparative data between humans and rabbits do not exist in the case of transscleral penetration of drugs to the vitreous after subconjunctival and retrobulbar injections.

C. Intraocular Kinetics

1. Aqueous Humor

The aqueous humor of rabbits and humans is formed in the ciliary processes. Aqueous humor flows from the posterior chamber to the anterior chamber and it is drained via the trabecular meshwork or uveoscleral route (24). The volume of the aqueous humor is 0.25–0.30 mL in rabbits and 0.10–0.25 mL in humans (depending on age) (24). The chemical composition of aqueous humor (mostly electrolytes with very little protein) is fairly similar in both species. The protein concentration is 0.55 mg/mL in rabbits and 30 mg/mL in humans (9). These concentrations are negligible compared to protein concentration in plasma. Thus, in the uninflamed eye, protein binding is not a major factor in the pharmacokinetics of the aqueous humor.

The aqueous turnover rate is 3.0–4.7 µL/min in rabbits (13,48) and 2.0–3.0 µL/min in humans (49); i.e., 1–2%/min in both species. The routes of outflow, however, are different. In rabbits, the aqueous humor is drained solely via chamber angle; the uveoscleral drainage is negligible (50). In monkey eyes, the trabecular route accounts for only 45–70% of the total aqueous humor drainage (51). In humans, the uveoscleral drainage route accounts for 5–20% of the total outflow (52). The influence of this factor on drug distribution is unknown.

In rabbits, steady-state volumes of drug distribution (V_{ss}) (e.g., clonidine) are close to 0.5 mL (53,54). The reported values for the terminal elimination phase volumes of distribution (V_z) of flurbiprofen and pilocarpine are about 0.6 mL (48,53,55). However, an also much higher value (1.8 ml) for pilocarpine has been reported (56). These values indicate that drugs distribute from the aqueous humor to the surrounding tissues. Ocular volumes of drug distribution in humans are not known. Geometrically, the human eye is slightly larger than the rabbit eye (24).

Although aqueous humor turnover is often considered to be the major route of drug elimination from the aqueous humor, the values of drug clearance from the aqueous humor of rabbits are higher (about 15 μL/min) (53,54,56) than the rate of aqueous humor turnover, suggesting additional routes of drug elimination. It is possible, especially for small lipophilic molecules, to gain access to the uveal blood circulation across the blood-aqueous barrier. Consequently, clearance of intracamerally injected pilocarpine from the aqueous humor in rabbits was much faster than clearance of inulin (48). Clearance of inulin was close to the rate of aqueous humor turnover, suggesting that no inulin was eliminated via uveal blood flow (48).

Owing to the properties of the blood-aqueous barrier (57), intraocular clearance is expected to be dependent on the lipophilicity and molecular weight of the drug.

2. Anterior Uvea

Drugs distribute from the aqueous humor to the anterior uvea of the eye easily. Consequently, the iris and ciliary body belong kinetically to the same compartment with aqueous humor in albino rabbits (24,56).

The anterior uvea of New Zealand white rabbits and humans differs in two important respects. In contrast to the albino rabbit, the human iris and ciliary body contain melanin pigmentation and the ciliary muscle is more prominent in the human eye (13,24,43). The latter feature may influence the pharmacodynamics of drugs like pilocarpine (59).

Ocular pigmentation has considerable effects on intraocular pharmacokinetics (9,24). Comparisons of the pigmented and albino rabbits have revealed striking differences in their intraocular kinetics. The melanin pigment of the anterior uvea binds many ophthalmic drugs (e.g., pilocarpine, timolol, atropine) (60–64). Melanin binding retards drug elimination from the iris and ciliary body, which leads to increased and prolonged drug levels (61,63). For example, timolol concentrations in the albino rabbit iris-ciliary body fall rapidly at a first-order rate of 0.6 h^{-1}, but in pigmented iris ciliary body, the rate of elimination is several times slower and the peak concentrations much higher than in the nonpigmented tissue (61). Interestingly, drug response is prolonged also; e.g., mydriasis by atropine (60) and miosis by pilocarpine (65). On the other hand, at lower doses, peak pilocarpine response was decreased compared to the albino rabbit (65). Pilocarpine was bound to melanin pigment so that in the proximity of the receptor less drug was available. Despite the decreased peak response, the duration of the miotic response was prolonged with a small pilocarpine dose (65).

Melanin binding is important also in clinical ocular pharmacokinetics (5). Patients with heavily pigmented irides need higher doses of, e.g., timolol, in order to achieve similar decreases in intraocular pressure (66). Ocular pigmentation prolongs the presence of the drug in the anterior uvea and it explains at least partly the discrepancy between the short presence of the drug in the aqueous humor compared to its final duration of action in the human eye (e.g., timolol, pilocarpine, atropine). For example, the human pupillary responses to pilocarpine and homatropine are prolonged in brown-eyed patients compared to blue-eyed patients (5).

In conclusion, clinically more meaningful pharmacokinetic results can be obtained if pigmented rabbits are used instead of albino rabbits.

3. Posterior Segment

After topical administration only very low drug concentrations are achieved in the vitreous (24). However, pharmacokinetics in the vitreous are important in the treatment of proliferative vitreoretinopathy (67) and endophthalmitis (68). The rabbit is the most commonly used animal model for vitreous kinetics.

Intravitreal drugs may eliminate across the blood-retinal barrier and via the anterior chamber (e.g., penicillins) or only via the anterior route (e.g., gentamicin) (24). Anterior elimination is preferred, because it will provide more homogeneous drug distribution in the vitreous and longer half-life (24). The existing data do not allow firm conclusions about the validity of the rabbit as an animal model. However, there are similarities in the posterior segment kinetics of fluorescein in humans and rabbits (69). Owing to the larger size of the human eye and more tight anterior path for drug elimination, longer half-lives for intravitreal drugs are expected in humans (24).

The rabbit is also a commonly used model for the aphakic vitrectomized eye (68). In this case, the rapid drug elimination from the vitreous is a problem. The pharmacokinetics of aphakic vitrectomized human and rabbit eyes have not been compared.

D. Drug Metabolism

In the case of drugs susceptible to enzymatic degradation, interspecies differences may cause differences in the ocular pharmacokinetics. The ocular tissues of the rabbit contain, e.g., acetyl cholinesterase (70), butyryl cholinesterase (70), carboxyl cholinesterase (70), catechol-O-methyl transferase (71), monoamine oxidase (71), N-acetyl transferase (72), aryl hydrocarbon hydroxylase (73), and aminopeptidases (74). It has been shown that the esterase activities in the cornea and iris-ciliary body vary considerably depending on the age and race (New Zealand white or pigmented) of the rabbits (75,76). Pigmented and older rabbits have higher esterase activities in ocular tissues (75). Consequently, the choice between albino and pigmented rabbits has great impact on the results of ocular pharmacokinetic studies. This is the case for pilocarpine (76,77) and ester prodrugs (78,79).

The enzyme activities of the human ocular tissues are not known as well as in the rabbit. It is known, however, that esterase activity in human corneal epithelium, corneal stroma, and iris-ciliary body is 1.6–4.2-fold compared with New Zealand white rabbits and it is also greater than the esterase activity in the ocular tissues of pigmented rabbits (9). Esterase activity in human eyes is also evidenced by the efficacy of the ester prodrugs of epinephrine and nadolol in human eyes (79). These drugs must be cleaved by the esterases and release the parent drug to be active.

E. Pharmacodynamic-Kinetic Studies

Pharmacodynamic responses are often used as a bioassay to compare the concentration profiles of the ocularly applied drugs in the eyes of rabbits (65) or humans (5). Usually, this approach is used when the drug response is easily quantitated, as in the case of miosis (65,80) and mydriasis (80,81).

Sometimes the responses are compared per se (25,35). It must be remembered, however, that drug responses are not linearly related to the drug concentrations in the aqueous humor or anterior uvea (5,82,83). Receptor-mediated drug response is always a saturable process which is a function of drug concentration (82,83). Maurice and Mishima (5,24) have developed equations relative to miotic, mydriatic, and cycloplegic drug responses to the eye. These equations relate the response to the maximum attainable effect by the drug and to the initial situation. This approach has been used, for example, in the cases of pilocarpine (23,65) and tropicamide (80,84). The calculation gives a closer estimate of the shape of the concentration profile and allows determination of the apparent absorption and elimination coefficients but it does not provide the actual concentrations. The actual in vivo drug concentrations have not been compared with corresponding drug responses until recently when Chien and Schoenwald (83) correlated the phenylephrine concentrations in the rabbit aqueous humor to the mydriasis. Interestingly, the concentration-response relationship changed during the time course of drug distribution after a single dose. This indicates a changing responsiveness of the system.

To some extent ocular pharmacokinetics of miotics and mydriatics can be followed in rabbits and humans by observing drug responses. Especially for screening purposes and for comparisons between dosage forms, it is a very useful approach that can save the lives of many laboratory animals. However, the actual concentration versus drug response relationship in the living eye is not known for most drugs.

F.   Role of Systemic Circulation

Systemic absorption of ocularly applied drugs has gained increased attention owing to the systemic side effects of ophthalmic drugs (85,86). This is a concern especially in children (87). The systemic absorption of ocularly applied drugs in humans can be quantitated only if sensitive enough analytical methods are available. This is not always the case, and the rabbit is the most commonly used animal model for the studies of the systemic absorption of ocularly applied drugs.

The systemic absorption of the ocularly applied drug takes place mostly from the conjunctiva of the eye and nasal mucosa (88,89). The nasal mucosa is highly permeable in both species, as indicated by the very high systemic bioavailabilities of nasally administered drugs (90–92). In rabbits, typically 50–100% of the ocularly instilled dose is absorbed to the systemic circulation (88,89), whereas only few percent is absorbed to the eye (9,24).

The lacrimal sac has an important indirect role in the systemic drug absorption in humans, because it regulates the solution transit to the nose (18,26,93). In the case of solution overflow from the lacrimal sac, the solution is drained to the nasal cavity (18,26,93). The access of the ocularly instilled solutions to the nose and, consequently, their systemic absorption vary substantially with instilled solution volume, position, and blinking (26,94). Owing to the small lacrimal sac (13) and the low blinking frequency (24), the variability in the ocular surface to nose transit times is expected to be less in rabbits than in humans.

In spite of the anatomical and physiological differences, the rabbit is a reasonable model for systemic absorption studies of ocularly applied drugs. In both species (88,89, 94–96), ophthalmic drugs are rapidly absorbed to the systemic circulation, as suggested by the early times of peak drug concentrations. The systemic bioavailabilities of ophthalmic drugs in humans, however, are not known because no comparisons to intravenous administration have been made.

Also, in ocular absorption studies, the major portion of the instilled dose may be absorbed to the systemic circulation from the conjunctiva and nose of the rabbit. Although the exchange of the solutes between the systemic circulation and ocular tissues is limited by the blood-aqueous and blood-vitreous barriers (24), a small part of the drug in plasma may gain access to the ocular tissues. Consequently, it is often recommended that in ocular absorption studies eye drops should be administered only unilaterally to the rabbit (9). In this way the systemic drug load and systemic entry of drug to the eyes is minimized but the need for rabbits is doubled.

Owing to the smaller body size of rabbits, the systemic entry of ocularly applied drugs to the eyes is probably greater in rabbits than in humans. Timolol concentrations in the untreated rabbit eye were 1–10% of those in the treated eye (61). Thus, the error in ocular absorption studies due to the ocular drug distribution via systemic circulation is not necessarily significant.

For intravenously given antibiotics, the drug concentrations in the aqueous humor are typically 5–20% of the concentrations in plasma at steady-state both in rabbits and in humans (24). The rabbit appears to be an adequate model for drug penetration from the systemic circulation to the eye.

G. Conclusions

Recognizing the complexity of the ocular pharmacokinetics, it is obvious that the resulting drug concentrations after eye drop administration are affected by several factors. Drug concentrations in the aqueous humor of the human and rabbit eye were compared only in few cases: pilocarpine (97), prednisolone acetate (98), timolol (99,100), fluorescein (1,24), gentamicin (4,101,102), and chloramphenicol (103,104). In most of these cases, the drug concentrations in the human aqueous humor were similar or lower than in the rabbit. Nevertheless, the lower concentrations were in the same range in both species. Substantial concentration differences were observed in cases of gentamicin and chloramphenicol (24). The occurrence of smaller concentrations in human eyes is probably due to the faster preocular clearance.

In most cases, the conscious rabbit is a reasonable model for ocular pharmacokinetic studies. It is important, however, to know its limitations as a model of the human eye.

III. ANESTHETIZED RABBIT AS AN ANIMAL MODEL

Anesthetized rabbits are used frequently in ocular pharmacokinetic studies because many experimental procedures require general anesthesia. These procedures include, for example, steady perfusion of the cornea or conjunctiva with a drug solution through a cylinder that is attached to the conjunctival surface surrounding the rabbit cornea (8,105,106). This method allows the utilization of the steady-state kinetic equations that are simpler to use than the equations for non–steady-state conditions (106). Also, intracameral injections of drugs in the determination of ocular volume of drug distribution require general anesthesia (48), as well as the continuous sampling of drug from the vitreous with a microdialysis probe (107). It is important to realize, however, that general anesthesia interferes with many factors that may be important in ocular pharmacokinetics.

Instilled eye drops are drained from the unanesthetized ocular surface faster than from the anesthetized eye (28). Both induced lacrimation and normal tear turnover are suppressed in anesthetized rabbits (16,28). This led to the increased ocular absorption of fluorometholone (108), pilocarpine (28), and ethoxzolamide (29). General anesthesia increases the ocular bioavailability and this should be taken into account when the results are scaled to the human eye. In contrast, the systemic absorption of ocularly applied timolol was not affected by the general anesthesia (90).

General anesthesia may also affect many intraocular physiological factors in humans and laboratory animals. A more extensive list of the related literature has been compiled by Bartels (30). The factors influenced include the rate of aqueous humor formation and intraocular pressure. The effects of anesthetics are not always similar: Barbiturates and halothane decrease the intraocular pressure in animals and humans (30), whereas ketamine increases it in rabbits (29). The new veterinary sedative medetomidine (109,110) decreases intraocular pressure, presumably by its alpha$_2$-receptor–stimulating activity (111).

The effects of these intraocular effects on intraocular pharmacokinetics are not known. It is known, however, that anesthesia may influence drug responses. Despite the increased ethoxzolamide levels in the anesthetized rabbits, ketamine abolished the intraocular pressure–decreasing activity of the drug (29).

IV. OTHER ANIMAL MODELS

Although several different animal species are used in ocular drug-response studies, animals other than rabbits have been rarely used in ocular pharmacokinetic experiments.

Camber (112) has used pig corneas in drug permeability studies. However, the pig is a more suitable animal model for in vitro than in vivo experiments.

Monkeys have been occasionally used in ocular pharmacokinetic studies (113–115). The expense of these animals prohibits their wider use. As an animal model for noninvasive drug response studies, the monkey is a suitable model.

Other possible animals for ocular pharmacokinetic studies include cats, dogs, rats, and mice. The eyes of small rodents are too small for testing of different delivery systems, whereas dogs and cats might be too expensive for invasive ocular pharmacokinetic studies.

REFERENCES

1. Adler, C. A., Maurice, D. M., and Paterson, T. M. (1971). The effect of viscosity of the vehicle on the penetration of fluorescein into the human eye, *Exp. Eye Res., 11*:34.
2. Nagataki, S. (1975). Human aqueous humor dynamics, *Jpn. J. Ophthalmol., 19*:235.
3. Trueblood, J. H., Rossomondo, R. M., Carlton, W. H., and Wilson, L. A. (1975). Corneal contact times of ophthalmic vehicles, *Arch. Ophthalmol., 93*:127.
4. Utermann, D., Matz, K., and Meyer, K. (1977). Gentamicinspiegel in Kammerwasser des Menschen nach parenteralen, subkonjunktivaler und lokaler Applikation, *Klin. Monatsbl. Augenheilk., 171*:579.
5. Mishima, S. (1981). Clinical pharmacokinetics of the eye, *Invest. Ophthalmol. Vis. Sci., 21*:504.
6. Tang-Liu, D. D. S., and Burke, P. J. (1988). The effect of azone on ocular levobunolol absorption: Calculating the area under the curve and its standard error using tissue sampling compartments, *Pharm. Res., 5*:238.
7. Lee, V. H. L., and Robinson, J. R. (1979). Mechanistic and quantitative evaluation of precorneal pilocarpine disposition in albino rabbits, *J. Pharm. Sci., 68*:673.
8. Ahmed, I., and Patton, T. F. (1987). Disposition of timolol and inulin in the rabbit eye following corneal versus non-corneal absorption, *Int. J. Pharm., 38*:9.
9. Lee, V. H. L., and Robinson, J. R. (1986). Topical ocular drug delivery: Recent developments and future challenges, *J. Ocul. Pharmacol., 2*:67.
10. Mikkelson, T. J., Chrai, S. S., and Robinson, J. R. (1973). Altered bioavailability of drugs in the eye due to drug-protein interactions, *J. Pharm. Sci., 62*:1648.

11. Mishima, S., Gasset, A., Klyce, S., and Baum, J. (1966). Determination of tear volume and tear flow, *Invest. Ophthalmol., 5*:264.
12. Chrai, S. S., Patton, T. F., Mehta, A., and Robinson, J. R. (1973). Lacrimal and instilled fluid dynamics in rabbit eyes, *J. Pharm. Sci., 62*:1112.
13. Prince, J. H. (1964). *The Rabbit in Eye Research*, Charles C Thomas, Springfield, Illinois.
14. Ahmed, I., and Patton, T. F. (1984). Effect of pH and buffer on the precorneal disposition and ocular penetration of pilocarpine, *Int. J. Pharm., 19*:215.
15. Carney, L. G., and Hill, R. M. (1979). Human tear buffering capacity, *Arch. Ophthalmol., 97*:951.
16. Longwell, A., Birss, S., Keller, N., and Moore, D. (1976). Effect of topically applied pilocarpine on tear film pH, *J. Pharm. Sci., 65*:1654.
17. Mitra, A. K., and Mikkelson, T. J. (1982). Ophthalmic solution buffer systems. I. The effect of buffer concentration on the ocular absorption of pilocarpine, *Int. J. Pharm., 10*:219.
18. Hurwitz, J. J., Maisey, M. N., and Welham, R. A. N. (1975). Quantitative lacrimal scintillography. I. Method and physiological application, *Br. J. Ophthalmol., 59*:308.
19. Lutosky, S., and Maurice, D. M. (1986). Absorption of tears by the nasolacrimal system, In: *The Preocular Tear Film in Health, Disease, and Contact Lens Wear* (F. J. Holly, ed.), Dry Eye Institute, Lubbock, Texas, Chapt. 59.
20. Sorensen, T. B. (1984). Studies on tear physiology, pathophysiology and contact lenses by means of dynamic gamma camera and technetium, *Acta Ophthalmol., 167*(Suppl.):1.
21. Zaki, I., Fitzgerald, P., Hardy, J. G., and Wilson, C. G. (1986). A comparison of the effect of viscosity on the precorneal residence of solutions in rabbit and man, *J. Pharm. Pharmacol., 38*:463.
22. Chrai, S. S., Makoid, M. C., Eriksen, S. P., and Robinson, J. R. (1974). Drop size and initial dosing frequency problems of topically applied drugs, *J. Pharm. Sci., 63*:333.
23. Sugaya, M., and Nagataki, S. (1978). Kinetics of topical pilocarpine in the human eye, *Jpn. J. Ophthalmol., 22*:127.
24. Maurice, D. M., and Mishima, S. (1984). Ocular pharmacokinetics. *In: Handbook of Experimental Pharmacology vol. 69, Pharmacology of the Eye* (M. L. Sears, ed.), Springer-Verlag, Berlin-Heidelberg, p. 19.
25. Saettone, M. F., Giannaccini, B., Barattini, F., and Tellini, N. (1982), The validity of rabbits for investigations on ophthalmic vehicles: A comparison of four different vehicles containing tropicamide in humans and rabbits, *Pharm. Acta Helv., 57*:47.
26. Chavis, R. M., Welham, R. A. N., and Maisey, M. N. (1978). Quantitative lacrimal scintillography, *Arch. Ophthalmol., 96*:2066.
27. Birss, S. A., Longwell, A., Heckbert, S., and Keller, N. (1978). Ocular hypotensive efficacy of topical epinephrine in normotensive and hypertensive rabbits: Continuous drug delivery vs eyedrops, *Ann. Ophthalmol., 10*:1045.
28. Patton, T. F., and Robinson, J. R. (1976). Quantitative precorneal disposition of topically applied pilocarpine nitrate in rabbit eyes, *J. Pharm. Sci., 65*:1295.
29. Bar-Ilan, A., and Pessah, N. I. (1986). On the use of ketamine in ocular pharmacological studies, *J. Ocul. Pharmacol., 2*:335.
30. Bartels, S. P. (1984). Animal models useful in drug testing. *In: Glaucoma: Applied Pharmacology in Medical Treatment* (S. M. Drance and A. H. Neufeld, eds.). Grune & Stratton, Orlando, Florida, pp. 215–233.
31. Urtti, A., Sendo, T., Pipkin, J. D., Rork, G., and Repta, A. (1988). Application site dependent ocular absorption of timolol. *J. Ocul. Pharmacol., 4*:335.
32. DeSantis, L. M., and Schoenwald, R. D. (1978). Lack of influence of rabbit nictitating membrane on miosis effect of pilocarpine, *J. Pharm. Sci., 67*:1189.
33. Urtti, A., Pipkin, J. D., Rork, G., Sendo, T., Finne, U., and Repta, A. (1990). Controlled drug delivery devices for experimental ocular studies with timolol. 2. Ocular and systemic absorption in rabbits. *Int. J. Pharm., 61*:241.

34. Watsky, M. A., Jablonski, M., and Edelhauser, H. F. (1988). Comparison of conjunctival and corneal surface areas in rabbit and human, *Curr. Eye Res., 7*:483.

35. Saettone, M. F., Giannaccini, B., Teneggi, A., Savigni, P., and Tellini, N. (1982). Vehicle effects on ophthalmic bioavailability: the influence of different polymers on the activity of pilocarpine in rabbit and man, *J. Pharm. Pharmacol., 34*:464.

36. Saettone, M. F., Giannaccini, B., Ravecca, S., LaMarca, F., and Tota, G. (1984). Polymer effects on ocular bioavailability: the influence of different polymers on the activity of pilocarpine in rabbit and man, *Int. J. Pharm., 20*:187.

37. Benedetto, D. A., Shah, D. O., and Kaufman, H. E. (1975). The instilled fluid dynamics and surface chemistry of polymers in the preocular tear film, *Invest. Ophthalmol., 14*:887.

38. Saettone, M. F., Giannaccini, B., Guiducci, A., and Savigni, P. (1986). Semisolid ophthalmic vehicles. III. An evaluation of four organic hydrogels containing pilocarpine, *Int. J. Pharm., 31*:261.

39. Urtti, A., Periviita, L., Salminen, L., and Juslin, M. (1985). Effects of hydrophilicity of polymer matrix on in vitro release rate of pilocarpine and on its miotic activity in rabbit eyes, *Drug Dev. Ind. Pharm., 11*:257.

40. Maurice, D. M. (1955). Influence on corneal permeability of bathing solutions of differing reaction and tonicity, *Br. J. Ophthalmol., 39*:463.

41. Schoenwald, R. D., and Houseman, J. A. (1982). Disposition of cyclophosphamide in the rabbit and human cornea. *Biopharm. Drug Dispos., 3*:231.

42. Edelhauser, H. F., and Maren, T. H. (1988). Permeability of human cornea and sclera to sulfonamide carbonic anhydrase inhibitors, *Arch. Ophthalmol., 106*:1110.

43. Wolff, E. (1971). *The Anatomy of the Eye and Orbit*, 3rd ed. Blakiston, Philadelphia.

44. Francouer, M., Ahmed, I., Sitek, S., and Patton, T. F. (1983). Age-related differences in ophthalmic drug disposition III. Corneal permeability of pilocarpine in rabbits, *Int. J. Pharm., 16*:203.

45. Ahmed, I., Gokhale, R. D., Shah, M. V., and Patton, T. F. (1987). Physicochemical determinants of drug diffusion across the conjunctiva, sclera and cornea, *J. Pharm. Sci., 76*:583.

46. Conrad, J. M., and Robinson, J. R. (1980). Mechanisms of anterior segment absorption of pilocarpine following subconjunctival injection in albino rabbits, *J. Pharm. Sci., 69*:875.

47. Maurice, D. M., and Ota, Y. (1978). The kinetics of subconjunctival injections, *Jpn. J. Ophthalmol., 22*:95.

48. Conrad, J. M., and Robinson, J. R. (1977). Aqueous chamber distribution volume measurement in rabbits, *J. Pharm. Sci., 66*:219.

49. Brubaker, R. (1984). The physiology of the aqueous humor formation. In: *Glaucoma: Applied Pharmacology in the Medical Treatment* (S. M. Drance and A. H. Neufeld, eds.). Grune & Stratton, Orlando, Florida, p. 35.

50. Bill, A. (1966). The routes for bulk drainage of aqueous humor in rabbits with and without cyclodialysis, *Doc. Ophthalmol., 20*:157.

51. Bill, A. (1971). Aqueous humor dynamics in monkeys (Macaca irus and Cerephopithecus ethiops), *Exp. Eye Res., 11*:195.

52. Bill, A., and Phillips, C. I. (1971). Uveoscleral drainage of aqueous humor in human eyes, *Exp. Eye Res., 12*:275.

53. Schoenwald, R. D. (1990). Ocular drug delivery. Pharmacokinetic considerations, *Clin. Pharmacokinet., 18*:255.

54. Chiang, C. H., and Schoenwald, R. D. (1986). Ocular pharmacokinetic models of clonidine-^{3}H hydrochloride. *J. Pharmacokinet. Biopharm., 14*:175.

55. Tang-Liu, D. D. S., and Liu, S. (1987). Relationship between the ocular and systemic disposition of flurbiprofen: The effect of altered protein dynamics at steady state. *J. Pharmacokinet. Biopharm., 15*:387.

56. Miller, S. C., Himmelstein, K., and Patton, T. F. (1981). A physiologically based pharmacokinetic model for the intraocular distribution of pilocarpine in rabbits, *J. Pharmacokinet. Biopharm., 9*:653.

57. Raviola, G. (1977). The structural basis of the blood-ocular barriers. The ocular and cerebrospinal fluids. *Exp. Eye Res., 25*:27.

58. Gregersen, W. (1958). The tissue spaces in the human iris and their communication with the anterior chamber by way of iridic crypts, *Acta Ophthalmol., 36*:819.

59. Kaufman, P. L., Wiedman, T., and Robinson, J. R. (1984). Cholinergics. In: *Handbook of Experimental Pharmacology, Vol. 69, Pharmacology of the Eye* (M. L. Sears, ed.), Springer-Verlag, Berlin-Heidelberg, p. 149.

60. Salazar, M., and Patil, P. N. (1976). An explanation for the long duration of the mydriatic effect of atropine in eye, *Invest. Ophthalmol., 15*:671.

61. Salminen, L., and Urtti, A. (1984). Disposition of ophthalmic timolol in treated and untreated rabbit eyes, *Exp. Eye Res., 38*:203.

62. Araie, M., Takase, M., Sakai, Y., Ishii, Y., Yokoyama, Y., and Kitagawa, M. (1982). Beta-adrenergic blockers: Ocular penetration and binding to the uveal pigment, *Jpn. J. Ophthalmol., 26*:248.

63. Lee, V. H. L., and Robinson, J. R. (1982). Disposition of pilocarpine in pigmented rabbit eye, *Int. J. Pharm., 11*:155.

64. Salminen, L., Urtti, A., and Periviita, L. (1984). Effect of ocular pigmentation on pilocarpine pharmacology in the rabbit eye. I. Drug distribution and metabolism, *Int. J. Pharm., 18*:17.

65. Urtti, A., Salminen, L., Kujari, H., and Jäntti, V. (1985). Effect of ocular pigmentation on pilocarpine pharmacology in the rabbit eye. II. Drug response, *Int. J. Pharm., 19*:53.

66. Katz, I. M., and Berger, E. T. (1979). Effects of iris pigmentation on response of ocular pressure to timolol, *Surv. Ophthalmol., 23*:395.

67. Stern, W. H., Heath, T. D., Lewis, G. P., Guerin, C. J., Ericksson, P. A., Lopez, N. G., and Hong, K. (1987). Clearance and localization of intravitreal liposomes in the aphakic vitrectomized eye, *Invest. Ophthalmol. Vis. Sci., 28*:907.

68. Wingard, L. B., Zuravlev, J. J., Doft, B. H., Berk, B. H., and Rinkoff, J. (1989). Intraocular distribution of intravitreally administered amphotericin B in normal and vitrectomized eyes, *Invest. Ophthalmol. Vis. Sci., 30*:2184.

69. Cunha-Vaz, J. G., and Maurice, D. M. (1969). Fluorescein dynamics in the eye, *Doc. Ophthalmol., 26*:61.

70. Lee, V. H. L., Chang, S. C., Oshiro, C. M., and Smith, R. E. (1985). Ocular esterase composition in albino and pigmented rabbits: Possible implications on ocular prodrug design and evaluation, *Curr. Eye Res., 4*:1117.

71. Waltman, S., and Sears, M. L. (1964). Catechol-O-methyl transferase and monoamine oxidase activity in the ocular tissues of albino rabbits, *Invest. Ophthalmol., 3*:601.

72. Schoenwald, R. D., Campbell, D., Barfknecht, C., and Duffel, M. (1988). Acetylation of arylamines in ocular tissue homogenates of fast and slow acetylating rabbits, *Invest. Ophthalmol. Vis. Sci., 29*:438.

73. Shichi, H. (1984). Biotransformation and drug metabolism, In: *Handbook of Experimental Pharmacology*, Vol. 69, *Pharmacology of the Eye* (M. L. Sears, ed.), Springer-Verlag, Berlin-Heidelberg, p. 117.

74. Stratford, R. E., and Lee, V. H. L. (1985). Ocular aminopeptidase activity and distribution in the albino rabbit, *Curr. Eye Res., 4*:995.

75. Lee, V. H. L., Stratford, R. E., and Morimoto, K. W. (1983). Age-related changes in esterase activity in rabbit eyes, *Int. J. Pharm., 13*:183.

76. Lee, V. H. L., Hui, H. W., and Robinson, J. R. (1980). Corneal metabolism in pigmented rabbits, *Invest. Ophthalmol. Vis. Sci., 19*:210.

77. Sendelbeck, L., Moore, D., and Urquhart, J. (1975). Comparative distribution of pilocarpine in ocular tissues of the rabbit during administration by eyedrop and by membrane-controlled delivery systems, *Am. J. Ophthalmol., 80*:274.

78. Redell, M. A., Yang, D., and Lee, V. H. L. (1983). The role of esterase activity in the ocular disposition of dipivalyl epinephrine in rabbits. *Int. J. Pharm., 17*:299.

79. Lee, V. H. L., and Li, V. H. K. (1989). Prodrugs for improved ocular drug delivery, *Adv. Drug. Deliv. Rev., 3*:1.

80. Yoshida, S., and Mishima, S. (1975). A pharmacokinetic analysis of the pupil response to topical pilocarpine and tropicamide, *Jpn. J. Ophthalmol., 19*:121.

81. Schoenwald, R. D., and Smolen, V. F. (1971). Drug absorption analysis from pharmacologic data. II. Transcorneal biophasic availability of tropicamide, *J. Pharm. Sci., 60*:1039.

82. Wagner, J. G. (1968). Kinetics of pharmacologic response. I. Proposed relationships between response and drug concentration in intact animal and man, *J. Theoret. Biol., 20*:173.

83. Chien, D., and Schoenwald, R. D. (1990). Ocular pharmacokinetics and pharmacodynamics of phenylephrine and phenylephrine oxazolidine in rabbit eyes, *Pharm. Res., 7*:476.

84. Yoshida, S. (1976). Analysis of cycloplegic response to topical tropicamide, *Folia. Ophthalmol. Jpn., 11*:1009.

85. Salminen, L., and Huupponen, R. (1989). Systemic effects of ocular drugs. *Adv. Drug React. Acute Poison. Rev., 8*:89.

86. Munroe, W. P., Rindone, J. P., and Kershner, R. M. (1985). Systemic side effects associated with the ophthalmic administration of timolol, *Drug. Intell. Clin. Pharm., 19*:85.

87. Palmer, E. A. (1982). Drug toxicity in pediatric ophthalmology, *J. Toxicol. Cutan. Ocul. Toxicol., 1*:181.

88. Urtti, A., Salminen, L., and Miinalainen, O. (1985). Systemic absorption of pilocarpine is modified by polymer matrices, *Int. J. Pharm., 23*:147.

89. Chang, S. C., and Lee, V. H. L. (1987). Nasal and conjunctival contributions to the systemic absorption of topical timolol in the pigmented rabbit: Implications in the design of strategies to maximize the ratio of ocular to systemic absorption, *J. Ocul. Pharmacol., 3*:159.

90. Chang, S. C. (1987). Ph.D. Thesis, School of Pharmacy, University of Southern California, Los Angeles.

91. Hussain, A. A., Foster, T., and Hirai, S. (1981). Nasal absorption of propranolol in humans, *J. Pharm. Sci., 78*:1240.

92. McMahon, C., Hutchinson, L. E. F., and Hyde, R. (1987). Analysis of structural requirements for the absorption of drugs and macromolecules from the nasal cavity, *J. Pharm. Sci., 76*:535.

93. Amant, L. A., Hilditch, T. E., and Kwok, C. S. (1983). Lacrimal scintigraphy. III. Physiological aspects of lacrimal drainage, *Br. J. Ophthalmol., 67*:729.

94. Kaila, T., Huupponen, R., and Salminen, L. (1986). Effects of eyelid closure and nasolacrimal duct occlusion on the systemic absorption of ocular timolol in human subjects, *J. Ocul. Pharmacol., 2*:365.

95. Lahdes, K., Kaila, T., Huupponen, R., Salminen, L., and Iisalo, P. (1988). Systemic absorption of topically applied ocular atropine, *Clin. Pharmacol. Ther., 44*:310.

96. Kaila, T., Huupponen, R., Salminen, L., and Iisalo, E. (1989). Systemic absorption of ophthalmic cyclopentolate, *Am. J. Ophthalmol., 107*:562.

97. Krohn, D. L., and Breitfeller, J. M. (1979). Transcorneal flux of topical pilocarpine to the human aqueous, *Am. J. Ophthalmol., 87*:50.

98. Leibowitz, H. M., Berrospi, A. R., Kupferman, A., Restropo, G. V., and Galvis, V. (1977). Penetration of topically administered prednisolone acetate into the human aqueous humor, *Am. J. Ophthalmol., 83*:402.

99. Phillips, C. I., Bartholomew, R. S., Levy, A. M., Grave, J., and Vogel, R. (1985). Penetration of timolol eye drops into human aqueous humor: The first hour, *Br. J. Ophthalmol., 69*:217.

100. Schmitt, C. J., Lotti, V. J., and LeDouarec, J. C. (1980). Penetration of timolol into the rabbit eye, *Arch. Ophthalmol., 98*:547.

101. Bloomfield, S. E., Miyata, T., Dunn, M. W., Bueser, N., Stenzel, K. H., and Rubin, A. L. (1978). Soluble gentamycin ocular inserts as a drug delivery system, *Arch. Ophthalmol., 96*:885.

102. Ellerhorst, B., Golden, B., and Nabil, J. (1975). Ocular penetration of topically applied gentamycin, *Arch. Ophthalmol., 93*:371.

103. Beasley, H., Boltralik, J. J., and Baldwin, H. A. (1975). Chloramphenicol in aqueous humor after topical applications, *Arch. Ophthalmol., 93*:184.

104. Leopold, I., Nichols, A., and Vogel, A. W. (1950). Penetration of chloramphenicol USP into the eye, *Arch. Ophthalmol., 44*:22.

105. Doane, M. G., Jensen, A. D., and Dohlman, C. H. (1978). Penetration routes of topically applied eye medications, *Am. J. Ophthalmol., 85*:383.

106. Eller, M. G., Schoenwald, R. D., Dixson, J. A., Segarra, T., and Barfknecht, C. F. (1985). Topical carbonic anhydrase inhibitors III. Optimization model for corneal penetration of ethoxzolamide analogues, *J. Pharm. Sci., 74*:155.

107. Ben-Nun, J., Joyce, D. A., Cooper, R. L., Cringle, S. C., and Constable, I. J. (1989). Pharmacokinetics of intravitreal injection: assessment of a gentamycin model by ocular dialysis, *Invest. Ophthalmol. Vis. Sci., 30*:1055.

108. Sieg, J. W., and Robinson, J. R. (1974). Corneal absorption of fluorometholone in rabbits, *Arch. Ophthalmol., 92*:240.

109. Nevalainen, T., Pyhälä, L., Voipio, H. M., and Virtanen, R. (1989). Evaluation of anesthetic potency of medetomidine-ketamine combination in rats, guinea-pigs and rabbits, *Acta Vet. Scand., 85*:139.

110. Jalanka, H., Skutnabb, K., and Damsten, Y. (1989). Preliminary results on the use of medetomidine-ketamine combinations in the dog, *Acta Vet. Scand., 85*:125.

111. Reiman, J., Rouhiainen, H., Urtti, A., MacDonald, E., and Virtanen, R. (1990). Dexmedetomidine decreases intraocular pressure in normal and laser-induced glaucoma rabbits. 9th International Congress of Eye Research, Helsinki, Finland, abstract 732.

112. Camber, O. (1985). An in vitro model for determination of drug permeability through the cornea, *Acta Pharm. Suec., 22*:335.

113. Öhman, L., Edqvist, L., and Johansson, E. D. B. (1982). Absorption of topically applied hydrocortisone from the eye of the Rhesus monkey, *Acta Ophthalmol., 60*:106.

114. Barza, M., Kane, A., and Baum, J. (1978). Intraocular penetration of gentamycin after subconjunctival and retrobulbar injections, *Am. J. Ophthalmol., 85*:541.

115. Barza, M., Kane, A., and Baum, J. (1983). Pharmacokinetics of intravitreal carbenicillin, cefazolin, and gentamycin in rhesus monkeys, *Invest. Ophthalmol. Vis. Sci., 24*:1602.

7
Disease State Models

Lotta Salminen   *Tampere University Hospital, Tampere, Finland*

Arto Urtti   *University of Kuopio, Kuopio, Finland*

I. INTRODUCTION

Animal disease state models of human ocular diseases are an integral component of experimental vision research. Major advances in the ability to prevent, diagnose, and treat diseases of the eye during the last 2 decades have been possible owing to animal studies. Adequate care and humane treatment of laboratory animals are major concerns of the visual science community (see ARVO Resolution on the Use of Animals in Research), and alternatives to animal experimentation are sought continuously. However, animal research will of necessity continue to be of vital importance in the struggle against human blindness.

The induction and clinical follow-up of animal disease state models require basic ophthalmological knowledge and skills such as the use of the slit-lamp, ophthalmoscope, and tonometer. For an interested reader, several excellent textbooks on general ophthalmology and ocular pathology are available (e.g., see Refs. 1–3). Although animal disease state models have not been reviewed in detail, an abundant source of biochemical background on animal models of eye inflammation, corneal wound healing, cataract, and retinal degenerations are offered by two recent publications (4,5).

The topics selected to this chapter represent only a fraction of the total number of animal disease state models presented in the literature. The major part of this chapter is based on recent studies presented in major visual science journals, thus representing an overview of the currently used animal disease state models. Since a complete and detailed discussion of this vast field is beyond the scope of this text on ophthalmic drug delivery, the interested readers are encouraged to use the reference list in search for more in-depth information on induction, follow-up, and histological, cell biological, ultrastructural, immunocytochemical, biochemical, or genetic data of the disease state models.

II. CONJUNCTIVAL INFECTION AND INFLAMMATION

A. Bacterial, Viral, Chlamydial, and Parasitic Infections

In the guinea pig eye, a topically applied suspension of *Salmonella typhimurium* induced moderate to severe keratoconjunctivitis which resembled the keratitis of Reiter's syndrome

(6). A rabbit enterovirus 70 (EV70) model infection after topical application of EV70 closely mimicked human enteroviral conjunctivitis (7). An animal model of trachoma has been developed in cynomolgus monkeys by repeated ocular infections of *Chlamydia trachomatis* (8). A less expensive and for most laboratories a more easily accessible model was established in guinea pigs using conjunctival pockets under the abdominal skin; the pockets were infected with a *Chlamydia psittaci* strain (9). Chlamydial conjunctivitis in Hartley strain guinea pigs after ocular inoculation of *C. psittaci* was used to study the prophylactic effects of silver nitrate and erythromycin on chlamydial conjunctivitis. Silver nitrate did not have any prophylactic effect on the development of chlamydial conjunctivitis but erythromycin ointment prophylaxis 1 h or 2 h after inoculation with *C. psittaci* was statistically superior to placebo (10). *Toxoplasma gondii* parasites were inoculated onto the conjunctival epithelium of the guinea pig. The guinea pig conjunctiva was regarded as a suitable tissue for studying the pathogenesis of toxoplasmosis (11).

B. Allergic Conjunctivitis

The most predominant inflammatory reactions seen in the conjunctiva are of the allergic type. The animal models that have been developed demonstrate immediate and delayed hypersensitivity reactions (12).

Conjunctival inflammation has been induced in rabbits immunized with bovine serum albumin, and in sensitized guinea pigs by multiple topical administration of serum albumin (12,13). Delayed hypersensitivity reactions have been induced in the conjunctiva of guinea pigs sensitized with the intradermal injection of oxazolone with either Freud's incomplete or complete adjuvant and in sensitized guinea pigs by dropping tuberculin into the conjunctival sac (12–14). An antibody-mediated cytotoxic conjunctivitis was induced in neonatal rabbits by local or systemic administration of a murine monoclonal antibody against the basement membrane of the stratified squamous epithelium (15). A model of vernal conjunctivitis and contact lens–associated giant papillary conjunctivitis was induced in immunized guinea pigs using keyhole limpet hemocyanin (16).

Conjunctivitis in immunized rabbits, guinea pigs, and rats and histamine-induced ocular hyperemia has been followed in the tests of anti-inflammatory drug effects. Continuous hydrocortisone administration by means of an experimental ocular therapeutic system was more effective than eye drops in treating experimental conjunctivitis; salbutamol and terbutaline reduced the conjunctival microvascular permeability response to histamine and experimental immediate hypersensitivity; a combination of cimetidine and pyrilamine blocked histamine-induced ocular hypersensitivity; pretreatment with 2-deoxy-D-glucose or a combination of isoproterenol and diethylcarbamazine inhibited the immediate hypersensitivity reaction in the guinea pig conjunctiva; and disodium cromoglycate produced a dose-dependent inhibitory effect on the anaphylactic reaction in rat conjunctiva sensitized with mouse monoclonal immunoglobulin E (IgE) (17–21). Since chemical and biochemical studies on conjunctivitis suggest that leukotriens may be of pathological significance, considerable effort has been undertaken to find molecules that could modify the action of leukotriens on the ocular surface. Studies on LTD4 receptor antagonists and leukotriene synthesis inhibitors in allergic conjunctivitis have been summarized by Chan (22).

III. DISORDERS OF MEIBOMIAN AND LACRIMAL GLANDS

Meibomian gland dysfunction was induced in albino rabbits by the twice daily topical application of 2% epinephrine over a period of 6 months to 1 year (23,24). Two rabbit models of keratoconjunctivitis sicca were carried out by closing the lacrimal gland excretory duct and removing the nictitating membrane and harderian gland or by closing the lacrimal gland excretory duct (25). A murine model of Sjögren's syndrome with lacrimal gland inflammation was developed in autoimmune mice (26).

IV. CORNEAL INFECTION AND INFLAMMATION

A. Bacterial Keratitis

Quantitative models of bacterial keratitis have been developed in rats, rabbits, and guinea pigs (27,28). Corneas have been inoculated by a number of bacteria, e.g., *Staphylococcus aureus, Pseudomonas aeruginosa*, or *Streptococcus pneumoniae* either by an intrastromal injection or by topical application of the infective material after scratching the cornea with, e.g., a 26-gauge hypodermic needle. The amount of bacteria received by the cornea during the procedure is generally known; infectivity, inflammation, and response to therapy can be observed using a standard Draize scale, and the number of viable bacteria and leukocytes per cornea can be analyzed at the end of the experiment (27).

In a rat bacterial keratitis model, groups of animals received topical antibiotics and prednisolone. Prednisolone did not influence the effects of antibiotics, but steroid treatment alone increased the pseudomonas count 20-fold above the count in untreated eyes. A 1% gentamicin sulfate medication proved effective against bacterial keratitis (27). Ketorolac appears to be an anti-inflammatory agent that dose not worsen bacterial infection in a *P. aeruginosa* keratitis model in rabbits (28). In a similar rabbit model, collagen shields immersed in tobramycin were effective in the treatment of *Pseudomonas* keratitis (29). In rabbits, the incidence of contact lens–associated *P. aeruginosa* keratitis was significantly higher in eyes that had undergone lid closure after the placement of *Pseudomonas*-contaminated lenses than in open eyes with contaminated lenses (30). The ocular infectivity of several *P. aeruginosa* strains and the pathogenicity of *Acanthamoeba* keratitis were studied in mice and rat models, respectively (31,32).

B. Fungal Keratitis

Like bacterial inoculations, *Candida albicans* isolates have been introduced into the corneal stroma of the rabbit to induce *Candida* keratitis (33,34). The efficacy of several concentrations of topical amphotericin and natamycin was examined in the model (33,34).

C. Viral Keratitis

For primary or recurrent herpes simplex virus (HSV) keratitis models, the rabbit is the preferred animal model but monkeys and mice are also used. To produce an acute primary infection of HSV in the cornea, two drops of HSV-1, e.g., McKrae strain virus suspension (105 platelet-forming units) (PFUs) were instilled into the eye. After the inoculation, the cornea was gently abraded or the lids were held shut and gently massaged for about 30 s. The animal eyes were examined by means of the slit-lamp biomicroscope daily after the inoculation and the severity of the herpetic keratitis was graded by fluorescein staining (35–37).

Therapy of primary HSV keratitis in rabbits with idoxuridine-releasing ocular inserts showed that an application rate of 30 mg/h gave significantly better results than conventional treatment with idoxuridine drops and ointment while exposing the eye to 40% less drug (35). Natural human leukocyte interferon and recombinant leukocyte A interferon were tested for prophylactic and for therapeutic effects in reducing the severity of keratitis in rabbit and monkey eye keratitis models infected with McKrae strain herpes virus. In the rabbit eye, combined prophylactic and therapeutic administration of natural interferon mitigated the disease, whereas recombinant interferon had no effect. In monkeys, the two interferons acted similarly: Combined prophylactic and therapeutic administration reduced disease symptoms, whereas therapeutic administration alone had no effect (36). In the treatment of murine herpetic keratitis, the antiherpetic effect of glycoprotein inhibitors alone or in combination with trifluoridine was not better than that of trifluridine (37). In a rabbit acute herpetic keratitis model, topical diclofenac did not exacerbate acute herpes keratitis. Diclofenac-treated eyes displayed less or at least no more severe disease than did the eyes treated with topical prednisolone or flurbiprofen and shedding of virus into tears was not prolonged (38). Acyclovir release from collagen discs on the mouse cornea infected with HSV-1 strain F by corneal scarification was 23% in the first minute after application; after that acyclovir clearance was exponential with a half-life of 21 min. Treatment given three times a day reduced HSV-1 titer in tear film, corneal tissue, and trigeminal ganglia (39).

In a rabbit and mice model of herpetic stromal keratitis, a viral suspension was injected into the corneal stroma; in some experiments the animals were presensitized subcutaneously with the virus (40–42). Topical trifluridine and vidarabine, when given early and frequently suppressed the stromal keratitis, indicating that viral replication was important in initiating the disease (40). The severity of stromal keratitis was significantly decreased in eyes treated with combined cyclosporine-trifluridine, whereas trifluridine alone had no effect on the stromal disease (41). In mice, topical flurbiprofen did not exacerbate HSV-1 stromal keratitis but has limited anti-inflammatory efficacy in the treatment of this disease (42).

After HSV inoculation, the primary acute dendritic keratitis develops within a few days and within some weeks the keratitis subsides and no corneal abnormalities are present. However, the initial ocular infection is followed by latency in the autonomic and sensory ganglia of the head and neck, and various stimuli, including administration of adrenergic agents like epinephrine, are known to cause reactivation of viral shedding in the preocular tear film and often clinically detectable disease.

Human interferons α and γ analogs in rabbits lessened the frequency of ocular shedding episodes by iontophoresis of 6-hydroxydopamine plus topical epinephrine treatment (43). Adenosine-5'-monophosphate did not reduce spontaneous or induced HSV-1 ocular shedding in latently infected rabbits with strain McKrae (44). Intravenous cyclophosphamide and dexamethasone induced HSV-1 ocular shedding and recurrent herpes simplex corneal lesions in the eyes of rabbits latently infected with HSV-1 strain McKrae. Shedding was unaffected by trifluridine after timolol iontophoresis (45,46). In primates, transcorneal iontophoresis of adrenergic agents was shown to produce HSV-1 shedding but repeated inoculations with HSV-1 and repeated intramuscular injections of prednisolone were required (47).

D. Corneal Inflammation

In a rabbit model, intracorneal injection of laboratory-grade clove oil (about 0.03 mL) induces an inflammatory keratitis which can be suppressed by topical prednisolone or suprofen (48,49). Corneal inflammation after intrastromal injection of human serum albumin and lipopolysaccharide into the rabbit cornea were suppressed by dietary fish oil or by the intravenous administration of hydroxyurea (50,51).

V. CORNEAL TRAUMA

A. Keratectomy Wounds and Epithelial Abrasions

A variety of experimental approaches have been used to elucidate biological and biochemical changes during corneal tissue repair. Rabbit corneal wounds of various size, shape, and depth have been made with trephines, the Graefe knife, and other surgical instruments (53). In the wound model, ketoprofen inhibited prostaglandin (PG) synthesis in the conjunctiva and iris-ciliary body but indomethacin was more effective in inhibiting PG synthesis in the conjunctiva (54). Ketorolac did not impair wound healing as determined by corneal tensile strength, whereas dexamethasone resulted in a significant impairment of wound healing (55). Epidermal growth factor enhanced the wound strength of full-thickness corneal wounds and accelerated the healing (56,57). Early epithelialization of a central scrape wound was decreased by topical nonsteroidal anti-inflammatory agents and prednisolone and enhanced by human epidermal growth factor (58,59). N-Heptanol and iodine vapor have been used for chemical débridement of corneal epithelium: topical retinoids, 5-fluorouracil, collagen shields, and beta adrenoceptors have been tested with this model (60–63).

B. Alkali Burns

Experimental alkali burns are produced by brief application of 2–4 N NaOH to the corneal surface. This results in immediate death of nearly all corneal cells, and although the epithelium ultimately regenerates, the cornea develops a sterile ulcer (5). The role of the plasminogen activator/plasmin system, systemic tetracycline treatment, epidermal growth factor, or ascorbate/citrate treatment, and a thiol peptide, which all inhibit corneal collagenase in vitro, have been tested in the rabbit alkali-induced corneal ulceration model (64–69). The clinical parameters of central corneal alkali burn injuries were standardized by applying five NaOH concentrations on uniformly soaked 7-mm filter paper discs to rabbits (70).

C. Thermal and Cryogenic Lesions

Healing of corneal ulceration after a thermal burn model in rabbits was decreased by ascorbic acid therapy. The corneal ulceration produced by a single 150°C-cautery application lasting 2 s was 4.5 mm in diameter and 2 mm from the corneoscleral limbus (71). In a cryodamage model, transcorneal freezing produced a 2-mm circular, central wound in the rabbit cornea; eicosanoid formation and corneal nerve changes were evaluated (72,73).

D. Corneal Edema and Endothelial Repair

Corneal edema was induced in guinea pigs and in rabbits by the intracorneal injection of phorbol myristate acetate or endotoxin and by contact lenses, respectively (74,75). After mechanical denudation of rabbit corneal endothelial cells, the healing process was followed by specular microscopy (76). Mild trauma was induced to rabbit corneal endothelial cells with a microglass tip and destruction of the central endothelium of the rat cornea was produced by mechanical injury, total débridement, or transcorneal freezing (77,78). One percent sodium hyaluronate protected in feline corneal endothelium against cell loss incurred by contact with intraocular lenses but not against cell loss incurred by penetrating keratoplasty (79).

E. Laser-Induced Trauma

A 193-nm excimer laser–induced corneal surface ablation and wound healing have been studied in rabbits. A 6-mm diameter area of the central rabbit cornea was ablated under various conditions of power, beam configuration, and exposure time. High repetition rates or prolonged exposures produced charring and prevented rapid epithelial wound closure (80). Dichlorotriazinyl aminofluorescein was used to dye the stromal bed after ablation (81).

F. Experimental Keratoplasty

Models of heterotopic full-thickness corneal transplantation in the rabbit, inbred mouse and rat, and orthotopic lamellar corneal transplantation in the inbred rat have been described (82,83). In the rabbit, allograft model cyclosporine in azone and cyclosporine containing collagen shields suppressed the rejection (84,85).

VI. CORNEAL NEOVASCULARIZATION

Neovascular growth into the cornea induced by silver nitrate cauterization was used in an experimental model to test potential anti-inflammatory drugs. Cauterization of the rat cornea with a silver nitrate applicator stick provided the stimulus for neovascularization, which was scored. For example, topical dexamethasone, prednisolone, and ketorolac lessened the severity and potentially damaging effects of the inflammation and neovascularization (86). Corneal neovascularization was reduced by photothrombic occlusion of neovascular vessels using intravenous rose bengal and argon laser irradiation (87). Heparin-cortisone pellets inhibited corneal vascularization in the rabbit in a surgical model (88). In the rabbit, endothelial cell–stimulating angiogenic factor from the human vitreous induced positive responses in the rabbit corneal pocket (89).

VII. CORNEAL CHANGES IN METABOLIC DISEASES

A. Diabetes Mellitus

In galactose-fed diabetic rats and dogs, aldose reductase inhibitors improved corneal epithelial healing and prevented corneal endothelial changes (90,91). In alloxan-induced diabetic rabbits, corneal endothelial morphology after 10 weeks of uncontrolled hyperglycemia showed increased corneal thickness, increased stromal hydration, and a decreased ability to recover from contact lens–induced corneal edema (92).

B. Vitamin A Deficiency

Vitamin A deficiency can be induced in rats by a vitamin A–deficient diet. Metabolic changes in the cornea of the vitamin A–deficient rat recovered to normal with vitamin A therapy (93). In the vitamin A–deficient rat, delayed epithelial wound healing was associated with an inflammatory cell layer and occurred in the absence of fibronectin (94).

C. Hypercholesterolemia

In an animal model of experimental lipid keratopathy, corneal changes were the result of increased lysosomal uptake of lipids from the extracellular space by the keratocytes (95).

VIII. GLAUCOMA

A. Water-Loading Hypertension

Water-loading tests have been used in rabbits to screen potentially useful ocular hypotensive drugs. The procedure is usually carried out by intragastric loading of water or by rapid intravenous infusion of glucose solution. In these models, experimental variability is caused by variations in the techniques (the amount of water, time of measurement, route of administration).

The ocular hypotensive effect of continuously delivered epinephrine was compared to that of pulsed doses provided by eye drops in normotensive and hypertensive rabbits after an intragastric water load of 60 mL water/kg rabbit body weight which induced transient elevation of intraocular pressure. Ocular hypertension induced by water load was significantly inhibited by continuous delivery of epinephrine at a rate of 3 or 6 µg/h or by 2% epinephrine eye drops (96). Trained albino rabbits were given loadings of fluids by different routes. An oral water load of 100 mL/kg body weight gave an elevation of the intraocular pressure (IOP) of about 12 mmHg. Smaller amounts gave a less pronounced IOP elevation. Intraperitoneal administration did not seem to increase IOP markedly. Rapid infusion of glucose 5% 15 mL/kg produced a transient and modest increase of the IOP (97). In another study, intraperitoneal water loading (60 mL/kg) provided an ocular hypertensive effect of longer duration than after oral or intravenous water loading in Dutch belt rabbits (98). The IOP elevation induced by delivering 30 mL/kg of distilled water by orogastric tube to pigmented rabbits was studied in normal eyes after retrobulbar infiltration anesthesia. The peak IOP elevation at 30 min after water administration was counteracted by retrobulbar anesthesia (99).

In testing of the prolonged-action drug delivery systems the major limitation of water-loading methods is their short duration of IOP elevation (1–2 h). Consequently, it is difficult to study the time course of drug responses with this model.

B. Laser-Induced Hypertension

Argon laser energy applied to the chamber angle of pigmented rabbits induced approximately in half of the laser-treated rabbits a secondary buphthalmos and sustained ocular hypertension. Histologic examination at 4 and 8 weeks after laser treatment demonstrated a wound-healing response resulting in closure of the intertrabecular spaces and obstruction of outflow to injected carbon particles (100). Chronic experimental laser-induced glaucoma in monkeys shares many features of human glaucomatous optic neuropathy and has been used in detailed morphological studies (101,102). Argon or Nd:YAG laser irradiation to the rabbit iris produced an IOP elevation which was inhibited by indomethacin or flurbiprofen and by apraclonidine, respectively (103,104).

C. Corticosteroid-Induced Hypertension

Weekly subconjunctival injections of 4 mg of repository betamethasone, repeated over 3 weeks, produced a sustained increase of IOP in 96% of the treated rabbits. The IOP was lowered by pilocarpine, propranolol, and clonidine (105). Subconjunctival betamethasone, cortisone, and triamcinolone also induced ocular hypertension in the rabbit. The most consistent elevation was observed with triamcinolone (106).

D. α-Chymotrypsin–Induced Hypertension

α-Chymotrypsin injected into the posterior chamber of albino or pigmented rabbits at least 8 months earlier induces an IOP elevation which has been widely used as an experimental model to screen antiglaucoma drugs (e.g., timolol, propranolol, epinephrine, isoproterenol, clonidine, and betaxolol) (107,108). Studies in monkeys suggest that α-chymotrypsin affects the glycoproteins of the cell membrane and as a result causes disorganization of the cytoskeleton, loss of loose adhesions, and breaks of cell processes in the outflow routes for aqueous humor (109).

E. Hereditary Glaucoma

A spontaneous glaucoma has been described in several breeds of dogs and in one strain of albino rabbits. Buphthalmos in rabbits is inherited as a semilethal-autosomal trait but its value as an animal model is limited, since it affects the general viability of the animal as well (110). Beagles, basset hounds, and cocker spaniels are prone to occasional cases of spontaneous glaucoma (110). Spontaneous glaucoma in the beagle was exhibited after 6 months of age by elevated IOP and open iridocorneal angles followed by secondary changes (111). An inherited eye disease leading to a secondary angle-closure glaucoma has been observed in turkeys of the Slate variety (112). Analysis of the proteins of the aging calf and cow trabecular meshwork lays a foundation for future work: The changes might simulate aging changes in humans (113).

F. Light-Induced Avian Glaucoma

Glaucoma can be induced in domestic chickens by the simple device of rearing the chickens under continuous light. This light-induced avian glaucoma was presented as an animal model system for human open-angle glaucoma and it has been demonstrated to be responsive to several antiglaucoma drugs (110).

G. Experimental Glaucoma Surgery

Glaucoma filtration surgery has been performed in rabbits and in glaucomatous monkeys to determine if fibroblastic proliferation occurring at the conjunctival scleral interface is interfered with by postoperative drugs to prevent filter failure. In rabbits, dexamethasone and D-penicillinamine but not 5-fluorouracil prolonged the duration of function of the filter surgery (114,115). In monkeys, bioerodible polyanhydride discs containing 5-fluorouridine extended the intraocular pressure–lowering effect of filtration surgery (116). Contact CW Nd:YAG laser-induced hypotension in the pigmented rabbit eye may not be directly due to cyclodestruction but may be related to the irritative response and extent of the neuro-epithelial defect irrespective of its distance from the limbus (117).

IX. CATARACT

A. Hereditary Cataract

Animal models for the study of cataractogenesis have been reviewed by Berman (5) and Zigler (118). In animal models of congenital cataract, the opacity is evident at birth (or eye opening) or it develops within the first few weeks of life. While the chances that any particular animal model directly corresponds to a human congenital cataract are small, it is likely that some biochemical processes in the human disease and animal models are similar (118). The Nakano mouse, Philly mouse, Fraser mouse, Strain 13/N guinea pig, miniature schnauzer dog, Scat (Suture cataract) in mice, and animal models of hereditary cataract secondary to other disease such as the Dahl salt-sensitive hypertensive rat, and the Royal College of Surgeons (RCS) rat have been summarized by Zigler (118). Such maturity-onset hereditary animal models as the Emory mouse, ICR rat, and senescence-accelerated mouse (SAM) were also discussed (118).

B. Induced Cataract

Cataract can be induced in vivo in many ways, including administration of a wide variety of chemical agents, exposure to ionizing or ultraviolet radiation, or generation of nutritional deficiencies (118).

The molecular basis of experimentally induced sugar cataracts, radiation cataracts, selenite cataract, cyanate cataract, and U18666A (a potent inhibitor of cholesterol biosynthesis) cataract and of some animal models of hereditary cataract have been summarized by Berman (5). Drugs have been tested for their possible cataractogenic or cocataractogenic potentials using animal cataract models (e.g., Ref. 119).

X. OCULAR INFLAMMATION

A. Immunogenic Uveitis

Active and passive immunogenic inflammatory reactions in the eye are induced by direct intraocular injection of the antigen in sensitized animals or antigen-antibody complex in nonsensitized animals (12). Acute anterior uveitis is produced in rabbits by injecting foreign protein, e.g., bovine or human serum albumin (BSA, HSA), into the vitreous body. The onset of inflammatory reactions in the model varies from 8 to 18 days and the vascular and cellular inflammatory reactions last for about 10 days (12,120). An alternative procedure to induce similar immunogenic ocular inflammation is to sensitize either the rat or rabbit by subcutaneous injection of BSA or ovalbumin at 3-day or weekly intervals. One week after the last injection, intraocular inflammation is induced by an intravitreal challenge of the antigen (12). Since local antibody formation and kinetics in the eye during the inflammation has a genetic background, many experimental models of clinical uveitis have a number of shortcomings (120).

Several attempts have been made to induce autoimmune uveitis with homologous or heterologous uveal and retinal antigen alone or together with Freund's complete adjuvant (12). A soluble antigen (S-antigen) was isolated and characterized from the photoreceptors of guinea pigs, rabbits, and bovine retina (121). Experimental autoimmune uveitis (EAU) in the guinea pigs, primates, and rats has been induced by subcutaneous injection of purified S-antigen in complete Freund's adjuvant, and its biochemical parameters have been analyzed (122–124). The EAU model has been used in numerous drug studies: ethylenediaminetetraacetic acid (EDTA), corticosteroids, cyclosporine A, cyclosporine G, quercetin, and adenosine produced a reduction of the inflammatory reaction (125–129). FK506, a new immunosuppressant isolated from the fermentation broth of *Streptomyces tsukubaensis*, effectively suppressed EAU in rats with lower doses than cyclosporine A. The drug was shown to induce an activation of T_s cells specific to S-antigen and the T_s cells might contribute, at least in part, to the uniquely prolonged and intensive immunosuppression by FK506 (130).

B. Nonimmunogenic Uveitis

Lens proteins are capable of producing an acute intraocular inflammation without prior sensitization. Whole lens protein extracts from albino rabbits were injected intracamerally into other albino rabbits. Within 2 h of the injection, the iris and ciliary body exhibit redness and congestion which will gradually subside after 48 h (131). Pretreatment of the eyes with indomethacin resulted in a marked reduction of inflammation induced by lens proteins; the effect was also obtained after systemic or topical administration of REV 5901, a lipoxygenase inhibitor, or after topical application of matrine, or after systemic administration of dimethyl thiourea or glutathione peroxidase (132–137).

Intraocular, intravenous, or footpad injection of phlogistic agents induce ocular inflammation. A single systemic dose of endotoxin (lipopolysaccharide) induced an acute inflammatory response in the uveal tract of rats (138). A single intraperitoneal injection of an aqueous suspension of group A streptococcal peptidoglycan-polysaccharide complex into Lewis rats induced a self-timing bilateral uveitis with associated perpetuating polyarthritis (139). Intravitreal injection of cachectin, primary mediator of shock in the setting of gram-negative septicemia, induced intraocular inflammation within 6 h (140). Prostaglandin E_2 and leukotriene B_4 levels were analyzed in the course of endotoxin-induced uveitis; after 6 h the levels began to rise rapidly (141). Endotoxin-induced ocular inflammation was not altered by fish oil dietary supplements but was significantly inhibited by dimethyl thiourea or platelet-activating factor (142–144).

Administering arachidonic acid topically produced a simple model for evaluating the effects of inhibitors on prostaglandins: In rabbits, aspirin, piroxicam, and indomethacin blocked lid closure and chemosis significantly (145). Topically administered S(+)-ibuprofen in a rabbit model of uveitis secondary to the intravitreal injection of human recombinant interleukin 1α was found to inhibit increased vascular permeability associated with this model (146). Topical application of diclofenac significantly reduced effects of traumatic uveitis in the rabbit eye, and topical administration of prostaglandin E_1 and F_2 prior to ocular trauma reduced the ocular inflammatory response (147,148). Infrared radiation was used to produce breakdown of the blood-retinal barrier in rabbits (149). Breakdown of the blood-aqueous barrier by mechanical, chemical, and thermal stimuli and the ocular response to injury have been discussed by Unger in an excellent review (150).

XI. VITREOUS AND RETINAL INFECTIONS

A. Bacterial Endophthalmitis

The clinical response, bacterial recovery, and histopathology of exogenous, bacterial endophthalmitis have been studied in monkey, rabbit, and guinea pig eyes after intracameral or intravitreal injection of aerobic or anaerobic bacteria.

Monkey eyes received a single injection of a suspension of 1000 or 10,000 *Staphylococcus aureus* organisms into the anterior chamber; extracapsular lens extraction with an intact posterior capsule or with a wide primary capsulectomy was performed 2 weeks earlier. Injection of 10,000 *S. aureus* organisms produced culture-positive endophthalmitis in eyes that had undergone posterior capsulectomy but it failed to produce endophthalmitis in eyes with intact posterior capsules (151).

Guinea pigs received intravitreal injections of *Pseudomonas aeruginosa*, and comparisons were made between bacterial counts from the vitreous of control of guinea pigs and experimental guinea pigs that underwent systemic decomplementation with cobra venom factor. Partially decomplemented guinea pigs showed impaired host defense to *P. aeruginosa* and the defense was restored as complement levels returned to normal (152).

Anaerobic bacterial endophthalmitis following intravitreal injection of *Fusobacterium necrophorum* was studied in rabbits: An inoculum of approximately 50 organisms produced endophthalmitis in 59% of injected eyes, whereas 1000 or more organisms produced endophthalmitis in 100% of injected eyes. The course and severity of disease seemed to be independent of the concentration of bacteria above a minimum inoculum size (153).

Endophthalmitis was produced in rabbits with cultures of *F. necrophorum*, *Propionibacterium acnes*, and *Peptostreptococcus magnus*. Relatively small inoculates of *F. necrophorum* caused severe, acute endophthalmitis with scleral perforation, whereas *P. acnes* and *P. magnus* produced a self-limited endophthalmitis (154). Anterior chamber inoculation of 2.5×10^6 *P. acnes* organisms produced chronic endophthalmitis which was more intense and prolonged in pseudophakic eyes (155).

In a rabbit model of aphakic bacterial endophthalmitis with *S. aureus*, eyes treated with intravitreal antibiotics and vitrectomy displayed significantly clearer media after therapy compared with eyes treated antibiotics alone (156).

Vitreous cefazolin levels were studied in a rabbit model of intraocular inflammation using heat-killed *S. epidermis* as the inducing organism. Inflammation, repeated antibiotic doses, and surgical status of the eye affected cefazolin levels: Cefazolin levels were well above the minimum inhibitory concentrations for organisms termed sensitive to cefazolin in inflamed phakic and inflamed aphakic/vitrectomized eyes (157).

B. Viral Retinitis

In 1924, von Szily demonstrated that inoculation of herpes simplex virus (HSV) into a ciliary body dialysis cleft of one eye in rabbits leads to uveitis and retinopathy in the contralateral, noninoculated eye (see references to Ref. 158). ICR white mice were inoculated with HSV-1 in the anterior chamber of one eye. Herpes simplex virus retinopathy developed in 91% of inoculated eyes and 88% of noninoculated eyes examined after the sixth postinoculation day. The retinopathy progressed in both eyes to total destruction of the retina by day 10. Viral infection of the retinal pigment epithelium occurred, but viral particles were seen only rarely in the underlaying choroid. According to the authors, the model may provide insight into the pathogenesis of HSV retinopathy in humans (158).

Unilateral inoculation of HSAV-1 (KOS strain) into the anterior chamber of BALB/c eyes produced an ocular disease with a distinctive differential pattern of retinal pathology. Specifically, the retina of the inoculated eye remained intact, whereas the contralateral retina became necrotic. Immunosuppression or lack of thymus resulted in bilateral retinal necrosis (159). Anterior chamber inoculation of 104 PFU of the MS strain of HSV-2 resulted in physiologic and morphologic changes in the retina of the inoculated and the uninoculated eyes (160). Secondary herpes simplex (HS) uveitis was induced in a rabbit eye that had recovered from primary HS uveitis by challenging it with an intravitreal injection of HSV antigen. Daily intramuscular injections of cyclosporine for 7 days prior to the intravitreal challenge with HSV antigen significantly suppressed the induction of secondary HS uveitis (161).

Retinal changes were investigated in healthy and immunosuppressed mice after intra-ocular inoculation of murine cytomegalovirus (MCMV). A 0.01-ml inoculum containing 105 PFU of MCMV was placed behind the lens in Swiss Webster mice. Part of the animals were immunosuppressed with cyclophosphamide given intraperitoneally at the time of inoculation and every 5 days thereafter. Uveal infection developed whether or not animals received cyclophosphamide, but retinal necrosis developed only in immunosuppressed mice (163). Intravitreal inoculation of 103 PFU of MCMV to BALB/c mice resulted in virus isolation from homogenates for 2 weeks and from cocultured specimens of the same eye up to 5 weeks after inoculation, indicating that MCMV in the eye became latent 2 weeks after the virus inoculation. Immunosuppressive treatment with daily intramuscular injection of cyclosporine and cortisone acetate 9 weeks after intravitreal MCMV inoculation resulted in isolation of infectious virus from about 22% of eye homogenates during a 3-week period, indicating in vivo reactivation of latent ocular MCMV (164).

C. Experimental Onchocerciasis

Infection of cynomolgus monkeys with microfilariae of *Onchocerca lienalis* was studied as a model for human onchocerciasis. Normal monkeys and immunized monkeys were given intracorneal/subconjunctival, intracameral, or intravitreal injections of microfilariae. Selected animals were given diethylcarbamazine (DEC) orally daily after the inoculation. The extent of the inflammatory reactions was not substantially altered by DEC treatment following intraocular injection of microfilariae (165). Hartley guinea pigs were injected with microfilariae of *O. lienalis* as a model for acute inflammatory responses to human *O. volvulus* infection. Administration of DEC and ivermectin did not alter the proportion of animals expressing autoantibody or the mean autoantibody titer (166).

XII. PROLIFERATIVE VITREORETINOPATHY

The cellular events of proliferative vitreoretinopathy (PVR) are migration of glial cells, pigment epithelial cells, and fibrocytes into the vitreous cavity, where they proliferate and undergo extensive transformation and dedifferentiation and interaction with endogenous membranous components of the vitreous, leading to the formation of vitreal, epiretinal, and subretinal membranes and traction retinal detachment (5).

Experimental PVR in the rabbit was induced by injecting homologous dermal fibroblasts into the vitreous. Autotransplantation of 250,000 tissue-cultured fibroblasts from rabbit rump skin into the vitreous cavity resulted in intravitreal strand formation and traction retinal detachment in 57% of treated eyes. A single intravitreal injection of 1 mg of dexamethasone alcohol inhibited fibroblast growth as judged by the significantly reduced number of retinal detachments (167). Intravitreal Adriamycin (doxorubicin) in a dose 10 nmol had the same effect: Adriamycin controlled fibroblast proliferation if given immediately after homologous dermal fibroblast injection (168). The effect of intravitreally injected triamcinolone was evaluated previously in a refined rabbit model of PVR in which the vitreous was compressed and partially detached from the retinal surface and small amounts of tissue-cultured homologous fibroblasts (25,000) were scattered over the vascularized part of the retina. Two milligrams of the corticosteroid reduced the incidence of retinal detachments from 90 to 56%. Large doses of triamcinolone had no additional effect (169). Intravitreal daunomycin and taxol effectively controlled PVR (170,171). Epiretinal membranes at the vitreoretinal interface were induced in the rabbit eye by injecting 0.05 ml of a 40% solution of autologous red blood cells into the center of the vitreous. Six weeks or more after cell injection, thin semitransparent membranes covering large and delicately folded posterior and peripheral retinal areas were found (172). Citrated rabbit plasma (0.2 mL) was injected intracamerally following paracentesis, resulting in fibrin clot formation within 3 h. The fibrin clots were stable for 4 days and then slowly lysed over the next 4 days. Approximately 24 h after clot formation, various concentrations of human tissue plasminogen activator (TPA) were injected intracamerally. The time taken for clot lysis was dose dependent, with 1800 IU of TPA producing clot lysis in 3 h. Tissue plasminogen activator also promoted clearance of postoperative intravitreal fibrin (173).

XIII. RETINAL DETACHMENT

Rhegmatogenous retinal detachments were created in cynomolgus monkeys, to study the outward and inward permeability of carboxyfluorescein across the blood-retinal barrier. It was concluded that outward flow of fluid across the blood-retinal barrier is a substantial contributor to carboxyfluorescein loss from the vitreous cavity following intravitreal injection (174). The absorption rate of subretinal serum in experimental nonrhegmatogenous retinal detachments in rabbits was not altered significantly by intravenous acetazolamide or mannitol (175).

XIV. RETINAL LIGHT DAMAGE

Cyclic light- and dark-reared rats were exposed to intense light for various periods and then rhodopsin-measured following recovery in darkness for up to 14 days. Animals were injected with ascorbic acid or ascorbate derivates at various doses prior to light exposure. The results showed that ascorbic acid administration elevated retinal ascorbate and reduced the loss of rhodopsin and photoreceptor cell nuclei resulting from intense light. L-Ascorbic acid, sodium ascorbate, and dehydroascorbate were equally effective in preserving rhodopsin (176). In a histopathological study, ascorbate ameliorated the photic injury of visible light in the rat retina (177). Albino rats were fed a basal diet either supplemented with or deficient in vitamin E. Each dietary group was divided into two light-treatment groups which were exposed to 12-h cyclic light of either 15 or 750 lux. Rats exposed to the bright-light condition suffered a pronounced loss of photoreceptor cells. Vitamin E deficiency did not enhance the effect of bright cyclic light in reducing photoreceptor cell densities (178).

XV. RETINAL VASCULAR DISEASES

A. Neovascularization

In pigmented rabbits, models of preretinal neovascularization have been developed: various concentrations (1–150 IU) of hyaluronidase were injected intravitreally and aspirated repetitively until the vitreous was partially liquified, or by repeated injection and aspiration of 1 IU hyaluronidase before injection of 250,000 homologous dermal fibroblasts (179,180). In monkeys, laser-induced subretinal neovascularization was treated with intravitreal steroids (181,182). The frequency of subretinal neovascularization in steroid-treated animals was significantly lower than in the control group of untreated animals (182).

B. Retinal Ischemia

In cats, branch retinal vein occlusion induced by transvitreal diathermy caused a significant decrease in preretinal oxygen tension in nonvitrectomized eyes; in vitrectomized eyes, the oxygen tension was not significantly reduced after branch vein occlusion (183). Intraretinal PO_2 profiles before, during, and after the occlusion of retinal circulation by a glass probe placed on the retinal vessels at the optic disc was measured in cats. Oxygen consumption differed in the regions measured (184). In rats, a suture was placed behind the globe closing the central retinal artery. Ischemia and reperfusion-induced damage was treated with superoxide dismutase or EGB 761. Both drugs significantly reduced the development of perfusion-induced retinal edema and significantly prevented the neutrophil leukocyte infiltration (185). A model for ischemic vasoproliferative retinopathy was induced in kittens reared in 80% oxygen for 65–72 h, after which they were returned to room air (186).

C. Diabetic Retinopathy

Spontaneously diabetic Bio-Breeding/Wistar rats and nondiabetic littermate controls were subjected to ultrastructural studies of the neural retina and retinal pigment epithelium. In diabetic rats, several progressive changes occurred the retinal pigment epithelium, Bruch's membrane, and retinal capillaries (187). In spontaneously diabetic Bio-Breeding/Worcester rats and streptozotocin-diabetic rats, changes in Bruch's membrane suggest that filtration through Bruch's membrane is altered in diabetes (188). In galactose-fed rats, blood flow was increased in the retina, choroid, and anterior uvea but not in the brain of rats fed for 3 weeks and 3 months versus controls and was normalized by sorbinil in the 3-week group (189). In Sprague-Dawley rats fed with diets containing 50% dextrin (control) or 50% galactose, tolrestat prevented retinal microvascular lesions in diabetic rats (190). Cats were rendered diabetic by partial pancreatectomy (191). Retinal capillary basement thickening observed in the diabetic cat was inhibited by sulindac treatment (191).

XVI. RETINAL DEGENERATIONS AND DYSTROPHIES

Several animal models with inherited retinal degenerations have provided histological, cell biological, ultrastructural, immunocytochemical, biochemical, and molecular genetic information of the diseases (5). Such models are the miniature poodle (192), the rd (retinal dystrophy) mouse (193), RCS (Royal College of Surgeons) rat (194), Wistar-Futh rat (195), rds (slow retinal dystrophy) mouse, Irish setter, collie, taurine deficiency in the cat and rat (5), and Abyssinian cat (196). None of the models have so far been used for drug studies.

REFERENCES

1. Pavan-Langston, D. (1988). *Manual of Ocular Diagnosis and Therapy.* Little, Brown, Boston.
2. Vaughan, D., Asbury, T., and Tabbara, K. F. (1989). *General Ophthalmology.* Appleton & Lange, Norwalk, Connecticut.
3. Yanoff, M., and Fine, B. S. (1990). *Ocular Pathology. A Color Atlas.* Imago Productions (FE) PTE, Singapore.
4. Bazan, N. G. (1990). *Lipid Mediators in Eye Inflammation.* Karger, Basel.
5. Berman, E. R. (1991). *Biochemistry of the Eye.* Plenum Press, New York.
6. Belfort, R., Toledo, M. R. F., Burnier, M., Smith, R. L., Silva, V. L., and Trabulsi, L. R. (1985). Experimental guinea pig ocular infection by Salmonella typhimurium, *Invest. Ophthalmol. Vis. Sci., 26*:591.
7. Langford, M. P., Yin-Murphy, M., Barber, J. C., Heard, H. K., and Stanton, G. J. (1986). Conjunctivitis in rabbits caused by enterovirus type 70 (EV 70), *Invest. Ophthalmol. Vis. Sci., 27*:915.
8. Taylor, H. R., Predergast, R. A., Dawson, C. R., Schachter, J., and Silverstein, A. M. (1981). An animal model for cicatrizing trachoma, *Invest. Ophthalmol. Vis. Sci., 21*:422.
9. Pham, R. T. H., Sung, M., Dawson, C. R., and Schachter, J. (1990). Chlamydial infection of subcutaneous conjunctival transplants in guinea pigs, *Invest. Ophthalmol. Vis. Sci., 31*:1367.
10. Sandstrom, I. K., Cummings, M., Johnson, P., Schachter, J., and Chandler, J. W. (1987). Prophylactic effects of silver nitrate and erythromycin on Chlamydia psittaci conjunctivitis, *Invest. Ophthalmol. Vis. Sci., 28*:1569.
11. Skorich, D. N., Chiappino, M. L., and Nichols, B. A. (1988). Invasion of the guinea pig conjunctiva by Toxoplasma gondii, *Invest. Ophthalmol. Vis. Sci., 29*:1871.
12. Bhattacherjee, P., and Paterson, C. A. (1990). Inflammatory mediators in models of immunogenic and nonimmunogenic inflammation on the anterior segment of the eye. *In: Lipid Mediators in Eye Inflammation* (N. G. Bazan, ed.). Karger, Basel, p. 65.
13. Dwyer, R. S. C., and Darougar, S. (1971). Models of immediate and delayed hypersensitivity in the guinea pig conjunctiva, *Trans. Ophthalmol. Soc. U.K., 91*:451.
14. Dwyer, R. S. C., Darougar, S., and Monnickendam, M. A. (1987). Responses to tuberculin in the guinea-pig eye as a model of cell mediated immune responses in the external eye, *Br. J. Ophthalmol., 71*:273.
15. Roat, M. I., Alstadt, S. P., Carpenter, A. B., Raj, N. S., and Thoft, R. A. (1990). Antibasement membrane antibody-mediated experimental conjunctivitis, *Invest. Ophthalmol. Vis. Sci., 31*:168.
16. Hann, L. E., Cornell-Bell, A. H., Marten-Ellis, C., and Allansmith, M. R. (1986). Conjunctival basophil hypersensitivity lesions in guinea pig, *Invest. Ophthalmol. Vis. Sci., 27*:1255.
17. Keller, N., Longwell, A. M., and Birss, S. A. (1976). Intermittent vs continuous steroid administration. Efficacy in experimental conjunctivitis, *Arch. Ophthalmol., 94*:644.
18. Stock, E. L., Dwyer, R. S. C., Jones, B. R., and Waters, J. A. (1985). Pharmacologic inhibition of immediate hypersensitivity in the guinea pig conjunctiva, *J. Ocul. Pharmacol., 1*:183.
19. Woodward, D. F., and Nieves, A. L. (1985). Topical anti-inflammatory activity of beta2-adrenoceptor agonist in the conjunctiva, *J. Ocul. Pharmacol., 1*:391.

20. Woodward, D. F., Johnson, L., Spada, C., and Chen, J. (1986). Effect of cimetidine and pyrilamine on histamine-induced ocular surface hyperemia, *J. Ocul. Pharmacol.,* 2:275.

21. Tanaka, H., Umemoto, M., Miichi, H., and Hayashi, S. (1987). Evaluation of an antiallergic (disodium cromoglycate) in rat conjunctiva using monoclonal IgE antibody, *Ophthalmic Res.,* 19:240.

22. Chan, C. C. (1990). Leukotriens and allergic conjunctivitis. *In: Lipid Mediators in Eye Inflammation* (N. G. Bazan, ed.). Karger, Basel, p. 41.

23. Jester, J. V., Nicolaides, N., and Smith, R. E. (1989). Meibomian gland dysfunction. I. Keratin protein expression in normal human and rabbit meibomian glands, *Invest. Ophthalmol. Vis. Sci.,* 30:927.

24. Jester, J. V., Nicolaides, N., Kiss-Palvolgyi, I., and Smith, R. E. (1989). Meibomian gland dysfunction. II. The role of keratinization in a rabbit model of MGD, *Invest. Ophthalmol. Vis. Sci.,* 30:936.

25. Gilbard, J. P., Rossi, S. R., Gray, K. L., Hanninen, L. A., and Kenyon, K. R. (1988). Tear film osmolarity and ocular surface disease in two rabbit models for keratoconjunctivitis sicca, *Invest. Ophthalmol. Vis. Sci.,* 29:374.

26. Jabs, D. A., Enger, C., and Predergast, R. A. (1991). Murine models of Sjögren's syndrome, *Invest. Ophthalmol. Vis. Sci.,* 32:371.

27. Badenoch, P. B., Hay, G. J., McDonald, P. J., and Coster, D. J. (1985). A rat model of bacterial keratitis. Effect of antibiotics and corticosteroid, *Arch. Ophthalmol.,* 103:718.

28. Fraser-Smith, E. B., and Matthews, T. R. (1988). Effect of ketorolac on Pseudomonas aeruginosa ocular infection in rabbits, *J. Ocul. Pharmacol.,* 4:101.

29. Hobden, J. A., Reidy, J. J., O'Callaghan, R. J., and Hill, J. M. (1988). Treatment of experimental Pseudomonas keratitis using collagen shields containing tobramycin, *Arch. Ophthalmol.,* 106:1605.

30. Aswad, M. I., Barza, M., and Baum, J. (1989). Effect of lid closure on contact lens-associated Pseudomonas keratitis, *Arch. Ophthalmol.,* 107:1667.

31. Hazzlett, L. D., Moon, M. M., Singh, A., and Rudner, X. L. (1991). Analysis of adhesion, piliation, protease production and ocular infectivity of several P. aeruginosa strains, *Curr. Eye Res.,* 10:351.

32. Badenoch, P. R., Johnson, A. M., Christy, P. E., and Coster, D. J. (1990). Pathogenicity of Acanthamoeba and a Corynebacterium in the rat cornea, *Arch. Ophthalmol.,* 108:107.

33. O'Day, D. M., Ray, W. A., Robinson, R. D., and Head, W. S. (1987). Correlation of in vitro and in vivo susceptibility of Candida albicans to amphotericin and natamycin, *Invest. Ophthalmol. Vis. Sci.,* 28:596.

34. O'Day, D. M., Ray, W. A., Robinson, R. D., Head, W. S., and Williams, T. E. (1991). Differences in response in vivo to amphotericin B among Candida albicans strains, *Invest. Ophthalmol. Vis. Sci.,* 32:1569.

35. Pavan-Langston, D., Langston, R. H. S., and Geary, P. A. (1975). Idoxuridine ocular insert therapy. Use in treatment of experimental herpes simplex keratitis, *Arch. Ophthalmol.,* 93:1349.

36. Sanitato, J. J., Varnell, E. D., Kaufman, H. E., and Raju, V. K. (1984). Differences in natural and recombinant interferon for herpes keratitis in two animal models, *Invest. Ophthalmol. Vis. Sci.,* 25:87.

37. Gordon, Y. J., Cheng, K. P., Araullo-Cruz, T., Romanowski, E., Johnson, B. J., and Blough, H. A. (1986). Efficacy of glycoprotein inhibitors alone and in combination with trifluridine in the treatment of murine herpetic keratitis, *Curr. Eye Res.,* 5:93.

38. Troudale, M. D., Barlow, W. E., and McGuigan, L. J. B. (1989). Assessment of diclofenac on herpes keratitis in rabbit eyes, *Arch. Ophthalmol.,* 107:1664.

39. Willey, D. E., Williams, I., Faucett, C., and Openshaw, H. (1991). Ocular acyclovir delivery by collagen discs: A mouse model to screen anti-viral agents, *Curr. Eye Res.,* 10:167.

40. McNeill, J. I., and Kaufman, H. E. (1979). Local antivirals in a herpes simples stromal keratitis model, *Arch. Ophthalmol.,* 97:727.

41. Boisjoly, H. M., Woog, J. J., Pavan-Langston, D., and Park, N. H. (1984). Prophylactic topical cyclosporine in experimental herpetic stromal keratitis, *Arch. Ophthalmol., 102*:1804.

42. Troudale, M. D., Goldstein, L., Stebbing, N., Peters, A. C. B., Schanzlin, D. J., and Robin, J. B. (1985). Human alpha and gamma interferon analogs in rabbits with herpetic keratitis, *Invest. Ophthalmol. Vis. Sci., 26*:1985.

43. Hendricks, R. L., Barfknecht, C. F., Schoenwald, R. D., Epstein, R. J., and Sugar, J. (1990). The effect of flurbiprofen on herpes simplex virus type 1 stromal keratitis in mice, *Invest. Ophthalmol. Vis. Sci., 31*:1503.

44. Hill, J. H., Haruta, Y., Yamamoto, Y., Jones, M. D., Wingate, H. L., and Jemison, M. T. (1987). Lack of efficacy of adenosine-5'-monophosphate against HSV-1 ocular shedding in rabbits, *J. Ocul. Pharmacol., 3*:1987.

45. Haruta, Y., Rootman, D. S., Xie, L., Kiritoshi, A., and Hill, J. M. (1989). Recurrent HSV-1 corneal lesions in rabbits induced by cyclophosphamide and dexamethasone, *Invest. Ophthalmol. Vis. Sci., 30*:371.

46. Rootman, D. S., Hill, J. M., Haruta, Y., Reidy, J. J., and Kaufman, H. E. (1989). Trifluridine decreases ocular HSV-1 recovery, but not herpetic lesions after timolol iontophoresis, *Invest. Ophthalmol. Vis. Sci., 30*:678.

47. Rootman, D. S., Haruta, Y., and Hill, J. M. (1990). Reactivation of HSV-1 in primates by transcorneal iontophoresis of adrenergic agents, *Invest. Ophthalmol. Vis. Sci., 31*:597.

48. Leibowitz, H. M., and Kupferman, A. (1979). Optimal frequency of topical prednisolone administration, *Arch. Ophthalmol., 97*:2154.

49. Leibowitz, H. M., Ryan, W. J., Kupferman, A., and DeSantis, L. (1986). Effect of concurrent topical corticosteroid and NSAID therapy of experimental keratitis, *Invest. Ophthalmol. Vis. Sci., 27*:1226.

50. Verbey, N. L., and van Haeringen, N. J. (1990). The influence of a fish oil dietary supplement on immunogenic keratitis, *Invest. Ophthalmol. Vis. Sci., 31*:1526.

51. Ando, E., Ando, Y., Inoue, M., Morino, Y., Kamata, R., and Okamura, R. (1990). Inhibition of corneal inflammation by an acylated superoxide dismutase derivate, *Invest. Ophthalmol. Vis. Sci., 31*:1963.

52. Trinkaus-Randall, V., Leibowitz, H. M., Ryan, W. J., and Kupferman, A. (1991). Quantification of stromal destruction in the inflamed cornea, *Invest. Ophthalmol. Vis. Sci., 32*:603.

53. Tervo, T., Tervo, K., van Setten, G. B., Virtanen, I., and Tarkkanen, A. (1989). Plasminogen activator and its inhibitor in the experimental corneal wound, *Exp. Eye Res., 48*:445.

54. Kulkarni, P. S., and Srinivasan, B. D. (1985). Anti-inflammatory effects of ketoprofen in rabbit corneal epithelial wound model, *Exp. Eye Res., 41*:267.

55. Waterbury, L., Kunysz, E. A., and Beuerman, R. (1987). Effects of steroidal and non-steroidal anti-inflammatory agents on corneal wound healing, *J. Ocul. Pharmacol., 3*:43.

56. Mathers, W. D., Sherman, M., Fryczkowski, A., and Jester, J. V. (1989). Dose-dependent effects of epidermal growth factor on corneal wound healing, *Invest. Ophthalmol. Vis. Sci., 30*:2403.

57. Leibowitz, H. M., Morello, S., Stern, M., and Kupferman, A. (1990). Effect of topically administered epidermal growth factor on corneal wound strength, *Arch. Ophthalmol., 108*:734.

58. Hersh, P. S., Rice, B. A., Baer, J. C., Wells, P. A., Lynch, S. E., McGuigan, L. J. B., and Foster, S. (1990). Topical nonsteroidal agents and corneal wound healing, *Arch. Ophthalmol., 108*:577.

59. Kitazawa, T., Kinoshita, S., Fujiya, K., Araki, K., Watanabe, H., Ohashi, Y., and Manabe, K. (1990). The mechanism of accelerated corneal epithelial healing by human epidermal growth factor, *Invest. Ophthalmol. Vis. Sci., 31*:1773.

60. Tseng, S. C. G., Hirst, L. W., Farazdaghi, M., and Green, W. R. (1987). Inhibition of conjunctival transdifferentiation by topical retinoids, *Invest. Ophthalmol. Vis. Sci., 28*:538.

61. Capone, A., Lance, S. E., Friend, J., and Thoft, R. A. (1987). In vivo effects of 5-FU on ocular surface epithelium following corneal wounding, *Invest. Ophthalmol. Vis. Sci., 28*:1661.

62. Robin, J. B., Keys, C. L., Kaminski, L. A., and Viana, M. A. G. (1990). The effects of collagen shields on rabbit corneal reepithelialization after chemical debridement, *Invest. Ophthalmol. Vis. Sci., 31*:1294.
63. Liu, G. S., Trope, G. E., and Basu, P. K. (1990). Beta adrenoceptors and regenerating corneal epithelium, *J. Ocul. Pharmacol., 6*:101.
64. Wang, H. M., Berman, M., and Law, M. (1985). Latent and active plasminogen activator in corneal ulceration, *Invest. Ophthalmol. Vis. Sci., 26*:511.
65. Seedor, J. A., Perry, H. D., and McNamara, T. F. (1987). Systemic tetracycline treatment of alkali-induced corneal ulceration in rabbits, *Arch. Ophthalmol., 105*:268.
66. Reim, M., Busse, S., Leber, M., and Schulz, C. (1988). Effect of epidermal growth factor in severe experimental alkali burns, *Ophthalmic Res., 20*:327.
67. Pfister, R. R., Haddox, J. L., and Lank, K. M. (1988). Citrate or ascorbate/citrate treatment of established corneal ulcers in the alkali-injured rabbit eye, *Invest. Ophthalmol. Vis. Sci., 29*:1110.
68. Haddox, J. L., Pfister, R. R., and Yuille-Barr, D. (1989). The efficacy of topical citrate after alkali injury in dependent on the period of time it is administered, *Invest. Ophthalmol. Vis. Sci., 30*:1062.
69. Ormerod, L. D., Abelson, M. B., and Kenyon, K. R. (1989). Standard models of corneal injury using alkali-immersed filter discs, *Invest. Ophthalmol. Vis. Sci., 30*:2153.
70. Burns, F. R., Gray, R. D., and Paterson, C. A. (1990). Inhibition of alkali-induced ulceration and perforation by a thiol peptide, *Invest. Ophthalmol. Vis. Sci., 31*:107.
71. Phan, T. M. M., Zelt, R. P., Kenyon, K. R., Chakrabarti, B., and Foster, C. S. (1985). Ascorbic acid therapy in a thermal burn model of corneal ulceration in rabbits, *Am. J. Ophthalmol., 99*:74.
72. Bazan, H. E. P. (1987). Corneal injury alters eicosanoid formation in the rabbit anterior segment in vivo, *Invest. Ophthalmol. Vis. Sci., 28*:314.
73. Chan, K. Y., Järveläinen, M., Chang, J. H., and Edenfiled, M. J. (1990). A cryodamage model for studying corneal nerve regeneration, *Invest. Ophthalmol. Vis. Sci., 31*:2008.
74. Chusid, M. J., Nelson, D. B., and Meyer, L. A. (1986). The role of the polymorphonuclear leukocyte in the induction of corneal edema, *Invest. Ophthalmol. Vis. Sci., 27*:1466.
75. Herse, P. R. (1990). Corneal edema recovery dynamics in the rabbit, *Invest. Ophthalmol. Vis. Sci., 31*:2003.
76. Matsuda, M., Sawa, M., Edelhauser, H. F., Bartels, S. P., Neufeld, A. H., and Kenyon, K. R. (1985). Cellular migration and morphology in corneal endothelial wound repair, *Invest. Ophthalmol. Vis. Sci., 26*:443.
77. Fukami, H., Laing, R. A., Tsubota, K., Chiba, K., and Oak, S. S. (1988). Corneal endothelial changes following minor trauma, *Invest. Ophthalmol. Vis. Sci., 29*:1677.
78. Tuft, S. J., Williams, K. A., and Coster, D. J. (1986). Endothelial repair in the rat cornea, *Invest. Ophthalmol. Vis. Sci., 27*:1199.
79. Bahn, C. F., Grosserode, R., Musch, D. C., Feder, J., Meyer, R. F., MacCallum, D. K., Lillie, J. H., and Rich, N. M. (1986). Effect of 1% sodium hyaluronate (HealonR) on a nonregenerating (feline) corneal endothelium, *Invest. Ophthalmol. Vis. Sci., 27*:1485.
80. Gaster, R. N., Binder, P. S., Coalwell, K., Berns, M., McCord, R. C., and Burstein, N. L. (1889). Corneal surface ablation by 194nm excimer laser and wound healing in rabbits, *Invest. Ophthalmol. Vis. Sci., 30*:90.
81. Goodman, G. L., Trokel, S. L., Stark, W. J., Munnerlyn, C. R., and Green, W. R. (1989). Corneal healing following laser refractive keratectomy, *Arch. Ophthalmol., 107*:1799.
82. Khodadoust, A. A. (1968). Penetrating keratoplasty in the rabbit, *Am. J. Ophthalmol., 66*:899.
83. Williams, K. A., and Coster, D. J. (1985). Penetrating corneal transplantation in the inbred rat: A new model, *Invest. Ophthalmol. Vis. Sci., 26*:23.
84. Newton, C., Gebhardt, B. M., and Kaufman, H. E. (1988). Topically applied cyclosporine in azone prolongs corneal allograft survival, *Invest. Ophthalmol. Vis. Sci., 29*:208.
85. Chen, Y. F., Gebhardt, B. M., Reidy, J. J., and Kaufman, H. E. (1990). Cyclosporine-containing collagen shields suppress corneal allograft rejection, *Am. J. Ophthalmol., 109*:132.

86. Mahoney, J. M., and Waterbury, L. D. (1985). Drug effects on the neovascularization response to silver nitrate cauterization of the rat cornea, *Curr. Eye Res., 4*:531.

87. Corrent, G., Roussel, T. J., Tseng, S. C. G., and Watson, B. D. (1989). Promotion of graft survival by photothrombic occlusion of corneal neovascularization, *Arch. Ophthalmol., 107*:1501.

88. Nikolic, L., Friend, J., Taylor, S., and Thoft, R. A. (1986). Inhibition of vascularization in rabbit corneas by heparin:cortisone pellets, *Invest. Ophthalmol. Vis. Sci., 77*:449.

89. Taylor, C. M., Kissun, R. D., Schor, A. M., McLeod, D., Garner, A., and Weiss, J. B. (1989). Endothelial cell-stimulating angiogenesis factor in vitreous from extraretinal neovascularizations, *Invest. Ophthalmol. Vis. Sci., 30*:2178.

90. Awata, T., Sogo, S., Yamagami, Y., and Yamamoto, Y. (1988). Effect off an aldose reductase inhibitor, CT-112, on healing of the corneal epithelium in galactose-fed rats, *J. Ocul. Pharmacol., 4*:195.

91. Datiles, M. B., Kador, P. F., Kashima, K., Kinoshita, J. H., and Sinha, A. (1990). The effect of sorbinil, an aldose reductase inhibitor, on the corneal endothelium in galactosemic dogs, *Invest. Ophthalmol. Vis. Sci., 31*:2201.

92. Herse, P. R. (1990). Corneal hydration control in normal and alloxan-induced diabetic rabbits, *Invest. Ophthalmol. Vis. Sci., 31*:2213.

93. Hayashi, K., Cheng, H. M., Xiong, J., Xiong, H., and Kenyon, K. R. (1989). Metabolic changes in the cornea of vitamin A–deficient rats, *Invest. Ophthalmol. Vis. Sci., 30*:769.

94. Frangieh, G. T., Hayashi, T., Teekhasaenee, C., Wolf, G., Colvin, R. B., Gipson, I. K., and Kenyon, K. R. (1989). Fibronectin and corneal epithelium wound healing in the vitamin A–deficient rat, *Arch. Ophthalmol., 107*:567.

95. Roth, S. I., Stock, E. L., Siel, J. M., Mendelsohn, A., Reddy, C., Preskill, D. G., and Ghosh, S. (1988). Pathogenesis of experimental lipid keratopathy. An ultrastructural study of an animal model system, *Invest. Ophthalmol. Vis. Sci., 29*:1544.

96. Birss, S. A., Longwell, A., Heckbert, S., and Keller, N. (1978). Ocular hypotensive efficacy of topical epinephrine in normotensive and hypertensive rabbits: Continuous drug delivery vs eyedrops, *Ann. Ophthalmol., 10*:1045.

97. Van Loenen, A. C., van Bijsterveld, O. P., and Nijkamp, F. (1984). Some aspects of water-loadings in rabbits, *Doc. Ophthalmol., 56*:345.

98. Flach, A. J., Peterson, J. S., and Donahue, M. E. (1985). Ocular hypertensive responses in pigmented rabbits following different methods of water-loading. *J. Ocul. Pharmacol., 2*:313.

99. Gual, A., Minteniig, G. M., and Belmonte, C. (1989). Intraocular pressure effects of water loading and venous compression tests in normal and denervated pigmented rabbits, *Exp. Eye Res., 48*:365.

100. Gherezghiher, T., March, W. F., Nordqvist, R. E., and Koss, M. (1986). Laser-induced glaucoma in rabbits, *Exp. Eye Res., 43*:885.

101. Gaasterland, D., and Kupfer, C. (1974). Experimental glaucoma in the rhesus monkey, *Invest. Ophthalmol., 13*:455.

102. Quigley, H. A., Sanchez, R. M., Dunkelberger, G. R., L'Hernault, N. L., and Baginski, T. A. (1987). Chronic glaucoma selectivity damages large optic nerve fibers, *Invest. Ophthalmol. Vis. Sci., 28*:913.

103. Gherezghirer, T., and Koss, M. C. (1989). Argon laser-induced ocular hypertension: Animal model of ocular inflammation, *J. Ocul. Pharmacol., 5*:7.

104. Sugiyama, K., Kitazawa, Y., and Kawai, K. (1990). Apraclonidine effects on ocular responses to YAG laser irradiation to the rabbit iris, *Invest. Ophthalmol. Vis. Sci., 31*:708.

105. Bonomi, L., Perfetti, S., Noya, E., Bellucci, R., and Tomazzoli, L. (1978). Experimental corticosteroid ocular hypertension in the rabbit, *Albrecht v. Graefe's Arch. Klin. Exp. Ophthalmol., 209*:73.

106. Hester, D. E., Trites, P. N., Peiffer, R. L., and Petrow, V. (1987). Steroid-induced ocular hypertension in the rabbit: A model using subconjunctival injections, *J. Ocul. Pharmacol.*, 3:185.

107. Vareilles, P., Silverstone, D., Plazonnet, B., Le Douarec, J. C., Sears, M., and Stone, C. A. (1977). Comparison of the effects of timolol and other adrenergic agents on intraocular pressure in the rabbit, *Invest. Ophthalmol. Vis. Sci.*, 16:987.

108. Himber, J., De Burlet, G., and Andermann, G. (1989). Effects of adrenergic agents on alpha-chymotrypsin-induced ocular hypertension in albino and pigmented rabbits: A comparative study. *J. Ocul. Pharmacol.*, 5:93.

109. Hamanaka, T., and Bill, A. (1988). Effects of alpha-chymotrypsin on the outflow routes for aqueous humor, *Exp. Eye Res.*, 46:323.

110. Lauber, J. K. (1987). Review: Light-induced avian glaucoma as an animal model for human primary glaucoma, *J. Ocul. Pharmacol.*, 3:77.

111. Samuelsin, D. A., Gum, G. G., and Gelatt, K. N. (1989). Ultrastructural changes in the aqueous outflow apparatus of beagles with inherited glaucoma, *Invest. Ophthalmol. Vis. Sci.*, 30:550.

112. De Kater, A. W., Smyth, J. R., Rosenqvist, R. C., and Epstein, D. L. (1986). The slate turkey: A model for secondary angle closure glaucoma, *Invest. Ophthalmol. Vis. Sci.*, 27:1751.

113. Russell, P., Garland, D., and Epstein, D. (1989). Analysis of the proteins of calf and cow trabecular meshwork: Developing of a model system to study aging effects and glaucoma, *Exp. Eye Res.*, 48:251.

114. McGuigan, L. J. B., Cook, D. J., and Yablonski, M. E. (1986). Dexamethasone, D-penicillinamine, and glaucoma filter surgery in rabbits, *Invest. Ophthalmol. Vis. Sci.*, 27:1755.

115. Lee, D. A., Leong, K. W., Panek, W. C., Eng, C. T., and Glasgow, B. J. (1988). The use of bioerodible polymers and 5-fluorouracil in glaucoma filtration surgery, *Invest. Ophthalmol. Vis. Sci.*, 29:1692.

116. Jammel, H. D., Leong, K. W., Dunkelburger, G. R., and Quigley, H. A. (1990). Glaucoma filtration surgery in monkeys using 5-fluorouridine in polyanhydride disks, *Arch. Ophthalmol.*, 1008:430.

117. Schubert, H. D., and Federman, J. L. (1989). The role of inflammation in CW Nd:YAG contact transscleral photocoagulation and cryopexy, *Invest. Ophthalmol. Vis. Sci.*, 30:543.

118. Zigler, J. S. (1990). Animal models for the study of maturity-onset and hereditary cataract, *Exp. Eye Res.*, 50:651.

119. Wegener, A., Maierhofer, O., Heints, M., and Hockwin, O. (1989). Testing possible cocataractogenic potential of befunolol (GlauconexR) with animal cataract model, *J. Ocul. Pharmacol.*, 5:45.

120. Van der Voet, J. C. M., Liem, A., Otto, A. J., and Kijlstra, A. (1989). Intraocular antibody synthesis during experimental uveitis, *Invest. Ophthalmol. Vis. Sci.*, 30:316.

121. Wacker, W. B., Donoso, L. A., Kalsow, C. M., Yankeelov, J. A., and Organisciak, D. T. (1977). Experimental allergic uveitis. Isolation, characterization, and localization of a soluble uveitopathogenic antigen from bovine retina, *J. Immunol.*, 119:1949.

122. Nussenblatt, R. B., Kuwabara, T., de Monasterio, F. M., and Wacker, W. B. (1981). S-antigen uveitis in primates. A new model for human disease, *Arch. Ophthalmol.*, 99:1090.

123. Mahlberg, K., Uusitalo, H., Palkama, A., and Tallberg, Y. (1987). Correlation between histopathological, clinical and biochemical parameters in S-antigen–induced experimental autoimmune uveitis in guinea-pigs, *Exp. Eye Res.*, 45:1157.

124. Mahlberg, K., Uusitalo, R., Palkama, A., and Tallberg, T. (1987). Phospholipase A_2, leukotriene C_4 and prostaglandin E_2 levels in aqueous humor of guinea pigs with experimental S-antigen induced autoimmune uveitis, *Curr. Eye Res.*, 2:321.

125. Mahlberg, K., Uusitalo, H., Uusitalo, R., Palkama, A., and Tallberg, T. (1987). Suppression of experimental autoimmune uveitis in guinea pigs by ethylenediamine, tetra-acetic acid, corticosteroids, and cyclosporine, *J. Ocul. Pharmacol.*, 3:199.

126. Dinning, W. J., Nussenblatt, R. B., Kuwabara, T., and Leake, W. (1987). The induction of tolerance by cyclosporine-G in experimental autoimmune uveitis in the Lewis rat, *J. Ocul. Pharmacol., 3*:135.

127. Nordmann, J. P., de Kozak, Y., le Hoang, P., and Faure, J. P. (1986). Cyclosporine therapy of guinea-pig autoimmune uveoretinitis induced with autologous retina, *J. Ocul. Pharmacol., 2*:325.

128. Romero, J., Marak, G. E., and Rao, N. (1989). Pharmacologic modulation of acute ocular inflammation with quercetin, *Ophthalmol. Res., 21*:112.

129. Marak, G. E., deKozak, Y., Faure, J. P., Rao, N. A., Romero, J. L., Ward, P. A., and Till, G. O. (1988). Pharmacologic modulation of acute ocular inflammation, *Ophthalmic. Res., 20*:220.

130. Kawashima, H., Fujino, Y., and Mochizuki, M. (1990). Antigen-specific suppressor cells induced by FK506 in experimental autoimmune uveoretinitis in the rat, *Invest. Ophthalmol. Vis. Sci., 31*:2500.

131. Chiou, G. C. Y., and Chang, M. S. (1990). Ocular inflammation induced by lens protein and its prevention. In: *Lipid Mediators in Eye Inflammation* (N. G. Bazan, ed.). Karger, Basel, p. 94.

132. Miyano, K., and Chiou, G. C. Y. (1984). Pharmacological prevention of ocular inflammation induced by lens proteins, *Ophthalmic Res., 16*:256.

133. Chiou, L. Y., and Chiou, G. C. Y. (1985). Ocular anti-inflammatory action of lipoxygenase inhibitor in the rabbit, *J. Ocul. Pharmacol., 1*:383.

134. Chuanng, C. Y., Xiao, J. G., and Chiou, G. C. Y. (1987). Ocular anti-inflammatory action of matrine, *J. Ocul. Pharmacol., 3*:129.

135. Chang, M. S., and Chiou, G. C. Y. (1989). Prevention of lens protein-induced ocular inflammation with cyclooxygenase and lipoxygenase inhibitors. *J. Ocul. Pharmacol., 5*:353.

136. Rao, N. A., Fernandez, M. A., Sevanian, A., Romero, J. L., Till, G. O., and Marak, G. E. (1988). Treatment of experimental lens-induced uveitis by dimethyl thiourea, *Ophthalmic Res., 20*:106.

137. Rao, N. A., Romero, J. L., Sevanian, A., Fernandez, M. A., Wong, C., Ward, P. A., and Marak, G. E. (1988). Anti-inflammatory effect of glutathione peroxidase on experimental lens-induced uveitis, *Ophthalmic Res., 20*:213.

138. Cousins, S. W., Guss, R. B., Howes, E. L., and Rosenbaum, J. T. (1984). Endotoxin-induced uveitis in the rat: Observations on altered vascular permeability, clinical findings, and histology, *Exp. Eye Res., 39*:665.

139. Wells, A., Paraarajasegaram, G., Baldwin, M., Yang, C. H., Hammer, M., and Fox, A. (1986). Uveitis and arthritis induced by systemic injection of streptococcal cell walls, *Invest. Ophthalmol. Vis. Sci., 27*:921.

140. Kulkarni, P. S., and Srinnivasan, B. D. (1988). Cachectin: A novel polypeptide induces uveitis in the rabbit eye, *Exp. Eye Res., 46*:631.

141. Csukas, S., Patersson, C. A., Brown, K., and Bhattacherjee, P. (1990). Time course of rabbit ocular inflammatory response and mediator release after intravitreal endotoxin, *Invest. Ophthalmol. Vis. Sci., 31*:382.

142. Rubin, R. M., Bennett, W. M., Elzinga, L., and Rosenbaum, J. T. (1988). Effects of a fish oil dietary supplement on endotoxin-induced ocular inflammation. *J. Occul. Pharmacol., 4*:259.

143. Fleisher, L. N., Ferrell, J. B., Olson, N. C., and McGahan, M. C. (1989). Dimethylthiourea inhibits the inflammatory response to intravitreally-injected endotoxin, *Exp. Eye Res., 48*:561.

144. Lin, N., Bazan, H. E. P., Braquet, P., and Bazan, N. G. (1991). Prolonged effect of a new platelet-activating factor antagonist on ocular vascular permeability in an endotoxin model of uveitis, *Curr. Eye Res., 10*:19.

145. Abelson, M. B., Butrus, S. I., Kliman, G. H., Larson, D. L., Corey, E. J., and Smith, L. M. (1987). Topical arachidonic acid: A model for screening anti-inflammatory agents, *J. Ocul. Pharmacol., 3*:63.

146. Tilden, M. E., Boney, R. S., Goldberg, M. M., and Rosenbaum, J. T. (1990). The effect of topical S(+)-ibuprofen on interleukin-1 induced ocular inflammation in a rabbit eye, *J. Ocul. Pharmacol., 6*:131.

147. Rowland, J. M., Ford, C. J., Della Puca, R. A., and Cash, W. D. (1986). Effects of topical diclofenac sodium in a rabbit model of ocular inflammation and leukotaxis, *J. Ocul. Pharmacol.*, 2:23.

148. Houng, P. F. J., Verbey, N., Thörig, L., and van Haeringen, N. J. (1986). Topical prostaglandins inhibit trauma-induced inflammation in the rabbit eye, *Invest. Ophthalmol. Vis. Sci.*, 27:1217.

149. Kurnik, R. T., Burde, R., and Becker, B. (1989). Breakdown of the blood-aqueous barrier in the rabbit eye by infrared radiation, *Invest. Ophthalmol. Vis. Sci.*, 30:717.

150. Unger, W. G. (1990). Review: Mediation of the ocular response to injury, *J. Ocul. Pharmacol.*, 6:337.

151. Beyer, T. L., Vogler, G., Sharma, D., and O'Donnell, F. E. (1984). Protective barrier effect of the posterior lens capsule in exogenous bacterial endophthalmitis: An experimental primate study, *Invest. Ophthalmol. Vis. Sci.*, 25:108.

152. Aizuss, D. H., Mondino, B. J., Sumner, H. L., and Dethlefs, B. (1985). The complement system and host defence against Pseudomonas endophthalmitis, *Invest. Ophthalmol. Vis. Sci.*, 26:1262.

153. Ormerod, D., Koch, K., Juarez, R. S., Edelstein, M. A. C., Rife, L. L., Finegold, S. M., and Smith, R. E. (1986). Anaerobic bacterial endophthalmitis in the rabbit, *Invest. Ophthalmol. Vis. Sci.*, 27:115.

154. Ormerod, L. D., Edelstein, M. A. C., Schmidt, G. J., Juarez, R. S., Finegold, S. M., and Smith, R. E. (1987). The intraocular environment and experimental anaerobic bacterial endophthalmitis, *Arch. Ophthalmol.*, 105:1571.

155. Nobe, J. R., Finegold, S. M., Rife, L. L., Edelstein, M. A. C., and Smith, R. E. (1987). Chronic anaerobic bacterial endophthalmitis in pseudophakic rabbit eye, *Invest. Ophthalmol. Vis. Sci.*, 28:259.

156. Talley, A. R., D'Amico, D. J., Talamo, J. H., Casey, V. N. J., and Kenyon, K. R. (1987). The role of vitrectomy in the treatment of postoperative bacterial endophthalmitis. An experimental study, *Arch. Ophthalmol.*, 105:1699.

157. Martin, D. F., Ficker, L. A., and Aguilar, H. A. (1990). Vitreous cefazolin levels after intravenous injection. Effects of inflammation, repeated antibiotic doses, and surgery, *Invest. Ophthalmol. Vis. Sci.*, 108:411.

158. Holland, G. N., Togni, B. I., Briones, O. C., and Dawson, C. R. (1987). A microscopic study of herpes simplex virus retinopathy in mice, *Invest. Ophthalmol. Vis. Sci.*, 28:1181.

159. Whittum-Hudson, J. A., and Pepose, J. S. (1987). Immunologic modulation of virus-induced pathology in a murine model of acute herpetic retinal necrosis, *Invest. Ophthalmol. Vis. Sci.*, 28:1541.

160. Hamasaki, D. I., Atherton, S. S., and Dix, R. D. (1990). HSV-2 alters retinal physiology and morphology bilaterally in mice, *Invest. Ophthalmol. Vis. Sci.*, 31:1056.

161. Oh, J. O., Minasi, P., Grabner, G., and Ohashi, Y. (1985). Suppression of secondary herpes simplex uveitis by cyclosporine, *Invest. Ophthalmol. Vis. Sci.*, 26:494.

162. Hayashi, K., Kurihara, I., and Uchida, Y. (1985). Studies of ocular murine cytomegalovirus infection, *Invest. Ophthalmol. Vis. Sci.*, 26:486.

163. Holland, G. N., Fang, E. N., Glasgow, B. J., Zaragosa, A. M., Siegel, L. M., Graves, M. C., Saxton, E. H., and Foos, R. Y. (1990). Necrotizing retinopathy after intraocular inoculation of murine cytomegaloviris in immunosuppresses adult mice, *Invest. Ophthalmol. Vis. Sci.*, 31:2326.

164. Rabinovitch, T., Oh, J. O., and Minasi, P. (1990). In vivo reactivation of latent murine cytomegalovirus in the eye by immunosuppressive treatment, *Invest. Ophthalmol. Vis. Sci.*, 31:657.

165. Donnelly, J. J., Taylor, H. R., Young, E., Khatami, M., Lok, J. B., and Rockey, (1986). Experimental ocular onchocerciasis in cynomolgus monkey, *Invest. Ophthalmol. Vis. Sci.*, 27:492.

166. Donnely, J. J., Xi, M. S., Haldar, J. P., Hill, D. E., Lok, J. B., Khatami, M., and Rockey, J. H. (1988). Autoantibody induced by experimental onchocerca infection. Effect of different routes of administration of microfilariae and of treatment with diethylcarbamazine citrate and ivermectin, *Invest. Ophthalmol. Vis. Sci., 29*:827.

167. Tano, Y., Sugita, G., Abrams, G., and Machemer, R. (1980). Inhibition of intraocular proliferations with intravitreal corticosteroids, *Am. J. Ophthalmol., 89*:131.

168. Sunalp, M. A., Wiedemann, P., Sorgente, N., and Ryan, S. J. (1985). Effect of Adriamycin on experimental proliferative vitreoretinopathy in the rabbit, *Exp. Eye Res., 41*:105.

169. Chandler, D. B., Rozakis, G., deJuan, E., and Machemer, R. (1985). The effect of triamcinolone acetonide on a refined experimental model of proliferative vitreoretinopathy, *Am. J. Ophthalmol., 99*:686.

170. Wiedemann, P., Sorgente, N., Bekhor, C., Patterson, R., Tran, T., and Ryan, S. J. (1985). Daunomycin in the treatment of experimental proliferative vitreoretinopathy, *Invest. Ophthalmol. Vis. Sci., 26*:719.

171. Van Bockxmeer, F. M., Martin, C. E., Thompson, D. E., and Constable, I. J. (1985). Taxol for the treatment of proliferative vitreoretinopathy, *Invest. Ophthalmol. Vis. Sci., 26*:1140.

172. Miller, B., Miller, H., and Ryan, S. J. (1986). Experimental epiretinal proliferations induced by intravitreal red blood cells, *Am. J. Ophthalmol., 102*:188.

173. Snyder, R. W., Lambrou, F. H., and Williams, G. A. (1987). Intraocular fibrinolysis with recombinant human tissue plasminogen activator. Experimental treatment in a rabbit model, *Arch. Ophthalmol., 105*:1277.

174. Tsuboi, S., and Pederson, J. E. (1987). Permeability of the blood-retinal barrier to carboxy-fluorescein in eyes with rhegmatogenous retinal detachment, *Invest. Ophthalmol. Vis. Sci., 28*:96.

175. Kawano, S., and Marmor, M. F. (1988). Metabolic influences on the absorption of serous subretinal fluid, *Invest. Ophthalmol. Vis. Sci., 29*:1255.

176. Organisciak, D. T., Wang, H., Li, Z. Y., and Tso, M. O. M. (1985). The protective effect of ascorbate in retinal light damage in rats, *Invest. Ophthalmol. Vis. Sci., 26*:1985.

177. Li, Z. Y., Tso, M. O. M., Wang, H., and Organisciak, D. T. (1985). Amelioration of photic injury in rat retina by ascorbic acid: A histopathologic study, *Invest. Ophthalmol. Vis. Sci., 26*:1589.

178. Katz, M. L., and Eldred, G. E. (1989). Failure of vitamin E to protect the retina against damage resulting from bright cyclic light exposure, *Invest. Ophthalmol. Vis. Sci., 30*:29.

179. Gottlieb, J. L., Antoszyk, A. N., Hatchell, D. L., Saloupis, P. (1990). The safety of intravitreal hyaluronidase. A clinical and histologic study, *Invest. Ophthalmol. Vis. Sci., 31*:2345.

180. Antoszyk, A. N., Gottlieb, J. L., Casey, R. C., Hatchell, D. L., and Machemer, R. (1991). An experimental model of preretinal neovascularization in the rabbit, *Invest. Ophthalmol. Vis. Sci., 32*:46.

181. Miller, H., Miller, B., and Ryan, S. J. (1986). The role of retinal pigment epithelium in the involution of subretinal neovascularization, *Invest. Ophthalmol. Vis. Sci., 27*:1644.

182. Ishibashi, T., Miki, K., Sorgente, N., Patterson, R., and Ryan, S. J. (1985). Effects of intravitreal administration of steroids in the subhuman primate, *Arch. Ophthalmol., 103*:708.

183. Stefansson, E., Novack, R. L., and Hatchell, D. L. (1990). Vitrectomy prevents retinal hypoxia in branch retinal vein occlusion, *Invest. Ophthalmol. Vis. Sci., 31*:284.

184. Wallow, I. H. L., Bindley, C. D., Linton, K. L. P., and Rastergar, D. (1991). Pericyte changes in branch retinal vein occlusion, *Invest. Ophthalmol. Vis. Sci., 32*:1455.

185. Szabo, M. E., Droy-Lefaix, M. T., Doly, M., Carre, C., and Braquet, P. (1991). Ischemia and perfusion-induced histologic changes in the rat retina. Demonstration of a free radical-mediated mechanism, *Invest. Ophthalmol. Vis. Sci., 32*:1471.

186. Kremer, I., Kissun, R., Nissenkorn, I., Ben-Sira, I., and Garner, A. (1991). Oxygen-induced retinopathy in newborn kittens. A model for ischemic vasoproliferative retinopathy, *Invest. Ophthalmol. Vis. Sci., 28*:126.

187. Vinores, S. A., Campochiaro, P. A., May, E. E., and Blaydes, S. H. (1988). Progressive ultrastructural damage and thickening of the basement membrane of the retinal pigment epithelium in spontaneously diabetic BB rats, *Exp. Eye Res., 46*:545.

188. Caldwell, R. B., Slapnick, S. M., and McLaughlin, B. J. (1986). Decreased anionic sites in Bruch's membrane of spontaneous and drug-induced diabetes, *Invest. Ophthalmol. Vis. Sci., 27*:1691.

189. Tilton, R. G., Chang, K., Weigel, C., Eades, D., Sherman, W. R., Kilo, C., and Williamson, J. R. (1988). Increased ocular blood flow and ^{125}I-albumin permeation in galactose-fed rats: inhibition by sorbinil, *Invest. Ophthalmol. Vis. Sci., 29*:861.

190. Robinson, W. G., Nagata, M., Laver, N., Hohman, T. C., and Kinoshita, J. H. (1989). Diabetic-like retinopathy in rats prevented with an aldose reductase inhibitor, *Invest. Ophthalmol. Vis. Sci., 30*:2285.

191. Mansour, S. Z., Hatchell, D. L., Chandler, D., Saloupis, P., and Hatchell, M. C. (1990). Reduction of basement membrane thickening in diabetic cat retina by sulindac, *Invest. Ophthalmol. Vis. Sci., 31*:457.

192. Anderson, R. E., Maude, M. B., Alvarez, R. A., Acland, G. M., and Aguirre, G. D. (1991). Plasma lipid abnormalities in the miniature poodle with progressive lid-cone degeneration, *Exp. Eye Res., 52*:349.

193. Danciger, M., Bowes, C., Kozak, C. A., LaVail, M. M., and Farber, D. B. (1990). Fine mapping of a putative rd cDNA and its co-segregation with rd expression, *Invest. Ophthalmol. Vis. Sci., 31*:1427.

194. Nir, I., Sagie, G., and Papermaster, D. S. (1987). Opsin accumulation in photoreceptor inner segment plasma membranes of dystrophic RCS rats, *Invest. Ophthalmol. Vis. Sci., 28*:62.

195. Lin, W. L., and Essner, E. (1988). Retinal dystrophy in Wistar-Furth rats, *Exp. Eye Res., 46*:1.

196. Narfström, K. (1985). Progressive retinal atrophy in the Abyssinian cat, *Invest. Ophthalmol. Vis. Sci., 26*:193.

8
Mathematical Models of Ocular Drug Transport and Disposition

Kenneth J. Himmelstein *University of Nebraska Medical Center, Omaha, Nebraska*

I. INTRODUCTION

The eye is one of the most highly structured organs on a macroscopic level in human (and mammalian) systems. The structures contained in the eye were developed evolutionarily to receive and transduce signals from visible light. Yet, these same structures are otherwise interesting, being one of the most fruitful domains in which to develop drug delivery strategies to manipulate and exploit in order to optimize therapeutic treatment. Because of the anatomy and physiology of the eye, there are significant opportunities for the chemotherapeutic treatment of the eye not possible with other tissues and organs that are more diffuse, less segregated with respect to function, or available to drugs only by the systemic circulation.

Notwithstanding the above, the eye, quite frankly, is a difficult target for drug delivery. This is because of the same reason that it offers so many possibilities: the structured and complex interrelationship of tissues, structures placed together in a highly interactive fashion with respect to transport, absorption, pharmacology, and elimination of drugs. A knowledge of the interrelationship of the various processes which affect and offer strategies for drug delivery is required for that effort to be successful.

The analysis of the complex nature of drug pharmacokinetics and pharmacodynamics in the eye is very much amenable to quantitative procedures, specifically mathematical modeling. Two distinct benefits accrue. First, the interrelationship between various serial and parallel processes can be assessed; and second, the lack of an understanding of unidentified processes can be determined by the inability to describe adequately the phenomena of interest. With this power, no longer are we left with only concepts of "rate-limiting processes" and "competing processes"—we can tell how much.

II. DRUG TRANSPORT AND ELIMINATION

To understand how drugs are transported to their site of action and eliminated on only a superficial level, consider the following processes which occur when a topical dosage form is placed in the cul-de-sac of the eye.

A. Anterior Area

1. Mixing of the dosage form with tear fluid
2. Elimination by tear drainage, a function of the instilled dosage form
3. Dilution by induced and natural tear production
4. Absorption by nonproductive routes, e.g., conjunctival absorption
5. Spillage
6. Ionization in an open buffered system
7. Protein binding
8. Metabolism and chemical degradation
9. Pharmacological effects such as vasodilation

B. Cornea

1. Surface interactions of drug between tear film and mucosal layer
2. Transport across the multilayered cornea by trans- and paricellular routes
3. Interactions with components of the cornea such as protein binding
4. Metabolism

C. Anterior Chamber

1. Transport through the aqueous humor
2. Distribution and uptake into tissues such as iris and lens
3. Elimination by aqueous humor turnover
4. Redistribution from tissues due to the transient nature and differing time constants in various tissues
5. Protein binding and metabolism
6. Pharmacological effects such as induced aqueous humor flow
7. Elimination by blood and aqueous humor flow

This incomplete listing of the processes which affect the pharmacokinetics of drugs in the eye after topical administration serves to demonstrate the complexity of the system. However, as stated above, ocular pharmacokinetics and pharmacodynamics are suitable for mathematical analysis, since the tissues and transport phenomena are distinct and identifiable. It is the purpose of this chapter to present some of the efforts to develop such descriptions, evaluate their success or failure, and to present areas of potentially fruitful future work.

III. MODELING GOALS AND STRUCTURE

In this chapter, the mathematical models developed to describe the transport and disposition of drugs in the eye after topical administration will be covered. These models have been developed because it is apparent that the factors which influence how a drug reaches, enters, and remains at the site of action can have as dramatic effect on the efficacy as the inherent pharmacological action. This is especially true of ophthalmic drugs since, because of rapid precorneal elimination and the barrier properties of the eye, only a small fraction of the administered dose reaches the site of action, usually in a rapidly transient mode.

Mathematical modeling of the local pharmacokinetics of ophthalmic drugs, like other modeling efforts, is done to determine whether or not the perceived interrelationships between various processes is responsible for the observed phenomena. Thus, it is possible to determine if all important processes are known and to determine what the relative importance of these processes are. If a representative model is available, then various scenarios such as controlled delivery, ocular retention, increased uptake by penetration enhancement, and other drug manipulations can be evaluated in a prospective manner to evaluate the approach before expensive and extensive laboratory work is undertaken.

In this chapter, only those models that have been developed based on a mechanism of action will be considered. Often in the course of drug development, the local concentrations of drug in the tear film or aqueous humor will be described by curve-fitted models. These models lack any predictive power, since although the curve fit may be called "compartmental," no significance can be placed on the parameters or model structure used. As an example, typical aqueous humor concentration-time profiles after a single topical dose can be fitted with a one-compartment with first-order absorption model. Since only the aqueous humor concentration is being fitted, the model lacks any power to describe the mechanism which makes up this gross description and, therefore, cannot be used in a predictive manner. As will be seen, the division between curve-fitted and mechanistic models is not clear-cut.

Two basic model forms have commonly been used for ophthalmic pharmacokinetic modeling: lumped and distributed parameter.

A. Lumped Parameter Models

Lumped parameter models are constructed by assuming that a given anatomical space is homogeneous with respect to drug concentration. The space represented may be any given area, from intracellular up through (in general) the whole body. Obviously the predictive power of these models depends on the soundness of this assumption. The power of this assumption is that no spatial dimension need be included in the model. Not only does this simplify the model conceptually, but also reduces the model from partial to ordinary differential equations for dynamic systems or from ordinary differential equations to algebraic equations for steady-state systems. In this chapter, the terms *compartment* and *homogeneous* (but identifiable) volume are used interchangeably.

B. Distributed Parameter Models

In distributed parameter models, spatial dimensions are included as independent variables. In exchange for the obviously increased mathematical difficulty, the ability to describe tissues and structures where the concentration of drug is significantly different over time scales is important to treatment. As will become clear, two areas where this is important for ocular pharmacokinetics are transcorneal transport with short transients in the precorneal area and transport in the lens, which tends to act as a sink structure. Each of these modeling approaches have utility in the description of ocular pharmacokinetics.

A. Model Principles

In order to avoid repetitive presentation of the models to be discussed in this section, the basic model structure common to all of the models is presented here. In the course of discussion of each example taken from the literature, the equation structure will be comparable to the form presented here and the actual equations reconstructed by reference to the particular schematic model representation.

1. Lumped Parameter Models

In many biological systems, volumes of interest can be treated as being homogeneous with respect to drug distribution. In these cases, a powerful simplifying assumption can be made: The tissue can be considered to be a volume where all of the events with respect to the drug are the same everywhere. This assumption allows the mass balances for the drug to be written as sets of ordinary differential equations which can be solved relatively easily compared to partial differential equations which result when spatial differences are included. The transport between and from these homogeneous tissues is described by transfer based on the bulk concentrations in the tissue or organ under study. The assumption is not limited to a given level of hierarchy: intra- and extracellular spaces, tissues, organs, and entire organisms can sometimes be treated by this approach. A differentiation must be made between lumped parameter models which describe the observed data. On one hand, some observed phenomenon, e.g., blood level of a drug, can be described by a series of lumped parameter equations which are not relative to known mechanistic processes. These models, which are not predictive, are commonly called compartmental models. A second class of models, while based on the same simplifying assumption of homogeneity, are termed physiological-anatomical, since they are based on knowledge of the various processes and extent, e.g., the correct anatomical volume, which govern the mass balances of the drug. Thus, each term in the equation can be associated with known events. Thus, the models may be predictive and are useful for testing the knowledge base concerning drug transport and elimination.

The eye, as noted above, is an organ for which a physiological-anatomical modeling approach is tailormade. Many of the structures in the eye are distinct on a macroscopic level and are placed in juxtaposition with each other such that drug-related events in one affect those in another in a complex and interrelated way. The line between compartmental analysis and physiological-anatomical modeling is not clear-cut however, since homogeneous regions, e.g., aqueous humor, lens, and precorneal area, are clearly identifiable, yet the transport and elimination processes may not be. As a result, it is not possible to point to the first physiologically based model or even to state unequivocally that a given model meets the definition given above. Nonetheless, we will attempt to do just that.

The basis for any mechanistic lumped parameter (homogeneous volume) pharmacokinetic model is the conservation of mass. In the case of metabolizable drugs, the species balance is constructed analogously.

$$\begin{array}{ccccccc} \text{rate of mass} \\ \text{accumulated} \end{array} = \begin{array}{c} \text{rate of mass in} \\ \text{by transport} \end{array} - \begin{array}{c} \text{rate of mass out} \\ \text{by transport} \end{array} - \begin{array}{c} \text{rate of} \\ \text{metabolism} \end{array}$$

That is, any mass in the open system must be conserved or accounted for by removal from the system. Systems of equations are then developed for each of the volumes and species of drug or metabolite. The equations form a coupled set, in general, since the transport from one tissue or compartment to another usually depends on the drug concentration in more than one compartment.

Translating the above word equation to the format most commonly employed, a typical mass or species balance takes the form

$$\frac{dV(t)C(t)}{dt} = \Sigma pf[C(t)] + \Sigma Q(t)C(t) + \Sigma kg[C(t)]$$

where V is the volume of the tissue, C is the concentration of drug in the tissue, p is the coefficient associated with molecular (diffusive) transport, Q denotes convective (flow) transport, and k the proportionally constant associated with metabolism. Time, t, is the independent variable. The functions f and g are defined by knowledge of the particular process. For example, if a metabolic process is enzymatically mediated, it may well take on a nonlinear form akin to a Michaelis-Menten expression. The summations are used to indicate that more than one of each type of process may be present.

The volume and flow rate terms are written as a function of time. As will be seen, these terms may vary owing to the physiology of the eye and its dependence on the drug of interest. The transport based on diffusion to and from each tissue is generally based on the transport mechanism describable by Fick's first law:

$$J = - \frac{DdC}{dx}$$

where J is the flux, and the right-hand side denotes that the flux is proportional to the instantaneous derivative with respect to position, x. This expression can be integrated at steady state to yield

$$\frac{\text{Amount}}{\text{Time}} = \frac{DA}{1}(C_1 - C_2)$$

where A is the area and 1 the distance over which the transport occurs between two characteristic concentrations. In biological systems, it is difficult to assess the separate parameters and DA/1 are often lumped into a single mass transfer coefficient, p. The units of p are volume/time, a clearance, and must not be confused with first-order rate constants. Similarly, the metabolic terms are constructed from functional forms which resemble typical homogeneous rate laws, but care must be taken to ensure consistent units when included in the mass balances.

From these basic expressions mechanistically derived sets of mass balances can be constructed to represent drug instillation, distribution, metabolism, and elimination. The individual models to be considered all use this starting point.

IV. PHYSIOLOGICALLY BASED MODELS FOR PILOCARPINE

In this section, the models which have been developed to describe the ocular distribution and elimination of pilocarpine after topical administration are considered.

A. Precorneal Flow and Volume

The first physiological-anatomically based model to describe ocular pharmacokinetics was constructed to describe the distribution of pilocarpine from the precorneal area into the aqueous humor (1). The model structure is shown in Figure 1. It is useful to examine some

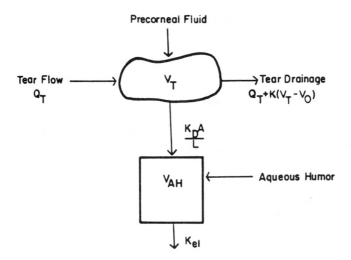

Figure 1. Model scheme. (From Ref. 1. Reproduced with permission of the copyright owner, the American Pharmaceutical Association.)

of the assumptions used—both stated and tacit—to reveal the extent to which a model can be predictive in the sense that all relevant mechanisms are included. This examination will then allow a more parsimonious approach with respect to model structure when reviewing other ocular pharmacokinetic modeling.

This model is nominally physiologically based, since it attempts to provide a description of clearly identifiable physiological volumes, the precorneal area and the aqueous humor. Both volumes are clearly candidates to be considered homogeneous, since they are composed of fluid volumes. In the case of the precorneal area, the volume is a direct function of the instilled volume of the dosage; this has been included in the model. Whether or not the two volumes are truly homogeneous with respect to drug concentration is certainly much more open to question. In each case, the liquid pool receives fresh fluid, either tears or aqueous humor. In the former case, the presence of either the drug or the extra instilled volume may well effect the tear production rate. In each case, the location of both the inflow and outflow streams is well defined. Only in the case of the tear film is there a mechanism for stirring. The real justification for homogeneity, however, lies in the time scales of the processes that depend on the homogeneity assumption compared to the time scale of the processes that "create" the homogeneity. If the time scale for mixing is rapid compared to the time scale of the processes that depend on homogeneity, no matter what their real values, then the assumption will be valid.

In the precorneal area of this model, two processes which depend on the homogeneity assumption are the corneal transport and the tear drainage. The time scale for each of these processes is slow compared to the blink rate (four/min) and, therefore, the model probably makes a reasonable assumption. It is not clear that the assumption holds for the aqueous humor, since the turnover is slow (1%/min), and the flow is laminar to and from the center of the chamber in the radial direction. Whether or not the assumption holds depends on the method of observation.

Experimentally, the aqueous humor is sampled in a mixing-cup fashion with time points relatively widely spaced (0.1/min), since the samples are obtained with difficulty and destructively. Therefore, in the sense of sampling times, all processes which affect the aqueous humor concentration are rapid enough to allow the assumption of homogeneity. As a result, it would be very difficult in practice to determine deviations from the assumption for this anatomical compartment.

Now consider the transport processes in this model as shown in Figure 1 and compare them to the processes actually present in the biological system. Let us go from the realistic to the simplistic; minor commissions and omissions of sin to the truly egregious. The tear drainage from the eye had previously been shown to be dependent on the volume of the instilled dosage. To be truly mechanistic, the model would have to be able to include the causal phenomena which led to the observed phenomenon; i.e., volume-dependent tear drainage. Since this information was not available, a correlation between flow and volume was determined by curve-fitting. As a result, the model thus lacks the ability to predict this relationship outside of the available data and is useful only within the range of sizes of drops and their frequency—one administration until complete drug washout occurs. Since this is not clearly pointed out, the model promises more than it can ultimately deliver. However, this sin of omission is not the least of the problems here caused by the over-promise of mechanistically based modeling.

It is assumed that the clearance from the aqueous humor can be lumped into a single first-order elimination. For the aqueous humor drainage, a clearly defined convective flow, this form is both theoretically and practically correct. The implications of lumping other elimination processes with it is not so clear.

First, there is the explicit assumption that the other processes, e.g., distribution to other tissues, is unimportant. There are three distinct implications with this assumption. First, it is clearly presumed that the mass balance is not affected by the mass that is obviously being distributed there. The assumption also precludes the reverse transport of drugs from these tissues to the aqueous humor as drug is cleared from the aqueous.

Second, it is tacitly assumed that the mass transport is rapid enough between the site of action, presumably the trabecular meshwork, and the aqueous humor. This raises a significant point: When the mass of drug in the effect tissue is small compared to the mass in the system, it is all but impossible to accurately model drug concentration in that tissue, since it will not have significant impact on the overall disposition of drug in the system. Thus, small changes in the parameters (real, such as an actual volume different from the literature value used in the model, or model related, such as poorly fitted parameters or stiff differential equations) lead to predicted concentrations vastly different than those observed. The utility of any model to yield pharmacodynamic insight hinges on this subtle point.

Finally, this assumption limits the time frame of application of the model as well as the concentration limitations, since open mass systems with only an initial mass input are dissipative. This is especially important if the model is to be used to extrapolate to long times and/or small drug masses. As pointed out by Miller et al. (2), this is precisely the case for pilocarpine after single-drop administration.

The next most important deviation from mechanistic modeling contained in this effort resides in the form of the transport between the precorneal and aqueous humor volumes. It is assumed that the mass transfer between these two areas is proportional to the bulk concentration difference of the two. It is known that the cornea is a complex, multilayered tissue which has the ability to contain a significant mass of drug itself. Thus, it is both unlikely that a lumped parameter model of the cornea is appropriate (see discussion of distributed parameter models below) as well as subject to the limitations noted above when a drug-containing tissue is excluded from the model. These two limitations are relatively straightforward. What is not readily apparent is how this assumption, together with crucial missing data, can lead to a model that has no real predictive value at all despite the stated goal of the effort.

The first-order–like drainage term in the precorneal area gives substantially the same form for drug concentration in the precorneal area as that which would be achieved if other elimination processes such as absorption were included. However, the mass transfer coefficient, KdA/L, for drug transport across the cornea is estimated in terms of the model. (As an aside, the naming of this adjustable parameter demonstrates a second propensity of mechanistic modelers: It is implied that the parameter can be adjusted to yield other results if a rational manipulation of the parameter based on measurable conditions were conducted, i.e., an adjustable parameter may actually have a mechanistic interpretation. That the authors never did so implied more worth to the model than actually is warranted.) Since precorneal concentrations were not available at the time of the modeling effort, the combination of one free adjustable parameter, KdA/L, and the presence of one differential equation, the precorneal area expression, for which no dependent variable data are available, leads to a system where the calculated precorneal concentrations can take on any values at all and still yield reasonable aqueous humor concentrations. Thus, the extra "mass balance" representing the precorneal area is not physiological at all but is really a second degree of freedom in the model system. In practice, the calculated precorneal concentrations are actually two or so orders of magnitude higher than the actual concentrations (3–5). That the model is "predictive" at all is based on the presence of two processes (drainage, included, and nonproductive absorption, not included) with approximately the same form and the presence of a second degree of freedom, the extraneous differential equation. While little damage was directly done, since the stated limitations of the model in the original paper practically precluded testing anything but interpolated results, it is clear that this model is unable to dispel the confusion concerning the mechanisms contributing to removal of drug from the precorneal volume. Figure 2 shows, however, that the model is able to demonstrate the effect of dose volume and concentration of pilocarpine after topical administration, at least in an interpolative sense.

After that critique, it is probably anticlimactic to suggest that several important and useful points did emerge from that effort. First, it illustrated that the aqueous humor concentration after single-drop administration of pilocarpine could well depend on the presence of processes in the precorneal area that depended on both the volume of the instilled dose as well as the concentration. Second, it illustrated that a quantitative description based on known transport processes could be used to study the pharmacokinetics in structured organs such as the eye.

B. A Comprehensive Precorneal Area Pharmacokinetic Model

Given the deficiencies of the physiological model noted above, particularly the lack of quantitation of precorneal area drug concentration, a model which included instilled volume effects as well as other factors was lacking. This void was remedied in the work of Lee and Robinson (3). Indeed, their paper is representative of how a mechanistically based mathematical model can be used to assess the level of understanding of a complex set of

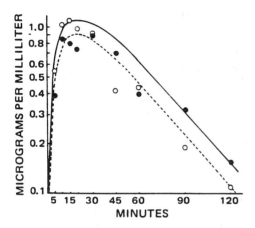

Figure 2.   Aqueous humor concentration time profile following administration of 25 μL of 1×10^{-2} M pilocarpine and 5 μL of 1.61×10^{-2} M pilocarpine. (From Ref. 1. Reproduced with permission of the copyright owner, the American Pharmaceutical Association.)

processes as well as lead to areas for new experimental observation. As a result, the work of Lee and Robinson is important as a model for the interaction of experimental and mathematical interaction to aid in understanding as well as the presentation of a comprehensive model of pilocarpine precorneal area disposition.

The authors (3) develop a comprehensive model of pilocarpine precorneal area disposition according to Figure 3. In this model, a four-area approach is used as shown. The cornea is viewed as a two-tissue structure with the ability both to contain drug and act as a barrier to transport, as was previously shown experimentally for this drug (6). Since the intent was to study the precorneal area, the receptor tissue was the third compartment composed of the stromal layer of the cornea and the aqueous humor. The fourth tissue was a volume of distribution, also observed experimentally (7). This latter volume represented a degree of freedom of the system which allowed fitting of the aqueous humor data very well. However, given the small contribution of the mass of drug in these areas compared to the mass of drug in the precorneal area, and given the intent of the study, the use of an arbitrary model structure for this portion should be viewed merely as minor fine tuning. To reject the success of this model to explore precorneal disposition on this small point would be (pilo)carping at best.

Mass balances for all four homogeneous compartments were written. The precorneal area included the variable volume and time-dependent drainage flow rate used previously (1). Also included was a nonproductive loss term which was assumed to be proportional to drug concentration. When examining the precorneal concentration of pilocarpine experimentally, the authors noted that while discernible when careful measurement was made, the effect of variable drainage and precorneal volume could be approximated as a time-averaged first-order loss, although with different constants when describing either precorneal area drug mass or concentration. The complete model using parameters measured independently in experimental systems where only one factor was present was tested to simulate the precorneal concentration of pilocarpine after single-drop administration. The complete model was unable to simulate the experimental result. In comparing the value of

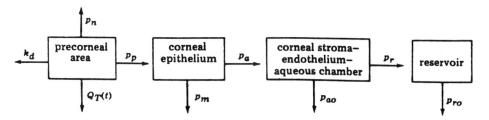

Figure 3. Model scheme. (From Ref. 3. Reproduced with permission of the copyright owner, the American Pharmaceutical Association.)

the nonproductive rate-loss constant attributable to conjunctival absorption with the overall time-averaged constant found experimentally, it was noted that there was not enough absorption by this route to account for the disposition of the drug in the face of all other known factors included such as volume reduction and time-dependent drainage. The authors then were able to demonstrate, based on this effort and on additional experimental data, that vasodilation but not induced lacrimation was a significant factor involved in precorneal disposition of pilocarpine. When the appropriate value for induced lacrimation was included, the model was able to calculate the precorneal and aqueous humor concentrations of pilocarpine, as shown in Figures 4 and 5.

In summary, the effort to realistically represent the multitude of competing processes present in the precorneal area of the eye is impressive; the various contributions of corneal and conjunctival absorption, tear turnover, instilled volume and induced drainage, induced lacrimation, and vasodilation are all included. Further, the basis for the inclusion of metabolism and protein binding is provided. This model still stands as the state of the art for precorneal pharmacokinetics.

As an aside, while alluding to the relative importance of precorneal factors for drug bioavailability, Lee and Robinson (3) did not explicitly demonstrate the influence of drainage and nonproductive absorption on corneal uptake of pilocarpine. This was left to others (5), who showed that while responsible for removal of a large fraction of the instilled mass of pilocarpine, the drainage mechanism did not significantly reduce the concentration of pilocarpine in the precorneal area. This reduction was primarily due to nonproductive absorption. As a result, since corneal absorption—and as a consequence local bioavailability—depends on the concentration present, the most important issue to improve the bioavailability of pilocarpine was to maintain a high concentration gradient for longer periods of time rather than the mere suppression of outflow. Employing these factors, the model is well able to represent the disposition of pilocarpine from the precorneal area.

V. A PHYSIOLOGICALLY BASED PHARMACOKINETIC MODEL FOR INTRAOCULAR DISTRIBUTION OF PILOCARPINE IN RABBITS

In previous models, the principal thrust was to develop a description for the precorneal area and its impact on aqueous humor concentration of drug. However, the distribution to other ocular tissues was either ignored (1) or lumped into a single, vaguely defined reservoir (3). This is justifiable based on mass balance considerations if the target tissue is the aqueous

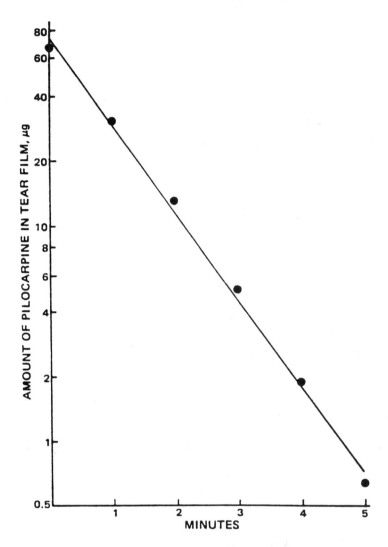

Figure 4. Simulated profile of pilocarpine concentration in the tear film. (From Ref. 3. Reproduced with permission of the copyright owner, the American Pharmaceutical Association.)

humor or if the other tissues do not significantly contribute to the mass balance. However, the target tissue may not be the aqueous humor; therefore, a model which takes into consideration distribution to and elimination from other ocular tissues can be of utility.

Miller et al. (4) have considered the intraocular pharmacokinetics of pilocarpine. Their model is shown in Figure 7. The cornea, aqueous humor, lens, and iris-ciliary body were each represented as homogeneous volumes. Mass transfer coefficients for each of the tissues was estimated from in vitro bathing experiments. In addition, since the bathing experiments were done, it was possible to estimate the equilibrium partition coefficient between tissue and aqueous humor. Thus, the forward and back rates of transport from each of the tissues are the same, and thermodynamic driving forces between the tissues are

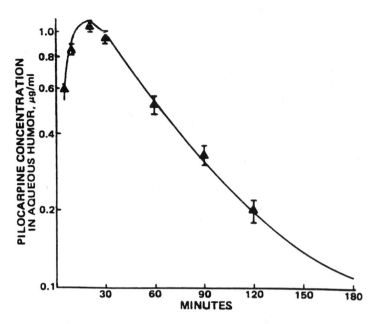

Figure 5. Simulation of pilocarpine in aqueous humor. (From Ref. 3. Reproduced with permission of the copyright owner, the American Pharmaceutical Association.)

included as an effective activity, C/PC, where C is the measured drug concentration in the tissue and PC is the ratio of drug concentration in the tissue to drug in the aqueous humor or tear film at equilibrium. A second refinement in the model was that it was possible to include the pharmacological effect of pilocarpine on aqueous humor outflow. The model does not include the precorneal considerations used by others to avoid the consequent numerical difficulties associated with a set of stiff differential equations. Instead, the precorneal concentration is included as a curve-fit forcing function.

The model was well able to represent the elimination of drug from interior ocular tissues, especially the aqueous humor and iris-ciliary body. That the model is less successful for the lens is probably due to the model considering the lens to be homogeneous. This is addressed further below. Combined with the detailed picture of the precorneal area provided by others (1,3,5–7), the macroscopic pharmacokinetics of pilocarpine is reasonably well described. Of particular interest is that most, if not all, of the parameters for these models are independently estimated from separate experimental determinations.

VI. PHYSIOLOGICALLY BASED MODELS FOR TIMOLOL OCULAR PHARMACOKINETICS

A very important drug for the treatment of glaucoma is timolol, a beta-blocker. The introduction of this compound in the late 1970s was concomitant with the development of physiologically based pharmacokinetic models for the eye. Models for this drug, then, were based on the prior efforts for pilocarpine. However, pointing out that a separate

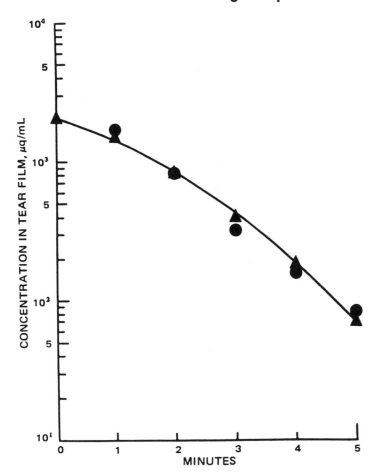

Figure 6. Simulated tear film concentration of pilocarpine. (From Ref. 5. Reproduced with permission of the copyright owner, the American Pharmaceutical Association.)

understanding of the pharmacokinetics must be gained for each particular drug, each of the models proposed has considerations which are peculiar to timolol.

Francoeur et al. (8) developed a model which includes the iris-ciliary body and aqueous humor as physiologically identified compartments. The uptake characteristics of these tissues as well as the cornea and lens were determined in in vitro and in vivo experiments. From these results, the authors made several observations, the most important of which is that the lens could not be treated as a homogeneous tissue over the time scale of interest for this compound. This, of course, is not surprising given the mass and structure of the lens compared to other ocular tissues. It is also consistent with the results of Miller et al. (4) for pilocarpine. As a result, instead of using a physiological compartment for the lens, experimentally determined concentrations of timolol in the lens after topical administration were fitted with a extrapolation from previous efforts on other drugs such as pilocarpine. As it is, the model is able to simulate systemic timolol blood levels after administration of timolol topically.

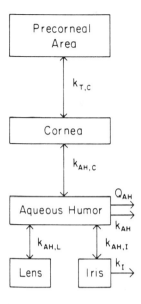

Figure 7. Model scheme. (From Ref. 4. Reprinted with permission of the copyright holder, the Plenum Publishing Co.)

Finally, the issue of how to tackle the inhomogeneous distribution of ophthalmic drugs was attacked initially be Ahmed et al. (10). In this effort, the lens is viewed as a one-dimensional slab geometry bathed on one side by the aqueous humor and the other by vitreous humor, both of which form time-variable boundary conditions for the slab by fitting experimentally determined timolol fluid concentrations. The main feature of the model was a position-dependent diffusivity justified by the perceived structure of the lens and the inability of a simple model to explain the observed results. Since the actual diffusivity-position relationship was hard to determine experimentally, an exponential polynomial functional form is assumed with two arbitrary parameters that are assumed to fit the diffusivity as a function of position. A suitable combination of parameters adequately represents a mixing-cup (i.e., a homogenized) average of the drug concentration in the lens as a function of time. Whether or not this is an adequate representation is not clear, since no experimentally available concentration profile is available for comparison. That being the case, it is easy to envision other structures and transport patterns which may also explain the observation such as two-dimensional diffusion. Be that as it may, the model does demonstrate that a complete understanding of ocular drug pharmacokinetics may well require distributed parameter approaches, especially for potent drugs with long durations of action.

VII. OCULAR PHARMACOKINETICS: STATUS AND PROSPECTS

While there have been a few other efforts (11–13) to describe comprehensive pharmacokinetics of the eye, the above models represent the main mechanistically based efforts which have demonstrated approaches available to describe ocular pharmacokinetics. The prospects for progress in this area are clearly open to question.

No single effort has been made to organize the complete pharmacokinetic profile of a drug in a single effort to give a comprehensive picture of known information, let alone accurately treat such questions as systemic uptake, pharmacodynamics, and local toxicity that is drug related. The closest effort has been the combined results of Lee and Robinson (3) and Miller et al. (4). Since the Lee-Robinson model of precorneal area accurately predicts precorneal concentrations of pilocarpine and the Miller model simulates well the interior of the eye using a forcing function that the precorneal model simulates, the job is done for pilocarpine. This begs the question of whether or not the effect compartment for pilocarpine, presumably the trabecular meshwork, can be incorporated in such a model. As a result, delivery systems for this drug—and this drug alone—can be evaluated with respect to delivery characteristics in a prospective manner. The existing results for timolol are anything but encouraging, being scarcely more advanced than pilocarpine was 10 years ago.

Why is this the case? For a mathematical model to be useful, it must represent the phenomena of interest well and then be used to test our current level of understanding. So far, only the efforts of Lee and Robinson (3) augmented by Thombre's observations have led to either an improved understanding of drug disposition or led to a further understanding of ways to improve ocular drug delivery. Until a major effort in the systematic understanding of drug disposition in the eye is made, most modeling efforts will continue to lack any comprehensive predictive power and the insight into the factors which can be exploited to achieve improved ocular delivery of drugs will be unavailable. It is very puzzling that we should continue to develop delivery systems without this insight.

REFERENCES

1. Himmelstein, K. J., Guvenir, I., and Patton, T. F. (1978). Preliminary pharmacokinetic model of pilocarpine uptake and distribution in the eye, *J. Pharm. Sci., 67*:603.
2. Miller, S. C., Gokale, R. D., Patton, T. F., and Himmelstein, K. J. (1980). Pilocarpine ocular distribution volume, *J. Pharm. Sci., 69*:615.
3. Lee, V. H. L., and Robinson, J. R. (1979). Mechanistic and quantitative evaluation of precorneal pilocarpine in albino rabbit eyes, *J. Pharm. Sci., 68*:673.
4. Miller, S. C., Himmelstein, K. J., and Patton, T. F. (1981). A physiologically based pharmacokinetic model for the intraocular distribution of pilocarpine in rabbits, *J. Pharmacokinet. Biopharm., 9*:653.
5. Thombre, A. G., and Himmelstein, K. J. (1984). Quantitative evaluation of topically applied pilocarpine in the precorneal area, *J. Pharm. Sci., 73*:219.
6. Sieg, J. W., and Robinson, J. R. (1976). Mechanistic studies on transcorneal permeation of pilocarpine, *J. Pharm. Sci., 65*:1816.
7. Conrad, J. M., and Robinson, J. R. (1977). *J. Pharm. Sci., 66*:219.
8. Francoeur, M. L., Sitek, S. J., Costello, B., and Patton, T. F. (1985). Kinetic disposition and distribution of timolol in the rabbit eye. A physiologically based ocular model, *Int. J. Pharmaceut., 25*:275.
9. Grass, G. M., and Lee, V. H. L. (1990). "A Stella model to predict aqueous humor and plasma drug concentrations from topically administration to the eye," Proceedings of the 17th International Symposium on Controlled Release of Bioactive Materials, *17*:299.
10. Ahmed, I., Francoeur, M. L., Thombre, A. G., and Patton, T. F. (1989). The kinetics of timolol in the rabbit lens: Implications for ocular drug delivery, *Pharm. Res., 6*:772.

11. Thombre, A. G., Masters Thesis, University of Kansas, 1981.
12. Tojo, K., Ohtori, A., and Yamamoto, Y. (1989). Proceedings of the 16th International Symposium on the Controlled Release of Bioactive Materials, *16*:113.
13. Tojo, K., and Ohtori, A. (1990). "In Vivo/In Vitro Correlation of Ocular Drugs," Proceedings of the 17th International Symposium on the Controlled Release of Bioactive Materials, *17*:301.

9
Conventional Systems in Ophthalmic Drug Delivery

Orest Olejnik *Allergan Pharmaceuticals, Irvine, California*

I. INTRODUCTION

The development of ocular therapeutic preparations has undergone notable changes over the course of many years. An informative historical chronicle was presented by Duke-Elder (1). The earliest accounts of ophthalmic treatment on record date back to the Mesopotamian era, circa 3000–4000 B.C. Stages in therapeutics were, to say the least, mystical. Treatment was mostly prophylactic, depending on preventing demons from entering the eyes, which was thought to be achieved through various rituals. It was not until the seventh century B.C. that vegetable drugs became common when powders, ointments, or washes mixed with water, milk, urine, or oil were used. The powders at that time were blown into the eye through reeds or tubes as a means of topical administration. One of the first therapeutic delivery systems, the collyrium, noted in the writings of Celsus (20 B.C. to A.D. 50), was apparently introduced by the Romans. This was not, as implied today a lotion, but rather a cake made of gum resembling a small bar of soap within which the drug was incorporated. For use, a small piece was taken and dissolved in water, oil, or other available liquid and applied to the eye. However, improvement in ocular delivery preparations and treatments did not occur for many centuries, with ocular therapeutics only finding meaningful value in the seventeenth century. Ophthalmology finally became of age.

Today, topical ophthalmic application is considered the preferred way to achieve therapeutic levels of drug agents used to treat ocular diseases. The conventional preparations for this route fall into several categories: solutions, suspensions, semisolids, and others. From a biopharmaceutical standpoint, their use has met some criticism over their efficiency as drug delivery systems (2,3). Bioavailability, particularly for ocular solutions, ranges from 1 to 10% of the total administered dose (4). This is due in part to the rapid precorneal clearance kinetics resulting from reflex tearing and blinking, where half-life times of instilled isotonic solutions approximate only 15 s in the human (5). While precorneal elimination must not be ignored, where it contributes to the overall disposition profile of an instilled drug, there are two major factors that can control a drug's effectiveness worth mentioning at this stage: rate of dissolution and rate of absorption (6). The first

177

is a function of the preparation type, principally applicable to insoluble or poorly water-soluble drugs that are frequently formulated as suspensions. Governed by the Noyes and Whitney equation (7), the rate of drug dissolution becomes a controlling factor in the absorption process (8).

The second factor that can control the effectiveness of a drug is the drug absorption rate, which determines the ability of the drug to reach the site of activity via a transport process involving the corneal membrane. Most drugs are absorbed by passive diffusion governed by physicochemical laws and influenced by the inherent properties of the cornea (9). Any drug disposition profile is obviously reflected by an interplay of the above two factors as well as the other factors involved whether they be considered major or minor (Fig. 1). Understanding these factors with respect to their contribution to the ocular behavior of a drug preparation places the scientist in a position to develop systems that better meet the needs of the patient.

While the pursuit of new and improved delivery systems continues, the traditional preparations remain ubiquitously used in today's ocular disease management. A number of reviews have covered various aspects of these dosage forms from formulation compounding to product evaluation (10–13). It is not the intent to repeat the subject matter of these informative articles, but rather to focus on current thinking and examine the opportunities in the way these preparations may evolve into superior delivery systems.

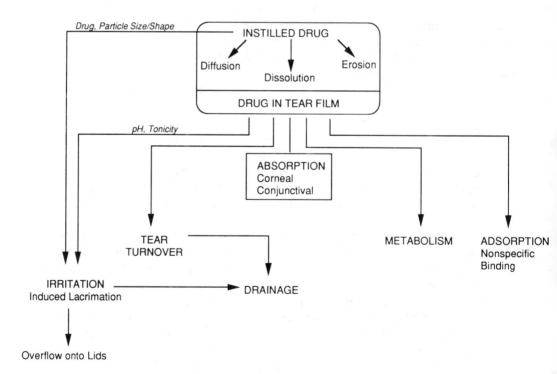

Figure 1.   Ocular disposition of ophthalmic formulations.

II. AQUEOUS SOLUTIONS

The majority of ocular preparations consists of a specifically formulated aqueous medium which acts as the drug carrier vehicle. The drug itself must be in a form that is not only stable within the formulation but well absorbed at the precorneal site. Essential elements in any absorption process must consider drug absorbability as a function of those physicochemical properties of the drug substance that would determine whether any changes in the physical and/or chemical characteristics of the substance could enhance or decrease drug penetration. An indication of the absorbability is obtained from molecular weight, solubility, partition coefficient, and pK_a data. Correlations between these factors and corneal drug penetration were determined for a series of beta-blocking agents (14). Changes in both molecular weight and degree of ionization showed an inverse relationship to permeability, although the ranges of these two parameters were narrow for the agents studied. Compounds with a molecular weight greater than 500 daltons offered poor corneal penetration where passive diffusion was no longer the predominant mode of drug transfer (15). However, this is not perceived as a major factor, since most ophthalmic drugs are lower in molecular weight (16). A greater degree of corneal penetration occurs when a greater presence of nonionized drug solutes exist (17). This effect is associated with phase partitioning activity of the drug substance (18). Both linear and parabolic relationships were considered, where a cut-off in drug activity was thought to be caused by a change in the linear relationship between biological activity and the hydrophobic character of a drug. This apparent switch from a linear to a parabolic relationship was indicative of the complexity of the corneal membrane. In particular for n-alkyl para-aminobenzoate ester homologs, the rate-limiting barrier of the lipophilic corneal epithelium was interpreted no longer to apply for the longer chain length homologs (19). Here the hydrophilic stroma became the significant barrier to drug penetration. Achieving good penetration through the epithelial layer was only inhibited by the stroma, resulting in lowered anterior chamber–drug concentrations. This obviously pointed to a need for optimization of the hydrophilic-lipophilic balance between drug and its biophase.

Corneal penetration enhancement can also be achieved by increasing the solution concentration of a drug. The driving force behind this is the concentration gradient described by Fick's first law of diffusion (20) which, as with phase partitioning, becomes self-limiting. At a certain point, the quantity of drug crossing the cornea decreases with increasing concentration, resulting in larger amounts of drug lost via the nasolacrimal drainage process. This was evident where topical pilocarpine varying in concentration was administered to monkeys and resulted in differing drug-aqueous humor recovery (21). The solution at 1% pilocarpine was found to be present at a higher concentration in the anterior chamber than either the 4 or 8% concentrations. Adopting this rationale for improving the bioavailability profile through increasing drug concentration should be closely evaluated not only on the merit of enhancing drug activity but also balancing it against any potential increase in drug side effects. Where the permeability characteristics of certain drug solutes are inconsistent with good drug absorption, this problem is sometimes overcome by selecting an active analog with different physicochemical properties such as one with a different pK_a or a salt form offering greater lipid solubility (7).

An alternative and often useful approach in aiding drug selection is through pharmaco-kinetic modeling; a model applicable in predicting the behavior of drugs when applied to the eye (9,22). Time-dependent modeling was used to simulate the kinetics of pilocarpine treatment to the eye (23). Building this model involved consideration of a number of processes: precorneal fluid dynamics, drug dynamics, drug binding, passive diffusion of the drug through the cornea, and finally the relationship between drug concentration and its pharmacological effect. Model elements for pupillary response to pilocarpine, for instance, are shown in Figure 2. The predicted model for miosis in this case correlated well with experimental data, allowing its use in examining drug effects with changing pharmacokinetic values.

Ocular bioavailability of drug solutes as a parameter for evaluating drug activity was also recently applied to show that conditions of maximum bioavailability existed (24). Moreover, formulation parameters could be selected that would provide the greatest advantages in improving drug availability in the human. Predictions from this model showed that high corneal permeability resultant of lipophilic compounds produced the highest bioavailability; drug bioavailability with high corneal permeability was relatively unaffected by drug volume; and utilizing small dosage volumes, the bioavailability improvement from drugs with low corneal permeability was increased by as much as four times.

Whatever process is applied in improving the effectiveness of an ophthalmic aqueous preparation, it is frequently assumed that the absorptive area of the cornea is completely available for drug transport to take place. In actuality, the precorneal distribution of instilled solution cannot be considered uniform. Sequential imaging through gamma scintigraphy of the ocular surface distribution of tear preparations in humans supports this claim (25). Histogram profiling was used to assess solution activity over the cornea, permitting a measure of evenness or range of distribution at a specific time (Fig. 3). Solution residence was predominantly over the inferior half of the cornea. While the overall effect on drug penetration was not addressed, the need for complete uniformity of drug-corneal coverage was evident. Limited emphasis has been placed on characterizing drug-solution behavior; perhaps a consequence of the lack of well-defined techniques that could provide both dynamic and quantitative data. Gamma scintigraphy may become an effective tool in this regard in the characterization of ocular solutions. The challenge in achieving acceptable levels of drug efficacy must now be focused on drug-corneal coverage and not just on promoting greater precorneal residence times and drug penetration through viscosity, pH, buffer, and drug modification approaches.

A. Vehicle Viscosity

Approaches to improving ocular drug bioavailability by decreasing precorneal clearance through solution viscosity enhancement have met with varying degrees of success. The more commonly used viscolyzing agents include polyvinyl alcohol (PVA) and derivatives of methylcellulose. Both PVA and methylcellulose solutions administered to rabbits were shown to decrease the clearance rate when compared with saline (5,26). With this effect on clearance, it is expected that activity of the drug in a viscous solution can increase overcoming the short duration of action normally found with simple aqueous solutions. An increase in the pharmacodynamic activity of pilocarpine in viscous 3.75% PVA administered to glaucomatous patients was shown (27). The extent of intraocular pressure lowering was found to be greater with a duration of efficacy increasing from 3 to 7 h. Other viscous solutions containing 0.2% tropicamide as the drug were compared and tested for mydriatic activity in both humans and rabbits. The viscosity of each preparation was

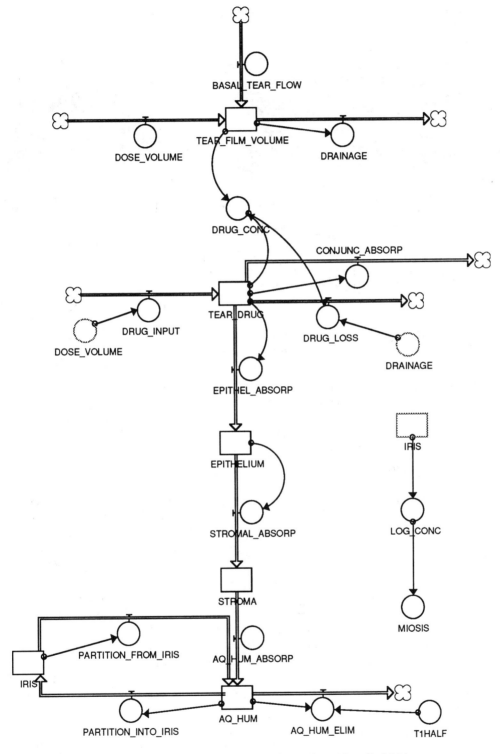

Figure 2. Ocular pharmacokinetic model for pilocarpine. (Adapted from Ref. 23.)

PRECORNEAL REGION

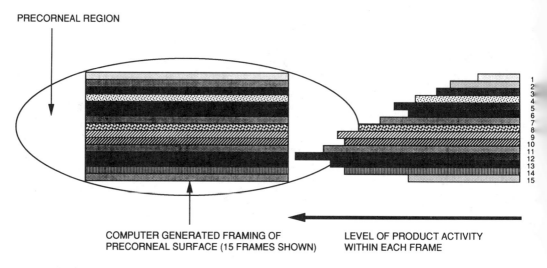

COMPUTER GENERATED FRAMING OF
PRECORNEAL SURFACE (15 FRAMES SHOWN)

LEVEL OF PRODUCT ACTIVITY
WITHIN EACH FRAME

Figure 3. Schematic representation of the precorneal distribution of an instilled preparation as evaluated by a method of histogram profiling. (Adapted from Ref. 25.)

adjusted to give an iso-viscous (70 cps) Newtonian solution or a pseudoplastic solution (apparent viscosity, 70 cps at 700 s^{-1}) (28). In each case, the bioavailability of the drug increased over its nonviscous phosphate buffered solution.

Natural polymers are being investigated for use as viscosity-inducing agents; namely, sodium hyaluronate and chondroitin sulfate. In their development as viscoelastic agents for endothelial cell protection during anterior segment surgery, claims were made that incorporation into topical formulations offered increases in product efficacy (29,30). These glycosaminoglycans represent an interesting class of compounds observed through their unique physicochemical properties and polyelectrolyte behavior (31). Chief among these is hyaluronic acid (HA), where its molecular weight can reach upwards of 10^7 D, the highest of all glycosaminoglycans. Its unusual rheological quality, producing a rapid transformation from a liquid to a solid character with increasing stress frequency, appears to be beneficial for topical vehicles (32). Quantitative gamma scintigraphy was used to determine the residence times of 0.2 and 0.3% sodium hyaluronate solutions and a polymer-free solution of buffered saline in patients with keratoconjunctivitis sicca (33). For the hyaluronate solutions, mean half-life times were 11.1 m and 23.5 m, respectively, compared to less than 1 m (50 s) for the buffered saline solution. The ability of each solution to coat the precorneal area was not comprehensively assessed, although tear film thickness was studied in the normal eye as a separate tear residence index.

Prolonged residence times for hyaluronate solutions indicate advantages for sustained delivery of drug compounds. The effect of adding HA to 1% pilocarpine hydrochloride showed a greater miotic response, an extended duration of action, and a larger area under the curve compared to pilocarpine alone (34). The pseudoplastic behavior of HA solution, where viscosity was higher at low shear rates, was thought to provide an improved distribution on the cornea during blinking. Viscosity enhancement through noncovalent and chain-chain interactions in which a crowding of the HA matrix occurs may also play a role (35). Conversely, since viscosity was higher at the resting phase, a slower drainage of the pilocarpine-HA combination would result.

It is of note that the rheological characteristics of a polymer are implicated in the retention pattern on the ocular surface (36). Each flow type (Table 1), with the exception of thixotropic systems, suggests advantages that are dependent upon key factors such as yield and shear. Where the flow properties of a viscous solution can influence precorneal behavior, selection of the correct system is more often based on rheological performance. Evidence for this was found in the evaluation of polymers on the bioavailability of tropicamide solution (28). Time profiles of the mydriatic responses indicated a preference for pseudoplastic systems rather than Newtonian systems. For PVA and polyvinyl-pyrrolidone solutions, a more uniform layer with good tear film mixing was indicated. Inconsistencies continue to occur when a rheological approach is adopted in selecting

Table 1. Viscosity Types and Their Expected Behavior in the Eye

Flow type	Characteristics	Potential ocular effects
Newtonian	Constant viscosity at constant temperature and pressure; viscosity independent of rate of shear	Drainage loss of drug solution should be inversely proportional to viscosity; due to shear independence, blinking should have no effect on viscosity and such systems should behave the same in rabbits and humans
Non-Newtonian Pseudoplastic	Stress increases more rapidly at low rates of shear than at high rates; the apparent viscosity decreases as shear stress (shear thinning) increases	If the system undergoes shear in the eye, this system would be poor; in humans, if blinking causes shear, the system will thin and drain from the eye; in rabbits, such a system will probably resemble a Newtonian system
Plastic	Resembles pseudoplastic system, but the rate of shear does not acquire a finite value until the stress exceeds a certain yield value	This system would be good as long as the yield value is not exceeded; in rabbits, this may be true, but in humans the system thins as with pseudoplastic once the yield value is exceeded
Dilatant	The opposite of pseudoplastic; the force increases faster than the rate of shear	If blinking in humans produces shear, the system will thicken; this system has good potential in humans, although the advantages of such a system would probably not be observed in rabbits
Thixotropic	A reversible and noninstantaneous decrease in apparent viscosity upon shear; the effect increases with the rate of shear; time-dependent shear thinning	Probably not a desirable situation in humans or in rabbits since the system will thin with time

Source: Adapted from Ref. 36.

the most suitable polymer; pseudoplastic solutions, for instance, have shown disadvantages in their abilities to provide a positive drug effect (37,38). Any benefits derived from rheological behavior are likely to involve other contributing factors relating to surface chemistry and biological interactions (39–41).

Changes in molecular weight of the viscolyzing polymer can affect drug performance. Pilocarpine solutions prepared from high molecular weight HA (4.6×10^6 D) resulted in a greater miotic response compared to lower molecular weight samples ($\leq 1.6 \times 10^6$ D) (42). At lower HA concentrations, the influence of molecular weight was found to be more pronounced (Table 2). This interrelationship between molecular weight and concentration was the interaction of two forces: compression and shear (43). The compression force represented the applied force perpendicular to the corneal plane, whereas the shear force was the applied force parallel to the corneal plane (Fig. 4). Each vector force contributed to the behavioral characteristics of the administered preparation, which altered depending on the viscosity—molecular weight of the HA system.

For simpler polymer solutions, optimum viscosities, at least for the rabbit eye, range from 12 to 15 cps (1.2 to 1.5 mPa) (44). Further increases in viscosity above this level do not appear to proportionally increase the drug concentration into the aqueous humor. At best, gradual increases in corneal residence with increasing PVA concentrations above 3.5% are expected (45). From a patient's perspective, increasing solution viscosity beyond 15 cps may have the effect of inhibiting product-tear mixing accompanied by distortion of the optical surface, producing visual disturbances for the patient (46). For this reason, a viscosity of less than 15 cps is indicated.

While viscosity enhancement has an important part to play in the precorneal dynamics of an instilled solution, the optimal viscosity for each agent must be identified through appropriate experimentation if these solutions are to be correctly used. It is no longer acceptable to consider viscosity as the primary element for achieving optimum bioavailability and patient comfort.

Table 2. Influence of Molecular Weight of Sodium Hyaluronate on Miotic Effect of 2% Pilocarpine HCl

Molecular weight sodium hyaluronate	Concentration of sodium hyaluronate (%)			
	0.125	0.25	0.50	0.75
0.6×10^6	2640[a] (404)[b]	3539 (750)	3900 (906)	3990 (857)
1.6×10^6	3246 (612)	4182 (955)	4304 (963)	4460 (882)
4.6×10^6	4492 (1004)	5072 (1230)	—	—

Source: Adapted from Ref. 42.

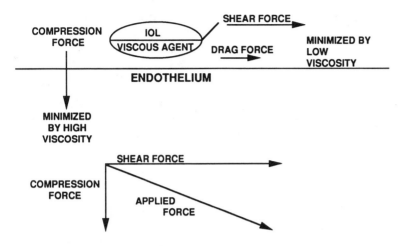

Figure 4. The applied force on an IOL can be represented by two vectors: the compression force and the shear force. High-viscosity agents transmit more of the shear force to the endothelial surface as a drag force. (Adapted from Ref. 43.)

B. pH

The pH of the tear fluid is of interest to the formulator in three ways: maintaining physiological pH upon solution administration, enhancing drug penetration through changes in the degree of drug ionization, and product stabilization. Varying values of normal tear pH are given in the literature ranging from pH 7.0 to 7.4 (47). Methods of measurement are often the cause of this variation, although improvements in the application of direct, noninvasive techniques in measuring tear pH in vivo are gaining favor. In the study by Norn (47), conjunctival fluid was measured with a microglass electrode. Among 41 binocularly normal persons, the pH was found to be 6.93 ± 0.26. Recently, measurement with a fluorescent probe resulted in a pH of 7.83 ± 0.1 for both open and closed eyes (48). In the same study (47), a more alkaline pH of 8.2 was established in the rabbit precorneal tear film. While it is not our purpose to discuss which of the measurement techniques are more accurate, a question clearly exists as to what is the true tear pH. Knowing actual in situ tear pH becomes critical under certain circumstances, since it can alter the penetrability of drug compounds. This is observed as a result of the pH-partition hypothesis (49), where it is widely accepted that certain compounds are only absorbed in appreciable quantities where the pH allows a significant fraction of the drug to remain in a nonionized and, therefore, lipid-soluble form. Deviations from a desired pH as a function of a compound's pK_a can significantly change its pharmacokinetic profile. Transcorneal flux of weak organic bases such as procaine were found to increase as the solution became more alkaline (50). Both aniline and pilocarpine were shown to increase in their transcorneal flux as a function of pH (51). A conversion to a greater percentage of the free base resulted in a greater lipid solubility. This strategy of pH manipulation for enhancing therapeutic drug levels is gaining greater attention despite obvious limitations, particularly with irritation caused through the use of acidic or alkaline drops (52). The premise is one of maximizing ocular absorption while minimizing systemic absorption. Ratios between ocular and systemic drug concentrations describe the relative safety of ophthalmic dosage forms.

Altering the solution pH of timolol (pK_a 9.2) from 6.2 to 7.5 increased its corneal penetration (53). Systemic bioavailability of timolol was not affected, although the systemic peak concentration was elevated through a faster rate of absorption. Raising the pH of the eye drops did not influence the actual ratio between ocular and systemic peak drug concentrations, since both ocular and systemic concentrations of timolol were increased. It illustrated that the therapeutic benefit cannot be realized by evaluating the ocular apparatus in isolation of the highly vascular systemic system. Both factors need consideration regardless of whether drug absorption is manipulated via a pH change or by some other physicochemical mechanism.

C. Buffers

While H^+ ion concentration as expressed in terms of pH can obviously influence drug absorption behavior, often neglected is the potential influence of the buffer type. Buffer components can inherently exert an effect on the corneal absorption of drugs. Increasing the concentration of a citrate buffer in pilocarpine eye drops was found to reduce the extent of absorption of the drug observed by changes in the miosis-time curves (54). At the maximum citrate buffer concentration studied, a fivefold reduction in miosis occurred. Pilocarpine nitrate solution at pH 4 in equimolar concentrations of acetate, phosphate, and citrate buffers was also evaluated through the effect of buffer capacity, buffering agents, average buffer capacity, and residual buffer capacity (55). The latter two parameters were applied to better elucidate the buffer functionality and ionization values on the in vivo time course of the tear fluid pH. Concentration and type of buffer used were considered key factors influencing the absorption efficiency of pilocarpine. The miotic agent was found to be less ocularly available from a phosphate buffered solution compared to an apparently strong acetate buffer (Fig. 5). Resistance to pH reequilibration near the pK_a of pilocarpine was attributed to the high residual buffer capacity of phosphate. Bioavailability appeared to be drastically reduced in the presence of citrate buffer, supporting the findings of others (54). A rapid pH reequilibration was found to be essential for optimal pilocarpine activity to occur, expressing the need for correct buffer selection.

D. Drug Enhancement

Where limitations to drug–corneal penetration are prevalent, techniques are often applied to improve the appropriate therapeutic effect. This is manifested through a variety of ways involving the use of drug penetration enhancers, drug modification, and other adjuncts. Clearly, the primary aim is in better targeting the drug to its receptor.

As potential drug penetration enhancers it is worthwhile mentioning the role of preservative agents which are used in most ophthalmic solutions and suspensions. Their primary purpose is to prevent the patient from administering microbiologically contaminated preparations into the eye. To date, no ideal antimicrobial agent exists that meets all of the criteria required for a preservative, as listed below (56):

Effective in low concentrations against a broad spectrum of organisms
Soluble in the formulation at the required concentration, nontoxic, and nonsensitizing
Compatible with a wide variety of drug compounds and excipients
Free of unacceptable organoleptic properties
Active with long-term stability over a wide pH and temperature range

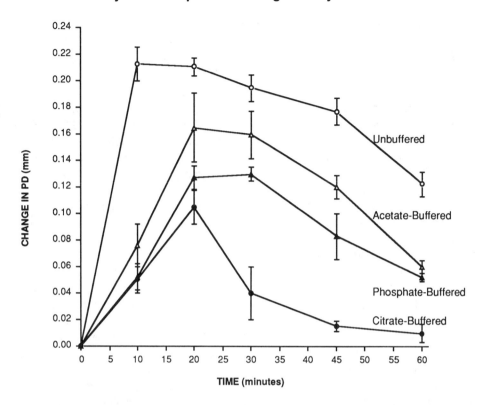

Figure 5. Miosis-time profiles: average changes in pupillary diameter after instillation of 1% pilocarpine nitrate in buffer test solutions. (Adapted from Ref. 55.)

Nonreactive with container components
Inexpensive

Agents that meet a sufficient number of these criteria are the quaternary ammonium compounds: e.g., benzalkonium chloride; mercurials, e.g., thimerosal; alcohols, e.g., 2-phenylethyl alcohol.

Since these agents influence the cell walls of microorganisms, it follows that they have the potential to act on biological membranes and altering membrane permeability. A consequence of this is an endeavor to increase drug penetration across the cornea through the utilization of preservatives (57). Appreciable increases in the penetration of fluorescein in normal human eyes, for instance, was found in the presence of chlorhexidine gluconate and benzalkonium chloride (58). Combinations with the local anesthetics oxybuprocaine and tetracaine showed greater corneal epithelial permeability in the presence of 0.01% w/v benzalkonium chloride; apparently due to its surfactant properties. It is no wonder that preservatives are used under the guises of drug penetration enhancers. Their potential benefits in this regard are often negated by their toxic effects. Unfortunately, endothelial degeneration is known to occur from the prolonged administration of topical medications containing benzalkonium chloride (59), although a single drop may rinse away without causing lasting or irreparable damage (60). In either case, it is accepted that the preservative exerts a profound effect upon the corneal tissue, which if understood and appropriately applied, can offer therapeutic advantages. This approach can also be extended to other agents, notably ethylenediaminetetraacetic acid (EDTA), an adjunct to benzalkonium chloride.

The mechanisms of EDTA for corneal drug penetration were examined where increases in the permeability of the cornea occurred (61). At 0.5%, EDTA was used to promote the transport of glycerol. This effect was considered to result from a decrease in the calcium concentration in "tight" epithelia, decreasing the transepithelial resistance to water-soluble compounds. In similar in vitro experiments at lower concentrations, 0.2 and 5.0 mM EDTA were devoid of any effects (62), suggesting a concentration dependence. The in vivo effects of EDTA were not investigated. It seems likely that the high concentration of divalent cations in the tear film would prevent EDTA from enhancing permeability. Increasing the EDTA concentration to a level that would bind all such ions would probably be toxic to the patient. However, an EDTA-drug combination does deserve some consideration in improving the bioavailability of poorly penetrating drugs.

While attempts toward improving the transport of drugs across the cornea through altering the corneal epithelium or increasing drug-corneal contact time have to a certain extent been successful; it is in the modification of the drug that has generated greater interest. One approach involves the concept of ion-pair formation, where the properties of the altered drug species such as ionic size, diffusivity, and partitioning behavior can differ from its respective free-drug ion (63). Ion-pair formation between the dianionic drug sodium cromoglycate and dodecylbenzyldimethylammonium chloride (DBDAC) was found to alter the extent and rate of corneal penetration of both ions upon coadministration. However, it was not determined whether the change in ocular penetration occurred via a transfer of an ion-pair species or whether the ionic interaction merely increased the availability of both ions to the surface of the corneal tissue. No consideration was given to the potential surfactant effect of DBDAC on the corneal membrane contributing to the observed penetration enhancement.

In the presence of a non–surface active ion-pairing agent, m-chlorobenzyltrimethyl-phosphonium chloride, the in vivo corneal uptake of chloramphenicol succinate was found to have significantly increased compared to its unassociated state (64). The data correlated well with in vitro findings, suggesting that ion-association effects can be used to increase the ocular penetration of drugs (65).

Other prodrug approaches were advocated, where again the physicochemical characteristics of a drug were altered. Detailed studies utilizing modified drug agents have been addressed elsewhere which show promise in increasing drug activity with decreasing drug side effects (66,67).

III. SUSPENSIONS

Biologically active drug compounds that are sparingly soluble in water are often formulated as suspensions. The drug is present in a micronized form, generally <10 μm in diameter, suspended in a suitable aqueous vehicle. Ophthalmic suspensions, particularly the steroids, are thought to be beneficial as delivery systems, since it is assumed that drug particles persist in the conjunctival sac and giving rise to a sustained release effect (68). To date, no definitive study has been reported on the precorneal residence profile of suspended drug particles in the human to show that this phenomenon occurs.

In the rabbit, the precorneal elimination of a saline suspension of serum albumin microspheres was shown to be rapid with total elimination occurring within minutes of instillation (45). There was no evidence of prolonged particle retention, although this might be related to the particle size studied (<1 μm in diameter). Other studies attempting to assess the in vivo performance of ocular suspensions were limited, providing no data on the actual residence profile of the suspended particles (69,70). In addition to particle-drug deposition, suspensions must also be quantitated by way of their solute concentration, drug potency, and solubility to better characterize their behavior (71,72), as well as other physical parameters; i.e., intrinsic solubility, dissolution rate, and particle size (73).

Increases in drug particle size were shown to influence bioavailability (74). Three suspensions of 0.1% tritiated dexamethasone were evaluated with varying mean particle sizes of 5.75, 11.5, and 22.0 μm. As the particle size increased, the in vivo dissolution rate decreased to the point that the particles were removed from the conjunctival sac before dissolution was complete. Both the rate and extent of dexamethasone penetration into the anterior chamber of the rabbit decreased.

To minimize any potential irritation to the eye, the particle size should be less than 10 μm. Increasing size significantly beyond this may well increase the elimination of the instilled suspensions through patient discomfort and tearing, producing a loss in drug activity. A 10 μm limit may not, however, be clear-cut, since other factors such as particle concentration, density, and shape may contribute to the patient comfort threshold. It would be expected that amorphous particles would offer greater comfort over their smaller crystalline counterpart, but the choice of a particulate system must be linked to the drug's bioavailability profile.

In another study, the dissolution rate of a sparingly soluble compound, fluorometholone, was considered (75). It was found that the use of an higher concentration of equivalent particle size did not improve the aqueous humor drug concentration-time profile. A saturated solution state for the fluorometholone already existed and adding further drug solid would not increase total solute concentration. Absorption of the drug in this case was at a maximum, restricted only by its inherent dissolution property. Comparisons of the results from aqueous dosing systems, saturated solutions/suspensions, and oleaginous/ointments, pointed to the fact that suspensions did not obey strict sustained-release principles. There was no evidence of a true plateau in the aqueous humor concentration-time profile. For the saturated aqueous solution, the drug was immediately available.

Different salt forms of the steroid prednisolone presented as either a solution or suspension showed similar aqueous humor-absorption profiles (6). A higher corneal concentration of the sodium phosphate salt form resulted from a higher concentration gradient when compared to its acetate homologue. Bioequivalence of the two salts was expected despite differences in their partition coefficients. However, the data did not parallel an intraocular penetration study of these steroids in humans (76).

Differing drugs and concentrations were compared after single 50 μL doses were administered to the patient. Relative mean peak concentration of prednisolone acetate in aqueous humor resulted in an order of magnitude 22–87 times greater than the other preparations studied. An attempt was made to explain this difference in terms of drug bioavailability and concentration effects.

Similar drug activities were not observed for the carbonic anhydrase inhibitor aminozolamide when two different vehicles were used (77,78). A lowering of intraocular pressure (IOP) in patients with ocular hypertension occurred when the aminozolamide was delivered in a carbomer gel (78). For an aqueous suspension and placebo, no difference in effect was observed with either a single- or multiple-drop study. Previous studies suggested that the retention of aminozolamide was a requirement if significant lowering of IOP was to occur through aqueous humor secretion reduction (79). The administration of the suspension form did not lend itself to prolonged ocular residence, limiting its effectiveness.

Irregularities in efficacy of drug suspensions, particularly for topical corticosteroids, was addressed as a result of inadequate dosing rather than possible variations in the physicochemical state of the suspension (80). Less than the maximum concentration of the corticosteroid of four medications was delivered (Fig. 6). Lack of compliance of patients in adequately shaking prednisolone acetate suspensions was a determinant factor contributing to poor drug levels available to the eye. It raises concern over the usefulness of suspensions as suitable ophthalmic preparations. However, the issue becomes more complicated and, in turn, challenging to the formulator. Accepting the premise that suspensions by their very nature do not deliver 100% of labeled drug owing to constant particle sedimentation; achieving a near solution state in which resuspendability is maximized and sedimentation rates minimized must remain the goal when suspension compounding is unavoidable.

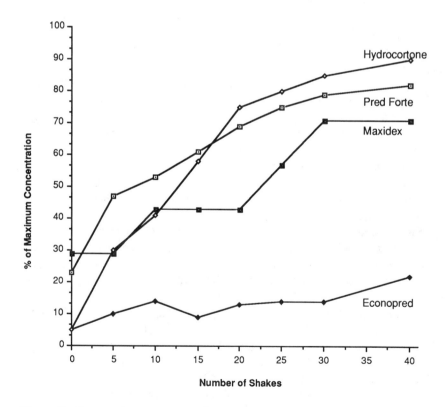

Figure 6. Percent of maximum corticosteroid concentration in relation to number of times bottle is shaken. (Adapted from Ref. 80.)

IV. SEMISOLIDS

The role of vehicles in achieving improved drug efficacy is exemplified with the use of semisolids, adding a further dimension to topical therapy (81). A wide variety of vehicular bases are used, which fall into two general categories: simple and compound bases.

Simple bases refer to a single continuous phase. These not only include the more commonly used bases such as white petrolatum and lanolin, but also include viscous gels, which are prepared from polymers such as PVA, carbopol, and methylcellulose, to name but a few.

Compound bases are usually of a biphasic type involving oil-aqueous systems, forming either oil-in-water or water-in-oil emulsions.

A drug in either a simple or compound type of base is thought to provide an increase in the duration of action for the following reasons: reduced dilution of the medication via the tear film, reduced drainage by way of a sustained release effect, and prolonged corneal contact time (82,83). However, the use of predominantly oily viscous preparations for ophthalmic use causes mixed feelings over their benefits to the patient. Most of the concerns have centered on vision interference, although it is recognized that enhanced bioavailability where sufficient drug is released offers a distinct clinical advantage.

The most commonly used semisolid preparations are ointments consisting of a dispersion of the solid drug in an appropriate vehicle base. The drug is channeled to the ointment-tear interface by the shearing action of the lids (84). As with aqueous suspensions, the onset of action depends on the inherent solubility and particle size and shape. Peak concentrations (Cmax) of the active drug in rabbit aqueous humor from administration of a fluorometholone ointment was found to be comparable to both a solution and a suspension (75). Time to peak concentration (Tmax) of the ointment occurred later with a significantly greater total bioavailability. Examining the response parameter–time curve for pilocarpine ointment revealed that its Tmax was also delayed compared to its simple aqueous solution. While the lag effect was similar to the fluorometholone ointment, the pilocarpine peak response parameter was clearly different.

Delays in Tmax may be attributed to the mode of drug release from the carrier base. Relationships governing the release rate of drugs from ointment bases were mathematically derived (85–87). The first of the equations describing the relationship refers to uniform solutions of drugs in ointments:

$$Q = g/A = 2C\frac{\sqrt{Dt}}{\pi}$$

where Q equals the amount of drug (g) released at time, t, per unit area (A) of contact, C equals the initial concentration of drug in the vehicle, and D equals the diffusion coefficient of the drug in the vehicle.

The second equation refers to suspension-type ointments where the drug is in a finely dispersed state:

$$Q = q/A = \sqrt{Dt(2C - Cs)Cs}$$

where C is the total drug concentration and Cs is the solubility of the drug in the ointment.

For ointments to fit these models, the following conditions must be met:

1. Only a single drug specie is dominant in the base
2. The diffusion coefficient remains constant both to time and position in the base

3. Only the drug is permitted to diffuse out of the base
4. Rapid removal of drug from the base-membrane interface into a "true sink"
5. Drug release is <30% that of solutions
6. C>>Cs for suspensions

A modified equation was proposed to overcome the concerns that D must be constant with respect to time and position (88). A relationship was shown to exist between the release rate and the concentration of drug dissolved in the base. This physical model was applied in evaluating in vitro the solubility of a drug in topical vehicles and by way of interactions between the drug and vehicles that might influence drug bioavailability (89). The model appeared useful when comparing observed and predicted rates of release of corticosteroids from ointments containing hydrophobic adjuvants (90). However, for ointments containing surfactant-emulsifying agents, these simplified models did not provide useful predictions where the calculated rates offered little help in predicting the observed rates. Surfactants orient at the oil-water interface, resulting in changes in the ointment surface layer (91). This effect was not considered in the mathematical expression and would explain the observed deviations.

Vehicle composition of semisolids influenced the ocular disposition of sodium cromoglycate; a drug used for allergic conjunctivitis where the target tissue was the conjunctiva (92). Three vehicles were investigated consisting of a water-soluble base (15% PVA in water), an absorption base (10% acetylated lanolin in a paraffin base), and an oleaginous base (a polyethylene and mineral oil blend). Drug disposition was monitored in the ocular fluids and tissues of the rabbit at specific time intervals 30, 60, and 240 min, using radiotracer techniques. At the earlier time points, all bases were judged to be equivalent in their performance. Differences occurred at the 240-min mark at which time the oleaginous base gave the highest concentration of the drug in the conjunctiva. The water-soluble PVA preparations resulted in significantly lower levels in the tears, conjunctiva, and cornea. Highest drug concentrations in the tear pool were achieved by the absorption base. Inclusion of only three time points limited a comprehensive evaluation of the pharmacokinetic profile of sodium cromoglycate in the bases studied; Cmax, Tmax, and $T^{1}/_{2}$ values would have proved valuable. Nevertheless, it was not surprising to find that the hydrophobic bases were better capable of maintaining a higher overall drug concentration.

This behavior was again observed over a 300-min period following the administration of two different vehicles containing sodium cromoglycate (93). At 6 h after administration of the drug-absorption base, concentration levels equaled or exceeded the concentration obtained with an aqueous solution 1 h postinstillation. Improved ocular retention occurred with the lipophilic preparation over its aqueous counterpart. These relative differences can also be expected to exist in humans. Studies involving pilocarpine suggested this to be true where rabbit data were extrapolated to the human (94). Assumptions on the ocular preparation behavior in the human based on species extrapolation should be viewed with caution. After all, there are notable differences in ocular physiology between these two species (Table 3). With a rapid blink rate in humans, it is expected that this factor alone results in different clearance rates which may change product performance when evaluated against the rabbit. Indeed, the mechanical shearing component resulting from blink rates was found to be critical when correlating in vitro release patterns with those in vivo (95). Shear facilitation occurs with every blink sequence, and the magnitude of the blink frequency can produce a more pronounced effect in the human than in the rabbit. It follows that in vivo

Table 3. Comparison of Precorneal Ocular Characteristics of Rabbits and Humans

Characteristic	Rabbit	Human
Lacrimal punctum/puncta	1	2
Nictitating membrane	Present	Absent
Blink rate	8–15 min	4–5 s
Tear flow	0.5–0.7 μL/min	0.5–2.2 μL/min
Tear volume	5–10 μL	5–10 μL
Solution drainage rate constant	0.545/min	1.45/min

Source: Adapted from Ref. 25.

human shear effects are critical in the evaluation of any semisolid system and cannot be ignored.

V. THERAPEUTIC LENSES

Inadequacies in drug delivery profiles of current ophthalmic preparations and the absence of an ideal ophthalmic delivery system have driven ophthalmologists in taking intermediary steps toward improving drug-ocular bioavailability. One approach is with the use of soft contact lenses for therapeutic purposes. It is generally accepted that soft contact lenses can act as a reservoir for drugs, providing improved release of the therapeutic agent. Most of the data generated were through in vitro or animal studies. Relatively few human studies have demonstrated a sustained-release effect by comparing the biological response to the effect observed in administering the basic aqueous preparation of the drug (96–98). This limited understanding in the manner drug preparations behave in the eyes of contact lens wearers, as well as utilizing drug-soaked contact lenses or corneal bandage shields, prevent one from making sound conclusions concerning the therapeutic benefits of these potential drug delivery systems. Complications are further protracted by the variety of lenses available in today's marketplace.

In determining pilocarpine's elimination from hydrophilic lenses, it has been shown that an interruption of drug flow produces a second release phase (99). Drug binding to the lens material was concluded to be the cause, although water structuring/binding might itself be implicated in this release phenomenon. While debates over the liquid structure of water continue, it leads one to speculate that the dipole nature of water or hydrogen bonds may indeed be responsible in influencing drug release. Using glucose and amino acids as tracer compounds, it was found that the water diffused 20–40 times slower in the hydrophilic material than in water alone (100). Gamma scintigraphy has shown that the diffusion of solutes and water through soft contact lenses is indeed a complex process and not solely dependent on molecular size (101). The hydration shell surrounding the molecule, chemical binding to lens material, and the chemical-mechanical composition of the polymer must each be considered. Prediction of the diffusion rates of solutes becomes very difficult, relying mostly on their determination through empirical means.

It is the collagen bandage shield that has found use as a delivery system that prolongs contact between a drug and the cornea (102). Drugs can either be incorporated into the collagen matrix, absorbed into the shield during rehydration, or applied topically over the shield in the eye. Since the shield is erodible, release of drug occurs gradually into the tear film, maintaining higher concentrations of drug than normally achieved through conventional preparations (103).

Again, it is the studies in animals that contribute to the belief in drug delivery superiority to the cornea and aqueous humor by way of the use of bandage shields compared to topical administration. Definitive data detailing reproducibility in the pharmacokinetic profile of the drug as well as its clinical significance in the human is lacking. Appropriate studies are of paramount importance before any superiority claims over existing preparations can ever be made.

VI. CONCLUSIONS

Impressive as the advances made over past years are, there continues to be no signs that they are ceasing. On the contrary, with the advent of micropharmaceutics promoting a better understanding of both drug delivery and drug transport mechanisms as they relate to the eye, revolutionary advances are still to come. How far these systems may develop to improve future therapies is difficult to predict and until such a time reliance on conventional ophthalmic preparations must continue. These preparations, while limited in providing ideal bioavailability profiles, do present opportunities for improvement that are well within the bounds of existing technology. A better appreciation of ocular product behavior coupled with formulation optimization can lead the way.

REFERENCES

1. Duke-Elder, S. (1975). The History of Ocular Therapeutics, *In: System of Ophthalmology,* Vol. 7, H. Kimpton, London, p. 461.
2. Shofner, R. S., Kaufman, H. E., and Hill, J. M. (1989). New horizons in ocular drug delivery, *In: New Ophthalmic Drugs* (T. J. Zimmerman and K. S. Kooner, eds.). *Ophthalmol. Clin. North Am.,* 2:15.
3. Shell, J. W. (1982). Ocular drug delivery systems—a review, *J. Toxicol. Cutan. Ocul. Toxicol.,* 1:49.
4. Lee, V. H. L. (1985). Topical ocular drug delivery: Recent advances and future perspective, *Pharm. Int.,* 6:135.
5. Zaki, I., Fitzgerald, P., Hardy, J. C., and Wilson, C. G. (1986). A comparison of the effect of viscosity on the precorneal residence of solutions in rabbit and man, *J. Pharm. Pharmacol.,* 38:463.
6. Olejnik, O., and Weisbecker, C. A. (1990). Ocular bioavailability of topical prednisolone preparations, *Clin. Therapeut., 12:2.*
7. Noyes, A. A., and Whitney, W. R. (1897). The rate of solution of solid substances in their own solution, *J. Am. Chem. Soc., 19:*930.
8. Kaplan, S. (1972). Biopharmaceutical considerations in drug formulation design and evaluation, *Drug Metab. Rev., 1:*15.
9. Maurice, D. M., and Mishima, S. (1984). Ocular pharmacokinetics. *In: Pharmacology of the Eye* (M. L. Sears, ed.). Springer-Verlag, New York, p. 19.
10. Hecht, G., Roehrs, R. E., and Shively, C. D. (1979). Design and evaluation of ophthalmic pharmaceutical products. *In: Modern Pharmaceutics* (G. S. Banker and C. T. Rhodes, eds.). Marcel Dekker, New York, p. 479.
11. Maurice, D. M. (1980). Factors influencing the penetration of topically applied drugs, *Int. Ophthalmol. Clin., 20:*21.
12. Chiou, G. C. Y., and Watanabe, K. (1982). Drug delivery to the eye, *Pharmacol. Ther., 17:*269.

13. Lee, V. H. L., and Robinson, J. R. (1986). Review: Topical ocular drug delivery: Recent developments and future challenges, *J. Ocul. Pharmacol., 2*:67.
14. Schoenwald, R. D., and Huang, H. S. (1983). Corneal penetration behavior of β-blocking agents: Physicochemical factors, *J. Pharm. Sci., 72*:1266.
15. Weld, C. B., Feindel, W. H., and Davson, J. (1942). The penetration of sugars into the aqueous humor, *Am. J. Physiol., 137*:421.
16. Benson, H. (1974). Permeability of the cornea to topically applied drugs, *Arch. Ophthalmol., 91*:313.
17. Conrad, J. M., Reay, W. A., Polcyn, E., and Robinson, J. R. (1978). Influence of tonicity and pH on lacrimation and ocular drug bioavailability, *J. Parent. Drug Assoc., 32*:149.
18. Lien, E. J., Alhaider, A. A., and Lee, V. H. L. (1982). Phase partition: Its use in the prediction of membrane permeation and drug action in the eye, *J. Parent. Sci. Technol., 36*:86.
19. Mosher, G. L., and Mikkelson, T. J. (1979). Permeability of the n-alkyl p-amino-benzoate esters across the isolated corneal membrane of the rabbit, *Int. J. Pharm., 2*:239.
20. Riggs, D. S. (1963). Transfer of substances by simple diffusion. *In: The Mathematical Approach to Physiological Problems* (D. S. Riggs, ed.). Williams & Wilkins, Baltimore, p. 181.
21. Asseff, C. F., Weisman, R. L., Podos, S. M., and Becker, B. (1973). Ocular penetration of pilocarpine in primates, *Am. J. Ophthalmol., 75*:212.
22. Gerlowski, L. E., and Jaim, R. K. (1983). Physiologically based pharmacokinetic modeling; principles and applications, *J. Pharm. Sci., 72*:1103.
23. Washington, C., Washington, N., and Wilson, C. G. (1990). Pharmacokinetic modelling using Stella on the Apple MacIntosh. Ellis Horwood, West Sussex, England, p. 73.
24. Keister, J. C., Cooper, E. R., Missel, P. J., Lang, J. C., and Hager, D. F. (1991). Limits on optimizing ocular drug delivery, *J. Pharm. Sci., 80*:50.
25. Olejnik, O., and Wilson, C. G. (1987). Use of gamma scintigraphy in the development of ophthalmic formulations. Gamma Scintigraphy Update, Excerpta Medica, p. 4.
26. Hardberger, R. E., Hanna, C., and Boyd, C. M. (1975). Effects of drug vehicles on ocular contact time, *Arch. Ophthalmol., 93*:42.
27. Davies, D. J. G., Jones, D. E. P., Meakin, B. J., and Norton, D. A. (1977). Effect of polyvinylalcohol on the degree of miosis and intraocular pressure reduction induced by pilocarpine, *Ophthalmol. Digest., 39*:13.
28. Saettone, M. F., Giannacini, B., Raveccu, S., La Marca, F., and Tota, G. (1984). Polymer effects on ocular bioavailability—the influence of different liquid vehicles on the mydriatic response of tropicamide in humans and in rabbits, *Int. J. Pharm., 20*:187.
29. Polack, F. M., and McNiece, M. T. (1982). The treatment of dry eyes with sodium hyaluronate, *Cornea, 1*:133.
30. Limberg, M. B., McCaa, C., Kissling, G. E., and Kaufman, H. E. (1987). Topical application of hyaluronic acid and chondroitin sulfate in the treatment of dry eyes, *Am. J. Ophthalmol., 103*:194.
31. Bettelheim, F. A. (1970). Physical chemistry of acidic polysaccharides. *In: Biological Polyelectrolytes* (A. Veis, ed.). Marcel Dekker, New York, p. 131.
32. Dea, I. C. M., Moorhouse, R., Rees, D. A., Arnott, S., Guss, J. M., and Balazs, E. A. (1973). Hyaluronic acid: A novel, double helical molecule, *Science, 179*:560.
33. Snibson, G. R., Greaves, J. L., Soper, N. D. W., Prydal, J. I., Wilson, C. G., and Bron, A. J. (1990). Precorneal residence times of sodium hyaluronate solutions studied by quantitative gamma scintigraphy, *Eye, 4*:594.
34. Camber, O., Edman, P., and Gurny, R. (1987). Influence of sodium hyaluronate on the miotic effect of pilocarpine in rabbits, *Curr. Eye Res., 6*:779.
35. Chakrabarti, B., and Park, J. W. (1980). Glycosaminoglycans: Structure and interaction, *CRC Revs.-Biochem., 8*:225.
36. Patton, T. F., and Robinson, J. R. (1975). Ocular evaluation of polyvinyl alcohol vehicle in rabbits, *J. Pharm. Sci., 64*:1312.

37. Saettone, M. F., Giannaccini, B., Tereggi, A., Sarigiri, P., and Telini, M. (1982). Vehicle effects on ophthalmic bioavailability: The influence of different polymers on the activity of pilocarpine in rabbit and man, *J. Pharm. Pharmacol., 34*:464.
38. Chrai, S. S., and Robinson, J. R. (1974). Ocular evaluation of methylcellulose vehicle in albino rabbits, *J. Pharm. Sci., 63*:1218.
39. Benedetto, D. A., Shah, D. O., and Kaufman, H. E. (1975). The instilled fluid dynamics and surface chemistry of polymers in the preocular tear film, *Invest. Ophthalmol. Vis. Sci., 14*:887.
40. Versura, P., Maltarello, M. C., Stecher, F., Caramazza, R., and Laschi, R. (1989). Dry eye before and after therapy with hydroxypropyl methylcellulose, *Ophthalmologica, 198*:152.
41. Saettone, M. F., Chetoni, P., Torracca, M. T., Burgalassi, S., and Giannaccini, B. (1989). Evaluation of muco-adhesive properties and *in vivo* activity of ophthalmic vehicles based on hyaluronic acid, *Int. J. Pharm., 51*:203.
42. Camber, O., and Edman, P. (1989). Sodium hyaluronate as an ophthalmic vehicle: Some factors governing its effect on the ocular absorption of pilocarpine, *Curr. Eye Res., 8*:563.
43. Hammer, M. E., and Burch, T. G. (1984). Viscous corneal protection by sodium hyaluronate, chondroitin sulfate, and methylcellulose, *Invest. Ophthalmol. Vis. Sci., 25*:1329.
44. Patton, T. F., and Robinson, J. R. (1976). Quantitative precorneal disposition of topically applied pilocarpine nitrate in rabbit eyes, *J. Pharm. Sci., 65*:1295.
45. Wilson, C. G., Olejnik, O., and Hardy, J. G. (1983). Precorneal drainage of polyvinyl alcohol solutions in the rabbit assessed by gamma scintigraphy, *J. Pharm. Pharmacol., 35*:451.
46. Eriksen, S. P. (1980). Physiological and formulation considerations on ocular drug bioavailability. *In*: *Ophthalmic Drug Delivery Systems* (J. R. Robinson, ed.). Academy of Pharmaceutical Sciences, Am. Pharm. Assoc., Washington, D.C., p. 55.
47. Norn, M. S. (1988). Tear fluid pH in normals, contact lens wearers, and pathological cases, *Acta Ophthalmol., 66*:485.
48. Chen, F. S., and Maurice, D. M. (1990). The pH in the precorneal tear film and under a contact lens measured with a fluorescent probe, *Exp. Eye Res., 50*:251.
49. Brodie, B. B. (1964). *Absorption and Distribution of Drugs* (T. B. Binns, ed.). Livingstone, Edinburgh.
50. Swan, K., and White, N. (1942). Corneal permeability: 1. Factors affecting penetration of drugs into the cornea, *Am.J. Ophthalmol., 25*:1043.
51. Hill, R. M., and Carney, L. G. (1980). Human tear responses to alkali, *Invest. Ophthalmol. Visual Sci., 19*:207.
52. Cogan, D., and Hirsch, E. (1944). The cornea: VII. Permeability to weak electrolytes, *Arch. Ophthalmol., 32*:276.
53. Kyyrönen, K., and Urtti, A. (1990). Effects of epinephrine pretreatment and solution pH on ocular and systemic absorption of ocularly applied timolol in rabbits, *J. Pharm. Sci., 79*:688.
54. Mitra, A. K., and Mikkelson, T. J. (1982). Ophthalmic solution buffer systems. I. The effect of buffer concentration on the ocular absorption of pilocarpine, *Int. J. Pharm., 10*:219.
55. Ahmed, I., and Chaudhuri, B. (1988). Evaluation of buffer systems in ophthalmic product development, *Int. J. Pharm., 44*:97.
56. Akers, M. J. (1984). Considerations in selecting antimicrobial preservative agents for parenteral product development, *Pharmaceut. Technol., 8*:36.
57. Marsh, R. J., and Maurice, D. M. (1971). The influence of non-ionic detergents and other surfactants on human corneal permeability, *Exp. Eye Res., 11*:43.
58. Ramselaar, J. A. M., Boot, J. P., van Haeringen, N. J., van Best, J. A., and Oosterhuis, J. A. (1988). Corneal epithelial permeability after instillation of ophthalmic solutions containing local anesthetics and preservatives, *Curr. Eye Res., 7*:947.
59. Gasset, A. R., Ishii, Y., Kaufman, H. E., and Miller, T. (1974). Cytotoxicity of ophthalmic preservatives, *Am. J. Ophthalmol., 78*:98.
60. Burstein, N. L. (1985). The effects of topical drugs and preservatives on the tear and corneal epithelium in dry eye, *Trans. Ophthalmol. Soc. U.K., 104*:402.

61. Grass, G. M., and Robinson, J. R. (1988). Mechanisms of corneal drug penetration I: *In vivo* and *in vitro* kinetics, *J. Pharm. Sci., 77*:3.
62. Green, K., and Tonjum, A. (1971). Influence of various agents on corneal permeability. *Am. J. Ophthalmol., 72*:897.
63. Wilson, C. G., Tomlinson, E., Davis, S. S., and Olejnik, O. (1981). Altered ocular absorption and disposition of sodium cromoglycate upon ion-pair and complex coacervate formation with dodecylbenzyldimethylammonium chloride, *J. Pharm. Pharmacol., 33*:749.
64. Olejnik, O., Davis, S. S., and Wilson, C. G. (1986). Ion-pairing: A method for overcoming the rabbit corneal epithelial barrier, *Invest. Ophthalmol. Vis. Sci., 275*:347.
65. Davis, S. S., Kinkel, J. F. M., Olejnik, O., and Tomlinson, E. (1981). Enhancement of drug distribution by ion-pair formation, *J. Pharm. Pharmacol., 335*:104P.
66. Chang, S.-C., Chien, D.-S., Bundgaard, H., and Lee, V. H. L. (1988). Relative effectiveness of prodrug and viscous solution approaches in maximizing the ratio of ocular to systemic absorption of topically applied timolol, *Exp. Eye Res., 46*:59.
67. Bundgaard, H., Buur, A., Chang, S.-C., and Lee, V. H. L. (1988). Timolol prodrugs: Synthesis, stability and lipophilicity of various alkyl, cycloalkyl and aromatic esters of timolol, *Int. J. Pharm., 46*:77.
68. Leibowitz, H. M., and Kupferman, A. (1975). Bioavailability and therapeutic effectiveness of topically administered corticosteroids, *Trans. Am. Acad. Ophthalmol. Otolaryngol., 79*:78.
69. Kupferman, A., Pratt, M. V., Suckewer, K., and Leibowitz, H. M. (1974). Topically applied steroids in corneal disease. III. The role of drug derivative in stromal absorption of dexamethasone, *Arch. Ophthalmol., 91*:373.
70. Green, K., and Downs, S. J. (1974). Prednisolone phosphate penetration into and through the cornea, *Invest. Ophthalmol. Vis. Sci., 13*:316.
71. Leibowitz, H. M., and Kupferman, A. (1980). Antiinflammatory medications, *Int. Ophthalmol. Clin., 20*:117.
72. Roberts, A. M., and Leibowitz, A. (1984). Corticosteroid therapy of ophthalmologic diseases, *Hosp. Pract., 19*:181.
73. Sieg, J. W., and Triplett, J. W. (1980). Precorneal retention of topically instilled micronized particles, *J. Pharm. Sci., 69*:863.
74. Schoenwald, R. D., and Stewart, P. (1980). Effect of particle size on ophthalmic bioavailability of dexamethasone suspensions in rabbits, *J. Pharm. Sci., 69*:391.
75. Sieg, J. W., and Robinson, J. R. (1975). Vehicle effects on ocular drug bioavailability. 1. Evaluation of fluorometholone, *J. Pharm. Sci., 64*:931.
76. McGhee, C. N. J., Watson, D. G., Midgley, J. M., Noble, M. J., Dutton, G. N., and Fern, A. I. (1990). Penetration of synthetic corticosteroids into human aqueous humour, *Eye, 4*:526.
77. Lewis, R. A., Schoenwald, R. D., and Barfknecht, C. F. (1988). Aminozolamide suspension: The role of the vehicle in a topical carbonic anhydrase inhibitor, *J. Ocul. Pharmacol., 4*:215.
78. Lewis, R. A., Schoenwald, R. D., and Barfknecht, C. F. (1986). Aminozolamide gel: A trial of topical carbonic anhydrase inhibitor in ocular hypertension, *Arch. Ophthalmol., 104*:842.
79. Putnam, M. L., Schoenwald, R. D., Duffel, M. W., Barfknecht, C. F., Segarra, T. M., and Campbell, D. A. (1987). Ocular disposition of aminozolamide in the rabbit eye, *Invest. Ophthalmol. Vis. Sci., 28*:1373.
80. Apt, L., Henrick, A., and Silverman, L. M. (1979). Patient compliance with the use of topical ophthalmic corticosteroid suspension, *Am. J. Ophthalmol., 87*:210.
81. Robin, J. S., and Ellis, P. P. (1978). Ophthalmic ointment, *Surv. Ophthalmol., 22*:335.
82. Norn, M. S. (1964). Role of the vehicle in the local treatment of the eye, *Acta Ophthalmol., 42*:727.
83. Sieg, J. W., and Robinson, J. R. (1977). Vehicle effects on ocular drug bioavailability II: Evaluation of pilocarpine, *J. Pharm. Sci., 66*:122.
84. McKeen, D. L. (1980). Aqueous formulations and ointments, *Int. Ophthalmol. Clin., 20*:79.
85. Higuchi, T. (1961). Rate of release of medicaments from ointment bases containing drugs in suspension, *J. Pharm. Sci., 50*:874.

86. Higuchi, W. I. (1962). Analysis of data on the medicament release from ointments, *J. Pharm. Sci., 51*:802.

87. Higuchi, T. (1963). Mechanisms of sustained-action medication. Theoretical analysis of rate of release of solid drugs dispersed in solid matrices, *J. Pharm. Sci., 52*:1145.

88. Koizumi, T., and Higuchi, W. I. (1968). Analysis of data on drug release from emulsions II: Pyridine release from water-in-oil emulsions as a function of pH, *J. Pharm. Sci., 57*:87.

89. Bottari, F., DiColo, G., Naniperi, E., Saettone, M. F., and Serafini, M. F. (1974). Influence of drug concentration on *in vitro* release of salicylic acid from ointment bases, *J. Pharm. Sci., 63*:1779.

90. Chowhan, Z. T., and Pritchard, R. (1975). Release of corticoids from oleaginous ointment bases containing drug in suspension, *J. Pharm. Sci., 64*:754.

91. Clayton, W. (1943). *Theory of Emulsions*, 4th ed. Blakiston, Philadelphia, p. 127.

92. Lee, V. H. L., Swarbrick, J., Redell, M. A., and Yang, D. C. (1983). Vehicle influence on ocular disposition of sodium cromoglycate in the albino rabbit, *Int. J. Pharmaceut., 16*:163.

93. Swarbrick, J., and Shrewsbury, R. P. (1984). The prolonged retention of sodium cromoglycate in the rabbit eye, *J. Pharm. Pharmacol., 36*:121.

94. Sugaya, M., and Nagataki, S. (1978). Kinetics of topical pilocarpine in the human eye, *Jpn. J. Ophthalmol., 22*:127.

95. Sieg, J. W., and Robinson, J. R. (1979). Vehicle effects on ocular drug bioavailability III: shear-facilitated pilocarpine release from ointments, *J. Pharm. Sci., 68*:724.

96. Aquavella, J. V., Jackson, G. K., and Guy, L. F. (1971). Therapeutic effects of Bionite lenses, *Ann. Ophthalm., 3*:1341.

97. Kaufman, H. E., Uotila, M. H., and Gasset, A. R. (1971). The medical uses of soft contact lenses, *Trans. Am. Acad. Ophthalmol. Otolaryngol., 75*:361.

98. Iwasaki, W., Kosaka, I., Momose, T., and Yasuda, T. (1988). Absorption of topical disodium cromoglycate and its preservatives by soft contact lenses, *CLAO J., 14*:155.

99. Hillman, J. (1975). Pilocarpine delivery by hydrophilic lens in management of acute glaucoma, *Trans. Ophthal. Soc. U.K., 95*:79.

100. Gumpelmayer, T. F., and Schwach, G. W. (1973). Diffusion properties of hydrophilic materials, *Am. J. Optom., 50*:904.

101. Sorenson, T. B. (1984). Studies on tear physiology, pathophysiology and contact lenses by means of dynamic gamma camera and technetium, *Acta Ophthalmol., 167*(Suppl.):8.

102. Bloomfield, S. E., Miyata, T., Dunn, M. W., et al. (1978). Soluble gentamicin ophthalmic inserts as a drug delivery system, *Arch. Ophthalmol., 96*:885.

103. Shofner, R. S., Kaufman, H. E., and Hill, J. M. (1989). New horizons in ocular drug delivery, *Ophthalmol. Clin. North Am., 2*:15.

10
Mucoadhesive Polymers in Ocular Drug Delivery

Ramesh Krishnamoorthy and Ashim K. Mitra
Purdue University, West Lafayette, Indiana

I. OVERVIEW: OCULAR DRUG DELIVERY SYSTEMS

A. Introduction

The search for novel ways of delivering therapeutically active agents has been the focus of attention in the past 2–3 decades. A better understanding of the biological constraints imposed by various routes of administration has enabled us to design newer dosage forms. Advances in the field of technology has improved to such a level that modern dosage forms can deliver drugs in a controlled manner over a long period of time; i.e., days to years. Passive, transcellular diffusion is the major mechanism of absorption of most drugs. The success of this type of Fickian diffusion requires that a concentration gradient be maintained over a period of time. However, it requires enhanced residence time of a dosage form at or around the site of administration. For any noninvasive route of administration, the need to prolong the duration of residence of the dosage form is evident. This is especially true in the area of ophthalmic drug delivery.

Patient acceptance is an important consideration, since the optimized ocular delivery system cannot be used if it is painful or discomforting to the patient. The cornea of the eye has one of the highest nerve densities in the human body and so patients perceive pain and discomfort at low thresholds of stimulation. Also, such stimuli may lead to increased blinking and lacrimation, resulting in rapid loss of drug. Thus, an effective ocular drug delivery device must be easy to use, comfortable to the patient, and yet must improve the therapeutic performance of the drug over the conventional dosage forms. These criteria justify the use of bioadhesive/mucoadhesive systems, where the dosage form adheres to the mucus and resides in the eye until the polymer dissolves or the mucin replaces itself.

The concept of mucoadhesives has been applied extensively to the area of controlled drug delivery for years. Relative ease of synthesizing polymers which could adhere to mucosal surfaces has attracted considerable attention. Some of the potential advantages of mucoadhesive devices include prolongation of drug release for both local and systemic types of delivery and improvement in the viability of nonparenteral, nonoral routes. Despite the application of mucoadhesives in various areas of drug delivery, our understanding of such systems is relatively incomplete.

The pioneering work of Hui and Robinson (1) demonstrated that the ocular bioavailability could be enhanced with bioadhesive polymers. Gurny et al. (2,3) and Saettone et al. (4) have further confirmed the beneficial properties of these polymers in improving ocular drug delivery through enhanced precorneal residence time. The research on mucoadhesives is still in its early stages and further advances are necessary to successfully translate the concept into practical application in controlled drug delivery. Depending on the physicochemical properties of the drug, some manipulation of the dosage form may be necessary to obtain a successful product. This chapter will address the issues of polymer structure and biophysical property relevant to ocular drug delivery. It will also delineate the progress made in the area and describe the challenges to be encountered in the future development of an ideal mucoadhesive ocular delivery system.

B. Potential Problems of Developing a Topical Ocular Drug Delivery System

During the course of developing a topical ocular drug delivery system, one must balance the desire to optimize drug delivery to the target tissue against the negative constraints imposed by the physical and physiological characteristics of the eye as well as by the components of a conventional ophthalmic dosage form. The tissues of the eye are protected from noxious substances present in the environment or systemic circulation by a number of mechanisms, most notably a tear secretion continuously flushing its surface, an impermeable surface epithelium, and egress systems clearing the ocular chambers of agents. From the ocular therapeutics point of view, it is very ironic that the same ocular physiological processes render the controlled or extended delivery of drugs to the eye a difficult task. They also act as primary barriers to achieving and maintaining an adequate or effective concentration of the drug in the intraocular fluids and tissues. The pathways of potential drug loss (e.g., induced lacrimation, a highly selective corneal barrier) upon instillation of a topical dose into the eye are shown in Scheme 1 (5,6). These difficulties are compounded

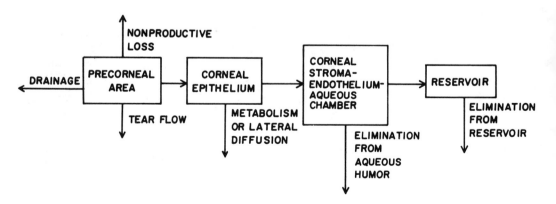

Scheme 1. Model for pilocarpine disposition in the aqueous humor following topical dosing. (From Ref. 5.)

by the structure of the globe itself, where many of its internal structures are isolated at a distance from the blood and from the outermost surface of the corneal epithelium. Figure 1 illustrates the barriers and diffusional resistances to ocular drug transport and the flow systems that regulate drug movement in the eye (7). A major problem, therefore, exists in ocular therapeutics relative to these structural obstacles and protective mechanisms. However, opportunities to bring about the desired biological response without creating local or systemic side effects must be ceased.

Topical application is by far the most common route of drug delivery to the eye, but more often than not, it fails to establish a therapeutic drug level for a desired length of time within the ocular tissues and fluids. There is a finite limit in the dose size (8) that can be applied to, and be tolerated by, the cul-de-sac. There is also a short time span of 1–2 min over which the applied dose is usually in direct contact with the absorptive surfaces of the eye (9,10). Introduction of the drug solution directly into the cul-de-sac results in its mixing with the tear fluid, which then bathes the entire corneal and conjunctival surfaces. This mode of topical instillation may be adequate only for the treatment of most external conditions of the eye and a few of the anterior segment ailments. Most of the anterior and posterior segment diseases are poorly controlled by pulsatile topical drug instillation. The extent of drug penetration into the anterior chamber is dependent upon the extent to which the drop is diluted by the tear fluid and the rate at which it is washed away by the tear flow. These physiological factors impart a high degree of variability in the extent of ocular drug absorption among individual patients and may result in large differences between the human and rabbit model, the principal animal species used in the study of ocular drug penetration (11,12). Normal fluid dynamics in the precorneal area of the eye has a significant influence on ocular drug disposition. The rate of drug loss may, however, be reduced to a considerable extent by progressively increasing the vehicle viscosity (13,14). In these cases, the surface spreading and adsorptive characteristics of added polymers have been postulated to exert an influence (15–18).

The earlier chapters in this book have already highlighted the various means of drug loss upon topic ocular drug administration. Tear turnover (10,19,20) and tear evaporation from the corneal surface (21) contribute to the rate of transport of drugs into the various ocular chambers. A factor such as pH, tonicity, or irritating drugs may stimulate and accelerate drug loss (22,23) and depending on the delivery system may cause the loss of the dosage form as well. Included in this realm are loss by metabolic degradation (24–28), protein binding (29–35), and other nonproductive loss mechanisms (36–39). The role of the cornea in ocular drug absorption has been discussed in depth by other authors (40–43). The corneal physiology, physicochemical properties of the active drug (44,45), and the final formulation (46–49) itself are some of the factors determining the efficiency of corneal penetration.

A component of the cornea that can be utilized to improve the residence time of instilled drug in the precorneal fluid is the mucin-glycocalyx domain (50). The mucin on the corneal surface is much less tightly bound and may provide adequate flexibility for entanglement or binding to appropriate polymer chains. Both mucin and glycocalyx are composed of glycoproteins, which are hydrophilic, anionic biopolymers capable of undergoing changes in viscosity and degree of hydration with changes in medium composition. Mucin constitutes a diffusional barrier to drug penetration. It has been postulated by Hui et al. (51) that prolongation in peak times for cimetidine and histamine concentrations in the aqueous humor was due to the sequestration of the drugs in the mucin layer. This

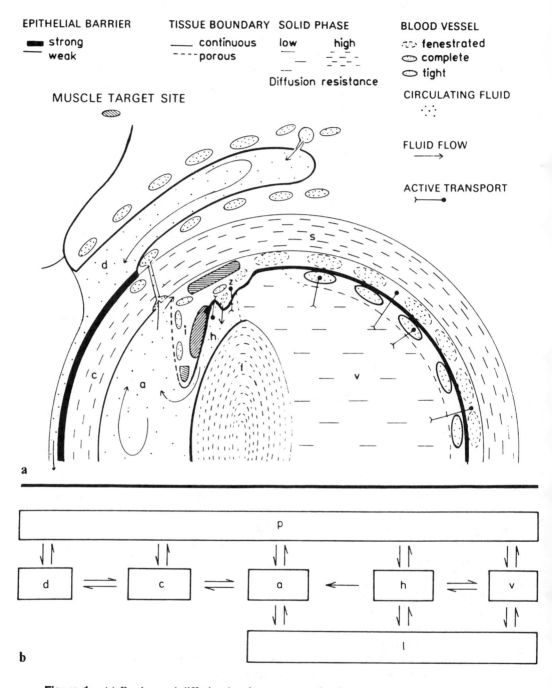

Figure 1. (a) Barriers and diffusional resistances to ocular drug transport and the flow systems that regulate drug movement. (b) Compartmental system used to model ocular pharmacokinetics: p, plasma; d, tear fluid; c, cornea; a, anterior chamber; h, posterior chamber; i, iris; l, lens; z, ciliary body; s, sclera; v, vitreous body.

finding suggests that the mucin-glycocalyx layer can be temporarily perturbed to alter ocular drug absorption. This perturbation can also be studied to understand the interactions between polymers used in ophthalmic formulations and mucin. Drug solution containing mucoadhesive polymers can be placed in the precorneal area. The polymer chains may then interact with the mucin layer of the corneal epithelium through noncovalent bonds.

C. Optimization of Ocular Drug Delivery Systems

Minimization of the negative influences exerted by the ocular physiological processes on the precorneal residence time and enhancement of corneal drug penetration are the primary objectives of an optimized ocular drug delivery system. The system must improve the fraction of the dose absorbed, must maintain the desired concentrations of the drug in the various segments of the eye, and above all must increase the drug's residence in the precorneal area for prolonged periods of time without causing any undesirable side effects. Specifically, the approaches to improve the optimization procedures should focus on reducing, if not totally eliminating, the precorneal loss mechanisms; should diminish the effects posed by the corneal barrier; and eliminate drug absorption into the conjunctiva. The last objective could be largely accomplished by maximizing corneal drug absorption. As a result, most approaches have been centered around improving drug residence time in the cul-de-sac, thereby modifying its pulse entry characteristics.

Increasing vehicular viscosity has been a popular way of trying to prolong drug residence time. However, that effect is not as significant as it was originally conceived and further increases are limited by the globes need for a smooth optical surface. Extremely viscous solutions have been studied for enhancing the ocular absorption of drugs but improvements available through viscosity increase alone are minimal; two- to threefold at best (17,52). An increase in viscosity above 10 cps provides little improvement in penetration; rather it causes interference with the vision.

The concept that all other conditions being kept equal, thicker solutions stay longer in the eye and produce greater penetration is generally true (53). Chrai and Robinson (13) have shown that increasing the solution viscosity 100-fold by the incorporation of methylcellulose caused a reduction in solution drainage by a factor of 10, although it increased the aqueous humor concentration only by a factor of 2. Saettone et al. (17) have demonstrated that the chemical nature of the polymer plays an integral role in improving the corneal drug absorption. This was attributed to the additional spreading effect and was also shown that these polymers attenuated the corneal membrane disruption (54). It is, however, unclear whether the attenuation in corneal membrane damage is due to the bulk mixing of the tear film (thereby disrupting the tear film stability) or due to an enhanced mixing in the mucin layer (54,55).

Another important consideration while employing the concept of increased vehicular viscosity to enhance absorption is to consider the lipophilicity of the drug in question (56). Lipophilic drugs tend to readily partition into the corneal epithelium and consequently any increases in the residence time of a solution would not increase in the amount of drug absorbed.

Alternate approaches to extend precorneal residence time include the various other dosage forms; i.e., suspensions, ointments, nanoparticles, gels, and matrices. The relative usefulness and applications of each system are detailed in Table 1. In this chapter, special

Table 1. Potential Topical Ocular Delivery Systems

Dosage form	Advantages	Disadvantages
Solutions	Convenience	Rapid drainage and loss of drug
		Not likely to be sustained
Suspensions	Patient compliance	Rapid loss of both solution and suspended solid
	Best for drugs with slow dissolution	Drug's properties decide product performance
Erodible insert	Flexibility in drug type and dissolution rate	Patient discomfort
		Requires patient insertion
	Need only be introduced into the eye and not removed	Movement of system around the eye
		Occasional product discharge
Nonerodible insert	Precise controlled rate of delivery	Patient discomfort
	Long delivery time	Patient placement and removal
	Flexibility for type of drug selected	Inadvertent loss of system from eye
Gel (includes in situ geling systems)	Instilled like ointment; comfortable	No rate control on diffusion
	Less blurred vision than ointment	Matted eyelids after use
		No true "sustaining" effect
Ointments	Flexibility in drug choice	Poor patient acceptance
	Improved drug stability	Drug choice limited by partition coefficient
	Good night time product	Possible oil entrapment

emphasis will be placed on the use of bioadhesives, namely, mucoadhesives, for ocular drug delivery.

II. MUCOADHESIVE DOSAGE FORMS

A. Rationale for the Use of Mucoadhesives

The mucoadhesives can provide a localized delivery of medicinal agents to a specific site in the body. The ability of mucoadhesives to provide an intimate contact of the delivery system with the absorbing corneal layer would undoubtedly improve ocular bioavailability. The intimate contact may result in high drug concentration in the local area and hence high drug flux through the absorbing tissue. The intimate contact may also increase the local permeability of high molecular weight drugs such as peptides and proteins (57).

Bioadhesion is a term which is widely used in the pharmaceutical literature. For drug delivery purposes, this term refers to the attachment of a drug carrier to a specific biological tissue. The majority of bioadhesives studied for drug delivery adhere to epithelial tissue and possibly to the mucosal surface of these tissues. Coating the external surface of the globe of the eye is a thin film of glycoprotein referred to as mucin. Therefore, such bioadhesion is also referred to as mucoadhesion. We shall take this opportunity to examine the structure and function of the mucus layer and its role in the process of mucoadhesion.

1. Physiology of the Mucus Layer

Mucus is a highly viscous secretion which forms a thin, continuous gel blanket adherent to the mucosal epithelial surface. It is continually secreted by either the goblet cells or specialized exocrine glands in various regions of the body (58). The major constituents of mucus are water (95%) and high molecular weight glycoproteins capable of forming slimy, viscoelastic gels (59,60). The mean thickness of the mucus layer varies from 50 to 450 μm in humans and about half as much in the rat (61). The exact composition of the mucus layer varies substantially depending on the anatomical location, the species, and the pathophysiological state (62). Mucus contains some nonmucin components which aid in its protective functions. Lipids and covalently bound fatty acids are frequently found in the mucin layer.

The mucus in the eye (Fig. 2) is mainly produced by the conjunctival goblet cells, which are most abundant in the inner canthral region and the lower fornix. The maximum number of such cells per unit area is found in the palpebral conjunctiva. On the surface of

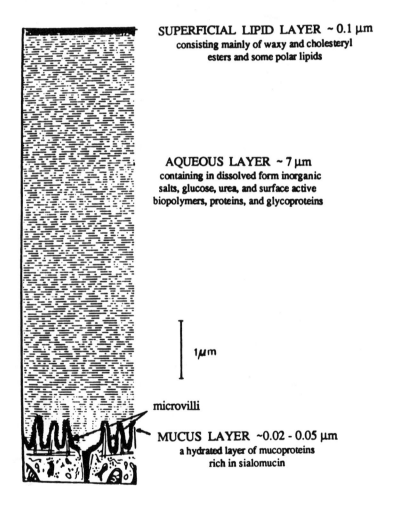

SUPERFICIAL LIPID LAYER ~ 0.1 μm
consisting mainly of waxy and cholesteryl esters and some polar lipids

AQUEOUS LAYER ~ 7 μm
containing in dissolved form inorganic salts, glucose, urea, and surface active biopolymers, proteins, and glycoproteins

1μm

microvilli

MUCUS LAYER ~0.02 - 0.05 μm
a hydrated layer of mucoproteins rich in sialomucin

Figure 2. Structure and composition of the tear film, illustrating the physicochemical properties of the mucus layer.

the mucosal tissue the mucin molecules are tightly packed. As one proceeds outward from the epithelial layer, the mucus layer becomes less densely packed with a corresponding lowering of viscosity and ion content. Neutral and acidic mucins are produced by the goblet cells. Once secreted onto the conjunctiva, the mucus is spread over the surface of the cornea by the upper eyelid.

The principal functions of the mucus layer are lubrication and protection of the underlying epithelial cells from dehydration and other challenges. Continuous secretion of mucus is necessary to compensate for the loss due to digestion, bacterial degradation, and solubilization of mucin molecules. Soluble mucus may form temporary unstirred layers atop the adherent mucus gel (61).

2. Composition of Mucin

Characteristically, the mucus is composed of a number of components: glycoproteins, proteins, lipids, electrolytes, inorganic salts, water, enzymes, mucopolysaccharides, among others. The mucin molecule consists of a polypeptide backbone which is attached to the pendant sugar groups at periodic intervals on the peptide chain. The molecular weights of these glycoproteins vary from 2×10^6 to 14×10^6 D (59). In general, a major portion of the peptide backbone is covered with carbohydrates grouped in various combinations. Galactose, fucose, N-acetylglucosamine, N-acetylgalactosamine, and N-acetylneuraminic acid (sialic acid) are typically found in the mucin molecules. These carbohydrates may constitute as much as 70–90% of the total mucin weight (63). The sugar molecules can carry sulfate residues via ester linkages. Each carbohydrate chain terminates in either a sialic acid ($pK_a = 2.6$) or with a L-fucose group. Hence, the mucin molecules behave as anionic polyelectrolytes at neutral pH (64). Because of the rather large number of sugar groups, the mucin molecule is capable of picking up almost 50–80 times its own weight in water. The oligosaccharides form a protective coat over the glycoprotein backbone by preventing the enzymatic action of proteases (65). Numerous sugar hydroxyl groups of mucin molecules have the potential to interact with other polymers by hydrogen bonds. The positions and relative amounts of amino acids in the glycoprotein backbone are important to the matrix structure of the mucus, since they confer to the overall tertiary structure and folding of the glycoprotein.

B. Mechanism of Mucoadhesion

The attachment of mucin to the epithelial surface may be considered as an interaction of a number of charged and neutral polymer groups with the mucin through noncovalent bonds. Understanding the mechanisms of mucoadhesion is fundamental to the development of mucoadhesives. One may view the entire process to be simply a physical entanglement—a currently accepted mechanism for the attachment of cross-linked polyacrylates to mucin (66). The polymer undergoes swelling in water which permits entanglement of the polymer chains with mucin on the epithelial surface of the tissue (67). The un-ionized carboxylic acid residues on the polymer form hydrogen bonds with the mucin molecule.

The mucoadhesion phenomenon has also been explained using the mechanisms of nonbiological adhesion, such as electron transfer (68), wetting (69–72), diffusion (67,73–76), adsorption (77–79), fracture (80,81), and mechanical interlocking theories (82). Although these theories provide some insights into the mechanisms of mucoadhesion, no one theory by itself has successfully explained the phenomenon of mucoadhesion. Considering the number of factors involved in this process, this is not surprising.

Understanding molecular interactions between mucin and mucoadhesives may provide a better hypothesis for mucoadhesion.

When two molecules coalesce, the interaction is composed of attractive and repulsive forces. The magnitudes of these two forces determine whether the molecules will interact or not. For mucoadhesion to occur, the attractive interaction should be larger than non-specific repulsion. Attractive interactions result from van der Waals forces, hydrogen bonding, electrostatic attractions, and hydrophobic bonding. Repulsive interactions occur as the result of electrostatic and steric repulsions. The theories relating to these phenomena are detailed elsewhere (83).

The bioadhesive process can be conceptualized as the establishment of intimate contact, by diffusion or network expansion, of the polymer chains, with subsequent interpenetration (67). This physical model is depicted in Figure 3. In swellable hydrogels, an expanded polymer is a necessary prerequisite for adhesion and this process may be further enhanced by viscoelastic deformation of the bioadhesive and substrate tissue by applied force or pressure.

When anionic polymers interact with anionic mucin, the maximum adhesion occurs at an acidic pH, indicating that it is the protonated form of the mucoadhesive that is responsible for the bioadhesion. Therefore, hydrogen bonding plays an important role in bioadhesion (84).

In addition, the expanded nature of both mucin and polymer networks permit mutual interpenetration. Interpenetration/interdiffusion of mucin and the adhesives results in an increased contact and henceforth physical entanglement of the two different macromolecules. The physical entanglement is time dependent and may be enhanced by

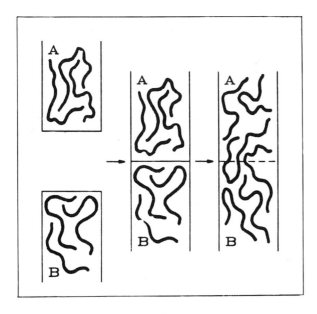

Figure 3. Schematic representation of the chain interpenetration during the bioadhesion of a polymer (A) with the mucus layer (B).

promoting intermolecular interactions between specific functional groups on the two polymers. Strong mucoadhesion depends on the moderate interactive forces between mucus and mucoadhesives which will allow diffusion and subsequent entanglements among polymer chains. A number of factors may affect interpenetration; i.e., chain segment mobility, chain entanglement, cross-linking density of the networks, swelling, porosity, and compatibility of adhesives and mucin.

While a number of polymers will attach to mucin through noncovalent and covalent bonds, the former is preferred, since the strength of attachment is sufficiently strong. The removal occurs primarily through mucin turnover. The strength of adhesion between polycarbophil (partial structure shown in Fig. 4) and mucin is sufficiently strong to resist rinsing. Forcible removal leads to rupture of mucin-mucin bonds and polymer-mucin bonds. The water-swellable yet water-insoluble systems are preferred as mucoadhesives, since predictable drug release from such systems would be easier to obtain. Moreover, toxicity concerns will also be less for an insoluble polymer. Table 2 lists some of the representative mucoadhesives.

C. Factors Relevant to Ocular Mucoadhesion

A number of variables can affect the performance of an ocular delivery system, especially when mucoadhesives are employed in the design of an ophthalmic vehicle. Satisfactory performance of a topical dosage form depends on a number of variables which include:

1. Experimental
2. Physiological
3. Dosage form effects

1. Experimental Variables

a. pH

The pH of the medium employed in the mucoadhesion studies has a profound effect on the performance of the delivery system. The effects of hydrophilicity and hydrogen bonding of polymers cannot be overemphasized in mucoadhesion considering the fact that common functional groups found in bioadhesive polymers, i.e., carboxyl, amide, and sulfate groups, are polar and have the ability to form hydrogen bonds. This property of the polymers in turn has been shown to correlate well with the degree of hydration, which can be controlled by adjusting the pH of the medium (85). The first systematic investigation of pH effects on mucoadhesive strength was undertaken using polycarbophil and rabbit gastric tissue (Fig. 5). The experiments revealed maximum adhesive strength at or below pH 3 and a complete loss in mucoadhesive property above pH 5. The results indicated that the

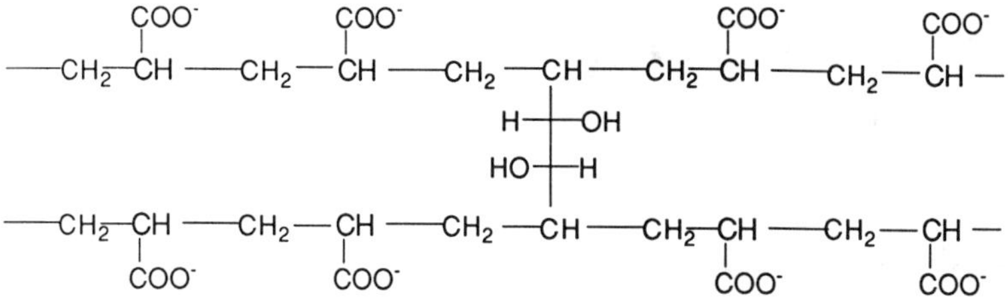

Figure 4. Partial structure of polycarbophil.

Table 2. Some Representative Mucoadhesives with Their Relative Mucoadhesive Performances

Substance	Adhesive performance
Carboxymethylcellulose	Excellent
Carbopol	Excellent
Carbopol and hydroxypropyl cellulose	Good
Carbopol base with white petrolatum/hydrophilic petrolatum	Fair
Carbopol 934 and EX 55	Good
Poly (methyl methacrylate)	Excellent
Poly acrylamide	Good
Poly (acrylic acid)	Excellent
Polycarbophil	Excellent
Homopolymers and copolymers of acrylic acid and butyl acrylate	Good
Gelatin	Fair
Sodium alginate	Excellent
Dextran	Good
Pectin	Poor
Acacia	Poor
Povidone	Poor
Poly (acrylic acid) crosslinked with sucrose	Fair

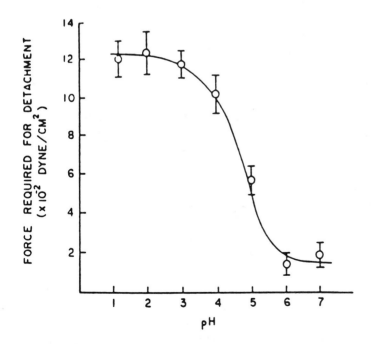

Figure 5. Effect of pH on in vitro bioadhesion of polycarbophil to rabbit gastric tissue.

protonated carboxyl groups rather than the ionized carboxylate anions interact with mucin molecules through numerous hydrogen bonds. At higher pH values, the chains are fully extended owing to electrostatic repulsion of the carboxylate anions. Since the mucin molecules are also negatively charged in this environment, electrostatic repulsion also occurs. Similar postulations have been forwarded by Nagai (86), where the interpolymer complex between hydroxypropylcellulose and carbopol 934 was observed below pH 4.5 (87).

At the physiological pH (pH 7.4) mucin is negatively charged owing to the presence of sialic acid groups at the terminal ends of the mucopolysaccharide chains (88). The preferential uptake of cationic liposomes by the cornea is probably evidence supporting the hypothesis of electrostatic interactions between the mucin and cationic mucoadhesives. In the case of anionic polymers, a hydrogen bonding mechanism is suggested for mucoadhesion.

At physiological pH, the hydration of the cross-linked polymers in the precorneal fluid is maximum, whereas the number of hydrogen bonds is comparatively low. Such loss in hydrogen bonding ability somewhat lowers the mucoadhesive strength in the precorneal fluid. However, the attachment is firm enough to provide some retention of the delivery system in the precorneal area.

b.   Contact Time

Almost all bioadhesive polymers are solvated in aqueous medium and owe their expanding networks to hydration and subsequent swelling. Also, this swelling would increase the flexibility and mobility of the polymer chains. Swelling is an important prerequisite for the interpenetration and entanglement; i.e., strong bioadhesion.

The initial contact time between mucoadhesives and the mucus determines the extent of swelling of the mucoadhesives and the interpenetration of polymer chains. The mucoadhesive strength has been shown to increase with an increase in the initial contact time (89,90). Nevertheless, one needs to consider the optimum contact time based on the tissue viability. In the case of mucoadhesives which need to be polymerized at the site of application, i.e., corneal, buccal, or nasal tissue, the initial contact time is critical for successful mucoadhesion (91).

Recent reports (92) suggest that the adhesive strength increases as the molecular weight of the bioadhesive polymer increases up to 100,000 D. For sodium carboxymethyl cellulose to function as an effective bioadhesive, the molecular weight should be in excess of 78,600 D (90). The adhesive force may be related to the critical macromolecular length required to produce entanglement and an interpenetrating layer.

c.   Selection of Model Substrate

An abundance of literature exists detailing the use of tissue samples for understanding the mechanism of mucoadhesion and bioadhesion of new materials. Gastric mucosa obtained from rabbits is the most common model tissue specimen cited in the literature. However, caution needs to be exercised in terms of extrapolation of these findings to any human clinical studies.

The handling and treatment of biological substrates during the testing of mucoadhesives is an important factor. Physical and biological changes may occur in the mucus gels or tissues under the experimental conditions (93–95), which may be of major concern in optimizing the delivery system. The viability of the biological tissue needs to be confirmed by electrophysiology or histological examinations.

2. *Physiological Variables*

a. Mucin Turnover

The mucin turnover is expected to limit the residence time of the mucoadhesives. This is especially significant, since the mucoadhesive will eventually be detached from the surface of the eye owing to mucin turnover. However, the turnover rate may increase in the presence of the mucoadhesive dosage form. An increase in the rate of mucus production generates a substantial amount of the soluble mucin molecules which will interact with mucoadhesives before they have a chance to attach to the mucus layer. This phenomenon has been demonstrated to be true and unavoidable (96). The exact turnover rate of the mucus layer remains to be determined. Although the thickness of the mucus layer in contact with the epithelial cells is quite small, it is of similar magnitude to the estimated mean diffusional path on the corneal surface.

b. Choice of Animal Model

The most commonly used animal model for ocular studies has been the albino rabbit, because of its ease of handling, low cost, comparable size of the eyes to those of humans, and a vast amount of available information on its anatomy and physiology. This animal model seems to be less sensitive to ocular availability alterations from viscosity changes in topical vehicles than humans (97). Since the blink rate of rabbits (4 times/h) (98) is significantly less than that of humans (15 times/min), humans commonly require higher viscosities than rabbits to retain the drug on the corneal surface. A very important consideration in using the rabbit model for evaluation of mucoadhesives as an ophthalmic delivery device is the size of the drainage apparatus. Rabbits have one large punctum that is capable of accommodating a large particle, whereas humans have two small puncta in each eye. Cross-linked mucoadhesives must be cleared from the eye. Thus, the drainage opening is an important consideration.

A recent report (54) documented the species differences in the effect of polymeric vehicles on the corneal membrane disrupting action of benzalkonium chloride. The report suggested that the rabbit and human corneas differed in the mucin glycocalyx domains at their surfaces. In view of this report, more work needs to be done to delineate these differences. The animal model, which must be predictive of behavior of the ocular delivery systems in humans, plays an important role in the iterative process of design and evaluation of such systems. The lack of absolute predictability of the rabbit model relative to vehicle effects on ocular drug bioavailability may be attributed in part to the differences between rabbits and human subjects with respect to the anatomy and physiology of the precorneal area and the cornea itself.

c. Disease States

The physicochemical properties of the mucus are known to change during various pathological conditions such as the common cold, bacterial and fungal infections, and inflammatory conditions of the eye (99–101). The exact structural changes taking place in mucus under these conditions are not clearly understood. The problems presented by such a complex and changing biological milieu for potential adhesion represent a unique challenge to pharmaceutical scientists. If mucoadhesives are to be used in the diseased states, the bioadhesion property needs to be evaluated under identical experimental conditions.

Many physiological factors of normal and diseased eyes affect the performance of the delivery system. The rate of tear turnover and composition of the preocular tear film changes in various pathological conditions. The vehicles used in the formulation may also contribute to direct stimulation of the epithelial layers of the cornea or conjunctiva and cause release of enzymes, glycoproteins, or immunological factors. In pathologies involving mucus-secreting epithelial cells, hypersecretion is more common than hyposecretion. Mucus hyposecretion results in disruption of the tear film and dry spot formation. An excess of mucus occurs in a number of disease states such as neuroparalytic keratitis and keratoconjunctivitis sicca. Under these conditions, the degree of sulfation of the mucin layer is also known to increase (63). Blinking mixes the secretions and removes tear film debris. In addition, the dosage form location will contribute to the composition and rate of tear secretion in a variety of ways. Thus, in both normal and diseased eyes, the effects of the adhesive dosage form on ocular physiology may determine the ultimate therapeutic outcome.

3. Dosage Form Effects

a. Extent of Drug Incorporation

The drug may be loaded onto the polymer matrix in a variety of ways. The most common approach is to incorporate the drug into mucoadhesive drug delivery systems as shown in Figure 6. For water-soluble polymers, it is possible to employ the mucoadhesive as a typical polymer to coat or to laminate a device. The contact time in such cases is rate limited by the dissolution of the polymer. Such systems, however, suffer from the disadvantage of having a short shelf life, because of the undesirable release of the drug in the aqueous environment (moisture) of the storage container.

The cross-linked mucoadhesives need to become hydrated to function as an effective mucoadhesive. In such cases, the adhesive often detaches itself from the rate-controlling drug delivery device and causes a premature release of the drug, especially with water-soluble drugs. One solution to such a problem is through incorporation of a sparingly soluble drug inside the mucoadhesive polymer. The device can slowly provide drug release until dissolution is complete. This approach may be used for sparingly soluble salts and lipophilic prodrugs of highly water-soluble drugs.

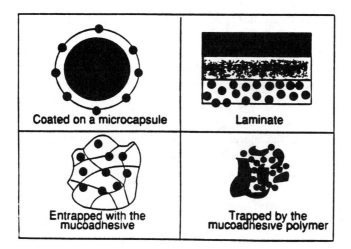

Figure 6. Approaches to incorporate drug into mucoadhesive drug delivery systems. Top panel: (•) mucoadhesive. Bottom panel: (•) drug.

Achieving high consistent loading of compounds into mucoadhesives continues to be a significant problem. A combination of a phase change and mucoadhesive concept may be used in some cases. For example, polycarbophil exhibits large changes in viscosity with pH and ionic strength. Thus, drugs either alone or with a small quantity of lipid can be suspended with the polycarbophil at the proper pH and ionic strength. When such a suspension is placed in the tear pocket of the eye, it rapidly gels, trapping the drug. The newly formed gel then releases the drug slowly over prolonged periods of time.

b.   Vehicular Effects

A delivery system which would allow the drug to remain associated with a vehicle possessing enhanced precorneal retention may, therefore, provide for an attractive ocular drug delivery system. Most attention has been directed toward the influence of solution viscosity, although it has been shown that the maximum ocular availability increase obtained in rabbits by increasing the viscosity of the vehicle is approximately twice that from a simple aqueous solution (63). The viscosity effect of mucoadhesives on ocular delivery, therefore, needs to be addressed.

According to Swan (102), maintaining the lubricity and viscosity of the precorneal film is as important as maintaining the isotonicity and pH of the ophthalmic solutions. When aqueous solutions are instilled in the eye, the integrity of the precorneal film is altered. However, when 1% methylcellulose solution is instilled into the eye, it spreads evenly over the surface of the globe, imparts viscosity to the precorneal film, and causes minimal alteration in the integrity of the precorneal film. The viscosity of the methyl-cellulose solution prevents it from being washed rapidly from the eye and maintains the normal physiology; i.e., lacrimation. A combination of these effects increases contact time, which prolongs the absorption of drugs like homatropine (103).

Increasing contact time with methylcellulose ophthalmic vehicles has been found to be proportional to its viscosity for up to about 25 cps. This effect has been found to level off at 55 cps (18). In humans, a significant reduction in the drainage rates was observed with higher concentrations of polyvinyl alcohol (5.85%) and with 0.9% hydroxypropyl methyl-cellulose (97). However, it appears that in order to achieve the substantial reduction in drainage rate, abnormally high viscosities are required.

Physicochemical parameters of the viscosity-imparting agents, other than those related to viscosity effects, may also influence the corneal retention as well as ocular bioavailability from an ophthalmic product. Benedetto (104) examined this effect using an in vitro model of the corneal surface, and suggested that polyvinyl alcohol but not hydroxypropyl methylcellulose would significantly increase the thickness of the corneal tear film. However, such effects are considered to be only minimal.

Increasing the contact time in the precorneal area appears to be governed by both the mucoadhesive agent as well as the viscosity effects of the polymer. Thus, in designing the ocular drug delivery systems using mucoadhesives, one needs to find a vehicle that imparts good mucoadhesive strength as well as high viscosity at a low concentration.

III.   CURRENT STATUS OF MUCOADHESIVES IN OCULAR DRUG DELIVERY

The successful development of newer mucoadhesive dosage forms for ocular delivery still faces a considerable challenge. Particularly important among these are the determination of the exact nature of the interactions occurring at the tissue-mucoadhesive interface and the development of an ideal, nontoxic, nonimmunogenic mucoadhesive for clinical application. Moreover, a better understanding of the exact physical structure of mucin molecules by computational chemistry may aid in the calculation of the mucoadhesive strength.

The pioneering work of Hui and Robinson (1) illustrated the utilization of bioadhesive polymers in the enhancement of ocular bioavailability of progesterone (Fig. 7). Subsequently, several natural and synthetic polymers have been screened for their ability to adhere to mucin epithelial surfaces; however, little attention has been paid to their use in ophthalmic drug delivery.

Saettone et al. (4) undertook a study evaluating the efficacy of a series of bioadhesive dosage forms for ocular delivery of pilocarpine and tropicamide. From this study, hyaluronic acid emerged as the most promising mucoadhesive agent. The biological analysis data, however, revealed that the physicochemical properties of the drug itself had an impact on the efficacy of the delivery system.

To retard rapid drug loss from the precorneal area, various devices have been tested. Some of the potential candidates have been:

1. An erodible insert of polyvinyl alcohol film for the ocular delivery of pilocarpine (105)
2. Poly(vinyl methyl ether-maleic anhydride) matrices containing timolol (106)
3. Polycyanoacrylate nanoparticles to improve the corneal penetration of hydrophilic drugs (107)
4. An aqueous dispersion with limited water solubility (108)

The aqueous dispersion upon instillation into the eye generated an apparent opaque mass which adhered to and stayed in the lower fornix for extended periods of time. The slow

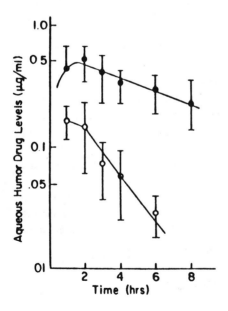

Figure 7. Progesterone levels in aqueous humor following topical administration of 0.3% suspension of progesterone—entrapped polymer (●) and 0.3% suspension of progesterone without polymer (○).

dissolution of the polymer itself and diffusion of pilocarpine out of the polymeric matrix probably controls the availability of the drug for ocular absorption (109).

Similar results of pilocarpine ocular availability enhancement due to precorneal retention through mucoadhesion has been reported by Saettone et al. (10). This group investigated the use of a series of bioadhesive polymers, including hyaluronic acid, polygalacturonic acid, mesoglycan, and carboxymethylchitin.

The biomaterials for ocular use have been mainly synthetic polymers. Some natural biopolymers, such as collagen and hyaluronic acid, have also been examined. Of these, hyaluronic acid offers attractive possibilities (111–114). Some of the materials indicated as "ocular mucoadhesives" are mentioned below.

A. Naturally Occurring Mucoadhesives

Collagen and fibrin have been used as erodible inserts for the long-term delivery of pilocarpine to the eye (115,116). The utility of these macromolecules in ophthalmic drug delivery depends largely upon their attachment capability to the drug molecules and their interaction with the glycocalyx domain of the corneal surface for maximum mucoadhesion. Among these, lectins and fibronectin are most promising.

The role of lectins as cellular-recognition mediators has been explored in great details in the field of cellular biology. Lectins belong to a class of proteins of nonimmune origin that bind carbohydrates specifically and noncovalently (117). The most commonly studied lectin is the one derived from tomatoes. This particular lectin has been found to be nontoxic, binds specifically to the sialic acids (a major component of the mucus glycoproteins), and is transported into the cells by endocytosis (118). Such properties could be useful for the delivery of therapeutic agents into the ocular chambers.

Fibronectin is a glycoprotein and a component of the extracellular matrix. The pentapeptide backbone of this substance has been identified as having a cell-attachment property (119). Purified fibronectin has been reported to lessen the healing time of corneal ulcers (120). It has also been used in conjunction with hyaluronic acid for decreasing the healing time.

B. Synthetic Mucoadhesives

As discussed earlier, the potential of a mucoadhesive agent is determined by a number of parameters; i.e., chain length, configuration, and molecular weight. The extent of corneal adhesion of some neutral polymers has been reported to be comparable to that of natural mucins. Lemp and Szymanski (15) measured the extent of corneal adsorption of water-soluble polymers onto the epithelial surface. Among the polymers, 1.4% polyvinyl alcohol, 0.5% hydroxypropyl methyl cellulose, and 2% hydroxyethyl cellulose vehicles have shown comparable corneal adhesion to that of mucin. The study concluded that ocular therapeutic agents would be well absorbed from topical formulations containing such polymers. Since only marginal improvements (two- to threefold) in ocular bioavailability was seen with these agents, the adsorbed polymers were either unable to hold the drug or were being rapidly removed from the surface by the bathing tears. Other water-soluble polymers like polyacrylic acid also improved the ocular bioavailability of pilocarpine, albeit by a factor of two.

A polymer most effective as a mucoadhesive will be the one which can form an extended and hydrated network to allow for greater interpenetration and subsequent physical entanglement. These kinds of networks may be formed by:

1. Physical intertwining of the polymers
2. Bridging of the polymer chains
3. Cross-linking of the polymer chains

Thus, cross-linked polyacrylic acid has been shown to have an excellent mucoadhesive property, causing significant enhancement in ocular bioavailability (1). A partially esterified acrylic acid polymer was successful in prolonging the therapeutic effect of topically applied pilocarpine (121). Urtti et al. (35) also indicated that the use of a poly-acrylamide and a copolymer of acrylamide (N-vinyl pyrrolidone and ethyl acrylate) as a matrix which resulted in a threefold increase in the ocular bioavailability of pilocarpine.

Similarly, cyanoacrylates have been used in the field of ophthalmology to seal corneal perforations and ulcers, to stop leakage of aqueous or vitreous humor, and to protect against external contamination (122,123). These agents have a potential as effective ocular mucoadhesive agents provided the monomer polymerization could be controlled.

IV. WHAT IS IN STORE FOR THE FUTURE?

A multidisciplinary approach will be necessary to overcome the challenges associated with the development of ocular mucoadhesives. A nonbiodegradable adhesive is adequate for topical use to treat perforations and ulcerations. However, the use of a nontoxic bio-degradable surgical adhesive is deemed necessary for long-term use in ocular drug delivery. Mucoadhesives can make an important contribution in this area. An ideal ocular mucoadhesive would be site specific, durable for the desired period of time, biodegradable, and above all nontoxic, nonimmunogenic, and nonirritant. It would be even better if the adhesive could serve as absorption enhancers (for therapeutic protein and peptide drugs) and/or as enzyme inhibitors.

REFERENCES

1. Hui, H. W., and Robinson, J. R. (1985). Ocular delivery of progesterone using a bioadhesive polymer, *Int. J. Pharm., 26*:203.
2. Gurny, R., Ibrahim, H., Aebi, A., Buri, P., Wilson, C. G., Washington, N., Edman, P., and Camber, O. (1987). Design and evaluation of controlled release systems from the eye, *J. Controlled Release, 6*:367.
3. Gurny, R., Boye, T., and Ibrahim, H. (1985). Ocular therapy with nanoparticle systems for controlled drug delivery, *J. Controlled Release, 2*:353.
4. Saettone, M. F., Chetoni, P., Torracca, M. T., Burgalassi, S., and Giannaccinni, B. (1989). Evaluation of mucoadhesive properties and in vivo activity of ophthalmic vehicles based on hyaluronic acid, *Int. J. Pharm., 51*:203.
5. Lee, V. H. L., and Robinson, J. R. (1979). Mechanistic and quantitative evaluation of pilocarpine disposition in albino rabbits, *J. Pharm. Sci., 68*:673.
6. Himmelstein, K. J., Guvenir, I., and Patton, T. F. (1978). Preliminary pharmacokinetic model of pilocarpine uptake and distribution in the eye, *J. Pharm. Sci., 67*:603.
7. Maurice, D. M., and Mishima, S. Ocular pharmacokinetics: *In: Pharmacology of the Eye* (M. Sears, ed.). Springer-Verlag, Berlin, 1984, p. 19.

8. Chrai, S. S., Makoid, M. C., Eriksen, S. P., and Robinson, J. R. (1974). Drop size and initial dosing frequency problems of topically applied ophthalmic drugs, *J. Pharm. Sci., 63*:333.

9. Blanksma, S. S., Schwietzer, N. M. J., Beekhuis, H., and Piers, D. A. (1977). Testing of lacrimal drainage with the aid of a gamma ray emitting radiopharmaceutical (^{99M}TcO$_4$–). *Doc. Ophthalmol., 42*:381.

10. Chrai, S. S., Patton, T. F., Mehta, A., and Robinson, J. R. (1973). Lacrimal and instilled fluid dynamics in rabbit eyes, *J. Pharm. Sci., 62*:1112.

11. Sugaya, M., and Nagtaki, S. (1978). Kinetics of topical pilocarpine in the human eye, *Jpn. J. Ophthalmol., 22*:127.

12. Saettone, M. F., Giannaccinni, B., Barattini, F., and Tellini, N. (1982). The validity of rabbits for investigating on ophthalmic vehicles: A comparison of four different vehicles containing tropicamide in humans and rabbits, *Pharm. Acta Helv., 57*:47.

13. Chrai, S. S., and Robinson, J. R. (1974). Ocular evaluation of methylcellulose vehicle in albino rabbits, *J. Pharm. Sci., 63*:1218.

14. Lee, V. H. L., Swarbrick, J., Stratford, R. E., and Morimoto, K. W. (1983). Disposition of topically applied sodium cromoglycate in the albino rabbit eye, *J. Pharm. Pharmacol., 35*:445.

15. Blaug, S. M., and Canada, A. T. (1965). Relationship of viscosity, contact time and prolongation of action of methylcellulose containing ophthalmic solutions, *Am. J. of Hosp. Pharm., 22*:662.

16. Adler, C. A., Maurice, D. M., Paterson, M. E. (1971). The effect of viscosity of the vehicle on the penetration of fluorescein into the human eye, *Exp. Eye Res., 11*:34.

17. Lemp, M. H., and Szymanski, E. S. (1975). Polymer adsorption at the ocular surface, *Arch. Ophthalmol., 99*:134.

18. Saettone, M. F., Giannaccinni, B., Ravecca, S., La Marca, F., and Tota, G. (1984). Polymer effects of ocular bioavailability: The influence of different liquid vehicles on the mydriatic response of tropicamide in humans and in rabbits, *Int. J. Pharm., 20*:187.

19. Mishima, S., Gasset, A., Klyce, S. D., and Baum, J. L. (1966). Determination of tear volume and tear flow, *Invest. Ophthalmol. Vis. Sci., 5*:264.

20. Mishima, S., and Maurice, D. M. (1961). The effect of normal evaporation on the eye, *Exp. Eye Res., 1*:46.

21. Mishima, S. (1965). Some physiological aspects of the precorneal tear film, *Arch. Ophthalmol., 73*:233.

22. Conrad, J. M., Reay, W. A., Polcyn, R. E., and Robinson, J. R. (1978). Influence of tonicity and pH on lacrimation and ocular drug bioavailability, *J. Parent. Drug. Assoc., 32*:149.

23. Holly, F. J., and Lamberts, D. W. (1981). Effect of nonisotonic solutions on tear film osmolality, *Invest. Ophthalmol. Vis. Sci., 20*:236.

24. Sendelbeck, L., Moore, D., and Urquhart, J. (1975). Comparative distribution of pilocarpine on ocular tissues of the rabbit during administration by eyedrops or membrane controlled delivery systems, *Am. J. Ophthalmol., 80*:274.

25. Makoid, M. C., and Robinson, J. R. (1979). Pharmacokinetics of topically applied pilocarpine in the albino rabbit, *J. Pharm. Sci., 68*:435.

26. Lee, V. H. L., Hui, H. W., and Robinson, J. R. (1980). Corneal metabolism of pilocarpine in pigmented rabbits, *Invest. Ophthalmol. Vis. Sci., 19*:210.

27. Lee, V. H. L., and Robinson, J. R. (1982). Disposition of pilocarpine in the pigmented rabbit eye, *Int. J. Pharm., 11*:155.

28. Schoenwald, R. D., and Houseman, J. A. (1982). Disposition of cyclophosphamide in the rabbit and human cornea, *Biopharm. Drug Dispos., 3*:231.

29. Mikkelson, T. J., Chrai, S. S., and Robinson, J. R. (1973). Altered bioavailability in the eye due to drug-protein interaction, *J. Pharm. Sci., 62*:1648.

30. Mikkelson, T. J., Chrai, S. S., and Robinson, J. R. (1973). Competitive inhibition of drug protein interaction in the eye fluids and tissues, *J. Pharm. Sci., 62*:1942.

31. Lazare, R., and Horlington, M. (1975). Pilocarpine levels in the eyes of rabbits following topical administration, *Exp. Eye Res., 21*:281.

32. Lyons, J. S., and Krohn, D. L. (1975). Pilocarpine uptake by pigmented uveal tissue, *Am. J. Ophthalmol., 75*:885.

33. Chrai, S. S., and Robinson, J. R. (1976). Binding of sulfisoxazole to protein fraction of tears, *J. Pharm. Sci., 65*:437.

34. Salazar, M., Shimada, K., and Patil, P. N. (1976). Iris pigmentation and atropine mydriasis, *J. Pharmacol. Exp. Ther., 197*:79.

35. Urtti, A., Salminen, L., Kujari, H., and Jäntti, V. (1984). Effect of ocular pigmentation on pilocarpine pharmacology in the rabbit eye. II. Drug response, *Int. J. Pharm., 19*:53.

36. Makoid, M. C., Sieg, J. W., and Robinson, J. R. (1976). Corneal drug absorption: An illustration of parallel first order absorption and rapid drug loss of drug from absorption depot, *J. Pharm. Sci., 65*:150.

37. Patton, T. F., and Robinson, J. R. (1976). Quantitative precorneal disposition of topically applied pilocarpine nitrate in rabbit eyes, *J. Pharm. Sci., 65*:1295.

38. DeSantis, L. M., and Schoenwald, R. D. (1978). Lack of influence of nictitating membrane on miosis effect of pilocarpine, *J. Pharm. Sci., 67*:1189.

39. Ahmed, I., and Patton, T. F. (1985). Importance of the noncorneal absorption route in topical ophthalmic drug delivery, *Invest. Ophthalmol. Vis. Sci., 26*:584.

40. Grass, G. M., and Robinson, J. R. (1988). Mechanism of corneal drug penetration. I: In vitro and in vivo kinetics, *J. Pharm. Sci., 77*:3.

41. Grass, G. M., and Robinson, J. R. (1988). Mechanism of corneal drug penetration. II. Ultrastructural analysis of potential pathways for drug movement, *J. Pharm. Sci., 77*:15.

42. Grass, G. M., Cooper, E. R., and Robinson, J. R. (1988). Mechanism of corneal drug penetration. III: Modeling of molecular transport, *J. Pharm. Sci., 77*:24.

43. Grass, G. M., and Robinson, J. R. (1984). Relationship of chemical structure to corneal penetration and influence of low viscosity solution on ocular bioavailability, *J. Pharm. Sci., 73*:1021.

44. Kishida, K., and Otori, T. (1980). A quantitative study on the relationship between transcorneal permeability of drugs and their hydrophobicity, *Jpn. J. Ophthalmol., 24*:251.

45. Schoenwald, R. D., and Huang, H. S. (1983). Corneal penetration behavior of β-blocking agents. I: Physicochemical factors, *J. Pharm. Sci., 72*:1266.

46. Tonjum, A. M. (1974). Permeability of horseradish peroxidase in the rabbit corneal epithelium, *Acta Ophthalmol., 52*:650.

47. Godbey, R. E. W., Green, K., and Hull, D. S. (1979). Influence of cetylpyridinium chloride on corneal permeability to penicillin, *J. Pharm. Sci., 68*:1176.

48. Keller, N., Moore, D., Carper, D., and Longwell, A. (1980). Increased corneal permeability induced by the dual effect of transient tear film acidification and exposure to benzalkonium chloride, *Exp. Eye Res., 30*:203.

49. Grass, G. M., Wood, R. W., and Robinson, J. R. (1985). Effect of calcium chelating agents on corneal permeability, *Invest. Ophthalmol. Vis. Sci., 26*:110.

50. Nichols, B. A., Chiappino, M. L., and Dawson, C. R. (1985). Demonstration of the mucus layer of the tear film by electron microscopy, *Invest. Ophthalmol. Vis. Sci., 26*:464.

51. Hui, H. W., Zelenick, L., and Robinson, J. R. (1984). Ocular disposition of topically applied histamine, cimetidine and pyrilamine in the albino rabbit, *Curr. Eye Res., 3*:321.

52. Saettone, M. F., Giannaccinni, B., Teneggi, A., Savigni, P., and Telleni, N. (1982). Vehicle effects on ophthalmic bioavailability—the influence of different polymers on the activity of pilocarpine in rabbit and man, *J. Pharm. Pharmacol., 34*:464.

53. Sieg, J., and Robinson, J. R. (1975). Vehicle effects on ocular drug bioavailability. I: Evaluation of fluorometholone, *J. Pharm. Sci., 64*:931.

54. Saettone, M. F., Giannaccinni, B., Guiducci, A., La Marca, F., and Tota, G. (1985). Polymer effects on ocular bioavailability. II: The influence of benzalkonium chloride on the mydriatic response of tropicamide in different polymeric vehicles, *Int. J. Pharm., 25*:73.

55. Holly, F. J., and Lemp, M. A. (1977). Tear physiology and dry eyes, *Surv. Ophthalmol., 22*:69.

56. Lee, V. H. L., and Carson, L. W. (1985). Possible mechanisms for the retention of topically applied vitamin A (retinol) in the albino rabbit eye, *J. Ocul. Pharmacol., 1*:297.
57. Harris, D., and Robinson, J. R. (1990). Bioadhesive polymers in peptide drug delivery, *Biomaterials, 11*:652.
58. Schacter, H., and Williams, D. (1982). Biosynthesis of mucus glycoproteins, *Adv. Exp. Med. Biol., 144*:3.
59. Marriot, C., and Gregory, N. P. (1990). Mucus physiology and pathology. *In: Bioadhesive Drug Delivery Systems* (V. Lenaerts and R. Gurny, eds.). CRC Press, Boca Raton, Florida, p. 21.
60. Allen, A. (1981). The structure and function of gastrointestinal mucus. *In: Basic Mechanisms of Gastrointestinal Mucosal Cell Injury and Protection* (J. W. Harmon, ed.). Williams & Wilkins, Baltimore, p. 351.
61. Allen, A., and Carrol, N. J. H. (1985). Adherent and soluble mucus in the stomach and duodenum, *Dig. Dis. Sci., 30*:55s.
62. Gandhi, R. B., and Robinson, J. R. (1988). Bioadhesion in drug delivery, *Indian J. Pharm. Sci., 50*:145.
63. Marriot, C., and Hughes, D. R. L. (1989). Mucus physiology and pathology. *In: Bioadhesion: Possibilities and Future Trends* (R. Gurny and H. E. Junginger, eds.). Wissenschaftliche Verlagsgesseelschaft, Stuttgart, p. 29.
64. Johnson, P. M., and Rainsford, K. D. (1978). The physical properties of mucus: Preliminary observations on the sedimentation behavior of porcine gastric mucus, *Biochim. Biophys. Acta, 286*:72.
65. Phelps, C. F. (1978). Biosynthesis of mucus glycoproteins, *Br. Med. Bull., 34*:43.
66. Robinson, J. R. (1989). Ocular drug delivery. Mechanism(s) of corneal drug transport and mucoadhesive delivery systems, *S.T.P. Pharma, 5*:839.
67. Mikos, A. G., and Peppas, N. A. (1986). Systems for controlled release of drugs. V. Bioadhesive systems, *S.T.P. Pharm., 2*:705.
68. Derjaguin, B. V., Toporov, Y. P., Mueler, V. M., and Aleinikova, I. N. (1977). On the relationship between the electrostatic and the molecular component of the adhesion of elastic particles to a solid surface, *J. Colloid Interface Sci., 58*:528.
69. Baier, R. E., Shafrin, I. G., and Zisman, W. A. (1968). Adhesion: Mechanism that assist and impede it, *Science, 162*:1360.
70. Helfand, E., and Tagami, Y. (1971). Theory of the interface between immiscible polymers, *Polym. Lett., 9*:741.
71. Helfand, E., and Tagami, Y. (1972). Theory of the interface between immiscible polymers. II. *J. Chem. Phys., 56*:3592.
72. Helfand, E., and Tagami, Y. (1972). Theory of the interface between immiscible polymers, *J. Chem. Phys., 57*:1812.
73. Peppas, N. A., and Buri, P. A. (1985). Surface, interfacial and molecular aspects of polymer adhesion on soft tissues, *J. Controlled Release, 2*:257.
74. Peppas, N. A., and Lustig, B. R. (1985). The role of crosslinks, entanglements, and relaxations of the macromolecular carrier in the diffusional release of biologically active materials: Conceptual and scaling relationships, *Ann. N.Y. Acad. Sci., 446*:26.
75. Reinhart, C. T., and Peppas, N. A. (1984). Solute diffusion in swollen membranes. II. Influence of crosslinking on diffusive properties, *J. Membr. Sci., 18*:227.
76. Peppas, N. A., and Reinhart, C. T. (1983). Solute diffusion in swollen membranes. Part I. New Therapy, *J. Membr. Sci., 15*:275.
77. Tabor, D. J. (1977). Surface forces and surface interactions, *J. Colloid Interface Sci., 58*:2.
78. Kinloch, A. J. (1980). The science of adhesion: I. Surface and interfacial aspects, *J. Mater Sci., 15*:2141.
79. Good, R. J. (1977). Surface free energy of solids and liquids: Thermodynamics, molecular forces and structure, *J. Colloid Interface Sci., 58*:398.

80. Ponchel, G., Touchard, F., Duchene, D., and Peppas, N. A. (1987). Bioadhesive analysis of controlled release systems. I. Fracture and interpenetration analysis in poly (acrylic acid) containing systems, *J. Controlled Release, 5*:129.

81. Mikos, A. G., and Peppas, N. A. (1988). Polymer chain entanglements and brittle fracture, *J. Chem. Phys., 88*:1337.

82. Wake, W. C. (1976). Theories of adhesion and adhesive action. *In: Adhesion and Formulation of Adhesives*. Applied Science, London, p. 65.

83. Israelachvili, J. N. (1985). *Intermolecular and Surface Forces*, Academic Press, New York.

84. Pritchard, W. H. (1971). The role of hydrogen bonding in adhesion, *Aspects Adhes., 6*:11.

85. Park, H., and Robinson, J. R. (1985). Physico-chemical properties of water insoluble polymers important to mucin/epithelial adhesion, *J. Controlled Release, 2*:47.

86. Nagai, T., and Machida, Y. (1985). Advances in drug delivery. Mucosal adhesive dosage forms, *Pharma. Int. Engl. Ed.*, August: 196.

87. Satoh, K., Takayama, K., Machida, Y., Suzuki, Y., Nakagaki, M., and Nagai, T. (1989). Factors affecting the bioadhesive properties of tablets consisting of hydroxypropyl cellulose and carboxy vinyl polymers, *Chem. Pharm. Bull., 37*:1366.

88. Gottschalk, A. (1960). *In: The Chemistry and Biology of Sialic Acid and Related Substances*, Cambridge University Press, London.

89. Leonard, F., Hodge, J. W., Jr., Houston, S., and Ousterhout, D. K. (1968). Alpha cyanoacrylate adhesive bond strengths with proteinaceous and non proteinaceous substances, *J. Biomed. Mater. Res., 2*:173.

90. Smart, J. D., Kellaway, I. W., and Worthington, H. E. C. (1984). An in vitro investigation of mucosal adhesive materials for use in controlled drug delivery, *J. Pharm. Pharmacol., 36*:295.

91. Leung, S. H. S., and Robinson, J. R. (1990). Polymer structure features contributing to muco-adhesion. II, *J. Controlled Release, 12*:187.

92. Chen, J. L., and Cyr, G. N. (1970). Compositions producing adhesion through adhesion, *In: Adhesive Biological Systems* (R. S. Manly, ed.). Academic Press, New York, Chapter 12.

93. Smart, J. D. (1991). An in vitro assessment of some muco-adhesive dosage forms, *Int. J. Pharm., 73*:69.

94. Park, K., and Park, H. (1990). Test methods of bioadhesion. *In: Bioadhesive Drug Delivery Systems* (V. Lenaerts and R. Gurny, eds.). CRC Press, Boca Raton, Florida, p. 43.

95. Wang, P. Y., and Forrester, D. H. (1974). Conditions for the induced adhesion of hydrophobic polymers to soft tissue, *Trans. Am. Soc. Artif. Int. Organs, 20*:504.

96. Teng, C. L. C., and Ho, N. F. L. (1987). Mechanistic studies in the simultaneous flow and adsorption of polymer coated latex particles on intestinal mucus. I: Methods and physical model development, *J. Controlled Release, 6*:133.

97. Zaki, I., Fitzgerald, P., Hardy, J. G., and Wilson, C. G. (1986). A comparison of the effect of viscosity in the precorneal residence of solutions in rabbit and man, *J. Pharm. Pharmacol., 38*:463.

98. Moss, R. A. (1987). The eyelids. *In: Adler's Physiology of the Eye: Clinical Applications*, 8th ed. (R. A. Moses and W. M. Hart, Jr., eds.), Mosby, St. Louis, p. 1.

99. Wright, P., and Mackie, I. A. (1977). Mucus in healthy and diseased eye, *Trans. Ophthalmol. Soc., U.K., 91*:1.

100. Hardy, J. G., Lee, S. W., and Wilson, C. G. (1985). Intranasal drug delivery by sprays and drops, *J. Pharm. Pharmacol., 37*:294.

101. Tabachnik, N. F., Blackburn, P., and Cerami, A. (1981). Biochemical and rheological characteristics of sputum mucus from a patients with cystic fibrosis, *J. Biol. Chem., 256*:7161.

102. Swan, K. C. (1945). Use of methylcellulose in ophthalmology, *Arch. Ophthalmol., 33*:378.

103. Mueller, W. H., and Deardorff, D. L. (1956). Ophthalmic vehicles: The effect of methylcellulose on the penetration of Homatropine hydrobromide through the cornea, *J. Am. Pharm. Assoc., 45*:334.

104. Benedetto, D. A., Shah, D. O., and Kaufman, H. E. (1975). Instilled fluid dynamics and surface chemistry of polymers in the preocular tear film, *Invest. Ophthalmol., 14*:887.
105. Saettone, M. F., Giannaccini, B., Chetoni, P., Galli, G., and Chiellini, E. (1984). Vehicle effects on the ophthalmic bioavailability: An evaluation of polymeric inserts containing pilocarpine, *J. Pharm. Pharmacol., 36*:229.
106. Finne, U., Salivirta, J., and Urtti, A. (1991). Sodium acetate improves the ocular/systemic absorption ratio of timolol applied ocularly in monoisopropyl PVM-MA matrices, *Int. J. Pharm., 75*:R1.
107. Losa, C., Calvo, P., Castro, E., Vila-Jato, J. L., and Alono, M. J. (1991). Improvement of ocular penetration of amikacin sulphate by association to poly(butylcyanoacrylate) nanoparticles, *J. Pharm. Pharmacol., 43*:548.
108. Vanderhoff, J., El-Asser, E. R., and Urgerstad, J. (1977). U.S. Patent Application #867031.
109. Robinson, J. R., and Li, V. H. K. (1984). Ocular disposition and bioavailability of pilocarpine from Piloplex® and other sustained release drug delivery systems. *In: Recent Advances in Glaucoma* (U. Ticho and R. David, eds.). Excerpta Medica, Amsterdam, p. 231.
110. Saettone, M. F., Giannaccinni, B., Guidicci, A., and Savigni, P. (1986). Semisolids ophthalmic vehicles. III. An evaluation of four organic hydrogels containing pilocarpine, *Int. J. Pharm., 31*:261.
111. Benditti, L. M., Kyyrönen, K., Hume, L., Topp, E., and Stella, V. (1991). Steroid ester of hyaluronic acid in ophthalmic drug delivery, *Proc. Int. Symp. Controlled Release Bioact. Mater., 18*:497.
112. Saettone, M. F., Giannaccinni, B., Torracca, M. T., and Burgalassi, S. (1987). "An Evaluation of the Bioadhesive Properties of Hyaluronic Acid." *Proceedings of the 3rd Eur. Congress on Biopharm. Pharmacokinetics*, Vol. I, Freiburg, April, p. 413.
113. Saettone, M. F., Chetoni, P., Torracca, M. T., Giannaccinni, B., and Ordello, G. (1986). Evaluation of Hyaluronic Acid as a Vehicle for Topical Ophthalmic Drugs, *Abstr. of Int. Symp. Ophthalmic Dosage Forms*, Pisa, Oct. 13–14.
114. Saettone, M. F., Chetoni, P., and Giannaccinni, B. (1985). Evaluation of hyaluronic acid as a vehicle for topical ophthalmic drugs, *Abstr. of 2nd. Int. Conference on Polymers in Medicine*, Capri, June 3–7.
115. Miyazaki, S., Ishii, K., and Takada, M. (1982). Use of fibrin film as a carrier for drug delivery: A long acting delivery system for pilocarpine into the eye, *Chem. Pharm. Bull., 30*:3405.
116. Bloomfield, S. E., Miyata, T., Dunn, M. W., Bueser, N., Stenzel, K. H., and Rubin, A. L. (1978). Soluble gentamicin ophthalmic inserts as a drug delivery system, *Arch. Ophthalmol., 96*:885.
117. McCoy, J. P., Jr. (1986). Contemporary laboratory applications of lectins, *Biotechniques, 4*:252.
118. Kilpatrick, D. C., Pusztai, A., Grant, G., Graham, G., and Ewen, S. W. B. (1985). Tomato lectins resist degradation in the mammalian alimentary canal and binds to intestinal villi without deleterious effects, *FEBS Lett., 185*:299.
119. Hynes, R. O., and Yamada, K. M. (1982). Fibronectins: Multifunctional modular glycoproteins, *J. Cell Biol., 95*:369.
120. Nishida, T., Ohashi, Y., Awanta, T., and Manabe, R. (1983). Fibronectin, new therapy for corneal trophic ulcer, *Arch. Ophthalmol., 101*:1046.
121. Ticho, U., Blumenthal, M., Zonis, S., Gal, A., Blank, I., and Mazor, Z. W. (1979). A clinical trial with Piloplex—a new long acting pilocarpine compound: Preliminary report, *Ann. Ophthalmol.*, April:555.
122. Refojo, M. F. (1982). Current status of biomaterials in ophthalmology, *Surv. Ophthalmol., 26*:257.
123. Refojo, M. F., Dohlman, C. H., and Koliopoulos, J. (1971). Adhesives in ophthalmology: A review, *Surv. Ophthalmol., 15*:217.

11
Ocular Inserts

Rajan Bawa *Bausch & Lomb, Rochester, New York*

I. INTRODUCTION

Existing ocular drug therapy systems are fairly primitive (1). This is because the development of improved ocular drug delivery systems is very challenging. Significant obstacles that need to be overcome are the rapid turnover rate of the tear film, which quickly flushes drugs out of the precorneal area, and the low permeability of corneal tissue (2). These factors make topical drug delivery to the eye extremely inefficient and, therefore, provide a strong motivation for developing *extended duration delivery systems* for ocular drug therapy.

The administration pattern of drugs given by conventional eye drops is pulse entry, as shown in Figure 1. This pattern is characterized by a transient overdose, followed by a relatively short period of acceptable dosing, in turn followed by a prolonged period of underdosing. The ocular and systemic side effects of some ophthalmic drugs are primarily related to overdosing (3,4).

In order to overcome the large drainage factor imposed by the eye and compensate, at least in part, for the low permeability of corneal tissue, several strategies have been explored to develop *extended-duration* drug delivery systems. These include boosting the eye drop viscosity or using ointments and gels as conventional improvements on eye drops. All these approaches, however, interfere with vision and fail to prolong precorneal drug residence time significantly (1,3). Other approaches include particulates (5) and liposomes (6), which will be discussed separately in this book, together with the Piloplex (7–9), which is a pilocarpine-polymer emulsion. To date, however, very few ocular products are available for once-daily or weekly therapy.

Utilization of the principles of *controlled release* as embodied by ocular inserts therefore offers an attractive alternative approach to the difficult problem of prolonging precorneal drug residence time. This is because the ultimate goal of an extended-duration ocular drug delivery system is to maintain an effective drug concentration in the target tissues and yet minimize the required number of applications consonant with the function of *controlled-release systems*.

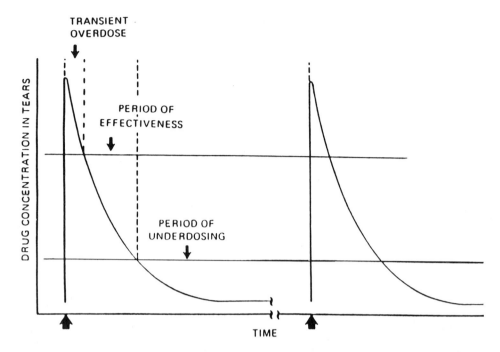

Figure 1. A typical ocular drug concentration-time profile for a drug given as eye drops.

II. RATIONALE FOR CONTROLLED-RELEASE OCULAR INSERTS

Controlled-release systems deliver a bioactive agent to a target site at a controlled concentration over a desired time interval. In practice, this is achieved by incorporating or encapsulating the agent (a drug, pesticide, or other bioactive material) into a carrier, generally a polymeric material.

Controlled-release formulations were first used in the agricultural industries for low molecular weight fertilizers and pesticides in the 1950s (10). In the mid 1960s, this concept was systematically applied to the medical field (11) for the development of nonprescription drugs. In the 1970s, the use of polymers as vehicles to deliver bioactive agents for prolonged time periods began to receive widespread attention (12). These applications included studies of vascular proliferation and bioassays of growth factors and drug delivery.

The significance of controlled-release systems for drug delivery stems from the fact that in order to effect therapy, drug concentration in the target tissue needs to be maintained between upper and lower bounds. The maximum represents the threshold above which the concentration of the drug is toxic and the minimum represents the limit below which the drug is ineffective. This is particularly necessary in the case of ocular tissues, as discussed earlier.

The rationale for controlled-release ocular inserts can best be appreciated by an inspection of Figure 2. The rate at which instilled solutions are removed from the eye

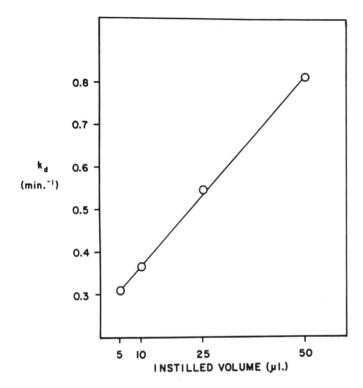

Figure 2. Relationship between the observed rate constant for decline in volume and volume instilled. (From Ref. 13.)

varies linearly with instilled volume. It follows, therefore, that if the drug is presented to the precorneal film as a solid in the form of an insert, the drainage rate can be minimized.

Furthermore, microdrops of a pilocarpine solution were administered to patients with glaucoma (14) on a nearly continuous basis to simulate a controlled-release system. The results clearly showed the therapeutic advantage of continuous controlled drug delivery.

Additionally, ocular inserts offer the potential advantage of improving patient compliance by reducing the dosing frequency.

However, in order to perform successfully as a controlled-release device, an ophthalmic insert raises a unique set of challenges that must be addressed. These are described in detail in the following section.

III. CRITERIA FOR SUCCESSFUL OCULAR INSERTS

In order for a controlled-release device to be considered satisfactory for use as an ocular insert, it must not only be capable of reproducible release kinetics but also must meet a unique set of criteria peculiar to ophthalmic applications.

This section comprises a detailed discussion of the desired criteria for a controlled-release ocular insert. These are the following:

1. Comfort
2. Lack of expulsion during wear
3. Ease of handling and insertion
4. Noninterference with vision and oxygen permeability
5. Reproducibility of release kinetics
6. Applicability to a variety of drugs
7. Sterility
8. Stability
9. Ease of manufacture

Although most of the above are unique to ocular devices, a few of the required attributes are common to controlled-release devices in general.

Detailed discussion of these criteria is important for two reasons. First, they provide a goal which, if achieved, can ensure the success of an ocular insert. Second, they provide a hallmark against which existing and experimental ocular inserts can be compared.

A. Comfort

Few tissues of the body are as sensitive to discomfort as the eye. Since the eye is a very important organ of the body, this extreme sensitivity can be viewed as a protective mechanism to prevent abrasion and injury to the eye, particularly the cornea.

In the context of ocular inserts, however, the foreign-body sensation, presents a challenge to be overcome. This is because of three reasons. Not only does discomfort lead to poor patient compliance, but the excessive lacrimation that accompanies irritation dilutes the drug and causes a reduction in its concentration. Furthermore, persistent irritation could cause the patient to rub the eye wearing the insert in an effort to alleviate the discomfort. This in turn may cause the expulsion of the insert from the eye.

Although it is practically impossible to eliminate the foreign-body sensation altogether, a properly designed ocular insert will seek to minimize the sensation caused by its insertion and wear. A factor that aids the use of ocular inserts is the adaptation to discomfort by the patient (15), particularly if the sensation is minimal.

B. Lack of Expulsion During Wear

In as much as the goal of a controlled-release ocular insert is to provide the requisite drug concentration to the eye, its expulsion from the eye during the stipulated period of its use is clearly undesirable.

Even if the previously discussed goal of acceptable comfort is met, an ocular insert may still be expelled from the eye. This is probably due to its excessive movement in the eye. Some movement of the insert is actually beneficial, since this allows turnover of the tear film from behind the insert. This in turn facilitates the supply of oxygen to the eye and eliminates the build-up of harmful metabolites such as carbon dioxide, which has been implicated in complications arising from improperly fitted contact lenses (16).

Accordingly, careful design of an ocular insert will allow it to move adequately without being subject to extreme movement. An improperly designed ocular insert can cause excessive excursions away from the eyeball and may result in its expulsion from the eye and consequent interruption in therapy.

C. Ease of Handling and Insertion

An ocular insert should be preferably easy to handle and insert in the eye. This is especially true for inserts that are to be self-administered by the patient. This has two benefits. First, ease of handling and insertion will improve patient compliance with the dosing regimen. Second, it will minimize the initial discomfort felt by the patient and consequent lacrimation immediately on insertion.

D. Noninterference with Vision and Oxygen Permeability

As the eye is a very important sensory organ, vital to day-to-day routine functions, it is important that an insert not interfere with vision unless absolutely necessary.

Ideally, a person wearing an insert should be able to forget that there is an insert in his or her eye while performing daily activities. Obviously, if there is a constant interference with vision, the wearer is likely to be distracted from daily activities.

Also, although the sclera is richly supplied with blood vessels, the cornea is avascular and obtains most of its required oxygen directly from the air. Oxygen deprivation leads to edema and poor corneal health (16). It follows, therefore, that an ocular insert should not block the access of oxygen to the cornea.

E. Reproducibility of Release Kinetics

The function of an ocular insert is to deliver the drug it contains in a reproducible and controlled manner. This is an attribute that an ocular insert shares with any other controlled-release device.

The factor that distinguishes ocular drug delivery is the fact that an ocular insert is placed in a largely aqueous environment. This is in contrast to transdermal patches or subcutaneous, vaginal, and rectal inserts. Furthermore, the tear film is subject to constant turnover and dilution. It is estimated (13,17) that drops in excess of 10 µL are eliminated from the eye in about 1–2 min after instillation.

Clearly, the ability of a controlled drug delivery device to perform reproducibly and for extended time periods under these conditions is severely challenged.

F. Applicability to a Variety of Drugs

Ophthalmic drugs vary considerably in their physicochemical properties. A large number of drugs used in the eye are highly water soluble. In addition, poorly water-soluble drugs, for example, steroids like fluorometholone (18), are also quite important. More recently, naturally occurring compounds like growth hormones are being explored for ophthalmic use (19).

It is reasonable to expect that once an ocular insert has successfully addressed criteria 1–4, discussed previously, for one drug, the resulting physical design can freely be applied to all new drugs. However, given the diversity of ophthalmic drugs, it is unreasonable to expect that a single universal polymer suitable for all present and future ocular drugs can be designed.

Rather, the physicochemical properties of the polymeric system have to be tailored to the unique properties of the drug to be delivered. It follows, therefore, that an ocular drug delivery system should preferably employ polymeric systems that easily allow variation in the range of available properties. This flexibility will permit their use with various drugs with minimal modification.

G. Sterility

It is a common practice to sterilize ophthalmic medications. This is true for conventional dosage forms like drops, ointments, and gels, as well as inserts.

A variety of sterilization techniques may be employed to sterilize drops, ointments, and gels. These include sterile fill (mainly for drops), autoclaving, and radiation sterilization (20). Of all these techniques, radiation sterilization is the one best suited to drug-containing ocular inserts.

It follows, therefore, that the polymer used as the matrix for the drug should be able to withstand the sterilization process, maintaining its mechanical integrity and biocompatibility.

H. Stability

Any drug dosage form whether it be oral, transdermal, parenteral, or ophthalmic is required to be stable. An ocular insert used for drug delivery is, therefore, no exception to this rule.

The point of differentiation between conventional dosage forms and controlled-release systems, when considering stability, is the presence of the polymer.

Just as the polymer used for the insert must be capable of sterilization, it should also be stable when exposed to heat and high humidity.

Also, it has been demonstrated by Bawa and Nandu (21) that the kinetics of drug release from polymeric systems can be affected by extended exposure to heat. Accordingly, the extent of these changes must be assessed when dealing with all polymeric systems, including those used as ocular inserts.

I. Ease of Manufacture

The criterion of ease of manufacture is important for any pharmaceutical dosage form, including ocular inserts. This is because it directly impacts on the manufacturing cost. A more complicated and inefficient process will generally result in wasted resources at a higher cost to the ultimate user of the pharmaceutical dosage form.

Over the years, processing machinery has been designed, built, and used to manufacture tablets, capsules, solutions, and ointments. This has resulted in the widespread availability of the necessary automated equipment, with several suppliers competing for market share. On the other hand, fabrication of controlled drug-release dosage forms remains, to date, a fairly specialized operation. The companies that fabricate these devices most often have proprietary specialized machinery and processes to do so.

Furthermore, the usage of controlled-release dosage forms in comparison with the conventional dosage forms is quite limited. Therefore, the degree of automation even within the companies that do possess the necessary technology may not have been developed to its full potential.

All these above factors contribute to a higher cost to the consumer than is potentially achievable. It could be argued that the therapeutic advantages of controlled-release systems would in most cases outweigh their usually higher cost. It is nevertheless important to consider, at the very least, means to design efficient processes wherever possible.

Following this discussion of the criteria desired for ocular inserts, we will shortly review systems presently available for use as ocular drug delivery inserts. However, before that discussion, it is worthwhile to compare the relative merits and drawbacks of the two broad classes of available controlled-release systems; i.e., erodible versus nonerodible, especially in the context of ocular therapy.

IV. ERODIBLE VERSUS NONERODIBLE SYSTEMS

The obvious appeal of erodible systems used in drug delivery systems stems mainly from the fact that these systems do not have to be removed from body tissues after the drug has been released. In general (10), it is desirable to have the polymer degradation process hydrolytically—rather than enzymatically—controlled, since in most body sites there is little patient to patient variation in water concentration.

Unfortunately, this general rule does not hold in the case of an ocular insert. In the eye, there is in fact significant patient to patient variability in the rate of tear production and turnover. In addition, the concentration of metabolic enzymes in the tear film of the eye also varies considerably from patient to patient.

It may, therefore, be anticipated that an erodible ocular insert is more prone to demonstrate variability in release kinetics from patient to patient than a nonerodible ocular insert. In the latter case, the release kinetics can be better controlled by manipulating mainly the physicochemical interactions of the polymer-drug combination rather than having to contend with the additional physiological variations imposed by the eye.

Another important advantage of ocular nonerodible inserts over erodible inserts manifests itself when a device is expelled from the eye.

If a nonerodible device is expelled and lost, it is obvious to the wearer that this has occurred. In that event, a new device can be inserted and therapy resumed. On the other hand, loss of an erodible device can be very confusing. As discussed above, erodible systems can have significantly variable erosion rates based on individual patient physiology and lacrimation patterns.

Therefore, in the latter case, the patient cannot definitively know whether the device was lost or merely eroded faster. The health care professional is, therefore, confronted with the option of advising the patient to replace the "lost" device and risking overmedication. Conversely, the patient could be advised to maintain the dosing regimen assuming that the device was "eroded" rather than lost, thus risking undermedication. Either option is clearly undesirable.

Last, the eye is in reality a very accessible site suitable for an *insert* compared to other body sites. Therefore, whereas erodible *implants* are probably preferred over nonerodible *implants* in sites accessible only by surgery such as subcutaneous or neural sites, the advantages of erodible inserts over nonerodible inserts for ocular therapy are not as intuitively obvious.

Suffice it to say that the advantage of greater convenience in administration afforded by erodible inserts has to be carefully weighed against the greater reliability of nonerodible inserts for each potential ocular application. The following section describes both non-erodible and erodible marketed systems.

V. REVIEW OF MARKETED OCULAR INSERTS

A. Nonerodible Systems

1. Contact Lenses

The primary use of contact lenses is for vision correction. In addition to this function, therapeutic soft contact lenses (27) are often used to aid in corneal wound healing. This is particularly true in patients with infectious corneal ulcers characterized by marked thinning of the cornea. An obvious extension of this latter use probably prompted physicians to investigate the use of contact lenses presoaked in drug solutions as potential drug delivery devices.

The use of presoaked hydrophilic contact lenses for ocular drug delivery has, therefore, been extensively examined (22–31) for a variety of drugs. These have included antibiotics, antiglaucoma agents, and polypeptides. However, the drug release from contact lenses is extremely rapid (32), most of the drug being released within the first 30 min, as shown by Figure 3 for pilocarpine nitrate release.

It can be shown (32) that the entire time course of release from this system can be represented adequately by two equations:

$$\frac{M_t}{M_\infty} = 4 \left(\frac{Dt}{l^2 \pi}\right)^{1/2} \tag{1}$$

which is valid for the first 60% of the drug released, and

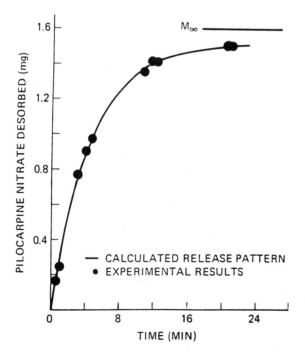

Figure 3. Release of pilocarpine nitrate from presoaked polyhydroxyethyl methacrylate contact lenses. (From Ref. 32.)

$$\frac{M_t}{M_\infty} = 1 - \frac{8}{\pi^2} \exp\left(-\frac{\pi^2 D t}{l^2}\right) \tag{2}$$

which is valid for the final 60% of the drug release. Both equations give nearly equal results for the middle 20% of the drug release. In these equations, M_t and M_∞ represent the mass of drug released at time, t, and the mass released after an infinite time, respectively; l is the lens thickness (modeled as a plane sheet); and D is the diffusion coefficient of the drug in the matrix, and is in the order of 1×10 E-6 cm^2/s.

In reality, the entire time course of the drug release from this system can be represented by the following single, more general equation (33):

$$\frac{M_t}{M_\infty} = 1 - \sum_{n=0}^{\infty} \frac{8}{(2n+1)^2 \pi^2} \exp\left\{-D_e(2n+1)^2 \frac{\pi^2 t}{4l^2}\right\} \tag{3}$$

as was done by Bawa et al. (34) for the controlled release of macromolecules from ethylene vinyl–acetate copolymer matrices. In this equation, the lens is considered to be a plane sheet with thickness 2l. The first two equations are "short" and "long" time solutions of the third equation.

The actual time taken for all the drug to elute out of the lens is dependent on various factors. These include the equilibrium water content of the hydrogel comprising the lens, its cross-link density, and the molecular weight of the drug. Use of a novel amino acid monomer (35) in the fabrication of a soft contact lens has demonstrated in vitro release times for these lenses presoaked with pilocarpine hydrochloride for longer periods than is possible for conventional contact lenses.

It is evident that the use of presoaked soft contact lenses to prolong the residence time of various hydrophilic drugs is likely to continue in limited cases. This is partly due to the fact that the use of presoaked contact lenses allows the physician the flexibility of choosing a drug and its concentration. Additionally, there are few other devices presently available that are suitable for extended ocular drug delivery.

Unfortunately, as discussed above, the residence time of drugs using commonly available presoaked lenses is not significantly prolonged. In addition, commonly used preservatives, such as benzalkonium chloride, have a greater affinity for the hydrophilic contact lens material than for the aqueous drug solutions that are used for presoaking the lenses. These are, therefore, concentrated in the lens to levels that can be toxic to corneal epithelium (24).

An alternate approach to presoaking soft contact lenses in drug solutions is to incorporate the drug either as a solution or a suspension of solid particles in the monomer mix. Next, the polymerization step is carried out to fabricate the contact lens (35–37). If spincasting is used as the processing step, the solid particles can be confined to the lens periphery where they do not interfere with vision. This technique has demonstrated the promise of longer times of release (up to 180 h) as compared to soaked lenses. Furthermore, the problem of concentration of preservatives is eliminated, since the drug without any added preservatives is incorporated into the lens.

In summary, when evaluated against the criteria that were set forth in Section III, contact lenses fall short of the ideal in the areas of comfort (in non–contact lens wearers) and difficulty of handling and insertion (particularly in the case of presoaking with drug solutions).

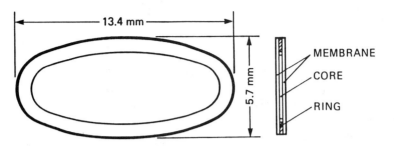

Figure 4. Dimensions of diffusional Ocusert drug delivery device. (From Ref. 32.)

Also, though contact lenses are sterile when supplied by the manufacturers, the presoaking step used by most practitioners usually results in a nonsterile device. Additionally, contact lenses are fit on the cornea and thus necessarily do adversely affect the transport of oxygen to it.

2. The Ocusert®

The Ocusert is a flat, flexible elliptical device consisting of three layers, as shown in Figures 4 and 5. Two outer layers of ethylene vinyl–acetate enclose the inner core of pilocarpine gelled with alginate (38). A retaining ring of ethylene vinyl–acetate, impregnated with titanium dioxide for visibility encloses the drug reservoir circumferentially.

The Ocusert is marketed in two sizes, Ocusert Pilo-20 and Ocusert Pilo-40, representing two different release rates (20 and 40 µg/h), as shown in Figure 6. The higher release rate for Ocusert Pilo-40 is achieved by making its rate-controlling membranes thinner and by use of the flux enhancer, di(2-ethylhexyl)phthalate. Both systems are used for the continuous delivery of pilocarpine for a week for the treatment of chronic glaucoma.

The satisfactory kinetic behaviour of the Ocusert relies on the unique solubility properties of pilocarpine free base. This drug is miscible in both water and organic

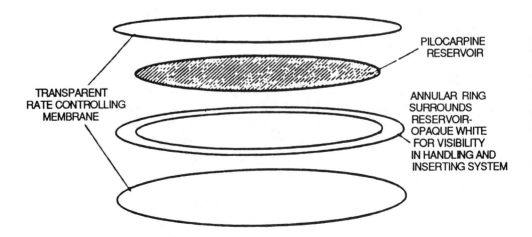

Figure 5. Exploded view of the Ocusert.

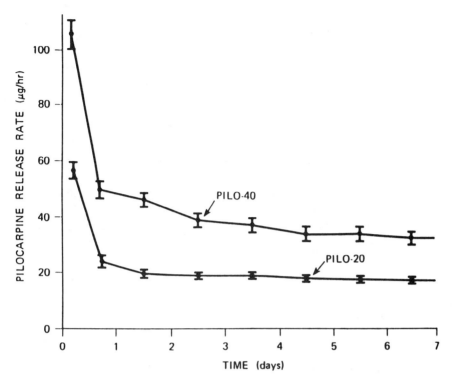

Figure 6. In vitro time course of the rate of release of pilocarpine from the two ocular therapeutic systems. The difference in the rates of release by the two systems is achieved by making the EVA membranes of the 40 μg/h system thinner than those of the 20 μm/h system and by use of the flux enhancer, di(2-ethylhexyl) phthalate. (From Ref. 38.)

solvents, exhibiting both hydrophilic and lipophilic character. It can, therefore, permeate the hydrophobic rate-controlling membranes, whereas water is excluded from the device.

The release rate, J, is derived from Fick's first law, yielding the following expression:

$$J = \frac{ADKC_s}{1} \tag{4}$$

where A is the surface area of the membrane, K is the distribution coefficient of the drug, 1 is the membrane thickness, and C_s is the drug solubility. The drug concentration outside the device is assumed to be negligible. Since all terms on the right-hand side of the above equation are constant, so is the release rate of the device.

An evaluation of the Ocusert against the criteria that were described in Section III indicates that foreign body sensation, expulsion, and difficulty of handling and insertion (requiring good manual dexterity) are problem areas of the Ocusert (39).

Also, release of drugs other than pilocarpine from this device could require significant modification of the polymers comprising the rate-controlling membranes. Only limited details are available for the release of other drugs such as chloramphenicol and hydrocortisone from the Ocusert system (32).

Finally, it may be surmised that the manufacturing process of the Ocusert is fairly involved. The rate controlling membranes, the titanium dioxide ring, and the drug-containing reservoir are probably fused together in an additional processing step after being separately fabricated. If, as is common with transdermal devices, the final elliptical shape of the Ocusert is cut out of sheets of material, there is probably some waste material discarded as "flash."

B. Erodible Systems

Over the years, several erodible drug delivery systems have been conceived and tested for ophthalmic use. These have included pilocarpine-containing carboxymethylcellulose wafers (40,41) and polyvinyl alcohol discs (42,43) or rods (44). Also, wafers of collagen-containing gentamicin sulfate (45–47) have indicated some promise in extending its ocular residence time as compared to conventional treatments (Fig. 7). In addition, erodible ocular inserts comprising hydrophobic polycarboxylic acids have been described as well (48).

Despite all these efforts, there are only three erodible devices that have been marketed to date. These will be discussed in the following section.

1. The Lacrisert®

The Lacrisert is a sterile, rod-shaped device made of hydroxpropyl cellulose without any preservatives that is used for the treatment of dry eye syndromes. It was introduced by Merck, Sharp & Dohme in 1981 (49). The device weighs 5 mg and measures 1.27 mm in diameter with a length of 3.5 mm (50). Figure 8 is a photograph of the edges of the device

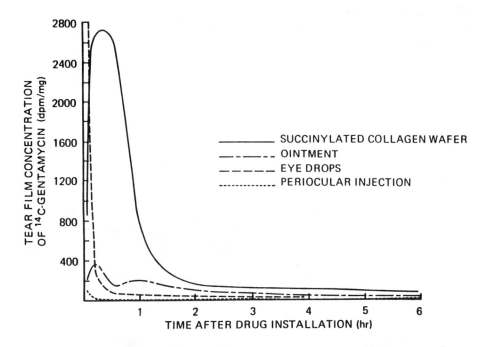

Figure 7. Medication in tear film plotted as concentration (disintegrations per minute per milligram, dpm/mg) of ^{14}C-gentamicin sulfate vs time. (From Ref. 45.)

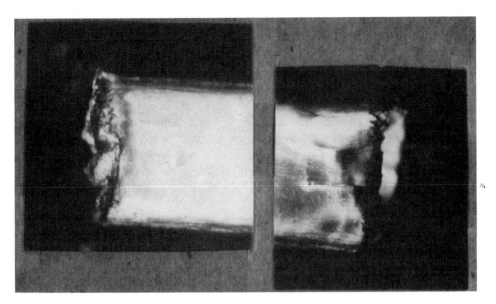

Figure 8. Photomicrograph of the edges of the Lacrisert. Magnification: 75×

magnified 75 ×. It is placed in the inferior cul-de-sac of the eye with the help of an applicator. Figure 9 shows the applicator and the device.

The probable forerunner of this insert was reported by Merck Sharpe & Dohme as a water-soluble delivery system for ocular medications (51). This insert was oval or rod-shaped and weighed either 12, 18, or 24 mg. The material of which the device was composed was not identified. Two years later, the Merck Sharpe & Dohme–Chibret

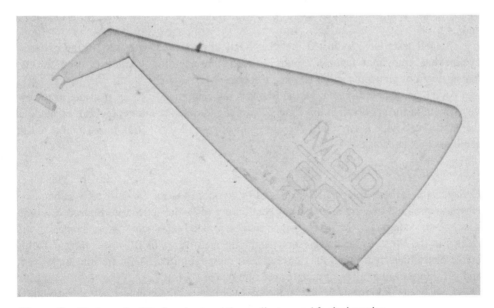

Figure 9. Photograph of the Lacrisert and the applicator used for its insertion.

Research Institute reported (52) the effect of an unmedicated cellulosic insert on tear breakup time in rabbits. The effect of the insert was greater in magnitude and duration than artificial tear solutions.

Although early reports (53,54) indicated that the insert was preferred over artificial tear solutions by patients with dry eye, a later study (49) concluded that the insert was not well received owing to subjective blurring of vision and ocular irritation. Matting of the eyelids has also been reported. The reason for the conflicting reports is probably patient selection. The earlier studies (53,54) used patients with Sjögren's syndrome, Stevens-Johnson syndrome, and loss of the lacrimal gland.

Based on the above discussion, it appears reasonable to conclude that the Lacrisert is useful in the treatment of patients with keratitis sicca whose symptoms are difficult to control with artificial tears alone.

It is probable that the ocular irritation demonstrated by some patients is due, at least in part, to the somewhat cumbersome insertion procedure using the applicator as recommended in the package insert. The patient is asked to entrap the 3.5-mm long device in the prongs of the insert and then transfer the device from the applicator into the lower cul-de-sac. This operation does require a fair degree of manual dexterity.

2. The SODI

The SODI (Soluble Ocular Drug Insert) is a small oval wafer which was developed by Soviet scientists for cosmonauts who could not use eye drops in weightless conditions (55). The SODI was brought to the West by Diversified Tech Inc., which negotiated exclusive rights to market the technology. At this time, it has been tested in Europe, the United States, and Saudi Arabia.

The SODI is a small oval wafer of polyacrylamide impregnated with drug. Figure 10 is a photograph of the SODI being inserted into a patient's eye. Its dimensions are 9 mm × 4.5 mm with a thickness of 0.35 mm.

Figure 11 is a schematic of the concentration profile, in tears, of a drug delivered by the SODI. It is claimed that the drug-release process can be varied to last between 12 and 24 h.

Clinical tests have indicated that the SODI impregnated with pilocarpine or tetracycline has compared favorably with the conventional drop treatments used for the management of glaucoma and trachoma, respectively.

As the published literature on the SODI is rather limited, it is not possible to review this system in further detail at this time. The only additional comment that can be made is that since the device is cut out of cast sheets of drug-loaded material, this would result in some wastage as "flash."

3. Collagen Shields

Collagen shields were originally developed by Fyodorov in the Soviet Union as bandage lenses to promote healing after radical keratotomy (57). Subsequently, Bausch & Lomb acquired the company—Medtech, which had negotiated with the Soviets to market the shields in the West. There are presently three different types of BioCor collagen shields marketed by Bausch & Lomb Pharmaceuticals, Tampa, Florida. These are BioCor-12, -24, and -72, representing different times of dissolution (in hours).

It has been demonstrated (58) that the use of collagen shields promotes corneal healing and provides lubricity to the eye.

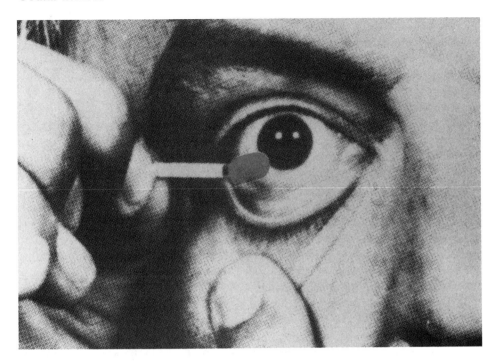

Figure 10. Photograph of the SODI being inserted into a patient's eye. (From Ref. 56.)

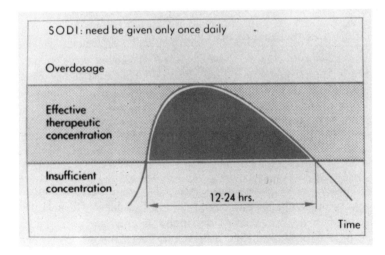

Figure 11. Schematic of the concentration profile in tears of a drug delivered by the SODI. (From Ref. 56.)

The corneal shields are composed of porcine scleral collagen with a 14.5-mm diameter, a 9.0-mm back curve, and about a 0.1-mm thickness at the center. Exposure to ultraviolet light for different time periods induces varying degrees of cross linkage (58). This in turn results in shields available with the different dissolution rates. Finally, the shields undergo a sterilization step by gamma-irradiation.

Much in the same fashion as the soft contact lenses discussed before, collagen shields soaked in aqueous drug solutions have been used by clinicians. Accordingly, antibiotics such as tobramycin (59–62) and gentamicin and vancomycin (63) have been shown to have their residence time in the rabbit eye increased as compared to the traditional eye drops. In addition, steroids such as prednisolone acetate (64) and dexamethasone (65) have demonstrated similar results.

Not surprisingly, the relatively rapid "dose-dumping" effect observed earlier for soft contact lenses is repeated when collagen shields are used instead (63). Most of the drug is released quite rapidly (in about an hour), although some extended release is observed in the case of vancomycin (up to 6 h). So even though the shield itself may not dissolve until a much later time, it is depleted of the drug quite rapidly (61).

The earlier work using collagen wafers with gentamicin sulfate incorporated in them (45–47) during the fabrication process is akin to similar work discussed before using soft contact lenses (35–37). Even this method when applied to the collagen material, however, does not prolong the release time appreciably.

Presoaked contact lenses and collagen shields can, therefore, be compared and contrasted, since they are similar drug delivery devices. They manifest an interesting example of the debate of erodible versus nonerodible ocular inserts, as discussed in Section IV. In both cases, although they are supplied sterile by the manufacturers, the soaking step results in a nonsterile device being placed in the eye.

The potential advantage of using collagen shields over contact lenses lies in the fact that since the former are erodible, they do not have to be removed. However, this advantage does have to be weighed carefully in view of the fact that collagen is capable of eliciting an inflammatory response (66) when used in ocular tissues. There are indications that this response can be avoided if the terminal peptides on the collagen responsible for its antigenicity are cleaved (67).

Also, it has been reported that the use of presoaked collagen shields yielded tobramycin concentrations in aqueous humor that were higher (59) than the levels obtained using presoaked soft contact lenses. In this study, the lenses used contained 38.6% water, whereas the collagen shield typically can contain up to about 90–95% water. The somewhat higher tissue concentrations attained by the collagen shields are, therefore, not unusual. The shields obviously were able to imbibe and release more drug solution than were the lenses. If, on the other hand, a higher water content lens had been used (68), one might expect the results to be closer for the two cases.

An evaluation of the collagen shields against the criteria discussed in Section III will indicate much of the same comments as were made previously with regard to contact lenses. The notable points of differentiation are as follows (58). The shields when used as surgical adjuncts without presoaking can cause discomfort if they are not properly hydrated. Also, shields produce a reduction in visual acuity when placed on the eye. Finally, if the shields are not used in conjunction with antibiotics, there is the potential for secondary infection.

Finally, in the following section is discussed the Minidisc, an effective and versatile prolonged-release ocular drug delivery system (69). Although the Minidisc has not yet been marketed, extensive and multifaceted investigations have been conducted on it. These will be described in the next section.

VI. THE MINIDISC

At the very outset of the developmental efforts on the Minidisc, it was recognized that criteria 1–4, discussed earlier in Section III, were virtual prerequisites for a successful ocular insert. As will be recalled, these were comfort, lack of expulsion, ease of handling and insertion, and noninterference with vision and oxygen permeability.

Accordingly, several designs were conceived, tested, and rejected before the Minidisc geometry was arrived at. One interesting design concept that initially appeared to demonstrate some promise was a contoured annulus. This can most easily be visualized as a contact lens with the center missing!

Figure 12 is a photograph of the annulur device on a human eye. In contrast to a contact lens, this device clearly would not interfere with vision and oxygen permeability. Unfortunately, when devices loaded with drug were tested on rabbit eyes, they caused significant discomfort. This was primarily due to the fact that the blinking action of the lids (although infrequent in rabbits) caused some movement of the inner edge of the annulus against the

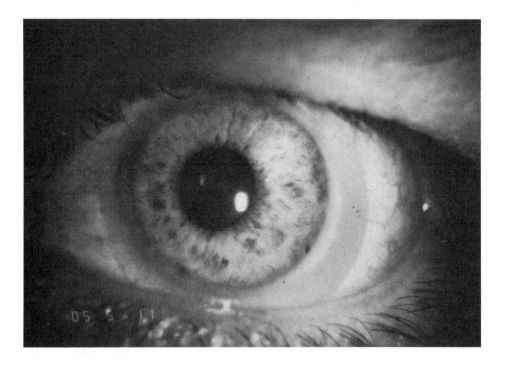

Figure 12.   Photograph of an annular device on a human eye. The device was stained with sodium fluorescein in order for it to be visualized better.

corneoscleral junction. This was clearly undesirable, since this junction is richly supplied with sensitive nerve endings.

Finally, an optimum design configuration for the ocular insert was arrived at and was dubbed the "Minidisc," depicted in Figure 13. Broadly stated, the Minidisc is shaped somewhat like a miniature contact lens (hence the name) with a convex front curve and a concave back curve. The latter is placed against the eye, using the forefinger and a technique similar to contact lens insertion. Unlike a contact lens, however, the diameter of the minidisc is between 4 and 5 mm. This allows the device to be easily placed behind the lower or upper eyelid without compromising comfort, vision, or oxygen permeability. The manual dexterity required is also less than for contact lens insertion. This is because contact lenses have to be carefully positioned on the cornea, whereas the Minidisc can be placed anywhere against the conjunctiva behind the lid. Figure 14 is a photograph of a Minidisc containing gentamicin sulfate on a human eye. The lower lid has been pulled down slightly in order to reveal the Minidisc, which is normally hidden behind the lid.

Extensive human clinicals were conducted using devices unloaded with drug to iterate to the optimum curves of the front and back surfaces of the Minidisc (70). Thus, not only was comfort maximized but dislodgment from the eye was minimized as well. This latter was accomplished without strong adherence of the Minidisc to a particular localized area of the conjunctiva that would have been undesirable (16).

Additionally, handling and insertion studies were conducted comparing the Lacrisert and the Minidisc (71) formed of the same material; i.e., hydroxypropyl cellulose. The 24 subjects used were not wearers of contact lenses, so as to eliminate any bias due to the similarity in shape between the Minidisc and a contact lens. Furthermore, the patients were

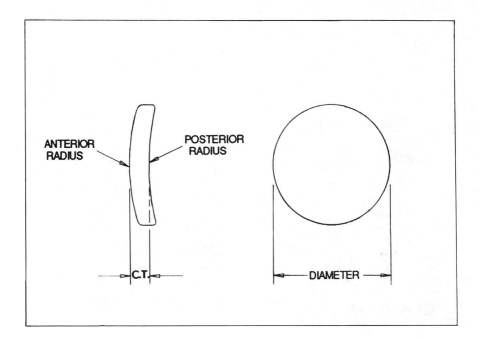

Figure 13. Schematic representation of the Minidisc device geometry. The anterior and posterior curves are shown. C.T. = center thickness.

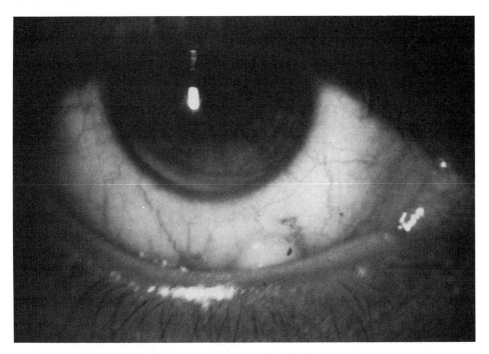

Figure 14. Photograph of a hydrophobic Minidisc on a human eye. The device contained 10% w/w gentamicin sulfate. The lower lid has been pulled down to reveal the upper portion of the device, which is normally concealed behind the lid.

of varying ages. The mean time required for patients to insert the Lacrisert was 39.5 s versus 16.6 s for the Minidisc of the same weight. The patients were allowed only three attempts to insert either device. Six of the 24 patients were unable to insert the Lacrisert, whereas all 24 patients were able to insert the Minidisc of the same weight.

Based on these studies, it was inferred that a good working design for the ocular insert had been achieved with which to conduct further investigations. It is of interest to note that the symmetric circular design of the Minidisc, in contrast with an elliptical or rod shape, eliminates the need to align a particular geometric axis of the device with the eyelid margin. This probably aids its easy insertion.

Concurrent to the above investigations, the idea was conceived that if during the fabrication process itself, a hydrophobic drug is incorporated into a hydrophilic matrix or a hydrophilic drug is incorporated into a hydrophobic matrix, one may effect controlled release of the drugs. On superficial reflection on the mechanism of action of these two "mirror-image" systems, one might conclude that one renders the other obvious.

In reality, however, the fundamental principles governing these two systems are quite different. In the case of the hydrophilic matrix, the dissolution rate of the hydrophobic drug in the aqueous environment of the matrix is expected to be the rate-controlling step in the drug-release process. In addition, the hydrophilic matrix probably competes with the drug for the available water, thus further slowing the drug-release kinetics. On the other hand, the dissolution rate of the hydrophilic drug incorporated into a hydrophobic matrix is probably not rate controlling, especially for highly water-soluble drugs. Instead, diffusion of the drug through the microporous network of the polymer or through macropores produced during the fabrication process is probably the rate-controlling step for drug release.

To test this general concept, a drug with very low solubility in water—sulfisoxazole—was incorporated into a hydrophilic matrix and a drug with a very high aqueous solubility—gentamicin sulfate—was incorporated into a hydrophobic matrix. These two extreme cases, representing nonerodible Minidiscs, will be discussed in the section that follows.

A. Nonerodible Minidisc

1. Hydrophilic Minidisc

In this embodiment, sulfisoxazole, a poorly water-soluble sulfur drug used in the treatment of bacterial infections such as trachoma, was incorporated into Soflens monomer mix. The Soflens monomer mix contains mainly Hema (hydroxymethyl methacrylate) with EGDMA (ethylene glycol dimethacrylate) used as a cross-linking agent. This mix is used to manufacture soft contact lenses with an equilibrium water content of 38.6%.

The drug was jetmilled and suspended as a solid dispersion in the liquid monomer mix at a loading concentration of 40% w/w. The suspension was then polymerized by inducing free radical polymerization initiated by ultraviolet light at room temperature (69). The front curve of the device was obtained by contact with a spinning mold, whereas the back curve was generated by a lathing operation.

On exposure to an aqueous solution, these devices demonstrated extended release for about 168 h, as shown in Figure 15, where the points represent the experimental data. If the system is modeled, as was done before for contact lenses, using the general Fickian diffusion equation (equation 3) (for the entire time course), we obtain the solid curve drawn in Figure 15, with a value of D, the diffusion coefficient, in the order of $5 \times E\text{-}9 \ cm^2/s$. Clearly, the deviation from experiment is significant, particularly for the latter time points.

This anomalous behavior is not particularly surprising in view of the fact that both diffusion and mechanical relaxation of the initially glassy matrix probably affect the drug-release kinetics but neither completely predominates (72). Also confounding the issue is the nature of water (free, bound, and interfacial) discussed in the literature (73,74).

In addition, many other parameters play a role in the transport properties of hydrogels. Among these are cross-linker type and content (75) and hydrophilicity of the comonomers used (76).

The mathematical modeling of the kinetics of diffusion of poorly water-soluble drugs from initially glassy matrices has been investigated by several researchers (77–81). However, in most cases, the matrices were loaded after prefabrication without drug. Additionally, loadings as high as 40% are seldom used. Most often drug loadings are confined to a few percent by weight of the matrix. Clearly, this area needs to be more thoroughly investigated.

Returning to the system under discussion, the cytotoxicity of the 40% sulfisoxazole system was thoroughly examined both by tissue culture techniques (82) and by insertion in the eyes of albino rabbits. The hydrophilic Minidisc was found to be biocompatible.

Next, the Minidisc was inserted into the eyes of three normal human volunteers and removed after varying amounts of time. For each time point, the residual drug left in the

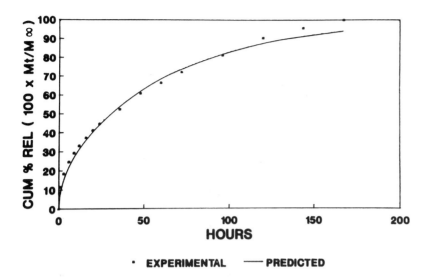

• EXPERIMENTAL —— PREDICTED

Figure 15. In vitro kinetics data of the polyhema (hydrophilic) Minidisc containing 40% w/w sulfisoxazole, plotted as cumulative percent release vs time. Each point represents an average of three groups with three devices per group. Standard deviations (not shown) are less than 5% of the mean values. The solid curve represents a Fickian unsteady-state model using equation 3 as explained in the text.

devices was eluted out in an aqueous solution and its quantity determined. Next, by mass balance, the amount of drug released into the tear film was calculated for each time point.

The results are shown in Figure 16. It is interesting to note from this illustration that 100% of the drug was released in about 72 h even though the in vitro kinetics indicated that the drug release lasted for 168 h. It may be possible that tear components increase the solubility of sulfisoxazole in the tear fluid, thus accelerating its release rate. Another, even more interesting feature of Figure 16 is the fact that the drug release appears to follow zero-order kinetics, yielding a straight line when plotted against time even though the in vitro kinetic data was highly nonlinear.

Finally, the eyes of albino rabbits were severely infected with *Staphylococcus aureus*. In this study, the commercially available solution form of the drug (Gantrisin = 4% sulfisoxazole) administered three times daily was compared to a single administration of the Minidisc. Negative controls (no treatment) were used as well. Daily Draize scores were used to compare the rate of healing for the three groups (69). Although the induced condition tended to resolve spontaneously, from Figure 17 it is evident that in the group receiving a single administration of the Minidisc the infection resolved the fastest.

As the range of applicability of the hydrophilic Minidisc is limited to drugs of low water solubility, such as steroids like fluorometholone and dexamethasone, this system is not suitable for most ophthalmic drugs, which are typically highly water soluble. For these drugs, therefore, a hydrophobic polymer capable of releasing hydrophilic drugs for extended time periods is required. This leads us to a discussion of the nonerodible, hydrophobic Minidisc in the next section.

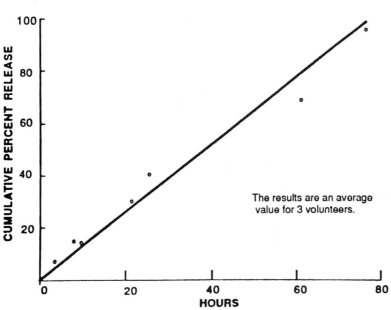

Figure 16. In vivo kinetics data of the polyhema (hydrophilic) Minidisc containing 40% w/w sulfisoxazole, plotted as cumulative percent release vs time. Each point represents an average of three data points, collected by mass balance. The devices were worn by normal human volunteers.

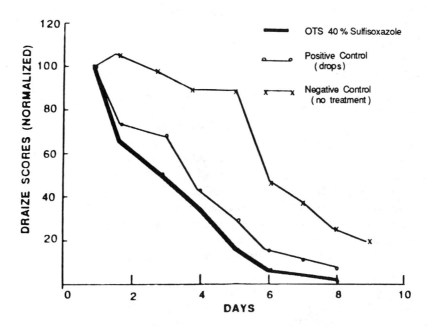

Figure 17. Normalized Draize scores plotted as a function of time for three sets of infected rabbits. A single administration of the polyhema (hydrophilic) Minidisc containing 40% w/w sulfisoxazole is compared with a standard drop regimen and negative controls.

2. Hydrophobic Minidisc

To investigate the fundamental aspects of hydrophilic drug release from a hydrophobic polymer matrix, the drug gentamicin sulfate (Fig. 18) was selected. This was because of its high solubility in water and its practical importance as a broad-spectrum antibiotic. This aminoglycoside has been widely used to combat bacterial infections in humans. It is expected that extended release of this drug in the predominantly aqueous environment of the tear film represents a formidable challenge. Since, as discussed earlier, a large number of drugs used in ocular therapy are water soluble, the choice of gentamicin sulfate is especially appropriate. Furthermore, this drug has potential side effects if delivered at high dosage levels, including ototoxicity and renal damage (83), thereby providing additional practical justification for its controlled release.

Unfortunately, hydrophobic matrices that are biocompatible to ocular tissues are relatively uncommon. In almost all reports, the polymer chosen, usually silicone or ethylene vinyl–acetate, appears to reflect its commercial availability rather than its biocompatibility (84). Additionally, the matrix fabrication process itself could potentially damage the drug. For instance, to incorporate the drug into a silicone matrix, the drug is mixed with elastomer and then typically polymerization is initiated by applying heat. This process

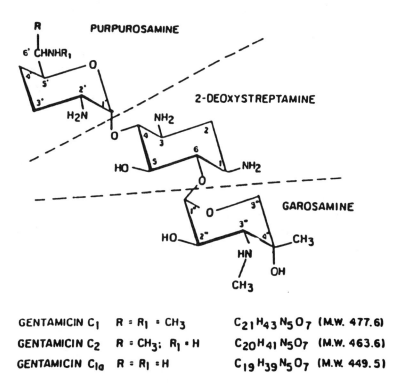

GENTAMICIN C_1	R = R_1 = CH_3	$C_{21}H_{43}N_5O_7$ (M.W. 477.6)
GENTAMICIN C_2	R = CH_3; R_1 = H	$C_{20}H_{41}N_5O_7$ (M.W. 463.6)
GENTAMICIN C_{1a}	R = R_1 = H	$C_{19}H_{39}N_5O_7$ (M.W. 449.5)

Figure 18. The structure of the gentamicin complex. This aminoglycoside is a mixture of basic water-soluble antibiotics, each consisting of three amino sugars—purpurosamine, 2-deoxystreptamine, and garosamine. In addition, depending on the nature of R_1 and R_2, the individual molecule in the mixture is classified as C_1, C_2, C_{1a}, C_{2a}. A separate structure for C_{2a} is not shown because this is a stereoisomer of C_2.

takes a long time (about 30 min) during which a heat-labile drug will be degraded. Thus, there is a strong motivation to use polymers that polymerize at room temperature.

Of all the silicones that are commercially available, many are not capable of being copolymerized with other hydrophobic or hydrophilic monomers like the acrylates and methacrylates. Such copolymerization is essential to provide the proper level of wettability for retention in the eye with a minimum of irritation. Furthermore, employing ethylene vinyl-acetate copolymers in the fabrication of controlled-release systems often necessitates the use of volatile and potentially toxic solvents such as methylene chloride (12). This makes removal of the residual solvents an imperative. In summary, the use of commonly available commercial polymers does not provide sufficient flexibility to "tailormake" polymer properties to allow for specific tissue or drug compatibility.

On the other hand, a suitable, predominantly hydrophobic polymer matrix may be designed based on a proprietary Bausch & Lomb (Contact Lens Division, Rochester, New York) prepolymer M_2D_x (85) containing flexible dimethylsiloxane groups along the chain. The structure of this prepolymer is shown in Figure 19. The silicone component of the prepolymer allows a high oxygen diffusivity, which (as discussed earlier) is a key concern when dealing with ocular tissues. Also, the methacrylate end groups allow this prepolymer to be copolymerized with various amounts of hydrophilic and hydrophobic monomers. Further, the availability of this prepolymer in varying numbers of "D" units allows the mechanical properties of the polymer to be varied so as to yield a polymer that can range from being hard to soft.

After extensive research, a formulation using M_2D_{100} as the major component was designed. Besides the prepolymer, the monomer blend contains trimethylsiloxy methacryloyl propyl silane (a modulus booster) and methacrylic acid (a wetting agent). This monomer mix is capable of being ultraviolet (UV) cured by free radical polymerization at room temperature, thus obviating the exposure of the drug to heat and possible thermal degradation. The resulting polymer is soft and tough and, therefore, quite suitable for ophthalmic use.

The drug was jetmilled and suspended as a solid dispersion in the liquid monomer mix at the desired loading concentration. The suspension was then polymerized by inducing free radical polymerization initiated by UV at room temperature (69). Both the front and back curves of the device were obtained by contact with molds.

As discussed before, ocular inserts must be sterilized before they can be used. To determine if the polymer can withstand the sterilization process without serious mechanical

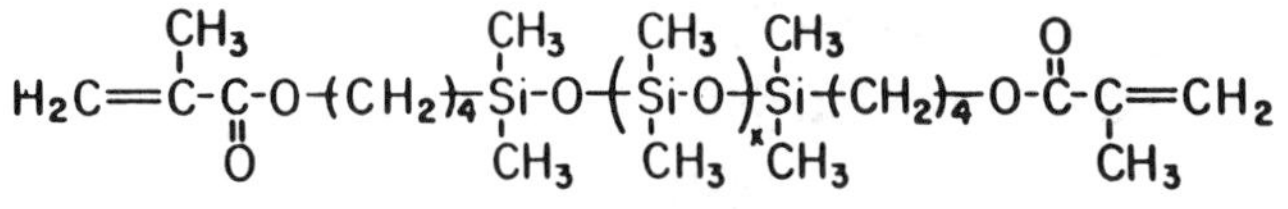

Figure 19. Chemical structure of α,ω-bis(4-methacryloxybutyl)poly(dimethylsiloxane) abbreviated as M_2D_x. D represents dimethylsiloxane and x represents the number of repeating D units in the prepolymer.

degradation, a series of experiments were conducted. First, Fourier transformed infrared (FTIR) analysis of the polymer films was performed using the multiple internal reflectance (MIR) technique before and after exposure to 2.5 Mrad of gamma-irradiation. The spectra for both sets of films were essentially the same as shown in Figure 20. Also, the mechanical properties of the nonirradiated and irradiated films were analyzed using an Instron at initial time and after being kept at 40°C for 3 months. Irradiation and heat treatment had no statistically significant effect on the mechanical properties of the polymer films.

In addition, the mechanical properties of films containing 10% w/w of gentamicin sulfate were evaluated before and after gamma-irradiation and exposure to heat at 40°C for 3 months (21). It was determined that the modulus, tensile strength, and percent elongation of the polymer-drug films are essentially unaffected by gamma-sterilization and heat exposure.

As the polymer could be required to be placed in the aqueous environment of the eye for extended periods of time, it is important to establish whether it can withstand hydrolytic degradation. This was done using a gravimetric technique (21). Several unloaded polymer films were prepared. Half of these were sterilized using gamma-irradiation at 2.5 Mrad. Next, 40 discs, each weighing 40 mg, were cut from each set (irradiated and nonirradiated). These were then placed in individual glass vials containing 7 ml of phosphate buffered saline (PBS) (pH 7.3 ± 0.1) and stored at 80°C for up to 14 days.

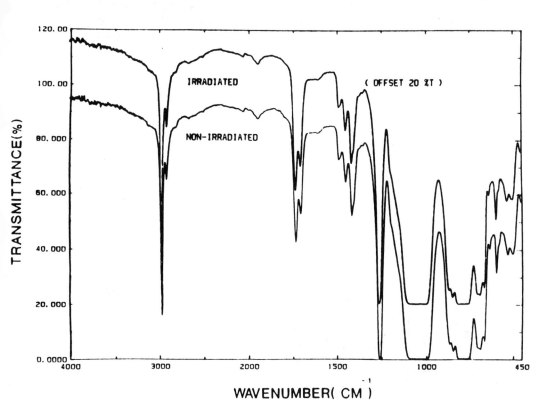

Figure 20. FTIR spectra, using the MIR technique, of M_2D_{100} based polymer investigating the effect of gamma-irradiation. No difference was observed between the two sets.

At selected time intervals (3, 5, 7, and 14 days), 10 discs were removed from each set, dried under vacuum at 80°C, and reweighed. The percent weight loss of each disc could thus be calculated. Figure 21 displays the results of these investigations. The polymer matrix was found to be quite stable in an aqueous environment.

Furthermore, no significant differences were observed between the weight-loss data for irradiated films compared to unirradiated films for up to 7 days. For the 14-day time point, the irradiated films exhibited a slightly higher weight loss. However, in both cases, the loss was <3.5% of the total weight.

Next, the cytotoxicity of the polymer before and after gamma-sterilization was evaluated using the tissue-agar overlay technique mentioned earlier (82). Both sets of films were found to be noncytotoxic. Additionally, drug-loaded devices containing up to 20% w/w loading were inserted in fully awake albino rabbit eyes for up to 5 days. Extensive histology testing indicated no toxicopathological effects.

Thus, it was established that a suitable polymeric system capable of withstanding the sterilization process had been designed. Also, the system was biocompatible and maintained its mechanical integrity. However, it is important for any pharmaceutical dosage form to determine the stability of the active ingredient.

High Pressure Liquid Chromatography (HPLC) investigations (21) confirmed that the polymerization process did not adversely affect the drug. However, exposure to heat for extended periods of time does result in a small amount of degradation. Figure 22 is a HPLC plot for a solution of the drug powder that serves as baseline information for Figure 23. Figure 23 is a HPLC plot for a sample of drug solution extracted from devices exposed to 40°C for 3 months. Comparisons of Figures 22 and 23 demonstrates a slight difference. Just

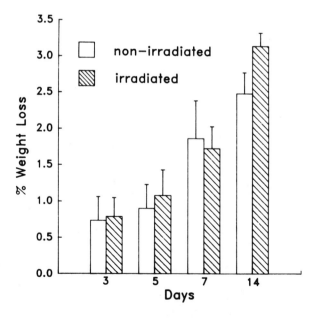

Figure 21. Comparison of weight loss data for irradiated and unirradiated polymer films as a function of time. The data represent the mean of 10 samples.

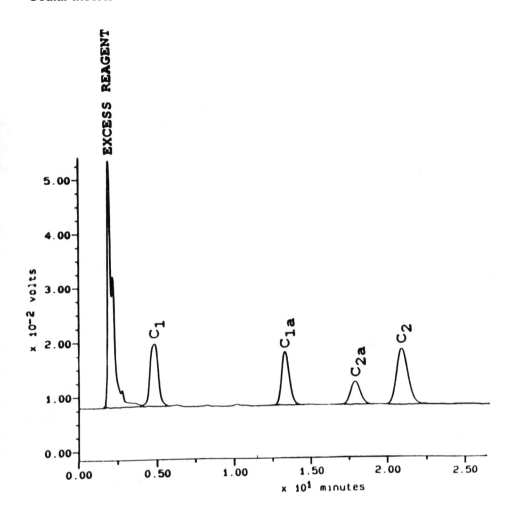

Figure 22. A representative HPLC chromatogram of a solution of gentamicin sulfate powder before incorporation into the polymer matrix. The four peaks marked C_1, C_{1a}, C_2, and C_{2a} are the naturally occurring components of the gentamicin complex.

to the left of the C_1 component, a small peak is observed in Figure 23 that is absent in Figure 22. Recent investigations have confirmed that this small peak is that of 2-deoxystreptamine, a degradation product of the drug. The amount of this product is very small, however, and is well within the 5% limit allowed by the U.S. Food and Drug Administration (FDA).

The kinetic data for release of the gentamicin sulfate from the Minidiscs is plotted in Figures 24, 25 and 26 as cumulative percent release versus time in hours. In all cases, drug release was monitored up to 408 h. It is apparent that the release rates are very reproducible as evidenced by the small standard deviations.

Figure 24 compares the release characteristics of devices before and immediately after gamma-irradiation. The shape of the two curves is somewhat different. Although 100% of the incorporated drug was released from the nonirradiated devices, only 94% of the drug

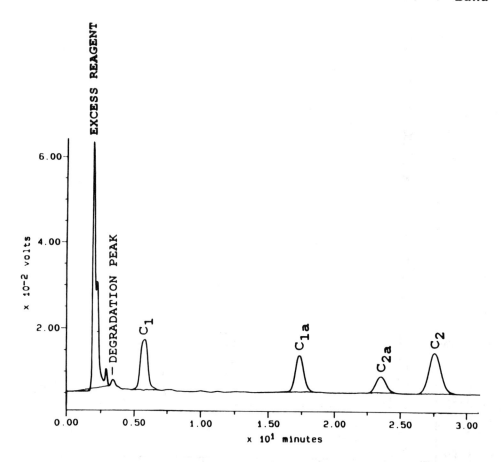

Figure 23. A representative HPLC plot of a sample extracted from polymer-drug devices after exposure to 40°C for 3 months. Notice the small degradation peak to the left of the C_1 component.

incorporated into the irradiated devices was able to leach out. Although the curves are comparable for most time intervals, their crossover behavior is interesting.

Figure 25 compares the release characteristics of irradiated devices stored for 3 months at 40°C with a comparable set that was analyzed immediately after irradiation. The devices exposed to the high temperature consistently demonstrated slower release kinetics.

Figure 26 compares the release characteristics of irradiated devices stored at either 23 or 40°C for a period of 3 months. Again a noticeable trend emerged. Exposure to heat for extended time periods caused a slowing down of the release rate and additional entrapment of the drug.

It is of interest, therefore, that although no statistically significant differences were observed in the macroscopic mechanical properties of polymer-drug films before and after gamma-irradiation or heat exposure, Figures 24–26 indicate that changes at the microscopic level do occur that influence the drug-release characteristics of the devices. This effect has to be recognized and accounted for by adding suitable overages or modifying the

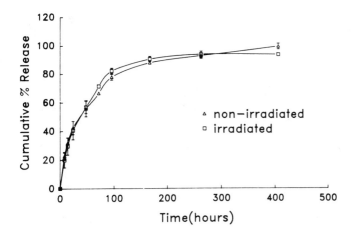

Figure 24. In vitro release kinetics of hydrophobic Minidiscs containing 10% w/w gentamicin sulfate before and after gamma-irradiation. Each datum point is the average of three groups, with 10 devices per group. Where the standard deviations are not shown, they lie within the area covered by the symbols. (From Ref. 21.)

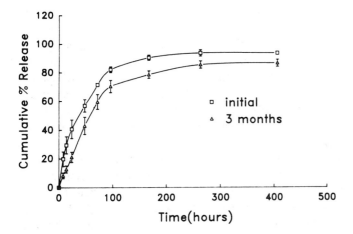

Figure 25. In vitro release kinetics of hydrophobic Minidiscs containing 10% w/w gentamicin sulfate after gamma-irradiation. Devices exposed to 40°C for 3 months are compared to devices immediately after irradiation. Each datum point is the average of three groups, with 10 devices per group. Where the standard deviations are not shown, they lie within the area covered by the symbols. (From Ref. 21.)

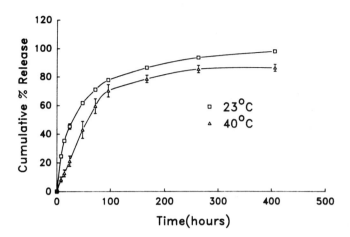

Figure 26. In vitro release kinetics of hydrophobic Minidiscs containing 10% w/w gentamicin sulfate after gamma-irradiation. Devices exposed to 40°C for 3 months are compared to devices stored at 23°C (room temperature) for 3 months also after irradiation. Each datum point is the average of three groups, with 10 devices per group. Where the standard deviations are not shown, they lie within the area covered by the symbols. (From Ref. 21.)

release kinetics of a polymer matrix when designing a device for a specific desired release rate.

At present, the exact nature of the changes causing this interesting behavior is unknown. However, it can be postulated that gamma-irradiation could be inducing additional cross-linking in the polymeric matrices (86). This in turn could account for the observed reduction in the diffusion of the drug from the matrix. The gamma-irradiation induced effect could be complemented by the application of heat, as indicated by Figures 25 and 26.

If, the system is modeled, as was done before for contact lenses, using the general Fickian diffusion equation (equation 3) (for the entire time course), we obtain the solid curve drawn in Figure 27, where the points represent the experimental data for hydrophobic Minidiscs containing 10% w/w gentamicin sulfate, assuming an average "slab" thickness of 0.6 mm. A diffusion coefficient of 1.28 E-9 cm^2/s can be obtained by "eye-balling" the fit, which appears quite good. This diffusion coefficient is more consistent with a diffusion coefficient through solid materials rather than liquids.

Unfortunately, this sourceless Fickian analysis is rather naive and does not adequately serve to explain more extensive and recent data collected on these polymeric systems (87).

Let us return for the moment, however, to the system under discussion. Minidiscs containing 10 and 30% w/w loading of gentamicin sulfate were inserted into the eyes of fully awake healthy albino rabbits. The tear fluid from these rabbits was analyzed at different periods of time up to 14 days employing a sensitive bioassay technique using agar plates seeded with *Staphylococcus epidermidis*. Commercially available 0.3% gentamicin sulfate drops were used three times a day as a control.

The results of the study with drops indicated an initially (5 min) high concentration of the drug in the tear fluid (1875 ± 875 ppm), with a quickly declining concentration

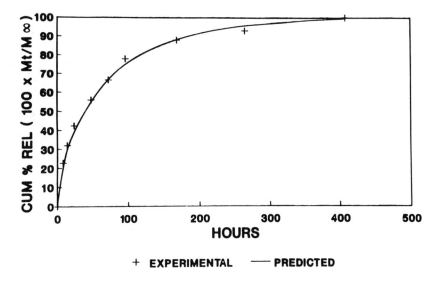

Figure 27. In vitro kinetics of the silicone (hydrophobic) Minidiscs containing 10% w/w gentamicin sulfate, plotted as cumulative percent release vs time. Each point represents an average of three groups with 10 devices per group. Standard deviations (not shown) are less than 15% of the mean values. The solid curve represents a sourceless Fickian unsteady-state model using equation 3, as explained in the text.

measured over 2.5 h (17 ± 9 ppm). In contrast, the 10% Minidisc attained a peak concentration of 219 ± 94 ppm at 4 h and maintained measurable tear concentrations above 2.5 ppm up to 341 h after a single-unit dose. The minimum inhibitory concentration of the drug for this assay is below 0.25 ppm.

Figure 28 is a scatter plot of the drug tear levels for the 30% loaded Minidisc in rabbit eyes.

Lastly, as was done in the case of the hydrophilic Minidisc, a study comparing the performance of the 10% loaded Minidisc with a negative control (no treatment) was conducted in infected rabbit eyes. As before, a single administration of the Minidisc resolved the bacterial infection much faster.

At present, preliminary human clinical data have been generated comparing the performance of the Minidisc with a standard drop regimen in the treatment of ocular bacterial infections. Initial results are encouraging.

Finally, let us evaluate the Minidisc against the criteria that were set forth in Section III. It is apparent that the Minidisc appears to have successfully met most of the criteria that are required for a successful ocular insert. These include comfort, lack of expulsion, ease of handling and insertion, noninterference with vision and oxygen permeability, reproducibility of release kinetics, sterility, and stability. Of course, it is quite conceivable that when more extensive clinical data are obtained, the physical and chemical design of the Minidisc may have to be refined in order to optimize and eliminate presently unknown problems.

Although not discussed earlier, the Minidisc is manufactured as a single unit in contrast with being cut out of a sheet. Accordingly, this manufacturing process lends itself

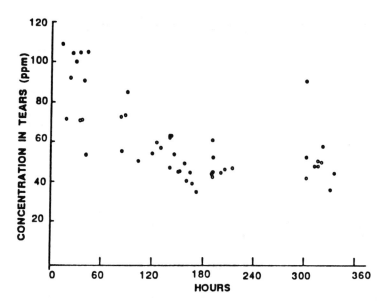

Figure 28. In vivo tear concentration profile of the silicone (hydrophobic) Minidisc containing 30% w/w gentamicin sulfate. Healthy, fully awake albino rabbits were used.

rather easily to automated polymerization, finishing, packaging, and sterilization operations. Waste is therefore minimized and the bioburden is kept quite low.

Figure 29 illustrates the effect of loading on the release kinetics of gentamicin sulfate from the Minidisc. It is evident that a fair amount of flexibility is possible with this parameter. Additionally, as discussed before, the prepolymeric system of which the Minidisc is comprised can be copolymerized with various hydrophobic and hydrophilic monomers quite easily. This enables the achievement of a high measure of flexibility in terms of release rates of gentamicin sulfate, in particular, and potentially other drugs as well.

Figures 30 and 31 illustrate the degree of flexibility possible with the M_2D_x chemistry. The release kinetics for both these figures is for flat circular discs of thickness significantly lower than the Minidisc. Figure 30 illustrates a family of x = 10 and Figure 31 a family of x = 180. In both illustrations, varying amounts of methacrylic acid have been added to a stock polymer mix that contains 10% w/w gentamicin sulfate. Altering the concentration of methacrylic acid from 0 to 16.8 wt% in M_2D_{10} for example, changes the time for 80% drug release from 8 to 72 h.

The data in Figures 30 and 31 has been plotted as ln of the fraction of drug remaining in the matrix versus time in hours rather than following the more conventional practice of plotting cumulative percent release versus time. This has specifically been done to elucidate the details of the kinetic mechanism. For instance, if the data are fit by a straight line on such a plot, they would indicate simple, unsteady-state Fickian diffusion. Rather, from Figures 30 and 31, a more complex mechanism of release is clearly indicated.

In the last section of this chapter, we now turn to the erodible Minidisc.

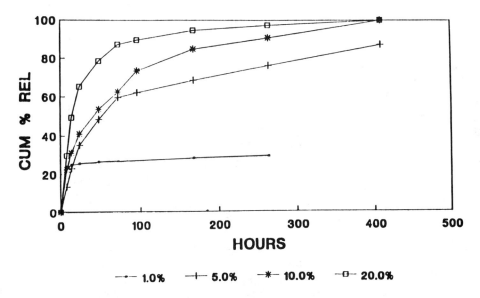

Figure 29. In vitro kinetic data for silicone (hydrophobic) Minidiscs containing gentamicin sulfate, demonstrating the effect of loading on the release rate.

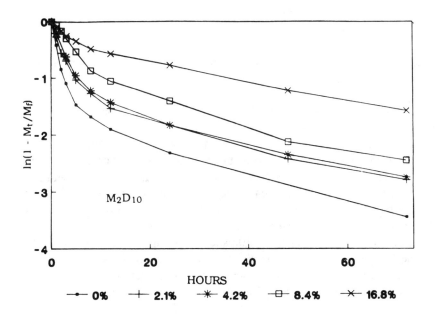

Figure 30. In vitro kinetic data for silicone (hydrophobic) flat discs demonstrating the effect of methacrylic acid content on the release kinetics of gentamicin sulfate from the M_2D_{10}-based system. Each point is the mean of three individual samples. The data are plotted as ln of the fraction retained vs time to demonstrate deviations from unsteady-state Fickian behavior.

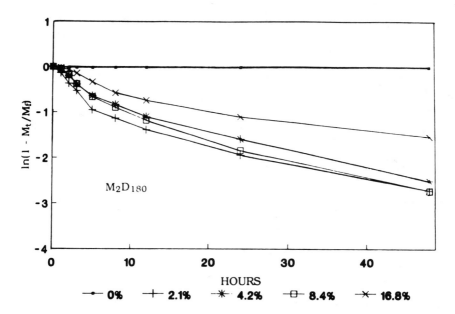

Figure 31. In vitro kinetic data for silicone (hydrophobic) flat discs demonstrating the effect of methacrylic acid content on the release kinetics of gentamicin sulfate from the M_2D_{180}-based system. Each point is the mean of three individual samples. The data are plotted as ln of the fraction retained vs time to demonstrate deviations from unsteady-state Fickian behavior.

B. The Erodible Minidisc

As mentioned earlier, once criteria 1–4 discussed in Section III are met by a device, the same geometry can conceptually be applied to other polymeric systems.

Accordingly, the Minidisc design can conceivably be used for erodible systems as well. The limitations obviously will be that of erodible systems versus nonerodible systems, as discussed in Section IV.

However, it was considered an interesting exercise to apply the Minidisc geometry to an existing marketed ocular system in order to overcome some of its design-related shortcomings. There are inferences in the literature (49) that the Lacrisert may benefit from design improvements. Therefore, erodible Minidiscs made of hydroxypropyl cellulose of the same weight (5 mg) as the Lacrisert were fabricated by a thermoforming process. In addition, 10-mg Minidiscs were formed as well.

A clinical evaluation was conducted in 10 patients wearing the standard Lacrisert in one eye and the 5-mg erodible Minidisc in the other eye. A similar study followed, using the same 10 patients, but comparing the standard Lacrisert versus the 10-mg Minidisc. Interestingly, the patients rated both sizes of the Minidisc equivalent in comfort to the 5-mg Lacrisert.

Not surprisingly, all devices demonstrated similar results with regard to matting of the eyelids and disturbance of vision.

Significantly, however, the patients found that both sizes of the Minidisc were easier to insert than the Lacrisert, with a slight preference toward the 10-mg Minidisc.

Although these results are somewhat limited, they do indicate that the Minidisc design can lend itself to the use of erodible polymeric matrices with some advantage. The drug-release characteristics of the erodible polymer, however, will necessarily dictate the performance of the Minidisc as an erodible controlled-release insert.

In summary, the Minidisc is an effective and versatile prolonged-release ocular drug delivery system with the advantage of less total drug being required. The Minidisc resolves patient compliance issues of comfort and dosing frequency with unique design features that are based on eye anatomical, physiological, and pharmacokinetic aspects of ocular drug disposition. Lastly, the Minidisc offers the flexibility of variable delivery rates, depending on the specific drug-polymer combination.

REFERENCES

1. Lee, V. H. and Robinson, J. R. (1986). Review: topical ocular drug delivery: Recent developments and future challenges, *J. Ocul. Pharmacol.*, 2(1):67.
2. Lee, V. H., and Robinson, J. R. (1979). Mechanistic and quantitative evaluation of precorneal pilocarpine disposition in albino rabbits, *J. Pharm. Sci.*, 68(6):673.
3. Shell, J. W. Ophthalmic drug delivery systems, *Surv. Ophthalmol.*, 29(2):117.
4. Trawick, A. B. (1985). Potential systemic and ocular side effects associated with topical administration of timolol maleate, *J. Am. Optom. Assoc.*, 56(2):108.
5. Harmia, T., Speiser, P., and Kreuter, J. (1987). Nanoparticles as drug carriers in ophthalmology, *Pharm. Acta Helv.*, 62:12.
6. Zeimer, R. C., Khoobehi, B., Neisman, M. R. and Magin, R. L. (1988). A potential method for local drug and dye delivery in the ocular vasculature, *Invest. Ophthalmol. Vis. Sci.*, 29(7):1179.
7. Ticho, U., Blumenthal, M., Zonis, S., Gal, A., Blank, I., and Mazor, Z. W. (1979). A clinical trial with Piloplex—a new long-acting pilocarpine compound: Preliminary report, *Ann. Ophthalmol.*, 11:555.
8. Ticho, U., Blumenthal, M., Zonis, S., Gal, A., Blank, I., and Mazor, Z. W. (1979). Piloplex, a new long-acting pilocarpine polymer salt. A: Long-term study, *Br. J. Ophthalmol.*, 63:45.
9. Mazor, Z., Ticho, U., Rehany, U., and Rose, L. (1979). Piloplex, a new long-acting pilocarpine polymer salt. B: Comparative study of the visual effects of pilocarpine and Piloplex eye drops, *Br. J. Ophthalmol.*, 63:48.
10. Langer, R., and Peppas, N. (1983). Chemical and physical structure of polymers as carriers for controlled release of bioactive agents: A review, *J. Macromol. Sci.*, 23:61.
11. Desai, S. J., Simonelli, A. P., and Higuchi, W. I. (1965). Investigation of factors influencing release of solid drug dispersed in inert matrices, *J. Pharm. Sci.*, 54:1459.
12. Langer, R., Hsieh, D. S. T., Peil, A., Bawa, R., and Rhine, W. (1981). Polymers for the controlled release of macromolecules: Kinetics, applications and external control, *Controlled Release Systems* (S. K. Chandrasekaran, ed.), *AIChe Symposium Series* 77(206):10.
13. Chrai, S. S., Patton, T. F., Mehta, A., and Robinson, J. R. (1973). Lacrimal and instilled fluid dynamics in rabbit eyes, *J. Pharm. Sci.*, 62(7):1112.
14. Lerman, S. (1970). Simulated sustained release pilocarpine therapy, *Ann. Ophthalmol.*, 2(8):435.
15. Mandell, R. B. (1971). Symptomatology and post-fitting care. *In: Contact Lens Practice: Basic and Advanced* (R. B. Mandell, ed.). Charles C Thomas, Springfield, Illinois, p. 222.
16. Smelser, G. K. (1952). Relation of factors involved in maintenance of optical properties of cornea to contact lens wear, *Arch. Ophthalmol.*, 47(3):328.
17. Chrai, S. S., Makoid, M. C., Eriksen, S. P., and Robinson, J. R. (1974). Drop size and initial dosing frequency problems of topically applied ophthalmic drugs, *J. Pharm. Sci.*, 63:333.
18. Sieg, J. W., and Robinson, J. R. (1974). Corneal absorption of fluorometholone in rabbits, *Arch. Ophthalmol.*, 92:240.

19. Hunt, T. K. (1984). Can repair processes be stimulated by modulators (cell growth factors, aniogenic factors, etc.) without adversely affecting normal processes?, *J. Trauma* 24(Suppl.):9.
20. *The United States Pharmacopeia*, 22nd Revision (1990). The United States Pharmacopeial Convention Inc., Rockville, Maryland, p. 1707.
21. Bawa, R., and Nandu, M. (1990). Physico-chemical considerations in the development of an ocular polymeric drug delivery system, *Biomaterials*, 11(9):724.
22. Maddox, Y. T., and Bernstein, H. W. (1972). An evaluation of the bionite hydrophilic contact lens for use in a drug delivery system, *Ann. Ophthalmol.*, 4(9):789.
23. Podos, S. M., Becker, B., Assef, C. F., and Hartstein, J. (1972). Pilocarpine therapy with soft contact lenses, *Precision Cosmet Digest*, 12:7.
24. Hillman, J. S. (1975). Management of acute glaucoma with pilocarpine-soaked hydrophilic lens, *Br. J. Ophthalmol.*, 58(7):674.
25. Mizutani, Y., and Miwa, Y. (1975). On the uptake and release of drugs by soft contact lenses, *Contact Intraocul. Lens Med. J.*, 1(1):177.
26. Ramer, R., and Gasset, A. R. (1974). Ocular penetration of pilocarpine: The effect of hydrophilic soft contact lenses on the ocular penetration of pilocarpine, *Ann. Ophthalmol.*, 6(12):1325.
27. Matoba, A. Y., and McCulley, J. P. (1985). The effect of therapeutic soft contact lenses on antibiotic delivery to the cornea, *Ophthalmology*, 92:1.
28. Friedman, Allen R. C., and Raph, S. M. (1985). Topical acetazolamide and methazolamide delivered by contact lenses, *Arch. Ophthalmol.*, 103(6):963.
29. Reccia, R., del Prete, A., Benusiglio, E., and Orfeo, V. (1985). Continuous usage of low doses of human leukocyte interferon with contact lenses in herpetic keratoconjunctivitis, *Ophthalmol. Res.*, 17(4):251.
30. Massimo, B., and Spitznas, M. (1988). Sustained gentamicin release by presoaked medicated bandage contact lenses, *Ophthalmology*, 95(6):796.
31. Jain, M. R. (1988). Drug delivery through soft contact lenses, *Br. J. Ophthalmol.*, 72:150.
32. Shell, J. W., and Baker, R. (1974). Diffusional systems for controlled release of drugs to the eye, *Ann. Ophthalmol.*, 6(10):1037.
33. Crank, J. (1975). *The Mathematics of Diffusion*, 2nd ed. Clarendon Press, Oxford, England, p. 48.
34. Bawa, R., Siegel, R. A., Marasca, B., Karel, M., and Langer, R. (1985). An explanation for the controlled release of macromolecules from polymers, *J. Controlled Rel.*, 1:259.
35. Bawa, R. (1987). Sustained-release formulation containing an amino acid polymer, United States Patent #4,668,506.
36. Bawa, R., and Deichert, W. G. (1987). Sustained-release formulation containing an amino acid polymer with a lower alkyl (C_1-C_4) polar solvent, United States Patent #4,713,244.
37. Bawa, R., and Ruscio, D. (1990). Sustained release formulation containing an ion-exchange resin, United States Patent #4,931,279.
38. Urquhart, J. (1980). Development of the Ocusert pilocarpine ocular therapeutic systems—a case history in ophthalmic product development. In: *Ophthalmic Drug Delivery Systems* (J. R. Robinson, ed.). American Pharmaceutical Association, Washington, D.C., p. 105.
39. Friederich, R. L. (1974). The pilocarpine Ocusert: A new drug delivery system, *Ann. Ophthalmol.*, 6:12.
40. Haddad, H. M. (1974). Solid state ophthalmic medication delivery method, United States Patent #3,845,201.
41. Haddad, H. M., and Loucas, S. P. (1975). Solid state ophthalmic medication delivery method, United States Patent #3,870,791.
42. Maichuk, Y. F. (1975). Ophthalmic drug inserts, *Invest. Ophthalmol.*, 14:87.
43. Grass, G. M., Cobby, J., and Makoid, M. C. (1984). Ocular delivery of pilocarpine from erodible matrices, *J. Pharm. Sci.* 73(5):618.
44. Bondi, J. V., and Harwood, R. J. (1988). Biosoluble ocular insert, United States Patent #4,730,013.
45. Bloomfield, S. E., Miyata, T., Dunn, M. W., Bueser, N., Stenzel, K. H., and Rubin, A. L. (1978). Soluble gentamicin ophthalmic inserts as drug delivery system, *Arch. Ophthalmol.*, 96:885.

46. Slatter, D. H., Costa, N. D., and Edwards, M. E. (1982). Ocular inserts for application of drugs to bovine eyes—in vivo and in vitro studies on the release of gentamicin from collagen inserts, *Aust. Vet. J.*, 59:4.

47. Punch, P. I., Slatter, D. H., Costa, N. D., and Edwards, M. E. (1985). Ocular inserts for application of drugs to bovine eyes—in vitro studies on gentamicin release from collagen inserts, *Aust. Vet. J.*, 62(3):79.

48. Heller, J., and Baker, R. W. (1974). Bioerodible ocular device, United States Patent #3,811,444.

49. LaMotte, J., Grossman, E., and Hersch, J. (1985). The efficacy of cellulosic ophthalmic inserts for treatment of dry eye, *J. Am. Optom. Assoc.*, 56(4):298.

50. Scrip, #666, February 10, p. 15 (1982).

51. Katz, I. M., and Blackman, W. M. (1977). A soluble sustained-release ophthalmic delivery unit, *Am. J. Ophthalmol.*, 83(5):728.

52. Gautheron, P. D., Lotti, V. J., and Le Douarec, (1979). Tear film breakup time with unmedicated cellulose polymer inserts, *Arch. Ophthalmol.*, 97:1944.

53. Katz, J. I., Kaufman, H. E., Breslin, C., and Katz, I. M. (1978). Slow-release artificial tears and the treatment of keratitis sicca, *Ophthalmology*, 85:787.

54. Lamberts, D. W., Langston, D. P., and Chu, W. (1979). A clinical study of slow-releasing artificial tears, *Ophthalmology*, 85:794.

55. New drug delivery system—more efficient treatment (1985). *Optician*, October 18, p. 6.

56. SODI—Soluble polymeric drug delivery system for ophthalmic applications, company brochure, Diversified Tech Inc., Salt Lake City, Utah.

57. Marmer, R. H. (1988). Therapeutic and protective properties of the corneal collagen shield, *J. Cataract Refract. Surg.*, 14:496.

58. Aquavella, J. V., Ruffini, J. J., and LoCascio, J. A. (1988). Use of collagen shields as a Surgical adjunct, *J. Cataract Refract. Surg.*, 14:492.

59. O'Brien, T. P., Sawusch, M. R., Dick, J. D., Hamburg, T. R., and Gottsch, J. D. (1988). Use of collagen corneal shields versus soft contact lenses to enhance penetration of topical tobramycin, *J. Cataract Refract. Surg.*, 14:505.

60. Poland, D. E., and Kaufman, H. E. (1988). Clinical uses of collagen shields, *J. Cataract Refract. Surg.*, 14:489.

61. Unterman, S. R., Rootman, D. S., Hill, J. M., Parelman, J. J., Thompson, H. W., and Kaufman, H. E. (1988). Collagen shield drug delivery: Therapeutic concentrations of tobramycin in the rabbit cornea and aqueous humor, *J. Cataract Refract. Surg.*, 14:505.

62. Hobden, J. A., Reidy, J. J., O'Callaghan, R. J., and Hill, J. M. (1988). Treatment of experimental pseudomonas keratitis using collagen shields containing tobramycin, *Arch. Ophthalmol.*, 106:1605.

63. Phinney, R. B., Schwartz, S. D., Lee, D. A., and Mondino, B. J. (1988). Collagen-shield delivery of gentamicin and vancomycin, *Arch. Ophthalmol.*, 106:1599.

64. Sawusch, M. R., O'Brien, T. P., and Updegraff, B. S. (1989). Collagen corneal shields enhance penetration of topical prednisolone acetate, *J. Cataract Refract. Surg.*, 15:625.

65. Hwang, D. G., Stern, W. H., Hwang, P. H., and MacGowan-Smith, L. A. (1989). Collagen shield enhancement of topical dexamethasone penetration, *Arch. Ophthalmol.*, 107:1375.

66. Peiffer, R. L., Safrit, H. D., White, E., and Eifrig, D. E. (1983). Intraocular response to cotton, collagen and cellulose in the rabbit, *Ophthalmic Surg.*, 14(7):582.

67. Ellis, D. A. F., Braig, F., and Rbertson, C. (1984). Collagen implant: An early assessment, *J. Otolaryngol.*, 13(4):267.

68. Waltman, S. R., and Kaufman, H. E. (1970). Use of hydrophilic contact lenses to increase ocular penetration of topical drugs, *Invest. Ophthalmol. Vis. Sci.*, 9:250.

69. Bawa, R., Dais, M., Nandu, M., and Robinson, J. R. (1988). "New extended release ocular drug delivery system—design, Characterization & Performance Testing of Minidisc Inserts," Proceedings of the 15th International Symposium on Controlled Release of Bioactive Materials, Controlled Release Society, Inc., Lincolnshire, Illinois, pp. 106a–106b.

70. Bawa, R., Nandu, M., Downie, W., and Robinson, J. R. (1989). "Recent Studies on the Continuing Characterization of Minidisc Inserts for Ocular Therapy," Proceedings of the 16th International Symposium on Controlled Release of Bioactive Materials, Controlled Release Society, Inc., Lincolnshire, Illinois, pp. 213–214.

71. Bawa, R., and Osborne, G. Unpublished data.

72. Korsmeyer, R. W. (1991). Diffusion controlled systems: Hydrogels. *In: Polymers for Controlled Drug Delivery* (P. J. Tarcha, ed.). CRC Press, Boca Raton, Florida, p. 27.

73. Jhon, M. S., and Andrade, J. D. (1973). Water and hydrogels, *J. Biomed. Mater. Res.*, 7:509.

74. Wisniewski, S., and Kim, S. W. (1980). Permeation of water-soluble solutes through poly(2-hydroxyethyl methacrylate) and poly(2-hydroxyethyl methacrylate) crosslinked with ethylene glycol dimethacrylate, *J. Membr. Sci.*, 6:299.

75. Gyselinck, P., Schacht, E. H., Van Severen, R., and Braeckman, P. (1983). Preparation and characterization of therapeutic hydrogels as oral dosage forms, *Acta Pharm. Techn.*, 29:9.

76. Drobnick, J., Spacek, P., and Wichterle, O. (1974). Diffusion of anti-tumor drugs through membranes from hydrophilic methacrylate gels, *J. Biomed. Mater. Res.*, 8:45.

77. Peppas, N. A., and Franson, N. M. (1983). The swelling interface number as a criterion for prediction of diffusional solute release mechanisms in swellable polymers, *J. Polym. Sci., Polym. Phys. Ed.*, 21:983.

78. Lee, P. I. (1987). Interpretation of drug release kinetics from hydrogel matrices in terms of time dependent diffusion coefficients. *In: Controlled Release Technology, Pharmaceutical Applications, ACS Symposium Series, #348* (P. I. Lee and W. R. Good, eds.). American Chemical Society, Washington, D.C., p. 71.

79. Klech, C. M., and Li, X. (1990). Consideration of drug load on the swelling kinetics of glassy gelatin matrices, *J. Pharm. Sci.*, 79:11, 999.

80. Vyavahare, N. R., Kulkarni, M. G., and Mashelkar, R. A. (1990). Zero order release from swollen hydrogels, *J. Membr. Sci.*, 54:221.

81. Vyavahare, N. R., Kulkarni, M. G., and Mashelkar, R. A. (1990). Zero order release from glassy hydrogels. I. Enigma of the swelling interface number, *J. Membr. Sci.*, 49:207.

82. Guess, W. L., Rosenbluth, S. A., Schmidt, B., and Autan, J. (1965). Agar diffusion method for toxicity screening of plastics on cultured cell monolayer, *J. Pharm. Sci.*, 54:10.

83. Leopold, I. H. (1984). Anti-infective agents. *In: Handbook of Experimental Pharmacology* 69 (M. L. Sears, ed.). Springer-Verlag, Berlin, p. 385.

84. Richardson, K. T. (1975). Annual review: Ocular microtherapy, *Arch. Ophthalmol.*, 93:1.

85. Deichert, W. G., Su, K. C., and VanBuren, M. F. (1979). Polysiloxane composition and contact lenses, U.S. Patent #4,153,641.

86. Bruck, S. D., and Mueller, E. P. (1988). Radiation sterilization of polymeric implant materials, *J. Biomed. Mater. Res. Appl. Biomater.*, 22:A2, 133.

87. Bawa, R. S., and Palmer, H. J. (1991). "Manipulating Release Kinetics of Gentamicin Sulfate by Altering Crosslink Length and Polarity of Novel Hydrophobic Matrices," Proceedings of the 18th International Symposium on Controlled Release of Bioactive Materials, Controlled Release Society, Inc., Lincolnshire, Illinois, pp. 692–693.

12
Corneal Collagen Shields for Ocular Delivery

James M. Hill, Richard J. O'Callaghan, Jeffery A. Hobden, and Herbert E. Kaufman
Louisiana State University Medical Center School of Medicine,
New Orleans, Louisiana

I. HISTORICAL ASPECTS

A. Soft Contact Lenses for Ocular Drug Delivery

Bandage soft contact lenses made of hydrophilic plastics are widely used to protect eyes with various problems, including nonhealing epithelial defects after corneal transplantation or refractive surgery and recurrent epithelial erosions after ocular herpes infection. Although these soft contact lenses may enhance healing while allowing the eye to remain open, their cost is relatively high. Also, the lenses must be fitted accurately and, usually, can be inserted and removed only in the ophthalmologist's office. Additionally, soft contact lenses may harbor ocular pathogens, a definite hazard to the healing eye.

The idea of using bandage soft contact lenses to deliver drugs to the cornea was proposed as far back as 1971, by Kaufman et al. (1). In this procedure, the hydrophilic lens was placed on the cornea and the drug was administered topically onto the surface of the lens. The contact lens was thought to act as a carrier vehicle, binding the drug and releasing it slowly, thereby increasing retention of the therapeutic agent in the tear film. Recently, however, Busin and Spitznas (2) and Matoba and McCulley (3) showed that hydrogel contact lenses hydrated with drug are nearly devoid of drug after only 1 or 2 h on the cornea. These lenses, therefore, are not the ideal approach to sustained, continuous ocular drug delivery.

B. Collagen Shields for Ocular Drug Delivery

Bloomfield et al. (4) were the first to suggest that collagen might provide a suitable carrier for sustained ocular drug delivery. Their study, published in 1978, showed that wafer-shaped collagen inserts impregnated with gentamicin produced the highest levels of drug in the tear film and tissue in the rabbit eye compared to drops, ointment, or subconjunctival injection.

Fyodorov (5) suggested substituting collagen for hydrophilic plastic in a contact lens–like shape. His purpose, however, was not drug delivery but the creation of a temporary protective device for the healing cornea. In the mid 1980s, Fyodorov and his colleagues (5,6) introduced the collagen shield for use as a bandage lens and showed that the shields enhance corneal epithelial healing after radial keratotomy and other anterior segment surgical procedures.

Numerous vision researchers saw the collagen shield as an extension of and improvement on Bloomfield's collagen inserts (4)—a potential new vehicle for the sustained administration of drugs to the cornea. Over the next several years, various drugs were incorporated into the collagen matrix of shields during manufacture, adsorbed to shields during rehydration, and/or applied in topical drops directly onto shields in situ. Studies in animal models (described below) showed that as the shields dissolved drug was released gradually into the tear film, resulting in increased contact time with the cornea and increased penetration into both the cornea and the aqueous humor. Clinical studies showed that collagen shields are easy to use in the ophthalmologist's office, prevent delay in beginning therapy, and maintain therapeutic concentrations of drug in the eye without the need for frequent topical instillation of drops.

Presently, new uses for collagen shields are appearing monthly in the literature. The development of this modality for drug delivery, however, is still in relative infancy and it remains to be seen where its permanent place in the ophthalmologist's armamentarium will be found.

II. COLLAGEN SHIELDS: PHYSICAL PROPERTIES

A. Properties of Collagen

The safety of collagen for human use is evidenced by its diverse general and biomedical applications. Collagen is a common constituent in soaps, shampoos, facial creams, body lotions, and food-grade gelatin. In medicine, collagen has been used in cardiovascular surgery, plastic surgery, orthopedics, urology, neurosurgery, and ophthalmology. The major medical application of collagen is catgut suture, which is derived from intestinal collagen (7).

Twenty-five percent of the total body protein in mammals is collagen; it is the major protein of connective tissue, cartilage, and bone. The secondary and tertiary structures of human, porcine, and bovine collagen are very similar, making it possible to use collagen derived from animal sources in the human body. Biologically, collagen is known to promote wound healing (7). Nearly all studies on collagen have shown very low or no immunogenicity (7). Of the 10 collagen types that have been characterized, types I, III, and V are the most desirable for biomedical applications because of their high biocompatibility and low immunogenicity.

A collagen molecule consists of three polypeptide chains, called α-chains, which form a helix connected by interchain hydrogen bonds. This domain of collagen, called tropocollagen, forms a rodlike unit, 2600 to 26,000 Å in length and 15 Å in diameter. The molecular weight of the tropocollagen is 300,000 D. Collagen has a characteristic amino acid sequence: glycine appears in approximately every third position. Proline and hydroxyproline make up approximately 25% of the total amino acid content. The hydroxyproline residues form interchain, noncovalent cross-linkages. Newly synthesized collagen contains only a few cross-linked tropocollagen fibers. However, with increased age, there is an increase in the percentage of cross-linking (7).

In the manufacture of collagen shields, the ability to control the amount of cross-linking in the collagen subunits by exposure to ultraviolet (UV) light is an important physicochemical property, because the amount of cross-linking is related to the dissolution time of the shield on the cornea. Other physicochemical properties of collagen that favor its use for ocular drug delivery involve the ability of the protein to act as an ion exchanger and the semipermeable nature of collagen membranes.

B. Properties of Commercial Collagen Shields

The collagen shield was designed to be a disposable, short-term therapeutic bandage lens for the cornea. It conforms to the shape of the eye, protects the corneal surface, and provides lubrication as it dissolves. Unlike the hydrophilic plastic bandage lenses, the collagen shield offers no refractive benefit; in fact, because it is not optically clear, it reduces visual acuity to the 20/80–20/200 range.

One commercially available shield, first introduced in 1986, is made from porcine scleral tissue (Bio-Cor, Bausch & Lomb Pharmaceuticals, Clearwater, Florida). To prepare these shields, the collagen is extracted and molded into a contact lens configuration. The shields are 14.5 mm in diameter with a 9-mm base curve and a thickness of 0.15–0.19 mm. Dissolution time, determined by UV irradiation during manufacture, varies from 12 to 72 h. The shields are sterilized by gamma-irradiation (8), then dehydrated and individually packaged for storage and shipping. The oxygen permeability, thickness, and water content of the Bio-Cor 24-h collagen shield have been described (9,10). These and other physico-chemical characteristics are given in Table 1.

Other commercially available shields (MediLens, Chiron Ophthalmics, Irvine, California; and ProShield, Alcon Surgical, Fort Worth, Texas) are prepared from bovine corium tissue. The preparation and characteristics of these shields are similar to those of the porcine lens; Table 1 shows some specific differences.

Table 1. Comparison of Characteristics of Two Commercially Available Collagen Shields

Characteristic	MediLens[a]	Bio-Cor 24[b]
Diameter (mm)	16	14.5
Base Curve (mm)	8.8	9.0
Dry Weight (mg)	5.7	6.6
Wet Weight (mg)	34.7	25.6
Water Content (mg)	29	19
Hydration (% H_2O)	83	74
Swelling (%)	608	380
Dk (O_2 permeability)	50	36
Surface pH	6.8	5.7
Visual Acuity	20/80	20/200
Wet Light Transmission (%)	93	93

[a]Data obtained from Chiron Ophthalmics, Irvine, California; shield composed of bovine corium. Alcon Surgical (Fort Worth, Texas) has a similar product called ProShield.
[b]Data obtained from Bausch & Lomb, Clearwater, Florida; shield composed of porcine sclera.

III. DRUG DELIVERY BY COLLAGEN SHIELDS: EXPERIMENTAL STUDIES

A variety of studies have described the pharmacokinetics of ocular delivery of dyes and drugs by collagen shields, as well as the use of the shields in the chemotherapy of various disorders. These studies are reviewed below and summarized in Tables 2 and 3 (11).

A. Fluorescein, a Water-Soluble Dye

To determine the ocular penetration of water-soluble compounds delivered by collagen shields, Reidy et al. (12) applied shields hydrated in a solution of sodium fluorescein to the normal eyes of volunteers and measured the fluorescence in the anterior chamber by photofluorometry. The shields delivered significantly larger amounts of dye to the aqueous humor at 2 and 4 h compared with drops of the same concentration instilled every 30 min over 4 h, as well as in comparison with daily wear soft contact lenses presoaked in 0.01% fluorescein. The collagen shields did not induce any damage to the corneal epithelium over a 2-h period. These results demonstrated that the collagen shield is superior to topical drops and some soft contact lenses in delivering fluorescein to the cornea and aqueous humor and suggested that collagen shields might also successfully deliver other water-soluble compounds, potentially including antibiotics, to the eye in amounts comparable to or greater than the amounts delivered by drops over the same period of time.

B. Antibacterial Agents

Ideally, chemotherapy for bacterial keratitis would deliver antibiotic rapidly to both the cornea and aqueous humor, produce concentrations of antibiotic significantly above the minimum inhibitory concentration (MIC) or minimum bactericidal concentration (MBC) of ocular pathogens, and sustain this high concentration for many hours. There are, however, numerous problems associated with achieving this ideal, and numerous approaches have been taken to solve these problems. One method involves the frequent application of topical drops every 3–5 min over 1–2 h. The concentration of these antibiotic drops is usually significantly increased (fortified) over the commercially available concentrations. Other approaches include the use of bandage soft contact lenses in combination with antibiotics and iontophoresis of antibiotics to the cornea. At present, there is no universally accepted procedure or therapeutic regimen for the treatment of bacterial keratitis.

Various investigators have examined the utility of the collagen shield for the delivery of antibiotics to the cornea and aqueous humor. At this writing, there have been six reports (13–18) on antibiotic delivery by collagen shields in rabbit eyes: three pharmacokinetic and three chemotherapeutic studies.

In one of the earliest pharmacokinetic studies, Unterman et al. (13) assessed the pharmacokinetics of tobramycin delivered to rabbit eyes by means of collagen shields. Collagen shields were hydrated in a solution of either 40 or 200 mg/mL of tobramycin and corneal and aqueous humor concentrations were determined at 2, 4, and 8 h after application. No toxicity was observed with shields hydrated in the 40 mg/mL solution at any time. Eight hours after application, the corneas with shields hydrated in the 200 mg/mL solution

Table 2. Studies of Collagen Shield Drug Delivery

Reference	Drug	Compared with Collagen Shield	Assay site	Overall Result with Collagen Shield
15	Gentamicin	Loading dose + frequent drops	Tears Cornea Aqueous	Comparable at all sites
15	Vancomycin	Loading dose + frequent drops	Tears Cornea Aqueous	Comparable at all sites
14	Tobramycin	Soft contact lens	Aqueous	Superior
13	Tobramycin	Subconjunctival injection	Cornea Aqueous	Comparable at both sites
20	Dexamethasone	Single drop	Cornea Aqueous Iris Vitreous	Superior at all sites
20	Dexamethasone	Frequent drops	Cornea Aqueous Iris Vitreous	Superior at all sites
20	Dexamethasone	Collagen shield + frequent drops versus frequent drops	Cornea Aqueous Iris Vitreous	Superior at all sites
21	Prednisolone	Single drop	Cornea Aqueous	Superior at both sites
12	Fluorescein	Frequent drops Soft contact lens	Anterior chamber	Superior to both
19	Amphotericin B	Frequent drops	Cornea Aqueous	Comparable at both sites
23	Cyclosporine A	Frequent drops	Cornea Aqueous	Superior Comparable
22	Heparin	Subconjunctival injection	Aqueous	Superior
25	Trifluorothy-midine	Drops	Cornea	Normal cornea, no difference
		Collagen shield + drops	Aqueous	Cornea with epithelial defect: Collagen shield + drops superior Collagen shield superior from 0–2 h Drops superior from 4–8 h

Source: Adapted from Ref. 11.

Table 3. Studies of Collagen Shield Drug Delivery in Rabbit Models of Disease

Reference	Experimental Model	Drug	Compared with Collagen Shield	Result
Sawusch et al.[17] (1988)	*Pseudomonas* keratitis	Tobramycin	Collagen shield + frequent drops versus frequent drops	Enhanced antimicrobial effect with collagen shield
Hobden et al.[16] (1988)	*Pseudomonas* keratitis	Tobramycin	Frequent drops Collagen shield + delayed drops versus second collagen shield	Comparable antimicrobial effect Comparable antimicrobial effect
Hobden et al.[18] (1990)	Aminoglycoside-resistant *Pseudomonas* keratitis	Ciprofloxacin Norfloxacin Tobramycin	Collagen shield with vehicle Collagen shield with water	Ciprofloxacin > norfloxacin for antimicrobial effect Tobramycin, vehicle, water—no effect
Chen et al.[24] (1990)	High-risk keratoplasty	Cyclosporine A	Drops Drops	Superior preventive effect on graft rejection Superior therapeutic effect on graft rejection
Hagenah et al.[29] (1990)	Epithelial wound healing	EGF, aFGF	Collagen shield alone Untreated corneas	aFGF and collagen shield alone superior to untreated EGF comparable to untreated

Source: Adapted from Ref. 12.

of tobramycin had some epithelial defects. At all times and with either hydration solution, the concentration of tobramycin in the cornea and aqueous humor exceeded the mean inhibitory concentration for most aminoglycoside-sensitive strains of *Pseudomonas*. These results suggested that collagen shields containing an antibiotic could serve as a vehicle for drug delivery and could be used for preoperative and postoperative antibiotic prophylaxis and the initial treatment of bacterial keratitis (13).

O'Brien et al. (14) compared collagen shields and soft contact lenses in pharmacokinetic studies of the ocular penetration of tobramycin. Three groups were compared: 1) eyes with collagen shields rehydrated in 3 mg/mL of tobramycin, 2) eyes with therapeutic soft contact lenses, and 3) eyes with neither lenses nor shields. Topical tobramycin (3 mg/mL) was applied to all eyes every 5 min for a total of six doses. Aqueous humor samples were taken 15 and 60 min following the last dose. At both times, the eyes with the collagen shields had a significantly greater concentration of tobramycin than the eyes with soft contact lenses or the eyes that received topical drops only.

Phinney et al. (15) were the first to report the delivery of two antibiotics in combination (gentamicin and vancomycin) to uninfected rabbit eyes using the collagen shield. Tear, corneal, and aqueous humor concentrations of each of the two antibiotics were generally higher than, or at least similar to, those achieved by frequent topical application. Combinations of antibiotics have the potential to cover a broad spectrum of infectious agents, but care must be taken to test for pharmacological compatibility to avoid potential therapeutic interference and/or toxicity.

In the chemotherapeutic studies, Hobden et al. (16) and Sawusch et al. (17) reported the efficacy of collagen shields rehydrated with tobramycin in the therapy of experimental *Pseudomonas* keratitis in rabbit eyes. Hobden et al. (16) demonstrated that collagen shields hydrated in 4% tobramycin were as efficacious as 4% topical drops given every 30 min over a 4-h period; the numbers of colony-forming units in both the shield-treated and drop-treated corneas were reduced by 4–5 logs. Also, eyes with antibiotic-hydrated collagen shields plus one topical application of tobramycin drops over the shield halfway through the 9-h experimental period were compared to eyes with shields in which the shield was replaced half way through the experimental period. No difference in the number of bacteria was seen. Additionally, these studies showed that the shield alone does not enhance bacterial growth; the number of bacteria was no greater in infected corneas treated with collagen shields hydrated in distilled water than in untreated control corneas. The overall results provided support for the efficacy and convenience of collagen shields rehydrated in a water-soluble antibiotic such as tobramycin for the treatment of *Pseudomonas* keratitis.

Hobden et al. (18) also reported the use of collagen shields hydrated with a fluoroquinolone for the chemotherapy of an aminoglycoside-resistant *Pseudomonas*. The fluoroquinolones used were norfloxacin (40 mg/mL) and ciprofloxacin (25 mg/mL), and the aminoglycoside control was tobramycin (40 mg/mL). For this experiment, *Pseudomonas* was made aminoglycoside resistant by conjugal transfer of a plasmid. The MICs were 31.25 μg/mL for tobramycin, 0.24 μg/mL for ciprofloxacin, and 0.48 μg/mL for norfloxacin. The colony-forming units from rabbit corneas treated with ciprofloxacin were reduced by 4 logs compared to corneas treated with collagen shields containing tobramycin or untreated corneas. Norfloxacin, which decreased the colony-forming units approximately 2 logs, was not as effective as ciprofloxacin. This is, to our knowledge, the first report of ocular delivery of fluoroquinolones by collagen shields.

C. Amphotericin B, an Antifungal Agent

In the only study of delivery of an antifungal agent by collagen shields to date, Schwartz et al. (19) compared the delivery of amphotericin B in collagen shields hydrated in a 0.5% drug solution with delivery by frequent topical drugs (0.15%) in uninfected rabbit eyes. Drops were applied every 5 min for first half hour and at hourly intervals thereafter. The corneas and aqueous humor were assessed at 1, 2, 3, and 6 h following the initiation of drug delivery. At 1 and 2 h after therapy began, drug levels in shield-treated corneas were significantly higher than levels in drop-treated corneas. At 3 h, the concentrations of the antifungal in corneal tissues were similar for both delivery methods. At 6 h, both groups had significant concentrations of antifungal, but the amount of drug was greater in the drop-treated corneas than in the shield-treated corneas. Drug levels in the aqueous humor did not differ between the two groups at any time. The results suggest that amphotericin B can be delivered to the cornea via collagen shields at a rate that is ultimately comparable with frequent drop delivery; studies in fungus-infected eyes are needed to demonstrate therapeutic efficacy. Given positive results in such studies, however, the advantages of collagen shields in the clinical setting would include convenience and assured compliance with the intensive therapy needed to eradicate this highly destructive infectious agent.

D. Anti-Inflammatory Agents

Hwang et al. (20) and Sawusch et al. (21) used collagen shields to enhance the penetration of anti-inflammatory agents. Hwang et al. (20) compared the delivery of radiolabeled dexamethasone to the cornea and aqueous humor in normal rabbit eyes by four methods: 1) single 0.1% dexamethasone drop, 2) hourly drops, 3) collagen shields hydrated in 0.1% dexamethasone, and 4) collagen shields hydrated in 0.1% dexamethasone followed by hourly topical 0.1% drops. Treatment with the drug-hydrated collagen shields plus hourly drops resulted in both peak and cumulative drug concentrations in the cornea and aqueous humor that were two- to fourfold greater than the concentration achieved by hourly drops alone. Collagen shields without accompanying drops yielded drug concentrations either equal to or greater than the peak and cumulative drug concentrations produced by hourly drops. The authors concluded that collagen shields significantly enhance dexamethasone penetration and would be useful for maximizing the delivery of this anti-inflammatory agent. They also suggested that the use of collagen shields would decrease the requirement for frequent topical drops, which would reduce the potential for systemic toxicity.

Sawusch et al. (21) compared collagen shields hydrated in 1% prednisolone, collagen shields receiving topical drops in situ, and topical application of 1% prednisolone drops alone. Corneal tissue and aqueous humor were assessed for radioactively labeled prednisolone-21-acetate 30 and 120 min after drug application. Both collagen shield delivery systems produced significantly greater drug levels than topical drops alone at both times. Thus, both of these reports (20,21) support the potential for collagen shield delivery of corticosteroid anti-inflammatory agents in the clinical setting.

E. Heparin, an Anticoagulant

Heparin, a large molecule with a molecular weight between 6000 and 20,000 D, has been studied experimentally as a possible agent for the reduction of postoperative fibrin formation after vitrectomy. The intravenous route of administration, however, is apparently associated with increased postoperative hemorrhage. In an attempt to discover a vehicle that would permit more localized drug delivery, Murray et al. (22) examined the pharmacokinetics and anticoagulation efficacy of heparin delivered by collagen shields. Twenty-four–hour collagen shields hydrated with radiolabeled heparin were applied to rabbit eyes and the amount of isotope in aqueous humor, cornea, and iris was measured at intervals from 15 min to 6 h thereafter. In general, the peak of radioactivity was detected in the cornea and aqueous humor 1 h after application. Also in this study, 12-h collagen shields hydrated with heparin were compared to subconjunctival heparin injection. The highest biological activity (increase in anticoagulant activity) was seen 30 min after application of the collagen shield, and there was still a significant amount of anticoagulant activity in the aqueous humor 6 h after application. At no time was any anticoagulant activity seen in the aqueous humor following subconjunctival injection.

The results of this study demonstrate that a high molecular weight compound such as heparin can be delivered by 12-h or 24-h collagen shields and can reach significant levels in the aqueous humor. This suggests that collagen shields hydrated with heparin might be effective in the prevention or treatment of fibrin formation in the aqueous humor.

F. Cyclosporine A, an Immunosuppressive Agent

Cyclosporine A has been used successfully to prevent graft rejection in many forms of transplantation. The side effects of systemic administration, however, are not negligible, and the systemic dose needed to provide sufficient drug in the cornea makes this route less than useful to prevent rejection of corneal transplants. Also, the drug penetrates the cornea poorly, frustrating efforts at topical administration.

Reidy et al. (23) demonstrated that collagen shields with 4 mg of cyclosporine A incorporated during manufacture delivered significantly higher concentrations of drug to the cornea and aqueous humor than an equivalent amount of cyclosporine A prepared in olive oil and given as 7-μL drops at 15-min intervals. Four hours after application of the collagen shield, the corneas contained almost 2500 ng of the drug and the aqueous humor contained about 250 ng. At all times, the concentration of drug in the aqueous humor was higher in rabbits receiving cyclosporine A via collagen shields compared to drops.

In an extension of the original studies, Chen et al. (24) showed that cyclosporine A–containing collagen shields suppress corneal allograft rejection. Rabbit eyes with penetrating keratoplasty grafts were placed in vascularized beds to enhance the possibility of graft rejection. The grafts were treated with equivalent amounts of cyclosporine A in collagen shields or in olive oil drops. The mean survival time of shield-treated grafts was significantly longer than that of drop-treated grafts. Grafts showing early signs of graft reaction treated with cyclosporine-containing shields showed reversal of the rejection process. The results of these two studies indicate that the collagen shield is an effective delivery system for cyclosporine A and that the drug delivered in this manner can both suppress the initiation of graft rejection and reverse a graft reaction in progress.

G. Trifluorothymidine, an Antiviral Agent

Gussler et al. (25) investigated the delivery of trifluorothymidine (TFT) in collagen shields and topical drops in normal rabbit corneas and corneas with experimental epithelial defects. Collagen shields hydrated in 1% trifluorothymidine and 1% topical drops were used. The eyes were treated with either collagen shields hydrated with TFT, TFT drops, or a combination of collagen shields and drops.

Rabbits with normal corneas showed no difference among the treatment groups in terms of TFT levels in the cornea or aqueous humor 30 min and 2, 4, and 8 h after application of the antiviral.

Among the groups of animals with experimental epithelial defects, the highest drug concentrations were found in the eyes treated with the combination of shields and drops. The second highest tissue concentrations were seen in the eyes treated with collagen shields hydrated in TFT. Treatment with drops alone produced lower concentrations of TFT than either treatment involving the collagen shields.

The authors suggested that this method of drug delivery may be useful to enhance the eradication of herpes simplex virus in eyes with epithelial defects; increased drug penetration would reduce the frequency of application from every 1 to 2 h, as is needed with drops, to every 3–4 h. The authors noted, however, the need for studies of corneal toxicity and efficacy in herpes-infected eyes before a definitive therapeutic regimen can be established.

H. Growth Factors

After Fyodorov first described the clinical use of collagen shields for the protection and enhancement of epithelial healing, a number of experimental studies were published in the United States confirming his findings. Frantz et al. (26) showed that rabbits eyes with 6-mm superficial keratectomies treated with collagen shields healed significantly faster than untreated eyes. Marmer (27) reported increased healing and decrease inflammatory reactions after radial keratotomy in rabbit eyes treated with collagen shields. Finally, Shaker et al. (28) reported that cat eyes treated with non–cross-linked porcine collagen shields had a significantly greater healing response than control (untreated) eyes. However, there was no difference in the slope of the healing curve, suggesting that the shield did not increase the speed of epithelial cell migration.

An extension of these studies combined the healing properties of collagen shields with delivery of growth factors in an attempt to influence the rate of reepithelialization. Hagenah et al. (29) used rabbit eyes with superficial keratectomies to examine the effect of collagen shields alone or in combination with epidermal growth factor (EGF) or acidic fibroblastic growth factor (aFGF) on epithelial wound healing. Eyes treated with collagen shields alone or collagen shields hydrated with aFGF healed significantly faster than untreated controls. Shields containing EGF had no apparent effect. Although it is apparent from this and other studies that the shields alone promote healing, the utility of growth factors in and of themselves, including optimal dosage, timing, and duration of application, is still uncertain. Therefore, even if the shields enhance the delivery of growth factors, it is not clear at this time how such enhanced delivery can be used to improve epithelial healing.

IV. CLINICAL STUDIES

Most of the clinical studies published so far describe only the effect of collagen shields on healing. Although some of the studies used shields hydrated in various drugs, no systematic evaluation of antibacterial or other chemotherapeutic efficacy in human eyes has been reported.

In one of the studies of corneal epithelial healing after anterior segment surgery, Aquavella et al. (30) reported the use of porcine collagen shields hydrated with ophthalmic drugs to treat patients following penetrating keratoplasty and cataract extraction. The drugs included tobramycin, gentamicin, pilocarpine, dexamethasone, and flurbiprofen. No adverse effects were noted. In another study by this group (31), collagen shields used as bandage lenses appeared to accelerate corneal reepithelialization after keratoplasty or other types of anterior segment surgery.

Poland and Kaufman (32) reported the use of collagen shields hydrated with tobramycin in patients who had cataract extraction, penetrating keratoplasty, epikerato-phakia, or nonsurgical epithelial healing problems. All surgical patients showed more rapid healing of epithelial defects. Acute nonsurgical epithelial problems with impaired healing also benefitted from the use of collagen shields. In contrast, chronic epithelial defects responded poorly. No infections were noted in any of the patients.

Similarly, Groden and White (33) found that 24-h porcine collagen shields did not contribute to healing of persistent (chronic) epithelial defects following penetrating keratoplasty. They defined a persistent defect as an epithelial erosion (noninfectious) that did not heal in 2 weeks with patching, frequent lubrication, and/or temporary tape tarsorrhaphy. Patients with such defects were assigned to either collagen shield treatment or treatment with a hydrophilic bandage soft contact lens. When none of the collagen shield-treated defects healed, this approach was abandoned and bandage contact lens treatment instituted for all patients. The authors suggested that a longer-lasting corneal shield (72 h dissolution time) might be more effective.

Marmer (27) described postsurgical healing in human eyes treated with porcine collagen shields after radial keratotomy. The patients who were treated with the collagen shields reported less glare and discomfort than patients who did not receive shields. Also, the eyes with shields showed less inflammatory reaction and edema.

In a different kind of healing study, Fourman and Wiley (34) reported the results of treating a glaucoma filter bleb leak with a 24-h collagen shield hydrated in 4 mg/mL of gentamicin. The shield was placed over the leaking site; the bleb leak was sealed within 2 days and remained sealed 2 months later.

V. CONCLUSIONS

Collagen is a protein that can be safely applied to the body for a variety of medical and cosmetic purposes. The creation of the collagen shield has provided a means to promote wound healing and, perhaps more importantly, to deliver a variety of medications to the cornea and other ocular tissues. Presently, the collagen shield is under development as a major tool for the practicing ophthalmologist. Testing of collagen shields for delivery of a wide variety of drugs is proceeding at a rapid rate in animal models. There are many indications that the shields deliver drugs as well as, if not better, than topical drops. The simplicity of use and the convenience afforded by shields make them an attractive delivery device. With continuation of research on a broad front, collagen shields could become a commonly employed technological improvement in ophthalmology.

REFERENCES

1. Kaufman, H. E. (1988). Guest editorial: Collagen shield symposium, *J. Cataract Refract. Surg.*, 14:487.

2. Busin, M., and Spitznas, M. (1988). Sustained gentamicin release by presoaked medicated bandage contact lenses, *Ophthalmology*, 95:796.

3. Matoba, A. Y., and McCulley, J. P. (1985). The effect of therapeutic soft contact lenses on antibiotic delivery to the cornea, *Ophthalmology*, 92:97.

4. Bloomfield, S. E., Miyata, T., Dunn, M. W., Bueser, N., Stenzel, K. H., and Rubin, A. L. (1978). Soluble gentamicin ophthalmic inserts as a drug delivery system, *Arch. Ophthalmol.*, 96:885.

5. Fyodorov, S. N., Moroz, Z. I., Kramskaya, Z. I., Bagrov, S. N., Amstislavskaya, T. S., and Zolotarevsky, A. V. (1985). Comprehensive conservative treatment of dystrophia endothelialis et epithelialis corneae, using a therapeutic collagen coating, *Vestn. Oftalmol.*, 101:33.

6. Ivashina, A. I. (1987). Radial keratotomy as a method of surgical correction of myopia. *In*: *Microsurgery of the Eye: Main Aspects* (S. N. Fyodorov, ed.), Mir Publishers, Moscow, p. 45.

7. Chvapil, M., Kronenthal, R. L., and van Winkle, Jr., W. (1973). Medical and surgical applications of collagen, *Int. Rev. Connect. Tissue Res.*, 6:1.

8. Artandi, C. (1964). Production experiences with radiation sterilization, *Bull. Parenteral Drug Assoc.*, 18:2.

9. Weissman, B. A., and Lee, D. A. (1988). Oxygen transmissibility, thickness, and water content of three types of collagen shields, *Arch. Ophthalmol.*, 106:1706.

10. Weissman, B. A., Brennan, N. A., Lee, D. A., and Fatt, I. (1990). Oxygen permeability of collagen shields, *Invest. Ophthalmol. Vis. Sci.*, 31:334.

11. Friedberg, M. L., Pleyer, U., and Mondino, B. J. (1991). Device drug delivery to the eye. Collagen shields, iontophoresis, and pumps, *Ophthalmology*, 98:725.

12. Reidy, J. J., Limberg, M., and Kaufman, H. E. (1990). Delivery of fluorescein to the anterior chamber using the corneal collagen shield, *Ophthalmology*, 97:1201.

13. Unterman, S. R., Rootman, D. S., Hill, J. M., Parelman, J. J., Thompson, H. W., and Kaufman, H. E. (1988). Collagen shield drug delivery: Therapeutic concentrations of tobramycin in the rabbit cornea and aqueous humor, *J. Cataract Refract. Surg.*, 14:500.

14. O'Brien, T. P., Sawusch, M. R., Dick, J. D., Hamburg, T. R., and Gottsch, J. D. (1988). Use of collagen corneal shields versus soft contact lenses to enhance penetration of topical tobramycin, *J. Cataract Refract. Surg.*, 14:505.

15. Phinney, R. B., Schwartz, S. D., Lee, D. A., and Mondino, B. J. (1988). Collagen-shield delivery of gentamicin and vancomycin, *Arch. Ophthalmol.*, 106:1599.

16. Hobden, J. A., Reidy, J. J., O'Callaghan, R. J., Hill, J. M., Insler, M. S. and Rootman, D. S. (1988). Treatment of experimental *Pseudomonas* keratitis using collagen shields containing tobramycin, *Arch. Ophthalmol.*, 106:1605.

17. Sawusch, M. R., O'Brien, T. P., Dick, J. D., and Gottsch, J. D. (1988). Collagen corneal shields in the treatment of bacterial keratitis, *Am. J. Ophthalmol.*, 106:279.

18. Hobden, J. A., Reidy, J. J., O'Callaghan, R. J., Insler, M. S., and Hill, J. M. (1990). Quinolones in collagen shields to treat aminoglycoside-resistant pseudomonal keratitis, *Invest. Ophthalmol. Vis. Sci.*, 31:2241.

19. Schwartz, S. D., Harrison, S. A., Engstrom, R. E., Bawdon, R. E., Lee, D. A., and Mondino, B. J. (1990). Collagen shield delivery of amphotericin B, *Am. J. Ophthalmol.*, 109:701.

20. Hwang, D. G., Stern, W. H., Hwang, P. H., and MacGowan-Smith, L. A. (1989). Collagen shield enhancement of topical dexamethasone penetration, *Arch. Ophthalmol.*, 107:1375.

21. Sawusch, M. R., O'Brien, T. P., and Updegraff, S. A. (1989). Collagen corneal shields enhance penetration of topical prednisolone acetate, *J. Cataract Refract. Surg.*, 15:625.

22. Murray, T. G., Stern, W. H., Chin, D. H., and MacGowan-Smith, E. A. (1990). Collagen shield heparin delivery for prevention of postoperative fibrin, *Arch. Ophthalmol.*, 108:104.

23. Reidy, J. J., Gebhardt, B. M., and Kaufman, H. E. (1990). The collagen shield: A new vehicle for delivery of cyclosporin A to the eye, *Cornea*, 9:196.

24. Chen, Y. F., Gebhardt, B. M., Reidy, J. J., and Kaufman, H. E. (1990). Cyclosporine-containing collagen shields suppress corneal allograft rejection, *Am. J. Ophthalmol.*, 109:132.

25. Gussler, J. R., Ashton, P., VanMeter, W. S., and Smith, T. J. (1990). Collagen shield delivery of trifluorothymidine, *J. Cataract Refract. Surg.*, 16:719.
26. Frantz, J. M., Dupuy, B. M., Kaufman, H. E., and Beuerman, R. W. (1989). The effect of collagen shields on epithelial wound healing in rabbits, *Am. J. Ophthalmol.*, 108:524.
27. Marmer, R. H. (1988). Therapeutic and protective properties of the corneal collagen shield, *J. Cataract Refract. Surg.*, 14:496.
28. Shaker, G. J., Ueda, S., LoCascio, J., and Aquavella, J. V. (1989). Effect of a collagen shield on cat corneal epithelial wound healing, *Invest. Ophthalmol. Vis. Sci.*, 30:1565.
29. Hagenah, M., Lopez, J. G., and Insler, M. S. (1990). Effects of EGF, FGF, and collagen shields on corneal epithelial wound healing following lamellar keratectomy, *Invest. Ophthalmol. Vis. Sci. Suppl.*, 31:225.
30. Aquavella, J. V., Ruffini, J. J., and LoCascio, J. A. (1988). Use of collagen shields as a surgical adjunct, *J. Cataract Refract. Surg.*, 14:492.
31. Aquavella, J. V., Musco, P. S., Ueda, S., and LoCascio, J. A. (1988). Therapeutic applications of a collagen bandage lens: A preliminary report, *CLAO J.*, 14:47.
32. Poland, D. E., and Kaufman, H. E. (1988). Clinical uses of collagen shields, *J. Cataract Refract. Surg.*, 14:489.
33. Groden, L. R. and White, W. (1990). Porcine collagen corneal shield treatment of persistent epithelial defects following penetrating keratoplasty, *CLAO J.*, 16:95.
34. Fourman, S. and Wiley, L. (1989). Use of a collagen shield to treat a glaucoma filter bleb leak, *Am. J. Ophthalmol.*, 107:673.

13
Particulates (Nanoparticles and Microparticles)

Jörg Kreuter *Institute of Pharmaceutical Technology, Johann Wolfgang Goethe University, Frankfurt/Main, Germany*

I. INTRODUCTION

One of the main problems in ophthalmic drug delivery is the rapid elimination of conventional eye drops from the eye. This process results in extensive drug loss. Consequently, usually only a small amount (1–3%) actually penetrates the cornea and reaches intraocular tissues (1,2). The reasons for this inefficient drug delivery include rapid tear turnover, lacrimal drainage, and drug dilution by tears (3). Consequently, most drug becomes systematically absorbed via the nose or via the gut after drainage from the eye. This excessive systemic absorption not only reduces the ocular bioavailability but also may lead to unwanted side effects and toxicity of the drug.

One of the possibilities of decreasing the elimination rate from the eye and hence increasing the amount of ocular absorption is drug delivery with particulate polymeric drug delivery systems. These systems may avoid some of the disadvantages of other delivery systems that also are designed to enhance ophthalmic drug bioavailability or to decrease the administration frequency. Inserts, for instance, can very effectively prolong the ophthalmic absorption times. Their use, however, is accompanied with much discomfort for the patient and, especially in elderly patients, uncircumventable difficulties with insertion and removal of the inserts can totally prevent their use. Proper application of ointments and sometimes viscous solutions leads to significant vision obscurence. In addition, viscous solutions may lead to problems during manufacture and administration. Liposomes are less stable than particulate polymeric drug delivery systems.

Particulate polymeric drug delivery systems include micro- and nanoparticles. The difference between these particles is based on their size. Particles in the micrometer size range >1 μm are called microparticles or microspheres, whereas those in the nanometer size range <1 μm (1000 nm) are called nanoparticles (4). This discrimination is useful because of their different biological and physicochemical behavior (5,6). Microparticles with a capsule wall enclosing a liquid or solid core are called microcapsules. With nanoparticles it is often difficult to determine if they are real capsules or if they are matrix-type particles (4,7–9). For this reason, the expression nanoparticles will be used for both possible nanoparticle types in this chapter.

The upper size limit for microparticles for ophthalmic administration is about 5–10 μm. Above this size, a scratching feeling in the eye can result after ocular application. A reduction in particle size improves the patient comfort during administration.

II. MANUFACTURING METHODS

The manufacturing methods for the production of microparticles are very numerous. Since microparticles have been used so far only rather rarely for ophthalmic drug delivery, these methods will not be described in this chapter. This topic is, however, extensively reviewed in a number of books (10–12).

Nanoparticles for ophthalmic drug delivery have been mainly produced by emulsion polymerization. In this process, a poorly soluble monomer is dissolved in the continuous phase (4). This continuous phase can be aqueous or organic. Additional monomer may be emulsified in emulsion droplets that are stabilized by emulsifiers. The polymerization is then started by chemical initiation or by irradiation with gamma-rays, ultraviolet (UV), or visible light. The location of the polymerization is in the continuous phase where dissolved monomer molecules react with each other and grow until particle formation by phase separation occurs. Additional monomer molecules diffuse to the resulting growing polymer particles and maintain the polymerization. The emulsion droplets mainly act as monomer reservoirs. In later stages, the emulsifiers stabilize the resulting polymer particles. It has to be noted that the nanoparticles are not formed by one single large polymer molecule but consist of a large number of macromolecules.

The materials that have been so far mainly used for ophthalmic nanoparticles are the polyalkylcyanoacrylates. These materials have the advantage that their polymerization can be carried out in an aqueous phase at room temperature without high-energy irradiation. The polymerization of these compounds is initiated by bases such as OH^- resulting from the dissociation of water. For this reason, in order to obtain nanoparticles, the pH of the polymerization medium has to be kept below 3. After the polymerization, the pH can be adjusted to the desired value. The drugs may be added before, during, or after the polymerization. Addition before or during polymerization generally leads to a larger extent of drug incorporation into the nanoparticles. In some cases, the drug may be bound covalently to the polymer. Addition of the drug after the polymerization can lead to more surface adsorption. Smaller drug molecules, however, frequently are sorbed into the polymer matrix, forming a solid solution of the drug in the polymer network. The degree of incorporation or association of the drug with the polymer depends on the physicochemical properties of the drug as well as of the polymer and on the production methods. Some drugs do not associate at all with some of the polymers, whereas some drugs lead to extremely high payloads.

As mentioned above, very often a solid solution of the drug in the nanoparticles is obtained (13). In these cases, a constant distribution coefficient between the nanoparticles and the surrounding phase results independent on the drug concentration until a saturation in one or mostly both phases is achieved.

Other methods and materials may be employed as well for the production of nanoparticles. The choice of the polymer material and of the appropriate manufacturing method mainly depends on the drug to be delivered.

A number of studies are concerned with the preparation and optimization of the loading of ophthalmic drugs to nanoparticles. Pilocarpine is still among the most important drugs for ocular delivery. Pilocarpine nitrate and to a lower degree pilocarpine base could be incorporated into or sorbed by polycyanoacrylate nanoparticles (14,15). The presence of electrolytes such as nitrate, chloride, and sulfate significantly increased the amount of sorption of pilocarpine. Because of its high ionic strength, sodium sulfate had the highest sorption-enhancing effect. Nonionic surfactants below their CMC, used after pretreatment of the nanoparticles by lyophilization alone or by washing and additional lyophilization prior to the sorption of pilocarpine, improved the adsorption behavior of this drug even more than electrolytes (14). The surfactants with the longest hydrocarbon chain length showed the best adsorption increasing effect. Incorporation of pilocarpine nitrate into polybutylcyanoacrylate nanoparticles at low temperatures (5°C) in a nitric acid medium yielded the highest loading (15).

Pilocarpine as well as timolol base were successfully incorporated into similar nanoparticles in a nitric acid polymerization environment (16,17). The drugs were solubilized by secondary solubilization with ether and polysorbate 80 1.6% as the emulsifier.

With another beta-blocker for the treatment of glaucoma, betaxolol, a very high sorption of up to 0.45 g drug/g nanoparticle polymer was observed by Marchal-Heussler et al. (18). These nanoparticles consisted of isobutylcyanoacrylate and were produced in a hydrochloric acid medium of pH 3 containing 0.8% dextran 7000 and 0.3% dextran sulfate.

III. BIODEGRADATION OF NANOPARTICLES

As will be shown later, nanoparticles are drained through the lacrimal duct but a certain percentage stays in the eyes for several hours or even longer. For this reason, nanoparticles for ophthalmic delivery should be biodegradable.

As mentioned before, polyalkylcyanoacrylates are so far mainly used as materials for ophthalmic nanoparticles. Polyalkylcyanoacrylates are rapidly biodegrade. Their degradation rate depends on the chain length of their ester side chain. This rate can be monitored by mixing different alkylcyanoacrylate monomers prior to polymerization (19).

The biodegradation pathway of nanoparticles in an environment containing esterases seems to be different than degradation without the presence of the esterases. While the latter pathway results in the slow breakdown of the polymer backbone (2), the presence of esterases leads to a cleavage of the ester side chain and the formation of the water-soluble polymer acid (21). As a result, the nanoparticles are rapidly eliminated from the body (22).

In vitro, in collected rabbit tears, an initial rapid degradation of even the more slowly degrading polyhexylcyanoacrylate nanoparticles was observed (2). Twenty percent of the particles degraded within 1 h, followed by a slower but rather constant degradation rate of about 2.5%/h over several hours. This decrease in the degradation rate is probably due to a decrease in the enzymatic activity in the in vitro setup.

IV. IN VITRO RELEASE CONSIDERATIONS

In vitro release experiments in the most cases precede studies in animals or humans. In these experiments, the drug concentrations are determined either directly in the fluid surrounding the drug delivery system, or the delivery system is separated from the sampling compartment by an artificial or biological membrane. For the determination of the release from nanoparticles, the second experimental setup is preferable because determination of the released drug in the surrounding fluid would require time-consuming separation of the nanoparticles from this fluid by ultracentrifugation or ultrafiltration prior to the drug concentration measurements. The long duration of these separation steps prevents the assessment of an exact release versus time profile. For this reason, the released amount has to be determined in the receiver compartment after permeation through a membrane. This process, however, although faster than the above-mentioned methods also is not instant and, therefore, again does not allow the totally accurate determination of rapidly releasing drug. Moreover, nanoparticles are slightly bioadhesive (23,24) and interact with certain membranes, so that the type of membrane used greatly affects the rate and nature of the release (25). For this reason, in vitro release experiments with nanoparticles very often bear no relevance to the release characteristics of nanoparticles in vivo. Consequently, in two studies with pilocarpine nanoparticles employing artificial membranes as well as bovine cornea, no correlations between in vitro release and in vivo effects in rabbits were observable (26,27).

V. OCULAR DISTRIBUTION OF PARTICLES

First attempts to address the problem of precorneal elimination of particles were made by Sieg and Triplett (28). These authors used [141]Ce-labeled polystyrene spheres of sizes of 3 and 25 μm. With the smaller spheres, the elimination rate in rabbits was dependent on the volume instilled into the eye, i.e., 25 and 50 μL, the larger volume being eliminated about twice as fast as the smaller volume. For both dose volumes a very rapid elimination phase was observed for the first 3 min with an elimination of 25 or 55%, respectively, of the dose. This rapid elimination phase was followed by a much slower phase. Consequently, the total elimination after 10 min amounted to 35 or 65%, respectively. No significant elimination was observable for the larger 25-μm particles over 20 min at both dosages (25 or 50 μL).

In another study with 30-μm sized polyphthalamide microcapsules containing encapsulated [99]technetium-labeled albumin, Beal et al. (29) observed that 60% of the instilled dose was still present after 90 min, whereas in an aqueous solution, 90% of the albumin was cleared within 10 min.

This decreased elimination rate of the large particles should be accompanied by a prolonged ophthalmic efficacy. However, our experiments with pilocarpine-loaded albumin particles and microspheres did not reveal such an effect (unpublished results). In contrast, with particles ranging in size between 500 and 20 μm, we observed a shorter duration of the miosis and of the intraocular pressure–reducing effect after installation of the larger particles.

The elimination and ophthalmic distribution of [14]carbon-polyhexylcyanoacrylate nanoparticles in rabbits was extensively studied by Wood et al. (2). The observed elimination kinetics from the tear film was not first order but was linear after plotting the log of the concentration over the square root of time. This unusual elimination kinetics is probably primarily due to the dilution of the tears by the instilled volume of the nanoparticle suspension. Normally, the tear volume is about 7 μL (30); the additional volume of the nanoparticle suspension was 25 μL (2). Nevertheless, from these data an approximate elimination half-life of 20 min was estimated (23). In another study involving [111]indium-oxime–labeled polybutylcyanoacrylate nanoparticles (30), a much shorter ocular residence half-life of only 10 min was observed. However, it has to be considered that in the study of Wood et al. (2), the nanoparticles were labeled with ^{14}C within the polymer chain, whereas in the second study, the ^{111}In was complexed by oxime, and this complex was bound to the nanoparticles by hydrophobic interactions. Instability of the label in the second study, therefore, seems to be the reason for the observed differences in the elimination rate.

The distribution of the ^{14}C-polyhexylcyanoacrylate nanoparticles in rabbit eyes was followed by Wood et al. (2) and Diepold et al. (24). Diepold et al. investigated not only the distribution in normal eyes but also in chronically inflamed eyes. Figure 1 shows the results of this study. The highest concentrations of up to 130 μg nanoparticles/g tissue were observed in the conjunctiva of normal eyes 10 min after instillation. This value represented 7% of the initial nanoparticle dose. About 1% adhered to the cornea and to the nictitating membrane at early times. The concentrations in all of these tissues decreased rather rapidly within the next 10 min and reached a plateau at a total of about 1% of the initial dose in all of these tissues together. This amount remained again in all of these tissues for several hours. Very little radioactivity permeated into the aqueous humor. This permeating radio-activity is probably due to degradation products of the nanoparticles and not due to intact particles, since unpublished studies by our group have shown that nanoparticles may be taken up by the first two cell layers of the cornea, whereas a deeper penetration or permeation through the cornea was not observable.

In inflamed eyes, the tissue concentrations were about three to five times higher than in normal eyes except on the conjunctiva at early time points. The inflammation in these experiments was induced by pretreatment with clove oil 24 h prior to the instillation of the nanoparticles. The observed considerably higher association of the nanoparticles with the inflamed tissues renders these particles very promising as targeted drug carriers to inflamed regions of the eye. This could considerably improve the therapeutic index of a number of anti-inflammatory, antibiotic, or antiviral drugs for ophthalmic delivery.

VI. PHARMACOLOGICAL ACTION OF DRUG-LOADED NANO- AND MICROPARTICLES

Among the first particulate system with pilocarpine that were developed was a cellulose acetate hydrogen phthalate (CAP) pseudolatex formulation introduced by Gurny (31,32). In this formulation, the pH of the nanoparticulate pseudolatex was maintained at 4.5 during storage. After instillation into the eye, the tear fluids rapidly rose the pH of the system to 7.2, causing a dissolution of the polymeric particles. The resulting polymer solution had a very high viscosity that prevented a rapid wash-out of the formulation. As a result, the action of pilocarpine was considerably prolonged. Consequently, the miosis time as well as the area under the curve (AUC) of the miosis versus time curve were increased by 50% in comparison to a solution. The pilocarpine was present in the pseudolatex suspension in form of the hydrochloride salt. A binding of the drug to the CAP pseudolatex was not necessary because the prolongation of the action in this system was not caused by a prolonged release of the pilocarpine from the nanoparticles but by a decreased elimination rate from the eye due to the formation of a very viscous solution after instillation.

The pseudolatex preparation was considerably more effective in rabbits than ophthalmic rods or a thermosetting gel (33). However, a solution of 0.125% hyaluronic acid, a strong bioadhesive substance, induced a significantly prolonged elimination of ^{99m}Tc-labeled sulfur colloids and of pilocarpine from rabbit eyes in comparison to the pseudolatex formulation (34).

Distribution of Poly-hexyl-2-cyano-[3-^{14}C]acrylate
Nanoparticles – Healthy/Inflamed Eye

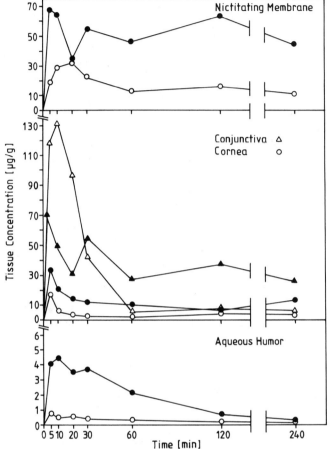

Figure 1. Concentration of ^{14}C-polyhexylcyanoacrylate nanoparticles in healthy (open symbols) or inflamed (closed symbols) rabbit eyes.

In another study by Vidmar et al. (35), poly(lactic acid) microcapsules containing micronized pilocarpine hydrochloride were prepared by a modified solvent deposition evaporation process. Microcapsules of a size between 63 and 100 μm were obtained after sieving. Freshly prepared microcapsules increased the miosis time in rabbits from 2 h with a pilocarpine solution to 4 h. However, after 3 days after preparation, no prolongation of the miosis time was observable anymore owing to the leakage of the encapsulated drug.

Binding of pilocarpine to polybutylcyanoacrylate nanoparticles by adsorption (26) or by partial incorporation (27) enhanced the miotic response by about 22 (26) or 33% (27). In the latter study by Diepold et al. (27) involving partially (15%) incorporated pilocarpine into polybutylcyanoacrylate nanoparticles, the aqueous humor levels as well as the intraocular pressure–lowering effects of the nanoparticles were measured in addition to the miotic response and compared to a solution. This study revealed very interesting effects obtained with the nanoparticles (Fig. 2): Although a considerable enhancement of the AUC determined as the pilocarpine aqueous humor concentrations versus time was observable with the nanoparticles (AUC = 200 μg ml^{-1} min) in comparison to the solution (AUC = 111 μg ml^{-1} min), the time period with higher pilocarpine concentrations in the aqueous humor lasted for less than 60 min. The miosis time, on the other hand, was prolonged from 180 to 240 min in comparison to the solution. The intraocular pressure–lowering effect was investigated in three rabbit models and its prolongation was even more pronounced. In these models, the intraocular pressure was increased artificially because pilocarpine has little effect on the pressure in normostatic eyes. The three models used were the water-loading model, the alpha-chymotrypsin model, and the betamethasone model. The results of this study concerning the duration of the intraocular pressure–lowering effect and the relative AUCs are shown in Table 1. Diepold et al. (27) concluded that the betamethasone model most closely resembles the course of the intraocular pressure curve in humans. As these data show, the duration of the intraocular pressure–lowering effects lasted over 9 h with the nanoparticles in all models. This long duration, and especially the differences in the curves between the nanoparticles and the solutions, cannot be predicted by the phar-macokinetics determined by the measurement of the aqueous humor concentrations of pilocarpine. In contrast, these differences suggest that different absorption pathways for pilocarpine may exist if the drug was delivered in the form of a solution or if it was bound to nanoparticles.

One of the drawbacks of the Diepold et al. (27) study was that the aqueous humor levels as well as the miosis data were determined in normostatic rabbits, whereas the

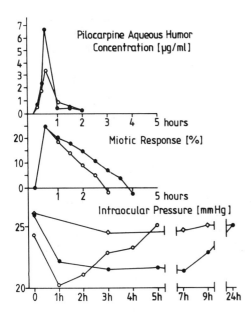

Figure 2. Pilocarpine aqueous humor concentration and miotic response in normal rabbits and intraocular pressure in betamethasone-treated rabbits after instillation of pilocarpine nitrate 1% (aqueous humor and miosis) or 2% (intraocular pressure) in the form of aqueous eyedrops ○ or bound to polybutylcyanoacrylate nanoparticles ●. Controls ◇. (From Kreuter, J., *J. Microencapsul.*, 5: 123.)

Table 1. Duration of activity and relative AUC (area under the activity vs time curve) of pilocarpine (2%) in three different rabbit models for the determination of the intraocular pressure.

Model	Duration (h)		Relative AUC	
	S	N	S	N
Betamethasone	5	>9	1	3.35
Alpha-chymotrypsine	>10	>10	1	1.28
Water loading	>9	>9	1	1.42

Pilocarpine nitrate was instilled into the eyes in the form of an eye drop solution (S) or incorporated into nanoparticles (N).
Source: Data from Ref. 27.

intraocular pressure was increased artificially in the three models. For this reason, we repeated this study and determined the aqueous humor concentrations as well as the miosis and the intraocular pressure after instillation of the nanoparticles and of the solution in the betamethasone model. Preliminary results are shown in Figures 3 and 4. Similar results were obtained as with the normostatic rabbits. The main difference in the two studies is that no significant differences were observed in the second study between the 30-min aqueous humor levels of both preparations. In addition, the miosis differences were less pronounced. The differences in the intraocular pressure remained, demonstrating the high reproducibility of the betamethasone model. These differences indicate that there is indeed a different pathway of absorption for pilocarpine delivered as a solution or bound to nanoparticles. The different absorption pathways seem to lead to different concentrations at the relevant receptor sites. The differences between the two pilocarpine formulations are especially significant, since it has to be taken into consideration that only 15% of the pilocarpine is bound to the nanoparticles, whereas 85% is contained in the solution form. Nevertheless, the low amount of nanoparticle-bound pilocarpine combined with the slow elimination of the particles from the eye leads to the observed significant effects. Improvement of the binding, therefore, may even enhance the effectivity of nanoparticles.

On the other hand, a study by Li et al. (36) demonstrates that a too efficient loading may reduce the drug delivery. Li et al. (36) sorbed progesterone to polybutylcyanoacrylate nanoparticles, yielding a solid solution with a polymer/water distribution coefficient of over 80.000. As a result, the drug was released too slowly and the nanoparticles were eliminated from the eye before effective progesterone delivery could take place.

Pilocarpine microspheres of a size of 30 μm using either albumin or gelatin as the matrix material were prepared by Leucuta (37). The production was carried out in both cases by emulsification of an aqueous solution of pilocarpine nitrate together with the macromolecule in sunflower oil. The formation of the microspheres was achieved by cross-linking with formaldehyde in the case of gelatin or heating to 150°C in the case of albumin. After this, the oil was removed by triplicate washing with ether. The AUC of the miosis versus time curve was enhanced 2.3-fold with the gelatin microspheres and even 3.3-fold with the albumin microspheres.

Other drugs delivered to the eye with particulate systems included ^{3}H-labeled hydrocortisone-17-butyrate-21-propionate (^{3}H-HBP) and betaxolol.

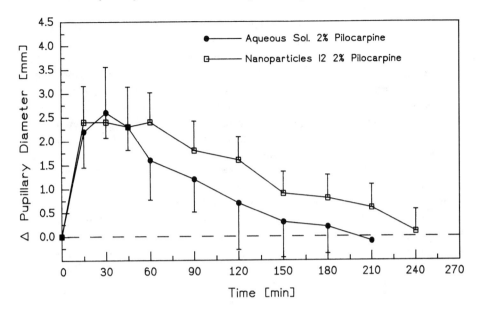

Figure 3. Miotic response of betamethasone-treated rabbits after instillation of pilocarpine nitrate 2% into the eyes. (Data generated by A. Zimmer and J. Kreuter.)

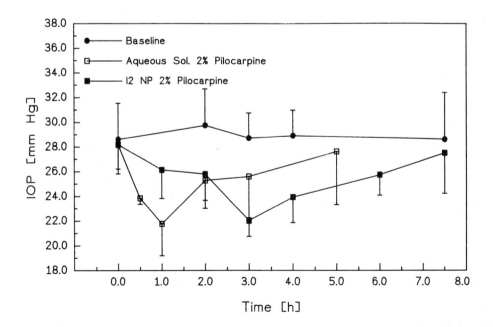

Figure 4. Intraocular pressure of betamethasone-treated rabbits after instillation of pilocarpine nitrate 2% into the eyes. (Data generated by A. Zimmer and J. Kreuter.)

The ^{3}H-HBP was incorporated into lipid microspheres (38). The concentrations of ^{3}H-HBP in the cornea, anterior sclera, and aqueous humor 1 h after instillation and in the cornea 3 h after instillation were significantly higher in the rabbits that obtained liquid microspheres than in the rabbit group that obtained the drug in the form of a suspension.

Betaxolol chlorhydrate was adsorbed to polyisobutylcyanoacrylate nanoparticles of a size of about 240 nm by Marchal-Heussler et al. (18), and the sorption isotherm, the drug release by dialysis, and the reduction of the intraocular pressure in alpha-chymotrysin-pretreated rabbits were determined. An S-shaped sorption isotherm resulted for all preparations tested. Although an optimal loading of 0.45 g drug/g nanoparticles was obtained with a preparation containing 0.8% dextran 70.000 and 0.3% dextran sulfate, an optimal reduction in the release rate and a better intraocular pressure reduction was observed with a preparation containing only 1% dextran 70.000. The latter preparation yielded a maximal loading of 0.25 g drug/g polymer. The release rate determined by dialysis of the latter preparation in comparison to the solution of the drug was reduced by 45%. The intraocular pressure–reducing effect also was most pronounced with the latter preparation. However, the difference to a commercial eye drop solution (Betopic®) was not statistically significant.

VII. TOXICITY

The materials most extensively studied as particulate carrier material for ophthalmic drug delivery are polybutylcyanoacrylate and albumin. Polybutylcyanoacrylate has been used as an artificial tissue and bone glue for over 20 years (39–42). It is well tolerated and significantly less histotoxic than other comparable tissue glues (43). Intact polybutylcyanoacrylate nanoparticles as well as their degradation products were tested by Couvreur et al. (44) in the Ames test. No mutagenicity was observed for the nanoparticles or their degradation products. The acute and subacute toxicity of polybutylcyanoacrylate nanoparticles also was tested by Couvreur et al. (44). These experiments demonstrated that the LD_{50} is above 500 mg/kg after intravenous injection. In the subacute toxicity tests, no significant effects on either the histological pattern of the tissues studied, the blood parameters, or on the body weight were observable after intravenous injection of polyisobutyl- and of polyhexyl-cyanoacrylate nanoparticles (23,44).

After ocular application of polybutylcyanoacrylate or polyhexylcyanoacrylate nanoparticles to rabbits, no reddening of the eyes or other adverse effects were observed even after multiple dosing. The ocular application of empty polybutylcyanoacrylate nanoparticles in saline to human volunteers did not cause any adverse reaction (23).

Albumin particles may be even better tolerated. Nanoparticles of this material in various forms in nuclear medicine have been used in humans for 20 years after intravenous injection and are very well tolerated. The possible danger of allergy induction seems to be reduced on account of the cross-linking process during their production.

VIII. CONCLUSIONS

Microspheres and nanoparticles represent promising drug carriers for ophthalmic application. The binding of drugs depends on the physicochemical properties of the drugs as well as of the nano- or microparticle polymer and also on the manufacturing process for these particles. After optimal drug binding to these particles, the drug absorption in the eye is enhanced significantly in comparison to eye drop solutions owing to the much slower ocular elimination rates of the particles.

Generally, smaller particles are better tolerated by the patients than larger particles. For this reason, especially nanoparticles may represent very comfortable ophthalmic prolonged-action drug delivery system. In preliminary unpublished patient studies, the patients were not able to distinguish between a pilocarpine eye drop solution and pilocarping polybutylcyanoacrylate nanoparticles.

In addition, polybutylcyanoacrylate nanoparticles were shown to adhere preferentially to inflamed eyes. Therefore, they represent very promising drug carriers for the selective targeting to inflamed parts of the eye.

REFERENCES

1. Patton, T. F., and Robinson, J. R. (1976). Quantitative precorneal disposition of topically applied pilocarpine nitrate in rabbit eyes, *J. Pharm. Sci.*, 65:1295–1301.
2. Wood, R. W., Li, V. H. K., Kreuter, J., and Robinson, J. R. (1985). Ocular disposition of poly-hexyl-2-cyano[3-^{14}C]acrylate nanoparticles in the albino rabbit, *Int. J. Pharm.*, 23:175–183.
3. Lee, V. H. L. and Robinson, J. R. (1979). Mechanistic and quantitative evaluation of precorneal pilocarpine disposition in albino rabbits, *J. Pharm. Sci.*, 68:673–684.
4. Kreuter, J. (1983). Evaluation of nanoparticles as drug delivery systems I: Preparation methods, *Pharm. Acta Helv.* 58:196–209.
5. Kreuter, J. (1983). Evaluation of nanoparticles as drug delivery systems II: Comparison of the body distribution of microspheres (diameter > 1 μm), liposomes, and emulsions, *Pharm. Acta Helv.*, 58:217–226.
6. Kreuter, J. (1983). Evaluation of nanoparticles as drug delivery systems III: Materials, stability, toxicity, possibilities of targeting, and use, *Pharm. Acta Helv.*, 58:242–250.
7. Birrenbach, G., and Speiser, P. P. (1976). Polymerized micelles and their use as adjuvants in immunology, *J. Pharm. Sci.*, 65:1763–1766.
8. Arakawa, M., and Kondo, T. (1980). Preparation and properties of poly(N,N-L-lysinediyltereph-thaloyl) microcapsules containing hemolysate in the nanometer range, *Can. J. Physiol. Pharmacol.*, 58:183–187.
9. Al Khouri Fallouh, N., Roblot-Treupel, L., Fessi, H., Devissaguet, J. Ph., and Puisieux, F. (1986). Development of a new process for the manufacture of polyisobutylcyanoacrylate nanocapsules, *Int. J. Pharm.*, 28:125–132.
10. Deasy, P. B. (1984). *Microencapsulation and Related Drug Processes*. Marcel Dekker, New York.
11. Widder, K. J., and Green, R. (eds.), (1985). *Methods in Enzymology*, Vol. 112, Academic Press, Orlando, Florida.
12. Donbrow, M. (ed.), (1992). *Microcapsules and Nanoparticles in Medicine and Pharmacy*, CRC Press, Boca Raton, Florida.
13. Kreuter, J. (1983). Solid dispersion and solid solution. In: *Topics in Pharmaceutical Sciences 1983* (D. D. Breimer, and P. Speiser, eds.). Elsevier, Amsterdam, pp. 359–370.
14. Harmia, T., Speiser, P., and Kreuter, J. (1986). Optimization of pilocarpine loading onto nanoparticles by sorption procedures, *Int. J. Pharm.*, 33:45–54.
15. Harmia, T., Speiser, P., and Kreuter, J. (1986). A solid colloidal drug delivery system for the eye: Encapsulation of pilocarpine in nanoparticles, *J. Microencapsul.*, 3:3–12.
16. Harmia-Pulkkinen, T., Tuomi, A., and Kristoffersson, E. (1989). Manufacture of polyalkylcyano-acrylate nanoparticles with pilocarpine and timolol by micelle polymerization: Factors influencing particle formation, *J. Microencapsul.*, 6:87–93.
17. Harmia-Pulkkinen, T., Ihantola, A., Tuomi, A., and Kristoffersson, E. (1986). Nanoencapsulation of timolol by suspension and micelle polymerization, *Acta Pharm. Fenn.*, 95:89–96.

18. Marchal-Heussler, L., Maincent, P., Hoffman, M., Spittler, J., and Couvreur, P. (1990). Anti-glaucomatous activity of betaxolol chlorhydrate sorbed onto different isobutylcyanoacrylate nanoparticle preparations, *Int. J. Pharm.*, 58:115–122.
19. Couvreur, P., Kante, B., Roland, M., and Speiser, P. (1979). Adsorption of antineoplastic drugs to polyalkylcyanoacrylate nanoparticles and their release in calf serum, *J. Pharm. Sci.*, 68: 1521–1524.
20. Leonhard, F., Kulkarni, R., Brandes, G., Nelson, J., and Cameron, J. (1966). Synthesis and degradation of poly(alkyl-α-cyanoacrylates), *J. Appl. Polym. Sci.*, 10:259–272.
21. Lenaerts, V., Couvreur, P., Christiaens-Leyh, D., Joiris, E., Rolland, M., Rollmann, B., and Speiser, P. (1984). Degradation of poly(isobutylcyanoacrylate) nanoparticles, *Biomaterials*, 5: 65–68.
22. Grislain, L., Couvreur, P., Lenaerts, V., Roland, M., Deprez-Decampeneere, D., and Speiser, P. (1983). Pharmacokinetics and distribution of a biodegradable drug-carrier, *Int. J. Pharm.*, 15: 335–345.
23. Kreuter, J. (1990). Nanoparticles as bioadhesive ocular drug delivery systems. *In: Bioadhesive Drug Delivery Systems* (V. Lenaerts and R. Gurny, eds.). CRC Press, Boca Raton, Florida, pp. 203–212.
24. Diepold, R., Kreuter, J., Guggenbuhl, P., and Robinson, J. R. (1989). Distribution of poly-hexyl-2-cyano[3-^{14}C]acrylate nanoparticles in healthy and chronically inflamed rabbit eyes, *Int. J. Pharm.*, 54:149–153.
25. Kreuter, J., Mills, S. N., Davis, S. S., and Wilson, C. G. (1983). Polybutylcyanoacrylate nanoparticles for the delivery of [^{75}Se]norcholestenol, *Int. J. Pharm.*, 16:105–113.
26. Harmia, T., Kreuter, J., Speiser, P., Boye, T., Gurny, R., and Kubis, A. (1986). Enhancement of the myotic response of rabbits with pilocarpine-loaded polybutylcyanoacrylate nanoparticles, *Int. J. Pharm.*, 33:187–193.
27. Diepold, R., Kreuter, J., Himber, J., Gurny, R., Lee, V. H. K., Robinson, J. R., Saettone, M. F., and Schnaudigel, O. E. (1989). Comparison of different models for the testing of pilocarpine eyedrops using conventional eyedrops and a novel depot formulation (nanoparticles), *Graefe's Arch. Clin. Exp. Ophthalmol.*, 227:188–193.
28. Sieg, J. W., and Triplett, J. W. (1980). Precorneal Retention of Topically Instilled Micronized Particles, *J. Pharm. Sci.*, 69:863–864.
29. Beal, M., Richardson, N. E., Meakin, B. J., and Davis, D. J. G. (1984). The use of polyphthalamide microcapsules for obtaining extended periods of therapy in the eye. *In: Microspheres and Drug Therapy, Pharmaceutical, Immunological and Medical Aspects* (S. S. Davis, L. Illum, J. G. McVie, and E. Tomlinson, eds.). Elsevier, Amsterdam, pp. 347–348.
30. Middleton, D. L., Leung, S. H. S., and Robinson, J. R. (1990). Ocular bioadhesive delivery systems. *In: Bioadhesive Drug Delivery Systems* (V. Lenaerts and R. Gurny, eds.). CRC Press, Boca Raton, Florida, pp. 179–202.
31. Gurny, R. (1981). Preliminary study of prolonged acting drug delivery system for the treatment of glaucoma. *Pharm. Acta Helv.*, 56:130–132.
32. Gurny, R. (1986). Ocular therapy with nanoparticles. *In: Polymeric Nanoparticles and Micro-spheres* (P. Guiot and P. Couvreur, eds.). CRC Press, Boca Raton, Florida, pp. 127–136.
33. Gruny, R., Boye, T., and Ibrahim, H. (1985). Ocular therapy with nanoparticulate systems for controlled drug delivery, *J. Controlled Rel.*, 2:353–361.
34. Gurny, R., Ibrahim, H., Aebi, A., Buri, P., Wilson, C. G., Washington, N., Edman, P., and Camber, O. (1987). Design and evaluation of controlled release systems for the eye, *J. Controlled Rel.*, 6:367–373.
35. Vidmar, V., Pepeljnjak, S., and Jalsenjak, I. (1985). The in vivo evaluation of poly(lactic acid) microcapsules of pilocarpine hydrochloride, *J. Microencapsul.*, 2:289–292.
36. Li, V. H. K., Wood, R. W., Kreuter, J., Harmia, T., and Robinson, J. R. (1986). Ocular drug delivery of progesterone using nanoparticles, *J. Microencapsul.*, 3:213–218.

37. Leucuta, S. E. (1989). The kinetics of in vitro release and the pharmacokinetics of miotic response in rabbits of gelatin and albumin microspheres with pilocarpine, *Int. J. Pharm.*, 54:71–78.

38. Komatsu, A., Ohashi, K., Oba, H., Kakehashi, T., Niizuma, T., Hirata, M., Mizushima, Y., Shirasawa, E., and Horiuchi, M. (1986). Studies of steroid eye-solution intraocular penetration with a lipid microsphere delivery system, *Nippon Ganka Kiyo*, 37:176–179.

39. Leonhard, F., Kulkarni, K., Nelson, J., and Brandes, G. (1967). Tissue adhesives and hemostasis-inducing compounds: The alkyl cyanoacrylates, *J. Biomed. Mater. Res.*, 1:3–9.

40. Matsumoto, T., Pani, K. C., Hardaway, R. M., and Leonhard, F. (1967). N-alkyl alpha cyano-acrylate monomers in surgery, *Arch. Surg.*, 94:153–158.

41. Häring, S. (1968). Klebstoff als Nahtersatz in der Chirurgie, *Fortschr. Med.*, 86:179–182.

42. Heiss, W. H. (1973). Gewebekleber, *Melsunger Med. Mitt.*, 47:117–135.

43. Pigisch, E. F., and Gottlob, R. (1970). Vergleichende Untersuchungen zur Histotoxizität eines Butyl-2-Zyanoacrylates und eines GRF-Klebers, *Z. Exp. Chirurg.*, 3:243–252.

44. Couvreur, P., Grislain, L., Lenaerts, V., Brasseur, F., Guiot, P., and Bienacki, A. (1986). Biodegradable polymeric nanoparticles as drug carriers for antitumor drugs. *In: Polymeric Nanoparticles and Microspheres* (P. Guiot and P. Couvreur, eds.). CRC Press, Boca Raton, Florida, pp. 27–93.

14
Advanced Corneal Delivery Systems: Liposomes

Nigel M. Davies* and Ian W. Kellaway *Welsh School of Pharmacy, University of Wales, Cardiff, Wales*

Jane L. Greaves and Clive G. Wilson[†] *Medical School, Queen's Medical Centre, Nottingham, England*

I. INTRODUCTION

Liposomes are vesicles composed of a lipid membrane enclosing an aqueous volume. These structures form spontaneously when a mixture of phospholipids are agitated in an aqueous medium to disperse the two phases. The vesicles may consist of many or few layers depending on the method of production but they share the property of a liquid crystalline bilayer, similar to the outer cell membrane. Drug can be entrapped either in the lipid or the aqueous phase; for an aqueous vehicle, the enveloping membrane provides a means of retarding drug release over a number of hours. Liposomes have been investigated as delivery systems for a variety of drugs administered by every route available and the literature is vast; for the purposes of this chapter, the data selected are pertinent to the eye, where the application has been more modest.

The potential advantages of liposomes in ocular drug delivery include their ability to control the rate of release of encapsulated drug, to protect the drug from the metabolic enzymes present at the tear/corneal epithelium interface, and their ability to form intimate contact with the corneal and conjunctival surfaces, thereby increasing the possibility of ocular drug absorption (1). The possibility of manipulation of permeability and encapsulation, together with their biodegradable and nontoxic nature, has stimulated interest into the use of liposomes as drug carriers for ocular delivery.

II. LIPOSOME STRUCTURE AND PROPERTIES

Liposomes or phospholipid vesicles consist of concentric phospholipid bilayers alternating with aqueous compartments. These vesicles form spontaneously by the addition of water to

Present affiliations:
*School of Pharmacy, University of Otago, Dunedin, New Zealand
[†]University of Strathclyde, Royal College, Glasgow, Scotland

certain films of phospholipids, a net result of the thermodynamically unfavorable inter-action of water with the alkyl chains and the attraction of the polar head groups of the phospholipids. Liposomes may be classified as multi- (MLVs) or unilamellar depending on the number of concentric alternating layers of phospholipid and aqueous spaces. Uni-lamellar vesicles may be further classed on the basis of size, with those smaller than 100 nm designated as small unilamellar vesicles (SUVs) and those of greater dimensions desig-nated as large unilamellar vesicles (LUVs). A liposomal preparation is usually abbreviated as a three-letter acronym with the lipid composition and mole ratio of lipids enclosed in brackets (2). For example, the idoxuridine-liposomes prepared by Smolin et al. (3) were multilamellar vesicles composed of phosphatidylglycerol, phosphatidylcholine, and cholesterol in a molar ratio of 1:4:5 and would therefore be abbreviated as MLV (PG/PC/CHOL, 1:4:5).

Phospholipids commonly used in the preparation of liposomes are phosphatidyl-choline, phosphatidylethanolamine, phosphatidylserine, phosphatidic acid, sphingo-myelins, cardiolipins, plasmalogens, and cerebrosides. Other substances such as sterols, glycolipids, organic acids or bases, membrane proteins, and synthetic polymers may be added to liposomes to vary their physical, chemical, and biological properties, including liposome size, charge, drug loading capacity (entrapment efficiency), and permeability.

Liposomes can be prepared by sonication of dispersions of phospholipids (4), reverse phase evaporation (5), solvent injection (6), detergent removal (7,8), or calcium-induced fusion (9). All of these methods can produce unilamellar liposomes but only the sonication method can produce multilamellar liposomes (Fig. 1). The advantages and disadvantages of each method has been reviewed by Szoka and Papahadjopoulos (2).

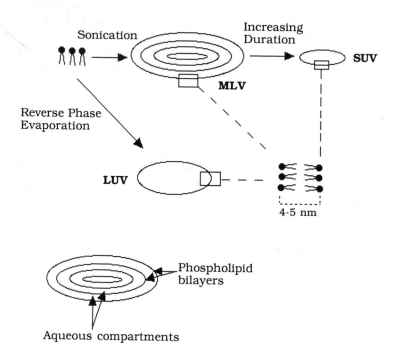

Figure 1. Two methods of liposome preparation. (Adapted from Ref. 1.)

Owing to their amphiphilic nature, liposomes can accommodate a variety of drugs with different physicochemical characteristics. Hydrophilic drugs (i.e., polar and ionic compounds) are encapsulated within the internal aqueous compartments, so that the in vitro encapsulation efficiency is equal to the ratio of the internal volume of the liposomes to the total volume. Lipophilic drugs, conversely, are usually associated with the lipid bilayers and, in general, the higher the lipid solubility of the drug, the greater the amount that can be intercalated within the hydrophobic phospholipid bilayers.

The rate of efflux of entrapped drugs from liposomes is governed by the physico-chemical characteristics of the drug in addition to the properties of the liposome membrane (10). Drugs with an extremely low or extremely high octanol-buffer partition coefficient exhibit prolonged liposomal retention (11). Molecules with log P values ranging from –0.3 to 1.7 are, in contrast, rapidly released. Lipophilic drugs are released by diffusive processes into the surrounding aqueous channels or vehicle. Before entering the aqueous solution, an energy obstacle must be overcome, which, coupled with any hydrophobic interactions between the diffusion material and the phospholipid are the rate-limiting factors in the diffusion of lipophilic materials from liposomes. In considering hydrophilic compounds, passage through the bilayer is probably the rate-limiting step for diffusion out of liposomes.

When fully hydrated, most phospholipids exhibit a phase change from the L-β-gel crystalline to the L-α-liquid crystalline state at a characteristic temperature called the transition temperature (Tc). Phospholipid bilayers become more permeable to entrapped materials above their phase transition temperature (12), and since the transition temperature of a lipid depends upon the fatty acid chain length, degree of unsaturation, and the polar head group structure, varying the phospholipid can give rise to different efflux rates. The addition of cholesterol into the lipid bilayer may also influence the rate of efflux of a solute. A decrease in efflux rate is observed if cholesterol is incorporated into liquid crystalline bilayers, whereas an increase in efflux results if it is incorporated into bilayers in the gel crystalline state (13). The nature of the phospholipid may also alter efflux with decreasing acyl chain length and degree of unsaturation causing an increase in the permeability of the bilayers (2). In addition, the presence of charged phospholipids in the bilayer may also affect efflux (12).

III. LIPOSOMES AS OPHTHALMIC DRUG DELIVERY SYSTEMS

The use of liposomes as an ophthalmic drug delivery system was first considered in the animal studies of Smolin et al. (3) who reported that in the treatment of acute and chronic herpetic keratitis in rabbits, idoxuridine entrapped within liposomes was more effective than a comparable therapeutic regimen of untrapped drug. The corneal penetration of idoxuridine was later shown to be significantly enhanced after liposomal entrapment (14). Schaeffer and Krohn (15) demonstrated that the corneal penetration of penicillin G, a water-soluble antibiotic, and the ocular bioavailability of indoxole, a lipophilic compound, were increased when vesicle formulations were compared to solutions of the respective drug. The bioavailability of both atropine base and atropine sulfate has also been shown to be slightly increased owing to liposomal entrapment when compared to drug solutions (16). However, the effect of drug entrapment within lipid vesicles on ocular availability seems inherently associated with the manner in which the entrapped drug interacts with the constituents of the vesicles. Singh and Mezei investigated the ocular delivery of both a lipophilic drug, triamcinolone acetonide (17), and a hydrophilic drug, dihydrostreptomycin sulfate (18), and reported the drug levels in the ocular tissues were increased for triamcinolone acetonide by more than twofold but aqueous humor levels were decreased by 15–20 times for dihydrostreptomycin sulfate. Stratford et al. (19) studied the ocular deposition of two model compounds, epinephrine and inulin, in rabbits. As a result of liposomal encapsulation, it was found that the concentration of epinephrine in the eye was reduced 1.5- to 3.0-fold as compared to a solution, whereas a 3- to 15-fold increase was observed for inulin. Benita et al. (20) encapsulated 0.2% pilocarpine into small multilamellar vesicles and compared it to 1 and 2% w/v pilocarpine solutions by measuring both changes in intraocular pressure and pupil diameter (Fig. 2). Preliminary results suggested that the liposome formulation was unable to enhance the corneal penetration of pilocarpine to reach satisfactory therapeutic levels when administered at lower concentrations than commonly used. Thus, it is clear from the disparity of the above investigations that mechanisms exist which may enhance the ocular drug uptake of certain types of liposome-entrapped drug from some types of liposomes.

The precise mechanism by which liposomes interact with cells is not fully understood and several mechanisms have been proposed (21), which include:

1. Intermembrane transfer
2. Contact release
3. Adsorption of the liposome to the cell surface via nonspecific means or specific ligands such as antibodies, hormones, and lectins
4. Fusion of the liposomes with the cell membranes
5. Endocytosis of the liposomes by the cell (Fig. 3)

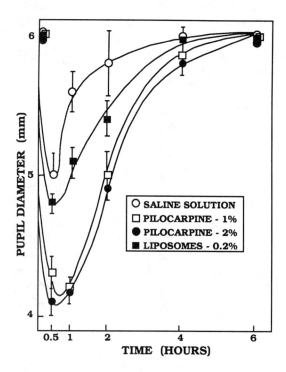

Figure 2.   Effect of different pilocarpine ophthalmic preparations on the pupil diameter of rabbits. (Adapted from Ref. 30.)

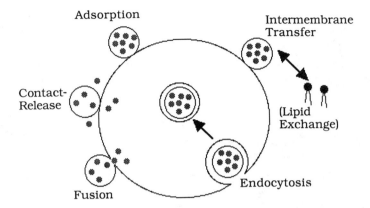

Figure 3. Mechanisms of liposome-cell interactions. (Adapted in part from Ref. 1.)

A. Intermembrane Transfer

Lipophilic materials situated in the liposome membrane can insert themselves into other membranes with which the liposome comes into contact provided that the distance between the two membranes is small enough to prevent materials being transferred from coming fully into contact with the bulk water phase during the process of transfer.

B. Contact-Release

Contact-release can occur when the membranes of the cell and the liposome, upon being brought together, experience perturbations as a result of that contact which increase the permeability of the liposome membrane, and possibly the cell membrane as well, to the solute molecules entrapped in the aqueous compartment of the liposome, bringing about leakage of solute from the liposome directly into the cell.

C. Adsorption

Liposome binding to the cell surface can occur with and without uptake. Not all liposomes which become associated with cells are subsequently taken up. In some cases, the liposomes may remain passively adsorbed on the cell surface indefinitely with complete retention of aqueous and lipid contents within the liposome separate from the cell. Adsorption may take place either as a result of physical attractive forces or as a result of binding by specific receptors to ligands on the vesicle membrane. It is thought that physical adsorption of liposomes may occur through binding to a specific cell surface protein. Adsorption is an essential prerequisite for ingestion of the liposome by cells.

D. Fusion

Close approach of liposomes and cell membranes can lead to fusion of the two, resulting in complex mixing of the liposomal lipids and those of the plasma membrane of the cell and release of the liposomal contents into the cytoplasm. In the case of a multilamellar vesicle, this will involve introduction of the internal membrane lamellae of the liposome intact into the cytoplasm so that similar interactions between liposomes and subcellular organelles can come into play. In vivo the process of fusion as a means inducing cellular uptake takes second place to phagocytosis. Under most circumstances liposomes are cleared far too rapidly from the blood stream by phagocytic cells for fusion events to occur. More favorable settings for fusion processes would be localized sites with low involvement of the reticular endothelial system such as the aqueous humor of the eye.

E. Phagocytosis/Endocytosis

Cells with phagocytic activity take liposomes up into endosomes, subcellular vacuoles formed by invagination of the plasma membrane. The endosomes then fuse with lysosomes to form secondary lysosomes, where cellular digestion takes place. Lysosomal enzymes break open the liposomes, the phospholipids being hydrolyzed to fatty acids, which can then be recycled and reincorporated into host phospholipid. The contents of the aqueous compartment are released, after which they will either remain sequestered in the lysosomes until exocytosis or will slowly leak out of the lysosome into the cell cytoplasm and gain access to the rest of the cell. Liposomes may also be taken up by receptor-mediated endocytosis; if liposomes are coated with low-density lipoproteins or transferrin, they will bind to the cells via surface receptors for these moieties, and will then be internalized via coated pits with subsequent ligand degradation or recycling. Thereafter, the liposomes may gain access to subcellular compartments other than lysosomes.

Studies by Machy and Leserman (22) and by Straubinger et al. (23) found that endocytosis was favored by negatively charged phospholipids and by unilamellar liposomes generally 0.1 μm or less in diameter. It was found that weakly acidic drugs, such as penicillin G, indomethacin, sodium cromoglycate, and the prostaglandins, partitioned out of the liposomes more readily than the weakly basic drugs, such as pilocarpine, epinephrine, dipivalyl epinephrine, and timolol.

Endocytosis is now considered by most investigators as being the dominant interaction between liposomes and cells (24). The cornea, however, has been demonstrated to exhibit poor phagocytic activity (25) and, as such, endocytosis is unlikely to be important in the interaction of vesicles with the corneal epithelium. In addition, Meisner et al. (16) demonstrated that the elimination profiles of atropine from various ocular tissues were similar when the drug was administered encapsulated within liposomes or in solution, an unexpected result should the drug remain associated with the vesicle when it reached the internal structures of the eye.

Fusion of phospholipid vesicles with cells normally requires special conditions of lipid fluidity and temperature. It is also more prominent in the presence of certain chemical agents (fusogens). Thus, the major mechanism of interaction between liposomes and the corneal epithelium would most probably be adsorption and/or lipid exchange (18). Alteration in the permeability of the cornea due to liposomes may again be discarded as a plausible explanation for enhanced pulsed entry, since it has been shown that the presence of "empty" lipid vesicles added to drug solutions does not enhance the availability of the drug (18,19).

IV. PRECORNEAL LIPOSOMAL CLEARANCE AND DRUG AVAILABILITY

Fitzgerald (26) studied the precorneal clearance of liposomes and reported that during the initial 10 min postinstillation, neutral liposomes were cleared at the same rate as the suspending buffer. Taniguchi et al. (27) studied the in vivo adsorption of $[^{14}C]$-dipalmitoyl-phosphatidylcholine vesicles onto the rabbit cornea and concluded that less than 0.1% of the phospholipid associated with the tissue, postulating that adsorption was not a mechanism of liposome-corneal interaction. Lee et al. (28) also studied the adsorption of liposomes onto the rabbit cornea and reported that the predosing of the eye with empty liposomes 30 min prior to the instillation of liposomes containing inulin vitiated the beneficial effects afforded by the liposome preparation, thus proposing liposome affinity for the corneal surface as a mode of interaction. These workers also speculated that the liposomes were merely in a loose association with the corneal surface, as evidenced by their low resistance to removal by rinsing the eye with saline. Thus, the low levels of phospholipid association observed by Taniguchi et al. (27) may have resulted from the removal of the vesicles from the corneal surface as the result of washing and blotting procedures employed prior to analysis.

Further evidence for adsorption being a mechanism of interaction between liposomes and the corneal surface arises from studies of the precorneal drainage of charged vesicles, where positively charged vesicles were found to exhibit a prolonged precorneal retention (15,29,30). At physiological pH, the corneal epithelium is negatively charged (31) and the electrostatic attraction may enhance adsorption. Studies have subsequently shown that positively charged vesicles can enhance the bioavailability of entrapped drugs over neutral or negatively charged vesicles (15,16,18).

Stratford et al. (19) calculated that the entire corneal surface would be covered by 1×10^8 liposomes, which amounted to 8% of the total number of liposomes instilled. Thus, only a small fraction of the liposomes instilled may be able to interact with the corneal surface, with excess draining into the nasolacrimal apparatus.

The capacity of vesicles, particularly positively charged vesicles, to exhibit prolonged corneal retention by adsorption onto the corneal surface would be expected to result in a delayed ocular adsorption of compounds, which exhibit prolonged efflux rates. To date, however, no delay in time to elicit maximum response nor any sustained release effect has been reported for drugs encapsulated within liposomes. The literature suggests that ocular delivery via liposomes may benefit lipophilic compounds to a greater extent than hydrophilic compounds (Table 1). The bioavailability of indoxole (15), triamcinolone acetonide (17), dexamethasone valerate (27), and atropine base (16) have all been enhanced by their entrapment within phospholipid vesicles. However, the bioavailability of the hydrophilic drugs pilocarpine (20) and dihydrostreptomycin sulfate (18) have been reduced when the drugs are encapsulated within liposomes. The only hydrophilic drug which has exhibited an enhanced corneal penetration when liposome entrapped is penicillin G (15). This increased corneal penetration, however, was only demonstrated in vitro where the liposomes suspension was allowed to remain in contact with enucleated corneas for 1 h; i.e., conditions dissimilar to those experienced in vivo.

The beneficial properties of liposomes in the ocular delivery of lipophilic compounds seems anomalous in view of the fact that such compounds are only released slowly from vesicles (11). Taniguchi et al. (32) studied the release of dexamethasone valerate from phospholipid vesicles and showed that less than 5% of the steroid was released from the vesicle over a 24-h period. However, the bioavailability of the lipophilic drug was enhanced owing to vesicle entrapment with no delay in the delivery of the drug to the ocular tissues. Thus, some mechanisms of direct transfer of drug from membrane (liposome) to membrane (cell) must exist, thereby facilitating drug transport across the cornea of

Table 1. The Influence of Drug Liposome Structure on Ocular Drug-Induced Effects

Drug	Liposome characteristics	Parameter examined	Effect	Reference
Idoxuridine	0.2 μm MLV Neutral PG:PC:C (1:4:5)	Control of herpes simplex keratitis in rabbits	Increased efficiency on encapsulation	3
Epinephrine	1.5 μM MLV Neutral PC:C (7:2)	Ocular drug disposition	Decreased transcorneal flux	19
Inulin	1.5 μm MLV Neutral PC:C (7:2)	Ocular drug disposition	Decreased transcorneal flux	19
Penicillin G	SUV and MLV Neutral PC:C (9:1)	In vitro corneal drug flux and uptake	For drug uptake: SUV > MLV	15
	SUV and MLV Negative PC:DCP:C (7:2:1)		For SUV: +ve> –ve> Neutral	
	SUV and MLV Positive PC:SA:C (7:2:1)			
Indoxole	MLV PC Neutral	In vivo aqueous humor drug concentration	Increased efficacy on entrapment	15
Triamcinolone Acetonide	5 μm MLV Neutral DPPC:C (11:5)	In vivo ocular drug disposition	Increased efficacy on entrapment	17

Drug	Liposome composition	Study	Comments	Ref.
Dihydrostreptomycin sulfate	MLV, LUV, and SUV Neutral DPPC:C (7:2) LUV and SUV Positive DPPC:C:SA (7:2:1)	In vivo ocular drug disposition	Reduced efficacy on liposome entrapment	17
Pilocarpine HCl	MLV Negative	In vivo IOP/Miosis	0.2% liposome formulation did not improve availability c.f. 2% solution	20
Dexamethasone	1 μm MLV Neutral PC	In vivo aqueous humor drug concentration	Dexamethasone valerate—increased efficacy on encapsulation Dexamethasone and palmitate ester—decreased efficacy on encapsulation	27
Atropine Base and Atropine sulfate	0.4–4.2 μm MLV Neutral DPPC:C (2:1) 0.4–4.2 μm MLV Negative DPPC:C:DCP (7:4:1) 0.4–4.2 μm MLV Positive DPPC:C:SA (7:4:1)	Mydriasis	Enhanced duration of action. +ve > –ve = Neutral	16

Abbreviations: PC = phosphatidylcholine; DCP = dicetylphosphate; DPPC = dipalmitoylphosphatidylcholine; SA = stearylamine; C = cholesterol; PG = phosphatidylglycerol; IOP = intraocular pressure.

compounds which are membrane associated. Meisner et al. (16) attributed the beneficial properties of liposomes to the inherent lipophilicity of the liposomal bilayers and the corneal epithelium which allowed for the increased pulsed entry of atropine.

Much research in recent years has concentrated on methods of increasing the precorneal residence of vesicular formulations. Schaeffer and Krohn (15) studied the interaction between different charged liposomes and the corneal epithelium in vitro. They concluded that the degree of association of liposomes with the corneal surface decreased in the order MLVs$^+$ > SUVs$^+$ > MLVs$^-$ > SUVs$^-$ > MLVs, SUVs. However, on incorporation of drug, SUVs$^+$ were found to enhance bioavailability to a greater extent than MLVs$^+$. At physiological pH, the corneal epithelium is negatively charged (–27.3 mV [31]). Therefore, these workers postulated that the enhanced interaction of positively charged liposomes with the cornea was due to an electrostatic attraction, with the superiority of the SUVs$^+$ in promoting bioavailability being attributed to the smaller size allowing for a closer apposition to the corneal epithelium.

Fitzgerald (26) investigated the effect of liposome charge and size on their precorneal clearance rates (Table 2). The MLVs were found to have a prolonged precorneal retention as compared to SUVs of the same composition with positively charged liposomes having a prolonged residence as compared to negatively charged or neutral liposomes (Fig. 4). Only negative and neutral SUVs were found to drain as quickly as the suspending buffer. The work also showed that the presence of liposomes may physically obstruct the drainage of the vehicle. Fitzgerald et al. (30) also compared the precorneal residence of small unilamellar liposomes and reverse phase vesicles (REVs) with positively or negatively charged or neutral surfaces with nanoparticles prepared from poly(butyl-2-cyanoacrylate). All were characterized and radiolabeled prior to use in vivo. Gamma-scintigraphy showed the drainage of the colloids from the cornea to be multiphasic in nature, with an initial rapid phase (150 s) followed by a slower phase. The inner canthal profile for all the particles were monophasic and exponential and were significantly slower ($P<0.05$, ANOVA) than solutions of the free isotopes. Positive surface charge significantly increased the residence of liposomes in the precorneal region, retention improving with a smaller mean particle size. The nanoparticles had similar drainage rates to the positively charged REVs, but had a slower clearance than negatively charged or neutral SUVs.

The reduced drainage rate of the liposomes was attributed to their affinity for the conjunctival membrane, a phenomenon also noted in the work of Singh and Mezei (18), who observed that the introduction of a positive charge enhanced the conjunctival but not the corneal absorption of dihydrostreptomycin sulfate. Singh and Mezei (18) consequently suggested that the initial electrostatic interaction between vesicles and the corneal epithelium, as demonstrated by the in vitro work of Schaeffer and Krohn (15) was not substantiated in vivo owing to the presence of the precorneal tear fluid.

Thus, a practical limitation of liposomes for topical drug delivery appears to be the lack of specificity of the vesicles for the cornea. However, this may be ameliorated by conjugating ligands, for which unique receptors are present on the corneal surface, to the liposomes. The use of "recognition" molecules has met with success in targeting liposomes to other cells. Procedures of this type have included the incorporation into vesicle membranes of glycoproteins, with the subsequent use of lectins to bind the glycoprotein to carbohydrate moieties associated with the surface of the target cell (33) and also the nonspecific binding of vesicles to the surface by antibodies directed against a target tissue (34). Indeed, the technology for producing monoclonal antibodies against insoluble antigen

Table 2. Initial (kd₁) and Basal (kd₂) Phase Kinetic Parameters of Drainage of Various Liposome Preparations from the Cornea of Rabbits (n=6)

Preparation	kd_1 (min^{-1})	t_{50} (min)	kd_2 (min^{-1})	t_{50} (min)
Egg lecithin				
MLV Neutral	0.12	5.2	0.012	48.1
MLV Positive	0.09	7.5	0.04	18.1
MLV Negative	0.02	3.4	0.06	11.8
REV Positive	0.21	3.3	0.02	45.0
DPPC				
MLV Neutral	0.2	3.5	0.072	9.6
MLV Positive	0.12	5.7	0.006	111.5
MLV Negative	0.15	4.6	0.042	16.5
SUV Neutral	0.61	1.1	0.140	4.9
SUV Positive	0.19	3.8	0.090	7.7
SUV Negative	0.65	1.1	0.130	5.2
[111]In-Oxine[a]	0.54	1.3	0.120	5.8
^{99m}Tc-DTPA[a]	0.51	1.4	0.150	4.6

[a]Marker solutions
Source: From Ref. 26.

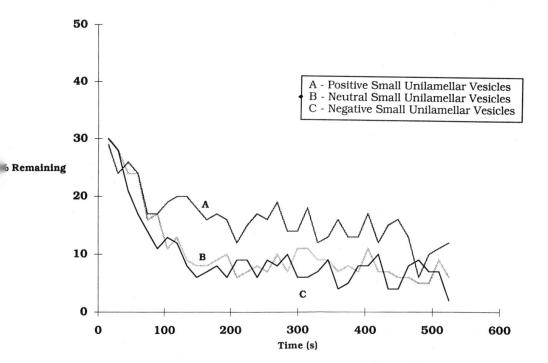

Figure 4. Mean drainage profiles of charged and uncharged small unilamellar DPPC vesicles from the rabbit cornea (n=6).

of the human corneal epithelium is available (35). Megaw et al. (36) investigated the possibility of binding lectin containing liposomes to the intraocular tissues of the dogfish and found that concanavalin A containing liposomes could be targeted to the lens capsule. Schaeffer et al. (15) incorporated mixed brain gangliosides into the membranes of phosphatidylcholine liposomes to provide receptor sites for wheat germ agglutinin, a plant lectin which had been previously shown to bind strongly to both the human and rabbit corneal epithelium. Pretreatment of isolated rabbit corneas with the lectin allowed for a 2.5-fold increase in the binding of ganglioside-containing liposomes. In addition, it was shown that under conditions of tear flow, ganglioside-containing liposomes with entrapped carbachol significantly enhanced drug flux across corneas pretreated with the wheat germ agglutinin.

More recently, Guo et al. (37) formulated vesicles containing between 20 and 50 mol% of a positively charged vesicle-forming lipid component, usually an amine-derived phospholipid of specific structure. These vesicles were shown to enhance precorneal retention with as much as 50% of the preparation remaining associated with the ocular tissues 60 min postadministration. Fitzgerald (26) studied the in vivo precorneal clearance rates of SUVs and MLVs in the presence of viscosity enhancing polymers; i.e., a 0.451 w/v solution of hydroxypropylmethylcellulose or 3.0% w/v solution of polyvinyl alcohol. Vesicles suspended in polymer solutions were retained on the corneal surface for a significantly longer period than those suspended in buffer. It was also demonstrated that MLVs suspended in polymer solutions were cleared from the corneal region at a similar rate to the suspending solution. Recent work in our laboratories (38,39) has concentrated on coating phospholipid vesicles with the mucoadhesive polymer, poly(acrylic acid) in order to enhance the precorneal retention of the vesicles. Vesicles coated with the acrylic acid–based polymers, Carbopol 934P and Carbopol 1342, were shown to exhibit significantly enhanced retention only when instilled at pH 5 (Fig. 5). Table 3 summarizes the main kinetic parameters of drainage of coated and uncoated vesicles from the rabbit cornea. The superiority of the formulation when instilled at the lower pH was attributed to the greater adhesion exhibited by the poly(acrylic acid)–based polymer to mucous membranes when the carboxyl groups of the polymer are protonated (40–42).

The influence of tear components on the stability of liposomes and the release of entrapped drug therein is a further factor which must be considered in the use of liposomes in ocular drug delivery. Stratford et al. (19) studied the release of both epinephrine and inulin from vesicles when incubated either in buffer or in a protein solution. The presence of protein was found to enhance the release of both compounds. Barber and Shelk (43) studied the release of both an entrapped water-soluble dye (6-carboxyfluorescein) and a high molecular weight protein (acetylcholinesterase) from multilamellar liposomes in the presence of rabbit tears, the presence of which was found to promote the release of both compounds.

Liposomes may also be administered either subconjunctively or intravitreously. Barza et al. (44) studied the pharmacokinetics of liposome-encapsulated gentamicin, free gentamicin, or a mixture of "empty" liposomes with free gentamicin. The liposomal form provided higher drug concentrations in the sclera and cornea up to 24 h after injection. The differences were 5- to 20-fold in the cornea. The authors concluded that liposome encapsulation extends the effect of a subconjunctival injection of antibiotics. Fishman et al. (45) studied the effect of liposome encapsulation on the pharmacokinetics of gentamicin after intravitreal injection. Concentrations of free and total gentamicin were found to be

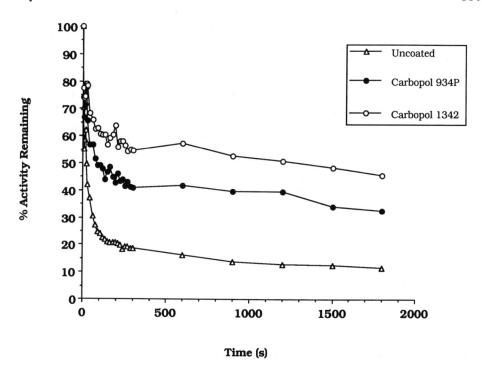

Figure 5. The precorneal clearance of poly(acrylic acid)–based polymer-coated MLV egg lecithin vesicles at pH 5.

Table 3. Corneal Clearance Parameters of Poly(acrylic acid)–based Polymer-coated and Uncoated Egg Lecithin Vesicles

Parameter	No coating	Carbopol 934P	Carbopol 1342
pH 7			
% remaining (1800s)[a]	10.87	14.66	15.48
AUC relative to no coating[b]	1.00	1.40	1.30
kd_1 (min^{-1})[c]	1.04	1.61	1.45
kd_2 (min^{-1})[d]	0.015	0.037	0.030
pH5			
% remaining (1800s)	11.59	32.68	45.67[e]
AUC relative to no coating	1.00	2.48[e]	3.30[e]
kd_1 (min^{-1})	2.10	1.42	1.23
kd_2 (min^{-1})	0.024	0.011	0.007

[a]% of instilled formulation remaining associated with the cornea at the termination of the experiment.
[b]Area under the % remaining—time profiles relative to that of the uncoated formulation.
[c]Initial rapid drainage phase kinetic parameter.
[d]Basal drainage phase kinetic parameter.
[e]Values statistically significant with respect to uncoated liposomes ($p<0.05$, Duncan's test).
Source; From Ref. 38.

significantly greater with liposome-encapsulated gentamicin than with the drug formulated in phosphate-buffered saline at 24, 72, 120, and 192 h. Similar results have been previously demonstrated for liposomal amphotericin B injected intravitreously in rabbits (46).

The concentration of free and liposome-bound cyclosporine in aqueous and vitreous humor of albino rabbits was measured by Alghadyan et al. (47). Using high performance liquid chromatography, aqueous and vitreous humor levels were measured at intervals of 24, 48, 96, and 192 hours after subconjunctival injections of 2.5 mg of free or liposome bound cyclosporine. The aqueous concentration reached therapeutic levels in both groups. The aqueous concentration was 1050 ng/ml in the group receiving free cyclosporine and 1438 ng/ml in the group receiving liposome-bound cyclosporine. The vitreous level was subtherapeutic in both treatment groups. After intravitreal injection of 100 mg of either free or liposome-bound cyclosporine, the half-life of free cyclosporine was about 6 h and that of liposome-bound cyclosporine was about 3 days, indicating that liposomes prolong the half-life of cyclosporine in the ocular environment (48). The retinal toxicity of intraocular liposome-bound cyclosporine was also assessed by the same group in albino rabbits by means of electrophysiology and histopathology. During a follow-up period of 1 month, no histopathological or electroretinographic changes were noted using concentrations of 100, 200, and 500 μg intravitreously (49).

Several studies report on the prolongation of vitreal levels of antiviral drugs following intravitreous injections of liposome-encapsulated drugs. Liposomal trifluorothymidine (trifluridine) (50) and ganciclovir (51) were examined in a rabbit model. Later, a combination liposome product of encapsulated ganciclovir and trifluridine (52) exhibited intravitreous drug levels above the mean inhibitory dose for many strains of virus belonging to the herpes simplex virus (HSV) family at 14 days postinjection.

V. NOVEL MECHANISMS FOR TARGETING LIPOSOMAL DRUG RELEASE

Ho et al. (53) and Norley et al. (54,55) used liposomes containing acyclovir combined with a monoclonal antibody to HSV glycoprotein D in attempting to target liposome-encapsulated antiviral agent specifically to herpes simplex virus–infected cells. These immunoliposomes were effective in binding to rabbit cornea cells and isolated mouse corneas in vitro although there are no data demonstrating binding of these immunoliposomes in vivo.

A new approach to targeting the release of drugs from liposomes involves the production of heat-sensitive liposomes coupled with a mechanism for raising the temperature locally at the target site. Zeimer et al. (56) used an argon laser to demonstrate that 85% of the carboxyfluorescein dye encapsulated in liposomes was released at 41°C. However, the energy required for liposome lysis slightly exceeded the maximum permissible exposure for humans. This novel ophthalmic delivery system may allow localized treatment to the retina without exposing the whole body to the toxic side effects of the drug if liposomes can be created that are stable at room temperature but are able to be dissolved with safety by short laser pulses. However, the use of laser energy to lyse the liposomes is not possible beyond a 1-mm depth of penetration in nontransparent ocular tissues. Some of the potential applications may include encapsulated urokinase, streptokinase, or tissue plasminogen activator for localized dissolving of clots in retinal vessels, as well as encapsulated anti-cancer agents for the treatment of retinoblastoma.

Khoobehi et al. (57) investigated the use of microwave irradiation for localized heating in vitro and in vivo. The in vitro study demonstrated that carboxyfluorescein (CF) can be released from liposomes in response to a localized temperature rise induced by microwave irradiation. In an in vivo study in rabbits, CF and the antineoplastic agent cytosine arabinoside were administered intravenously and selectively released by increasing the temperature of the ciliary body with microwaves. In the eyes receiving liposome-encapsulated dye, the average concentration of CF in the anterior chamber of the heated eyes was 8.0 times higher than in the anterior chamber of the unheated control eyes. In the eyes receiving liposome-encapsulated drug, the average concentration of cystine arabinoside in the aqueous humor of the heated eyes was 4.1 times higher than in the concentration in the contralateral unheated eye. Focused microwaves can be used to heat larger areas at greater depths compared with laser energy, thus allowing the treatment of tumors such as malignant melanoma with liposome-encapsulated antineoplastic agents while limiting systemic toxicity.

VI. CONCLUSIONS

Liposomes as drug carriers provide the possibility of controlled and selective drug delivery and improved bioavailability, although the potential of liposomes in ocular drug delivery appears greater for lipophilic than hydrophilic compounds. Liposomes can be easily prepared from nontoxic materials, which are nonirritant and do not obscure vision. Their surface properties can be altered to confer surface charges or ligands such as lectins to improve adhesion to cell surfaces (58). Their routine use in topical ocular drug delivery is presently limited by their short shelf life and by their limited drug loading capacity and by such obstacles as sterilizing the preparation. Nevertheless they offer the advantage of being completely biodegradable and relatively nontoxic.

It appears that liposomes have potential in ocular drug delivery, although future research is needed to elucidate the various parameters which may influence liposomal ocular drug delivery.

REFERENCES

1. Lee, V. H. L., Urrea, P. T., Smith, R. E., and Schanzlin, D. J. (1985). Therapeutic Review: Ocular drug bioavailability from topically applied liposomes, *Surv. of Ophthalmol.*, 29:335.
2. Szoka, F., and Papahadjopoulos, D. (1981). Comparative properties and methods of preparation of lipid vesicles (liposomes), *Ann. Rev. Biophy. Bioeng.*, 9:467.
3. Smolin, G., Okumoto, M., Feiler, S., and Condon, D. (1981). Idoxuridine-liposome therapy for Herpes simplex keratitis, *Am. J. Ophthalmol.*, 91:220.
4. Bangham, A. D., Standish, M. M., and Watkins, J. C. (1965). Diffusion of univalent ions across the lamellae of swollen phospholipids, *J. Mol. Biol.*, 13:238.
5. Szoka, F., Olson, F., and Heath, T. E. A. (1980). Preparation of unilamellar liposomes of intermediate size (0.1–0.2 µm) by a combination of reverse phase evaporation and extrusion through polycarbonate membranes, *Biochim. Biophys. Acta*, 601:559.
6. Batzri, S., and Korn, E. D. (1973). Single bilayer liposomes prepared without sonication, *Biochim. Biophys. Acta*, 298:1015.
7. Jackson, A. J. (1981). Intramuscular absorption and regional lymphatic uptake of liposome-entrapped inulin, *Drug Metab. Dispos.*, 9:535.

8. Zumbuehl, O., and Weder, H. G. (1981). Liposomes of controllable size in the range of 40 to 180 nm by defined dialysis of lipid/detergent mixed micelles, *Biochim. Biophys. Acta*, 640:252.

9. Papahadjopoulos, D., Vail, W. J., Jacobson, K., and Poste, G. (1978). Incorporation of macromolecules within large unilamellar vesicles (LUV), *Ann. NY. Acad. Sci.*, 308:259.

10. Juliano, R. L., and Stamp, D. (1979). Interaction of drugs with lipid membranes. Characteristics of liposomes containing polar and non-polar anti-tumor drugs, *Biochim. Biophys. Acta*, 586:137.

11. Defrise-Quertain, F., Chatelain, P., Ruysschaert, J. M., and Deimelle, M. (1980). Spin label partitioning in lipid vesicles. A model study for drug encapsulation, *Biochim. Biophys. Acta*, 628:57.

12. Alpar, O. B., Bamford, J. B., and Walters, V. (1981). The *in vitro* incorporation and release of hydroxocobalamin by liposomes, *Int. J. Pharm.*, 7:349.

13. Senior, J., and Gregoriadis, G. (1982). Stability of small unilamellar liposomes in serum and clearance from the circulation: the effect of the phospholipid and cholesterol components, *Life Sci.*, 30:2123.

14. Dharma, S. K., Fishman, P. H., and Peyman, G. A. (1986). A preliminary study of corneal penetration of ^{125}I-labelled idoxuridine liposome, *Acta Ophthalmol.*, 64:298.

15. Schaeffer, H. E., and Krohn, D. L. (1982). Liposomes in topical drug delivery, *Invest. Ophthalmol. Vis. Sci.*, 22:220.

16. Meisner, D., Pringle, J., and Mezei, M. (1989). Liposomal ophthalmic drug delivery 3. Pharmacodynamic and biodisposition studies of atropine, *Int. J. Pharm.*, 55:105.

17. Singh, K., and Mezei, M. (1983). Liposomal ophthalmic drug delivery system I. Triamcinolone acetonide, *Int. J. Pharm.*, 16:339.

18. Singh, K., and Mezei, M. (1984). Liposomal ophthalmic drug delivery system II. Dihydrostreptomycin sulfate, *Int. J. Pharm.*, 19:263.

19. Stratford, R. E. J., Yang, D. C., Redell, M. A., and Lee, V. H. L. (1983). Effects of topically applied liposomes on disposition of epinephrine and inulin in the albino rabbit eye, *Int. J. Pharm.*, 13:263.

20. Benita, S., Plenecassagne, J. D., Caves, G., Drouin, D., Le Hao Dong, P., and Sincholle, D. (1984). Pilocarpine hydrochloride liposomes: characterisation *in vitro* and preliminary evaluation *in vivo* in rabbit eye, *J. Microencapsulation*, 1:203.

21. New, R. R. C., Black, C. D. V., Parker, R. J., Puri, A., and Scherphof, G. L. (1990). Liposomes in biological systems. *In: Liposomes* (R. R. C. New, ed.). IRL Press at Oxford University, Oxford, England, p. 221.

22. Machy, P., and Leserman, L. D. (1983). Small liposomes are better than large liposomes for specific drug delivery *in vitro*, *Biochim. Biophys. Acta*, 730:313.

23. Straubinger, R. M., Hong, K., Friend, D. S., and Papahadjopoulos, D. (1983). Endocytosis of liposomes and intracellular fate of encapsulated molecules: Encounter with a low pH compartment after internalisation in coated vesicles, *Cell*, 32:1069.

24. Weinstein, J. N. (1984). Liposomes as drug carriers in cancer therapy, *Cancer Treat. Rep.*, 68:127.

25. Nilsson, S. E. G., and Latkovic, S. (1981). A difference in phagocytic capability between the corneal and conjunctival epithelium. *In: The Cornea in Health and Disease*, VIth Congress of the European Society of Ophthalmology (P. D. Trevor-Roper, ed.). Academic Press, New York, p. 21.

26. Fitzgerald, P. (1985). "An Assessment of the Precorneal Residence of Ophthalmic Drug Delivery Systems." Ph.D. Thesis, University of Nottingham, England.

27. Taniguchi, K., Itakura, K., Yamazawa, N., Morisaki, K., Hayashi, S., and Yamada, Y. (1988). Efficacy of a lipid preparation of anti-inflammatory steroid as an ocular drug delivery system, *J. Pharmacobiodyn.*, 11:39.

28. Lee, V. H. L., Takemoto, K. A., and Iimoto, D. S. (1984). Precorneal factors influencing the ocular distribution of topically applied liposomal inulin, *Curr. Eye Res.*, 3:585.

29. Fitzgerald, P., Hadgraft, J., and Wilson, C. G. (1987). A gamma scintigraphic evaluation of the precorneal residence of liposomal formulations in the rabbit, *J. Pharm. Pharmacol.*, 39:487.

30. Fitzgerald, P., Hadgraft, J., Kreuter, J., and Wilson, C. G. (1987). A gamma scintigraphic evaluation of microparticulate ophthalmic delivery systems: liposomes and nanoparticles, *Int. J. Pharm.*, 40:81.

31. Klyce, S. D. (1972). Electrical profiles in the corneal epithelium, *J. Physiol.*, 226:407.

32. Taniguchi, K., Yamazawa, N., Itakura, K., Morisaki, K., and Hayashi, S. (1987). Partition characteristics and retention of anti-inflammatory steroids in liposomal ophthalmic preparations, *Chem. Pharm. Bull.*, 35:1214.

33. Juliano, R. L., and Stamp, D. (1976). Lectin-mediated attachment of glycoprotein-bearing liposomes to cells, *Nature*, 261:235.

34. Gregoriadis, G., Neerunjun, D. E., and Hunt, R. (1977). Fate of a liposome-associated agent injected into normal and tumour-bearing rodents. Attempts to improve localization in tumour tissues, *Life Sci.*, 21:357.

35. Zam, Z. S., Das, N. D., Jones, P., and Stern, G. A. (1982). Hybridoma antibodies to insoluble antigens of the corneal epithelium, *Curr. Eye Res.*, 2:187.

36. Megaw, J. M., Takei, Y., and Lerman, S. (1981). Lectin-mediated binding of liposomes to the ocular lens, *Exp. Eye Res.*, 32:395.

37. Guo, L. S. S., Redemann, C. T., and Radhakrishnan, R. (1988). (Liposome Technology Inc.), Int. Pat. No. WO 88/00824.

38. Davies, N. M. (1990). "Mucoadhesive Polymers in Ocular Drug Delivery." Ph.D. Thesis, University of Wales, Cardiff, Wales.

39. Davies, N. M., Farr, S. J., Hadgraft, J., and Kellaway, I. W. (1989). The Influence of a Mucoadhesive Polymer Coating on the Precorneal Residence of Liposomes in Rabbit. *Proceedings of Inter. Symp. Control. Rel. Bioact. Mater.*, 16: p. 103.

40. Park, H., and Robinson, J. R. (1985). Physico-chemical properties of water insoluble polymers important to mucin/epithelial adhesion, *J. Controlled Rel.*, 2:47.

41. Kerr, L. J., Kellaway, I. W., Lewis, J. D., Kelly, D. R., and Parr, G. D. (1989). The Interaction of Polyacrylic Acid with Gastric Glycoprotein. *Proceed. Intern. Symp. Control. Rel. Bioactive. Mat.*, 16, p. 400.

42. Kerr, L. J., Kellaway, I. W., and Parr, G. D. (1989). The interaction of bioadhesive polymers with gastric glycoprotein, *J. Pharm. Pharmacol.*, 41:143P.

43. Barber, R. F., and Shek, P. N. (1986). Liposomes and tear fluid I. Release of vesicle entrapped carboxyfluorescein, *Biochim. Biophys. Acta*, 879:157.

44. Barza, M., Baum, J., and Szoka, F. (1984). Pharmacokinetics of subconjunctival liposome-encapsulated gentamicin in normal rabbit eyes, *Invest. Ophthalmol. Vis. Sci.*, 25:486.

45. Fishman, P. H., Peyman, G. A., and Lesar, T. (1986). Intravitreal liposome-encapsulated gentamicin in a rabbit model. Prolonged therapeutic levels, *Invest. Ophthalmol. Vis. Sci.*, 27:1103.

46. Tremblay, C., Barza, M., Szoka, F., Lahav, M., and Baum, J. (1985). Reduced toxicity of liposome associated amphotericin B injected intravitreally in rabbits, *Invest. Ophthalmol. Vis. Sci.*, 26:711.

47. Alghadyan, A. A., Peyman, G. A., Khoobehi, B., Milner, S., and Liu, K. R. (1988). Liposome-bound cyclosporine: Aqueous and vitreous levels after subconjunctival injection, *Int. Ophthalmol.*, 12:101.

48. Alghadyan, A. A., Peyman, G. A., Khoobehi, B., Milner, S., and Liu, K. R. (1988). Liposome-bound cyclosporine: Clearance after intravitreal injection, *Int. Ophthalmol.*, 12:109.

49. Alghadyan, A. A., Peyman, G. A., Khoobehi, B., and Liu, K. R. (1988). Liposome-bound cyclosporine: Retinal toxicity after intravitreal injection, *Int. Ophthalmol.*, 12:105.

50. Liu, K. R., Peyman, G. A., Khoobehi, B., Alkan, H., and Fiscella, R. (1987). Intravitreal liposome-encapsulated trifluorothymidine in a rabbit model, *Ophthalmology*, 94:1155.

51. Peyman, G. A., Khoobehi, B., Tawakol, M., Schulman, J. A., Mortada, H. A., Alkan, H., and Fiscella, R. (1987). Intravitreal injection of liposome-encapsulated ganciclovir in a rabbit model, *Retina*, 7:227.

52. Peyman, G. A., Schulman, J. A., Khoobehi, B., Alkan, H. M., Tawakol, M. E., and Mani, H. (1989). Toxicity and clearance of a combination of liposome-encapsulated ganciclovir and trifluridine, *Retina*, 9:232.

53. Ho, R. J. Y., Ting-Beal, H. P., Rouse, B. T., and Huang, L. (1988). Kinetic and ultrastructural studies of interactions of target-sensitive immunoliposomes with herpes simplex virus, *Biochemistry*, 27:500.

54. Norley, S. G., Guang, L., and Rouse, B. T. (1986). Targeting of drug loaded immunoliposomes to herpes simplex virus infected corneal cells: An effective means of inhibiting virus replication *in vitro*, *J. Immunol.*, 136:681.

55. Norley, S. G., Sendele, D., Huang, L., and Rouse, B. T. (1987). Inhibition of herpes simplex virus replication in the mouse cornea by drug containing immunoliposomes, *Invest. Ophthalmol. Vis. Sci.*, 28:591.

56. Zeimer, R. C., Khoobehi, B., Niesman, M. R., and Magin, R. L. (1988). A potential method for local drug and dye delivery in the ocular vasculature, *Invest. Ophthalmol. Vis. Sci.*, 29:1179.

57. Khoobehi, B., Peyman, G. A., McTurnan, W. G., Niesman, M. R., and Magin, R. L. (1988). Externally triggered release of dye and drugs from liposomes into the eye. An *in vitro* and *in vivo* study, *Ophthalmology*, 65:950.

58. Ketis, N. V., and Grant, C. W. M. (1982). Control of high affinity lectin binding to an integral membrane glycoprotein in lipid bilayers, *Biochim. Biophys. Acta*, 685:347.

15

Chemical Delivery Systems with Enhanced Pharmacokinetic Properties

Ronald D. Schoenwald *College of Pharmacy, University of Iowa, Iowa City, Iowa*

I. INTRODUCTION

Although there has been a tremendous increase in new therapeutic agents administered by systemic routes of administration over the last few decades, only recently has an awareness evolved that new drugs must be developed exclusively for the eye. In the past, new ocular drugs were discovered from screening programs of drugs intended solely for systemic use. At the same time, we have seen significant advances in more sensitive assay methodologies as well as an accumulation of scientific knowledge in physiological and physicochemical factors, permitting an improved delivery of ophthalmic drugs to the target site. In conjunction with improved assay methodologies, researchers have been able to detect low concentrations of drugs in many different tissues over time, concluding that pharmacokinetic processes in the eye are unique and must be considered apart from the pharmacokinetic behavior of drugs that are used systemically. Along with these factors, a specific need for ocular drugs has developed, partly because of an increase in the occurrence of eye diseases, but more importantly, because of innovations in diagnosis and treatment. In addition, market forces have intensified. In 1988, it was estimated that prescriptions written for ophthalmic use in individuals between the ages of 19 and 64 years old represent 15.7% of the total, a substantial increase over past years (1). A higher percentage of ophthalmic prescriptions would be expected in an older age group.

Over the past few decades, formulation approaches to improving corneal absorption have been successful in enhancing therapeutic activity (2–7). These studies have shown that improvement in ocular penetration has been achieved from better ocular retention of dosage forms (5–7). Ocular bioavailability for topical preparations is only approximately 1–7% (3,4); therefore, a relatively large margin for improvement is possible. Molecular modifications to a parent molecule that are correlated specifically to absorption or disposition phenomena as opposed to formulation approaches can also be expected to achieve significant enhancements in activity, as will be shown in this chapter.

II. IMPROVED CORNEAL ABSORPTION

Because of precorneal factors such as blinking, tearing, and rapid drainage of an instilled drop, the residence time for a conventional ophthalmic dose applied to the eye is about 3–5 min (8–10). Therefore, a rapid penetration rate is essential if a sufficient fraction of the dose is to reach the anterior chamber. The fraction absorbed has been accurately measured for a few drugs and has varied from less than 1% for the most hydrophilic drugs to 7% for the more lipophilic drugs (11–13). As a convenient research tool, the corneal permeability coefficient (CPC) can be used to assess the relative penetrability of drugs across the cornea independent of precorneal factors and the concentration studied.

$$\mathrm{CPC} = \frac{(\mathrm{flux})}{C_0 \, (360) \, A} \tag{1}$$

Equation 1 is often used to calculate CPC (cm/s) from flux studies of drug penetration across excised rabbit corneas (14), where C_0 is the initial concentration placed on the epithelial side of the cornea, A is the surface area exposed to drug, and 360 converts hours into seconds.

Although the human cornea consists of five layers, as shown in Figure 1, only three of the layers—the epithelium, stroma, and endothelium—are assumed to provide significant barrier resistance to penetration into the anterior chamber. The outer epithelium, which for most drugs provides the greatest resistance to penetration (15–18), consists of superficial layers of flat, tightly fitting squamous cells with underlying columnar cells comprising the remaining layers. Because of the lipophilic nature of the epithelium as well as its low porosity and high tortuosity, a rapidly penetrating drug must possess a log octanol/buffer (pH 7.65) partition coefficient (log PC) greater than 1 to attain optimal penetration.

The stroma consists of 78% water interspersed with geometrically arranged collagen fibrils. Therefore, because of its high porosity and low tortuosity, drugs are able to diffuse through the stroma with relatively little resistance at diffusional rates about one-fourth their diffusion rates in aqueous systems (3,14). Even though the endothelium is cellular in structure, it is only one cell thick and dose not provide significant resistance to the penetration of lipophilic drugs.

Table 1 lists CPC values across intact excised rabbit corneas for a wide range of drugs of ophthalmic interest, all calculated from the use of equation 1. Typically, CPC has been plotted against the partition or distribution coefficient* for each analog of a series so that optimal penetrability can be identified. Figure 1 represents a log-log plot of CPC and distribution coefficient (DC determined at pH=7.65) for an analog series of beta-blocking agents showing an increase in permeability with an increase in DC which approaches an upper limit or plateau region between log DC 1.5 and 2.5 (17). A similar upper plateau

---

*Partition coefficient is defined for a pH at which only un-ionized species exist, whereas distribution coefficient is defined at any pH for any proportion of ionized and un-ionized species.

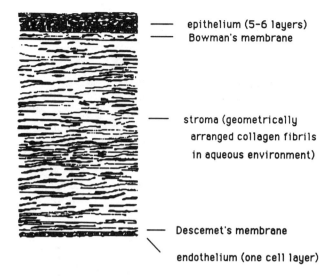

— epithelium (5-6 layers)
— Bowman's membrane

— stroma (geometrically
   arranged collagen fibrils
   in aqueous environment)

— Descemet's membrane

\ endothelium (one cell layer)

Figure 1. Cross-sectional area of the human cornea. (Schematic taken from Ref. 5.)

region has been identified for steroids (19), substituted benzothiazole-2-sulfonamides (20), and n-alkyl-p-aminobenzoate esters (21).

This upper plateau region occurs because of a limiting permeability of highly lipophilic drugs across the predominately aqueous stroma, the middle layer of the cornea. If stirring is not adequate in an in vitro chamber, a nonaqueous boundary layer adjacent to the epithelium may also contribute to a limiting permeability across the intact cornea (17). It is not clear what boundary layers significantly affect absorption in vivo; for example, the tear film may function as an external aqueous boundary layer for very lipophilic compounds (16).

At very low log DC values, between -1 and -2, a limiting plateau is also evident in Figure 2 (shown by a dotted line), which occurs because of parallel pore pathways through the cellular epithelium and endothelium. These pore pathways allow for very hydrophilic drugs to cross the cornea, albeit very slowly. Consequently, upper and lower limiting permeabilities of highly lipophilic and highly hydrophilic drugs prevent a continuous linear relationship between log CPC and log DC. Equation 2 represents the mathematical relationship between CPC and the octanol/buffer (pH 7.65) (14,17) distribution coefficient for an analog series of beta-blocking agents crossing an excised but intact rabbit cornea. Equation 2 does not include the possibility of a pore pathway for very hydrophilic drugs.

$$CPC = \frac{1}{h_1/[D_1 b_1 (DC)_1^a] + h_2/[D_2 b_2 (DC)_2^a] + h_3/[D_3 b_3 (DC)_3^a]} \tag{2}$$

In equation 2, h and D represent the effective thickness of the barrier and the diffusion coefficient, respectively. For any single corneal layer, where subscripts 1, 2, and 3 in equation 2 represent epithelium, stroma, and endothelium, a linear relationship exists between the biological partition coefficient (i.e., between drug and the biological membrane) and log DC with a slope equal to "a" and an intercept equal to (Db/h). As a

Table 1.   Corneal Permeability Coefficients (CPC) Across Excised Rabbit Corneas

Compounds of Ophthalmic Interest	CPC $(cm/s \times 10^{-6})$	Reference
[1,2,3]Thiadiazolo[5,4-h]-6,7,8,9-tetrahydroisoquinoline	78.8	18
6-Chloro-3-methyl-2,3,4,5-tetrahydro-1H-3-benzazepine	70.8	18
Bufuralol	72.4	17
4-Chloro-N-methylbenzenesulfonamide	65.1	70
Bevantolol	57.0	17
4-Chlorobenzenesulfonamide	54.6	70
O-Butyryl timolol	53.0	28
O-Propionyl timolol	48.9	28
5,8-Dimethoxy-1,2,3,4-tetrahydroisoquinoline	48.5	18
Propranolol	47.6	17
	30.9	28
6-Benzyloxy-2-benzothiazolesulfonamide	47.0	20
Penbutolol	44.9	17
Clonidine	44.0	13
	36.3	42
Ethoxzolamide	43.9	20
6-Chloro-2-benzothiazolesulfonamide	42.8	20
Testosterone	41.7	19
Desoxycorticosterone	39.8	19
4,6-Dichloro-2-benzothiazolesulfonamide	38.8	70
O-Acetyl timolol	38.3	28
Dexamethasone acetate	36.7	19
Prednisolone acetate	33.3	19
2-Benzothiazolesulfonamide	36.2	20
Crotexolone	30.2	19
Oxprenolol	25.1	17
O-Pivalyl timolol	24.4	28
alpha-Yohimbine	23.4	18
Ibuprofen	22.4	44
Metoprolol	22.0	17
Ibufenac	21.2	44
Yohimbine	18.4	18
Progesterone	17.8	25
	19.5	19
Pilocarpine	17.4	5
Fluorometholone	16.5	25
Levbunolol	16.4	17
Triamcinolone acetonide	15.9	25
4,7-Dimethyl-6-ethoxy-2-benzothiazolesulfonamide	13.7	20
Timolol	11.7	17
	18.2	28
Corynanthine	11.4	18
Cyclophosphamide	11.3	71
6-Quinoxalyinyl derivative of clonidine (AGN 190342)	9.8	42

Table 1. (Continued)

Compounds of Ophthalmic Interest	CPC (cm/s $\times 10^{-6}$)	Reference
Rauwolfine	9.2	18
2-Deoxyglucose	7.4	22
Chloramphenicol	6.8	5
6-Amino-2-benzothiazolesulfonamide	6.7	20
6-Nitro-2-benzothiazolesulfonamide	6.6	20
p-Hydroxyethoxy phenylacetic acid	6.2	44
Cocaine	6.1	16
2-(p-Isobutylphenyl) acetic acid	6.0	44
6-Hydroxy-2-benzothiazolesulfonamide	5.6	20
Dexamethasone	5.0	19
Nadolol diacetate	4.8	17
6-Acetamido-2-benzothiazolesulfonamide	4.7	20
1-Alpha-methyl-2-deoxy-glucose	4.6	22
Glycerin	4.5	25
Procaine	4.2	16
Methazolamide	4.2	70
Acetazolamide	4.1	70
Prednisolone	3.7	19
Hydrocortisone	3.5	25
	8.5	19
2-Benzimidazolesulfonamide	3.0	22
1-Alpha-ethyl-2-deoxy-glucose	2.9	22
Mannitol	2.4	25
N-Methylacetazolamide	2.3	70
7-Amino-6-ethoxy-2-benzothiazolesulfonamide	2.2	20
1-Alpha-cyclopropyl-2-deoxy-glucose	2.2	22
Tetrasodium edetate	2.1	25
Sulfacetamide	1.9	5
1-Alpha-isopropyl-2-deoxy-glucose	1.8	22
Sotalol	1.6	17
Tetracaine	1.5	16
6-Hydroxyethoxy-2-benzothiazolesulfonamide	1.5	20
Water	1.5	25
Cyclosporine	1.1	72
Cromolyn	1.1	25
Nadolol	1.0	14
Phenylephrine	0.94	18
Acebutolol	0.85	14
Atenolol	0.67	14
Tobramycin	0.52	5
p-Aminoclonidine	0.44	42

Averages of 4–10 determinations at pH 7.4–7.65 using the experimental procedure of Ref. 17; standard deviations range from 5–25% of mean.

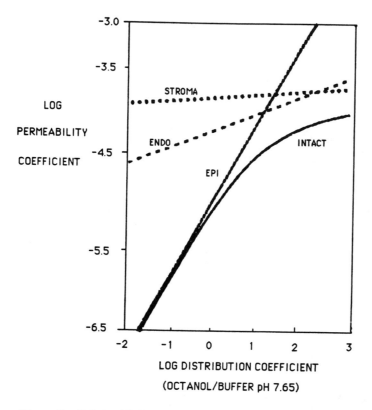

Figure 2. Relationship between log corneal permeability coefficient (CPC) and the log octanol/ buffer (pH 7.65) distribution coefficient (DC) for each anatomical barrier of the cornea. The solid line represents the apparent log CPC for an intact cornea and log DDC and is mathematically expressed by equation 2. (Graph constructed from data in Ref. 14.)

result of substitution of the biological PC for DC, equation 2 contains the constants "a" and "b," whose values can be experimentally obtained from the linear regression of each corneal layer. The solid line in Figure 2 is represented by equation 2 above.

Although equation 2 has been expanded to include additional terms accounting for pore pathways, specifically for beta-blocking agents, a comparison of the predicted line and experimental data was not conclusive (17). Experimental evidence for the existence of a lower limiting permeability is illustrated in Figure 3 for analogs of 2-deoxyglucose (22), a moderately active, but poorly penetrating antiviral. Molecular modifications were made to 2-deoxyglucose in the form of incremental additions of methylene units to the 1-alpha-hydroxy of 2-deoxyglucose to increase DC and allow for more extensive penetration through the cornea and into the anterior chamber. However, the changes that were made produced analogs with decreasing antiviral activity with an increase in DC; therefore, additional analogs in the series were not prepared. Although the range in log octanol/buffer (pH 7.65) for the six compounds is over 1.5 log units, from –2.13 to –0.54, they can be considered hydrophilic in partitioning behavior. The difference in their CPC, as observed from Figure 3, was found to be narrow (1.71 to 2.87×10^{-6} cm/s) and not statistically

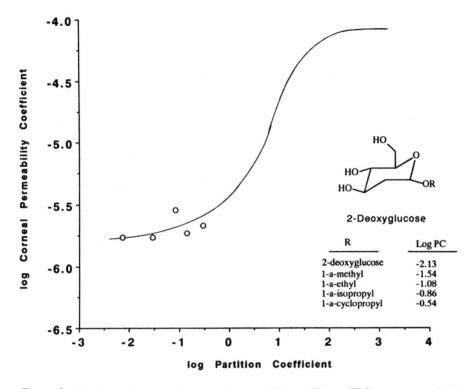

Figure 3. Relationship between log corneal permeability coefficient (CPC) across an excised intact rabbit cornea and the log octanol/buffer (pH 7.65) distribution coefficient (DC) for a series of analogs of 2-deoxyglucose. The solid line represents the expected relationship for the analog series extended into the lipophilic range. (Graph constructed from data in Ref. 22.)

different. A lower limit, likely by pore transport, would be expected to be independent of DC. A similar lower limit in corneal permeability has been observed for various carbonic anhydrase inhibitors (CAIs) when a log-log plot of first-order rate constants representing penetration across an excised cornea was constructed against their corresponding distribution coefficients (chloroform/buffer [pH 7.2]) (23).

Direct evidence for pore transport could be identified using microautoradiography; however, only indirect methods have been reported. Indirect methods identify changes in tissue structure, such as differential scanning calorimetry (DSC) (24) or scanning and transmission electron microscopy (SEM and TEM) techniques (25). For example, Grass and Robinson (25) used SEM and TEM to identify changes in the cellular junctions of the epithelium and endothelium of rabbit corneas. They added a calcium-chelating agent, ethylenediaminetetraacetic acid (EDTA), to solutions containing glycerol. When glycerol permeability was studied across rabbit corneas (both in vivo and in vitro), an increase in the size of cellular junctions was observed with an increase in EDTA concentrations. The increase in cellular junctions, which was measured by SEM and TEM, was also correlated to an increase in glycerol permeability. Precipitation of glycerol within the pore space was accomplished with the use of osmium tetroxide vapor, which further substantiated what researchers believe to be true; i.e., relatively small hydrophilic molecules (<350 MW) cross the cornea via pore pathway, whereas very lipophilic compounds preferentially cross lipophilic cell structures.

A. Use of Lipophilicity in Improving Absorption Across the Cornea

Physicochemical factors, such as pK_a, partitioning, and solubility, have a significant effect on the rate and extent of corneal absorption following topical application to the eye. Partitioning has been studied most extensively, as shown in Table 2, which lists the percentage resistance for drugs with a wide range of partitioning behavior across each of the three significant corneal layers. For hydrophilic drugs (based upon a octanol/buffer partitioning system where hydrophilic log DC < 0 and lipophilic log DC > 0), the

Table 2. Percent Resistance of Each Corneal Layer to Drug Penetration

Drug	Percent Resistant of Corneal Layers			
	Epithelium	Stroma	Endothelium	Log DC[a]
Lipophilic				
Bevantolol	7	44	49	2.2
Bufurolol	18	50	32	2.3
Penbutolol	1	48	53	2.5
Corynanthine	71	15	14	1.90
6-Chloro-3methyl-2,3,4,5-tetrahydro-1H-3-benzazepine	16	35	49	1.89
Yohimbine	12	20	68	1.77
Propranolol	7	45	48	1.6
Rauwolfine	71	8	21	1.17
Clonidine	60	20	20	1.03
[1,2,3]Thiadiazolo[5,4-h]-6,7,8,9-tetrahydroisoquinoline	42	35	22	0.53
Cyclophosphamide	72	10	13	0.4
Levobunolol	58	15	27	0.7
Metoprolol	48	18	34	0.3
Oxprenolol	45	21	34	0.7
Timolol	68	9	23	0.34
5,8-Dimethoxy-1,2,3,4-tetrahydroiso-quinoline	38	38	24	0.324
Acebutolol	91	1	8	0.2
Hydrophilic				
Atenolol	97	1	2	−1.52
Nadolol	95	1	4	−0.82
Phenylephrine	95	1	4	−1.0
Sotolol	95	1	4	−1.25
Tobramycin	95	1	4	<−2.0

[a]Log DC is the octanol/buffer (pH 7.65) distribution coefficient.
Source: Data from Refs. 14, 18, and 74.

epithelium provides the major resistance to corneal penetration, whereas the stroma and endothelium contribute minimally. As log PC becomes greater than 0, the stroma and endothelium become rate determining. Although a significant correlation exists ($p < 0.05$) between percent resistance of any layer and log DC, additional factors, such as molecular weight and pK_a, are other factors that could improve the correlation if included in an analyses. For example, corynanthine and rauwolfine are relatively large molecules (MWs of 355 and 327, respectively); consequently, their percent resistance across epithelium is large for drugs with such high lipophilicity.

Epinephrine penetrability has been improved about 10-fold by the formation of a prodrug, which is known as dipivefrin (a dipivalyl ester of epinephrine) and used clinically in concentrations of 0.5–2.0%. Figure 4 shows a dose-effect curve for topical administration of dipivefrin 0.005 to 0.5% to 10 patients with ocular hypertension. Concentrations above 0.025% significantly lowered intraocular pressure (IOP) and when administered twice daily over 31 days did not produce toxic side effects, as they can often occur with various salts of epinephrine. Systemic, and particularly ocular, side effects (allergic conjunctivitis) have been reduced with dipivefrin when compared to epinephrine (26). In the eye, the major clinical advantage from the use of a prodrug has been a reduction in dose with a concomitant lowering of side effects (27,28). Other drugs which have shown increased penetrability from prodrug formation are phenylephrine (29,30), timolol (31), pilocarpine (32,33), and idoxuridine (34).

Another advantage of prodrug formation is to transform an inactive or marginally active drug into a clinically useful agent. The tromethamine salt of prostaglandin $F_{2\alpha}$ has shown a minimal ability in lowering IOP in various species, including humans (35–37). Bito (36) established that the relatively low response was a consequence of inadequate penetrability across the epithelial barrier. Poor corneal penetration was remedied by

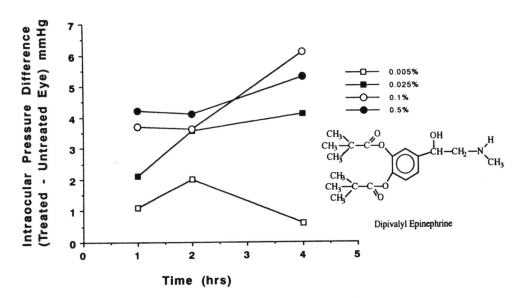

Figure 4.   Average intraocular pressure measurements (treated eye–fellow eye; mm Hg) over time for four topical doses of dipivalyl epinephrine solutions given to ten ocular hypertensive patients. (Graph constructed from data in Ref. 26.)

preparing an isopropyl ester of the parent drug which reduced IOP at much lower doses than prostaglandin $F_{2\alpha}$ in cat and human eyes (37).

Obviously, a prodrug must not only be capable of being converted metabolically in the eye to the active drug prior to reaching the target tissue but also have sufficient stability to provide an adequate shelf life. Larsen et al. (38) prepared model prodrugs of N-acyl sulfonamide derivatives; in particular, N-methyl-p-toluene sulfonamide showed ideal properties. It was water soluble, sufficiently stable at pH 4, and could be rapidly converted to the parent sulfonamide following corneal penetration.

A series of prodrug esters of timolol were prepared by Chien et al. (31) with a wide range of log DC values from 0 to 4.5 and compared in vivo following topical application to the intact rabbit eye. Figure 5 shows the results of measurements of aqueous humor concentrations of timolol at 20 min postdosing plotted against their respective log DC values. The relationship is a parabolic one for which timolol, the most hydrophilic of the series, has the lowest concentration. At the apex of the parabola is O-valeryl timolol with a log DC of about 2.8. As the series becomes more lipophilic, the aqueous humor concentrations of timolol are reduced with the most lipophilic ester, O-octanoyl timolol, showing aqueous humor concentrations of timolol only slightly higher than from dosing the parent compound. Because the epithelium of the cornea functions as a barrier to penetration as well as a site for the hydrolysis of esters, the shape of Figure 5 varies depending on which factor predominates. As chain length varies, the enzymatic hydrolysis rate also varies but in a linear fashion. Binding affinities as well as steric considerations for a homolog series interact to determine the rate of esterase-mediated hydrolysis rates (28).

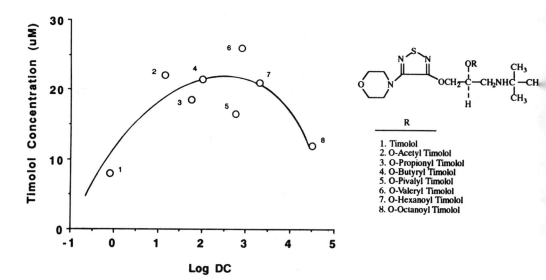

Figure 5. Relationship between timolol concentration in aqueous humor at 20 min following topical instillation of timolol ester prodrugs and their respective log distribution coefficient (DC) measured in octanol/buffer (pH 7.4). (Graph constructed from data in Ref. 31.)

B. Lipophilicity and Noncorneal Routes of Administration into the Anterior Chamber

It has always been assumed that the major route of drug entry into the anterior chamber is by corneal penetration. However, penetration across the conjunctiva and sclera may also be a significant route of entry into the anterior chamber. Ahmed and Patton (39) have shown that inulin (hydrophilic) and timolol (moderately lipophilic) can enter the iris-ciliary body in significant concentrations by either corneal or scleral pathways. In addition to entering the anterior chamber, once drug enters conjunctival and scleral tissue, uptake into fenestrated blood vessels can also occur. Maren and Jankowska (4) evoked this reasoning when two experimental CAIs, both of which inhibited carbonic anhydrase in vitro, were not effective when administered topically in lowering IOP in the rabbit.

Reduced systemic absorption resulting from uptake by blood vessels in the sclera was observed in a study by Ahmed et al. (41), who determined the barrier properties of both the sclera and the cornea for propranolol, timolol, nadalol, penbutolol, sucrose, and inulin. Overall permeability across the sclera was significantly higher than values obtained for the cornea for all drugs tested. However, the relative degrees of difference for the tissues varied with the partitioning behavior of the particular drug. For example, corneal resistance to inulin, the latter a polar compound with a high molecular weight, was much greater than scleral resistance. However, when timolol was compared, the resistance of each tissue was the same. The results of the study showed that the epithelium of the cornea provides a much greater barrier resistance to hydrophilic drugs than the outer layer of the sclera. For a more lipophilic drug, such as timolol, the sclera and cornea behave similarly with regard to barrier resistance.

Recent confirmation of these observations was reported in a study by Chien et al. (42) in which corneal versus scleral penetration were compared for clonidine, p-aminoclonidine, and a 6-quinoxalinyl derivative of clonidine (AGN 190342). A corneal well, fashioned from contact lens material, was secured to the corneoscleral junction using a cyanoacrylate adhesive. Drug solution was applied to either the cornea or to the sclera, depending on whether solution was placed inside or outside the well. Table 3 shows that when any of the

Table 3. Tissue Concentrations (ng/mL or ng/g) of Clonidine, AGN 190342, and p-Aminoclonidine Following Constant Concentration of 200 ng/mL Applied to Either the Corneal or Conjunctival Regions of the Rabbit Eye

Route	Conjunctiva	Cornea	Aqueous humor	Ciliary body
Corneal				
p-Aminoclonidine	0.230	8.03	0.55	0.17
AGN 190342	0.41	58.5	7.54	1.51
Clonidine	0.68	76.5	11.4	2.13
Conjunctival/scleral				
p-Aminoclonidine	5.99	1.46	0.038	0.312
AGN 190342	10.89	4.10	0.131	0.840
Clonidine	4.06	2.21	0.126	0.369

Source: Data from Ref. 48.

three derivatives of clonidine were maintained on the cornea of anesthetized rabbits for a duration of 60 min, drug concentration followed the trend: cornea > aqueous humor > ciliary body > conjunctiva. However, when drug was applied to the conjunctiva and excluded from the cornea, also for 60 min, the order became: conjunctiva > cornea > ciliary body > aqueous humor. From the corneal route clonidine and AGN 190342, which are similar in distribution coefficient (log Oct/buffer pH 7.4: 0.52 and 0.17, respectively), yielded nearly similar tissue concentrations. However, p-aminoclonidine, which is hydrophilic (log Oct/buffer pH 7.4: −0.96), yielded much lower tissue concentrations. When the drugs were applied exclusively to the conjunctiva, p-aminoclonidine yielded tissue concentrations that were less than the other two moderately lipophilic compounds but was considerably closer in value than when the three analogs were applied to the cornea. Maren and Jankowska (40) also indicated that lipophilic compounds diffuse rapidly through the conjunctival blood vessels and, therefore, are not ideal drug candidates for topical administration to the eye. These studies differentiated between sclera and cornea but do not suggest how a drug, once it enters the sclera, could be structurally designed to differentiate between uptake by vessels residing in the conjunctiva and subsequent penetration through the sclera and enter into the anterior chamber. Similarly, it is not clear what drug properties are necessary to encourage, or prevent, uptake by blood vessels in the iris-ciliary body, the location of the active site for many drugs distributed to that tissue but also a potential elimination pathway. Although more work must be completed with other analog series, it is becoming apparent that hydrophilic drugs gain access to anterior chamber tissues in higher concentrations than expected because of their ability to penetrate the conjunctiva/scleral pathway. Hitoshi et al. (43) reported that the conjunctiva and cornea are quite different in lipophilic character and that prodrugs could be designed selectively to reduce systemic absorption.

C. Use of Solubility in Improving Absorption Across the Cornea

For drugs with relatively poor permeability (i.e., those drugs in Table 1 below 10×10^{-6} cm/s), a high concentration must be instilled into the eye to compensate for the low permeability. A high concentration of drug permits a greater penetration rate than compared to a drug with limited solubility. This is observed mathematically from equation 3:

$$MPR = (CPC)\ (\text{Tear Solubility}) \tag{3}$$

where MPR is the maximum attainable penetration rate across the corneal barrier and tear solubility represents the solubility of drug under physiological conditions (20). Examples of drugs which are hydrophilic and, therefore, rely on high concentrations applied to the eye in order to improving penetrability include phenylephrine, epinephrine, and sulfacetamide. All of these drugs are very soluble and have been used clinically in concentrations of 2–10%. For those drugs which are highly potent and require only a small amount to reach the anterior chamber to be effective, such as, timolol, chloramphenicol, prednisolone acetate, fluoromethalone, dexamethalone, or tobramycin. It is not necessary to apply a high concentration.

From equation 3, it is obvious that if a drug is poorly soluble in the precorneal tear film, its penetration rate can be self-limited by a relatively low concentration gradient. This result is most evident with the molecular modification of nonsteroidal anti-inflammatory agents (NSAIDs), which are not as potent as steroids and have a low penetration rate at the pH of the tears owing to ionization. Improvements have been sought in their therapeutic effectiveness by the preparation of poorly soluble esters which were expected to penetrate rapidly. These lipophilic prodrugs of NSAIDs do not ionize in the tears and have poor aqueous solubility but convert to the parent drug by esterases, which are prevalent in the epithelium of the cornea. The NSAID prodrugs have not shown a significant increase in effectiveness, most likely because of a relatively low penetration rate. Although the lipophilic prodrug has a higher permeability coefficient than the original NSAID, the net effect on the penetration rate is apparently greater from the loss in solubility from formation of the prodrug than from the gain achieved from an increase in its CPC. The nonlinearity in the relationships between CPC and partitioning account for the nonequal offsetting effects.

The apparent lower limit to permeability theoretically allows for the design of a very soluble analog which could be instilled at a high concentration. This occurs because as solubility increases for a hydrophilic analog series, it is possible for the penetration rate to proportionately increase because CPC remains at a constant lower limit. However, there is at least one other factor that would limit this approach. As the concentration of drug increases, the instilled solution eventually becomes hypertonic and irritates the eye, promoting tearing and reducing bioavailability.

In addition to the potential advantage from an increased penetration rate, a water-soluble analog or prodrug, which is effective as a solution, has manufacturing and stability advantages when compared to an effective lipophilic but poorly soluble drug, because the latter must be formulated as a sterile suspension. A suspended drug must be micronized for use in the eye so that abrasions to the cornea are not likely to occur. However, a micronized powder intended for use in ocular suspensions presents difficulties in sterilization. Once formulated, it must not show appreciable particle size changes, caking, or poor resuspendability upon storage. Inadequate resuspendability of ophthalmic suspensions has been shown to occur with commercial prednisolone acetate products, potentially leading to errors in dosing (45).

In spite of the above-mentioned difficulties, slightly soluble steroids, indicated for anterior chamber inflammations, such as prednisolone acetate, fluoromethalone, or dexamethasone acetate, are highly effective when administered as suspensions. A self-limiting penetration rate, predicted for slightly soluble steroids in suspension, is offset in part by their high potency relative to NSAIDs and also by an improved extent of absorption because of better ocular retention of suspension dosage forms compared to solutions.

Ponticello et al. (46) and other Merck scientists (47,48) have reported on a new analog series of topically effective water-soluble CAIs, thienothiopyran-2-sulfonamides, which were developed expressly for the advantages in manufacturing but when first proposed were considered also to have possible advantages in bioavailability. Two of their analogs, MK-927 and L-671,152, have significantly reduced IOP in hypertensive, cynomolgus monkeys when administered as topical solutions. The former has also been administered as a single 50 μL instillation of a 2% solution to each of 24 patients with ocular hypertension. These analogs as well as the prodrugs reported by Larson et al. (38) achieve water solubility with the use of an ionizable amino substituent.

Figure 6 shows a mean peak decline of 77 mm Hg (−26.9%) in IOP occurring at 4.5 h after a topical dose of a 2% water-soluble derivative, MK-927 (49). Further analog modification has led to the development of L-662,583, a thiophene-2-sulfonamide, which also achieves water solubility from an ionizable amino functionality (50). Sugrue et al. (50) reported that it is more potent than MK-927 when expressed as $IC_{50}s$ (in vitro) but may not

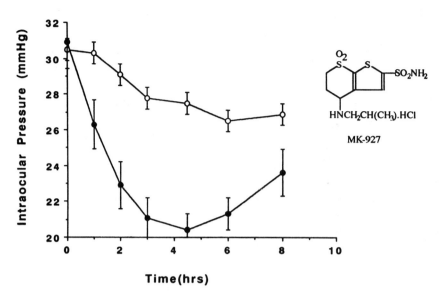

Figure 6. Comparison of mean IOP values measured over time for one drop of 2% MK-927 on the day of treatment and in the same eye on a pretreatment day. (Graph constructed from data in Ref. 49.)

be more effective in reducing IOP in hypertensive, cynomolgus monkeys when both are instilled at a concentration of 2%. The authors suggested that L-662,583 may not penetrate the cornea as well as MK-927. However, any benefit in penetration occurring from highly water-soluble analogs would be realized only with the application to the eye of a high concentration. The effect of higher concentrations for L-662,583 was not reported.

D. Correlation of Structural Parameters to Corneal Absorption

Clearly, modifications in chemical structure to produce a new analog series which is designed to improve absorption can be limited in approach when compared to prodrug modifications if potency, absorption, or disposition are negatively affected. On the other hand, if a portion of the molecule can be modified without affecting processes other than absorption, very specific information regarding drug design and pharmacokinetic processes can be obtained as compared to correlations of physicochemical parameters that are representative primarily of the properties of the entire molecule.

The contribution of partitioning and electronic properties of specific functional groups on the ocular penetration of the parent drug has been studied as a specific approach by Eller et al. (20). Their intention was to improve the pharmacological activity of CAIs by improving the ocular penetration of 2-benzothiazolesulfonamides. In order to more accurately define an optimally penetrating structure, the partitioning and electronic properties, pi and sigma$_p$, respectively, of various 6-substituents to benzene of the 2-benzothiazole sulfonamides was mathematically related to their corneal permeability. The analog series shown in Table 4, of which ethoxzolamide is a member, were all active when tested in vitro for their inhibitory activity against CA, indicating that the pharmacophore was not affected.

Table 4. Physicochemical Properties of Active Carbonic Anhydrase Inhibitors and Related Structures

Drug	pK_a	Solubility (mg/mL: pH)	IC50[a] (CA II: nM)
Acetazolamide	7.2	2.2 (7.8)	10.8
Methazolamide	7.3	5.9 (7.8)	21.2
Trifluoromethazolamide	6.6	35.0 (7.8)	20.0
Dichlorphenamide	8.3/9.8	0.7 (7.8)	55.6
Ethoxzolamide	8.1	0.015 (7.65)	4.1
6-Hydroxyethoxy-2-benzothiazolesulfonamide	7.9	0.31 (7.65)	11.6
Aminozolamide	8.0	0.27 (7.65)	14.7
L-650,719[b]	9.0	6.0 (8.1)	—
L-645,152[c]	—	—	2.2
MK-927[d]	—	20[e]	1.2
MK-417[f]	—	20[e]	0.54
L-662,583[g]	—	—	0.7
L-643,799[h]	7.8/9.26	0.7 (6.5)	6.0

[a]Comparisons of values to determine relative potencies cannot legitimately be made, since experimental conditions vary; nevertheless, large differences (i.e., 5–10×) likely indicate greater potency for the smaller value.
[b]6-Hydroxybenzo[b]thiophene-2-sulfonamide
[c](S,S-5,6-Dihydro-4H-4-ethylamine-6-methylthieno-(2,3b)-thiopyran-2-sulfonamide-7,7-dioxide hydrochloride
[d]d,1-5,6-Dihydro-4-(2-methylpropylamino)-4H-thieno-[2,3b]thiopyran-2-sulphonamide-7,7-dioxide hydrochloride
[e]Compounds were soluble in vehicle consisting of 0.5% aqueous hydroxyethylcellulose (75).
[f]The S + isomer of MK-927.
[g]5-(3-Dimethylaminomethyl-4-hydroxyphenylsulphonyl)thiophene-2-sulfonamide hydrochloride
[h]6-Hydroxy-2-benzothiazidesulfonamide

Ethoxzolamide is effective in lowering IOP when taken orally but not when instilled topically to the eye. It was hypothesized that if a significant improvement in the rate and extent of corneal absorption could be accomplished by an analog, then topical activity would result. Eller et al. (51) expanded equation 3 interrelating pK_a, DC, CPC, and solubility to pi and sigma$_p$ through a series of algebraic substitutions. Pi and sigma$_p$ are mathematically defined by equations 4 and 5:

$$pK_a = rho \ (sigma_p) + (pK_a)_H \tag{4}$$

$$log \ (DC)_X = c \ (pi)_X + log \ (DC)_H \tag{5}$$

where rho and c are equation parameters determined from regression analysis of the experimental data, the subscript H denotes the 6-hydrogen substituent as compared to any substituent (X) at the same 6 position on benzene of the 2-benzothiazole sulfonamide.

Figure 7 shows a three-dimensional view of the predicted MPR as a function of the electronic (sigma$_p$) and partitioning (pi) factors for substituents on the 6-substituted 2-benzothiazolesulfonamides. From this plot an optimal range of sigma$_p$ (–0.2 to 0.95) and pi (–0.8 to 0.95) values were identified (51). Pi and sigma$_p$ can be obtained from tables of values which exist for many substituent groups (52), so that once an optimal range is

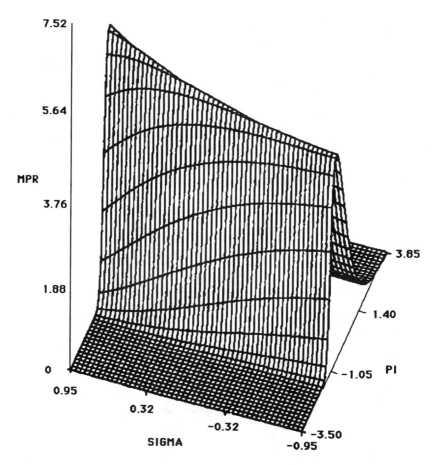

Figure 7. Three-dimensional view of the predicted maximal penetration rate (MPR) as a function of pi and sigma values for substituents on 6-substituted 2-benzothiazole sulfonamides. (Graph constructed from data in Ref. 51.)

established for a given series, substituents can be chosen which would be expected to show a significant improvement in penetration rate. Constraints, such as potential toxicity, availability of a synthetic pathway, and chemical stability, can limit the selection of a specific substituent in the optimal range. Nevertheless, the technique reduces the synthesis to a reasonably few compounds which are likely to show optimal penetrability.

Because of restricted pH and tonicity ranges required for an ophthalmic product, it could be beneficial to adjust the pK_a of a drug to a specific range. Substitutions affecting induction and/or resonance would affect penetration by altering the percent ionized at physiological pH. If the percent ionized is significantly high, then the rate and extent of absorption may be too low for a therapeutic effect to occur. Although manipulation of the pK_a to achieve improved absorption has not been attempted, one would have to be aware that changes in pK_a due to changes in structure could also impact on other phenomena (either known or unknown), such as potency or disposition of the drug within the eye.

III. IMPROVEMENT IN OCULAR DISTRIBUTION

In general, systemic distribution of a drug depends on blood flow, blood volume within tissues, partitioning, and binding. Blood flow and blood volume are physiological factors that are independent of a drug's structure, whereas partitioning and binding are specific to structure and indirectly determine duration and reservoir accumulation but often directly determine activity based upon binding to a specific receptor site.

In spite of the importance for drug to reach the target tissue in sufficient concentrations, little information is available for ocular drugs, or for that matter drugs intended for systemic use, regarding structural features that are responsible for optimizing distribution to the active site. Reasons may be related to a number of factors, such as indirect measurement of pharmacokinetic parameters that do not adequately describe the rate and extent of distribution as well as absorption or elimination. Further, the volume of distribution, which is an indirect measurement that indicates the extent to which drug distributes out of plasma, is also a relative measurement that does not differentiate between the active site and a reservoir site.

Whenever direct measurement of drug distribution is sought, difficulties arise in anatomically identifying the active site, surgically removing it from animal models without including adjacent tissue, extracting drug without interference from extraneous tissue substances and, of course, not having assay methodology available which is sufficiently sensitive to measure low concentrations.

There are relatively few studies identifying the relationship between physicochemical or structural parameters and the active site of ocular drugs. In one such study focusing on CAIs, Michelson et al. (53) studied the ocular pharmacokinetic properties of the topically active MK-927 and compared it to acetazolamide. They found that both CAIs had nearly equal IC_{50}s and also penetrated the cornea at nearly equivalent rates; however, only MK-927 was active when both CAIs were tested topically for a decrease in IOP in the rabbit eye. Consequently, their similarity in potency and absorption processes prompted other phenomena to be studied in order to explain their differences in activity when dosed topically. The authors hypothesized that a higher scleral penetration rate permitted MK-927, but not acetazolamide, to reach the iris-ciliary body without first entering the anterior chamber. Further studies, including distributive phenomena, such as partitioning and/or binding to target tissue, are required to identify more clearly the mechanism responsible for MK-927 to reach the target tissue in higher concentrations than acetazolamide.

In a series of studies (54–57) focusing on the IOP-lowering capability of 2-benzo-thiazolesulfonamide analogs, it was observed that only the poorly penetrating 6-amino and the 6-hydroxyethoxy analogs (see Table 5) were active in lowering IOP in high-pressure rabbit and monkey eyes when instilled topically. There was no relationship between corneal penetrability and topical activity. The ocular disposition of the poorly penetrating 6-amino analog was studied and showed that its topical activity was due to the formation, accumulation, and retention of an acetylated metabolite. The metabolite, a 6-acetamido analog, was synthesized and found to be active in inhibiting CA but not active when instilled topically into either the high-pressure–induced rabbit or monkey eye. The authors concluded that the metabolite, when formed at the active site by aryl N-acetyltransferase, was well retained but when dosed topically was not absorbed and/or distributed in sufficient concentrations to be active. For these analogs, potency and distribution were primary factors important in achieving topical activity; however, bioavailability, although not a primary factor, is apparently an important secondary factor. In these studies, scleral penetration rate was not measured and, therefore, could not be excluded as an additional mechanism to help explain the results.

The significance of scleral penetration as a more direct route to the iris-ciliary body has not been well documented for CAIs. However, Bar-Ilan et al. (58) reported on the ocular disposition of a new CAI (L-650,719) and found that it had moderate corneal penetration, water solubility (<0.2% at pH 8.1), and partitioning and high but not unusually high inhibitory activity against CA. Nevertheless, high concentrations of drug were found in the iris-ciliary body of the rabbit eye compared to aqueous humor concentrations following topical instillation of 0.5 mL of 0.25 to 1% suspensions maintained in the conjunctival sac for 10 min. The authors concluded that drug could be reaching the target site by the scleral as well as the corneal pathway.

Table 4 lists CAIs that have shown a significant lowering of IOP in the high-pressure–induced rabbit and/or monkey eye when dosed topically. At the present time, there are no clear indications why these agents are topically active compared to those which are not active. No doubt a number of factors must be optimized for activity to occur. Although Schoenwald and coworkers (51,54–57) have suggested that distribution is a key factor for topical CAI activity for one CAI (6-amino-2-benzothiazolesulfonamide), preferential scleral penetrability (in comparison to corneal penetration), as suggested by Merck scientists (4,46–49), is also a plausible explanation and may be occurring for a number of CAIs.

Evidence that this latter phenomena is primarily responsible for topical activity of CAIs comes from a recent comparison of corneal and scleral permeability across excised human and rabbit tissue for four CAIs (59). The two lipid-soluble compounds, methazolamide and ethoxzolamide, showed the same permeability rate in the two species, but the two hydrophilic compounds, benzolamide and bromacetazolamide, were 10-fold greater in permeability for human corneas. If these results can be extrapolated to other lipophilic and hydrophilic CAIs, it could be concluded that the pore pathway is more easily accessed in the human sclera as compared to rabbit sclera. If this is correct, a comparison of decline in IOP from topical instillation of these compounds in human eyes would show relatively greater activity than results from rabbit eyes. In reality, the opposite has occurred; results in human eyes have been less than expected from the rabbit or monkey results (50), which has been attributed to compensating factors for the human eye, such as a four- or fivefold greater blinking rate, a twofold greater tear turnover, and a twofold lower corneal/conjunctival area (2).

The CAIs are classified according to their pharmacological activity and not according to structure. Therefore, it is plausible that no single phenomena (e.g., SAR, physicochemical, pharmacokinetic) can be identified as the "most" significant because of the additive and/or compensating effect that significantly different structures (e.g., benzothiazoles, thiopyran, thiadiazoles) can have on a drug's therapeutic activity. Because of the considerable amount of work that has been generated in the development of a topically active CAI, various properties have been identified for topical activity based upon sufficient potency, distribution, and/or retention at the active site, adequate bioavailability, and lack of sensitization.

IV. IMPROVEMENT IN OCULAR ELIMINATION

Drugs are eliminated from internal tissues and fluids of the eye by metabolism, bulk aqueous humor turnover, and by systemic uptake by the highly vascular tissues of the anterior uvea (3). Although a number of enzyme systems have been identified with eye tissues (60–63), only esterases have been well studied; likely because of their importance to conversion of a prodrug to an active drug (15,28,31,32,64). Less information is known about other enzyme systems that are responsible for the elimination of drugs. Theoretically, it should be possible to prolong activity by reducing the rate of elimination, specifically by systemic uptake by vessels in the uvea. Whereas little if any research has been done to alter loss of drug by either blood or aqueous humor turnover, metabolic pathways have been studied as a tool in the design of new ophthalmic drugs.

A. Ophthalmic Drug Design Using Metabolic Pathways

Recently, Bodar and coworkers (65–67) have applied a knowledge of metabolic pathways to design new agents, many of which have been derived from drugs of ophthalmic interest. Referred to as soft drugs, these unique drugs have shown a marked improvement in ocular disposition and, most importantly, an improved therapeutic profile. Whereas prodrugs generally allow for control of the absorption process by conversion of an inactive drug into an active drug, soft drugs are designed to alter the drug's elimination profile. By studying the factors that affect the metabolic process, it has been possible to design a drug which would be converted from active drug into inactive drug, purposely either to extend or to shorten the drug's half-life.

For example, a soft analog of atropine has been prepared which when applied to the rabbit eye produced a much shorter duration of action than atropine; also, mydriasis in the fellow eye was absent, indicating that an inactive metabolite was rapidly formed (68). A potent mydriatic with a rapid onset and a short duration of action is advantageous because it allows the clinician to perform rapidly the procedure with the patient's vision returning to normal as soon as possible. Atropine is not often used to dilate the eye in ophthalmoscopy or other ocular procedures, because its cycloplegic and mydriatic effects can last as long as 1–2 weeks in susceptible patients (65). In another example, Wu et al. (67) studied the ophthalmic application of a series of soft drugs prepared from the acidic metabolite or metoprolol. The adamantylethyl ester was formulated as a 1% solution and compared to timolol for its ability to lower IOP in the normal rabbit eye. Compared to timolol, the adamantylethyl ester showed a prolonged and more significant reduction of IOP (Fig. 8) and, in a separate experiment, showed a reduced potential for systemic side effects based upon measurements conducted on rats with isoprenaline-induced tachycardia.

V. CONCLUSIONS

From the preceding discussion, it is apparent that molecular modifications to specifically improve the ocular pharmacokinetics of a drug should be considered during design of a new drug. Improvements of manyfold are possible, which in fact may be greater than one could achieve from formulation approaches. Nevertheless, one must be cautious in modifying chemical structure, since any number of phenomena may be adversely affected—potency, absorption, disposition, or toxicity. When structural-activity relationships have been well established, and it can be determined that only one pharmacokinetic process (i.e., ADME)

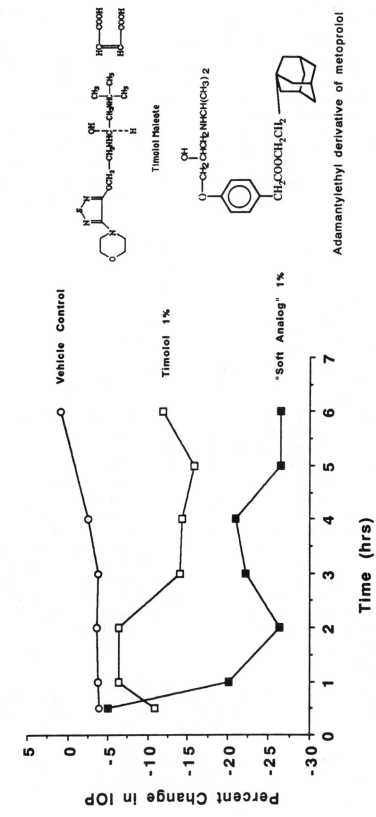

Figure 8. Percent change in IOP over time from topical administration of 1% solutions of timolol or a "soft" analog of metoprolol compared to vehicle in the high pressure induced (alpha-chymotrypsin) rabbit eye (n=4). (Graph constructed from data in Ref. 67.)

is responsible for a poor therapeutic profile, it should be feasible by the use of prodrug or analog modification to improve pharmacokinetic behavior.

REFERENCES

1. Anonymous (1990). When adults take medicine: Improper use, a national health problem. *In: Pharmacy Update* (E. Moran, ed.). American Pharmaceutical Association, Oct. 1, p. 5.
2. Lee, V. H. L., and Robinson, J. R. (1986). Review: Topical ocular drug delivery: Recent developments and future challenges, *J. Ocul. Pharmacol.*, 2:67.
3. Maurice, D. M., and Mishima, S. (1984). Ocular pharmacokinetics. *In: Pharmacology of the Eye* (M. L. Sears, ed.). Springer-Verlag, Berlin, pp. 19–116.
4. Plazonnet, B., Grove, J., Durr, M., Mazuel, C., Quint, M., and Rozier, A. (1987). Pharmacokinetics and biopharmaceutical aspects of some anti-glaucoma drugs. *In: Ophthalmic Drug Delivery Biopharmaceutical Technological and Clinical Aspects*, Vol. 11 (M. F. Saettone, M. Bucci, and P. Speiser, eds.). Liviana Press, Springer-Verlag, Berlin, pp. 118–139.
5. Schoenwald, R. D. (1985). The control of drug bioavailability from ophthalmic dosage forms. *In: Controlled Drug Bioavailability*, Vol. 3 (V. F. Smolen and L. A. Ball, eds.). Wiley, New York, pp. 257–306.
6. Burstein, N. L., and Anderson, J. A. (1985). Corneal penetration and ocular bioavailability of drugs. *J. Ocul. Pharmacol.*, 1:309.
7. Shell, J. W. (1985). Ophthalmic drug delivery systems, *Drug. Dev. Res.*, 6:245.
8. Chrai, S. S., Patton, T. F., Mehta, A., and Robinson, J. R. (1973). Lacrimal and instilled fluid dynamics in rabbit eyes, *J. Pharm. Sci.*, 62:1112.
9. Fraunfelder, F. T., and Meyer, S. M. (1987). Systemic side effects from ophthalmic timolol and their prevention. *J. Ocul. Pharmacol.*, 3:177.
10. Chrai, S. S., and Robinson, J. R. (1974). Ocular evaluation of methylcellulose vehicle in albino rabbits, *J. Pharm. Sci.*, 63:1218.
11. Patton, T. F., and Robinson, J. R. (1976). Quantitative precorneal disposition of topically applied pilocarpine nitrate in rabbit eyes. *J. Pharm. Sci.*, 65:1295.
12. Tang-Liu, D. D. S., Liu, S. S., and Weinkam, R. J. (1984). Ocular and systemic bioavailability of ophthalmic flurbiprofen, *J. Pharmacokinet. Biopharm.*, 12:611.
13. Chiang, C. H., and Schoenwald, R. D. (1986). Ocular pharmacokinetic models of clonidine-^{3}H hydrochloride, *J. Pharmacokinet. Biopharm.*, 14:175.
14. Huang, H. S., Schoenwald, R. D., and Lach, J. L. (1983). Corneal penetration behavior of beta-blocking agents II: Assessment of barrier contributions, *J. Pharm. Sci.*, 72:1272.
15. Camber, O., Edman, P., and Olsson, L. I. (1986). Permeability of protaglandin F_{2alpha} and prostaglandin F_{2alpha} esters across cornea in vitro. *Int. J. Pharm.*, 29:259.
16. Igarashi, H., Sato, Y., Hamada, S., and Kawasaki, T. (1984). Studies on rabbit corneal permeability of local anesthetics. *Jpn. J. Pharmacol.*, 34:429.
17. Schoenwald, R. D., and Huang, H. S. (1983). Corneal penetration behavior of beta-blocking agents I: physicochemical factors. *J. Pharm. Sci.*, 72:1266.
18. Chiang, C. H., Huang, H. S., and Schoenwald, R. D. (1986). Corneal permeability of adrenergic agents potentially useful in glaucoma, *J. Taiwan Pharm. Assoc.*, 38:67.
19. Schoenwald, R. D., and Ward, R. L. (1978). Relationship between steroid permeability across excised rabbit cornea and octanol-water partition coefficients, *J. Pharm. Sci.*, 67:786.
20. Eller, M. G., Schoenwald, R. D., Dixson, J. A., Segarra, T., and Barfknecht, C. F. (1985). Topical carbonic anhydrase inhibitors III: Optimization model for corneal penetration of ethoxzolamide analogues, *J. Pharm. Sci.*, 74:155.
21. Mosher, G. L., and Mikkelson, T. J. (1979). Permeability of the n-alkyl p-aminobenzoate esters across the isolated corneal membrane of the rabbit, *Int. J. Pharm.*, 2:239.

22. Ellingson, C. M., and Schoenwald, R. D. (1992). Rapid toxicological model for use in assessing ocular drugs, *Biopharm. Drug Dispos.*, (in press).
23. Maren, M. H., and Jankowska, L. (1985). Ocular pharmacology of sulfonamides: The cornea as barrier and depot. *Curr. Eye Res.*, 4:399.
24. Corbo, D. C., Liu, J. C., and Chien, Y. W. (1990). Characterization of the barrier properties of mucosal membranes, *J. Pharm. Sci.*, 79:202.
25. Grass, G. M., and Robinson, J. R. (1988). Mechanisms of corneal drug penetration II: Ultrastructural analysis of potential pathways for drug movement, *J. Pharm. Sci.*, 77:15.
26. Karback, M. B., Podos, S. M., Harbin, T. S., Mandell, A., and Becker, B. (1976). The effects of dipivalyl epinephrine on the eye, *Am. J. Ophthalmol.*, 81:768.
27. Goldberg, I., Kolker, A. E., Kass, M. A., and Becker, B. (1980). Dipivefren: Current concepts, *Aust. J. Ophthalmol.*, 8:147.
28. Chang, S. C., Bundgaard, H., Buur, A., and Lee, V. H. L. (1987). Improved corneal penetration of timolol by prodrugs as a means to reduce systemic drug load, *Invest. Ophthalmol. Vis. Sci.*, 28:487.
29. Schoenwald, R. D., Folk, J. C., Kumar, V., and Piper, J. G. (1987). In vivo comparison of phenylephrine and phenylephrine oxazolidine instilled in the monkey eye, *J. Ocul. Pharmacol.*, 3:333.
30. Chien, D. S., and Schoenwald, R. D. (1986). Improving the ocular absorption of phenylephrine, *Biopharm. Drug Dispos.*, 7:453.
31. Chien, D. S., Bundgaard, H., and Lee, V. H. L. (1988). Influence of corneal epithelial integrity on the penetration of timolol prodrugs, *J. Ocul. Pharmacol.*, 4:137.
32. Bundgaard, H., Falch, E., Larsen, C., and Mikkelsen, T. (1996). Pilocarpine prodrugs I. Synthesis, physicochemical properties and kinetics of lactonization of pilocarpic acid esters, *J. Pharm. Sci.*, 75:36.
33. Bundgaard, H., Falch, E., Larsen, C., Mosher, G. L., and Mikkelson, T. (1986). Pilocarpine prodrugs II. Synthesis, stability, bioconversion, and physicochemical properties of sequentially labile pilocarpine acid diesters, *J. Pharm. Sci.*, 75:775.
34. Narukar, M. M., and Mitra, A. K. (1989). Prodrugs of 5 lodo-2'-deoxyuridine for enhanced ocular transport, *Pharm. Res.*, 6:887.
35. Bito, L. Z., and Baroody, R. A. (1987). The ocular pharmacokinetics of eicosanoids and their derivatives. 1. Comparison of ocular eicosanoid penetration and distribution following the topical application of PGF 2alpha†, PGF 2alpha†-1-methyl ester, and PGF 2alpha†-1-isopropyl ester. *Exp. Eye Res.*, 44:217.
36. Bito, L. Z., Prostaglandins and other eicosanoids: Their ocular transport, pharmacokinetics, and therapeutic effects, *Trans. Ophthalmol. Soc. U.K.*, 105:162.
37. Kerstetter, J. R., Brubaker, R. F., Wilson, S. E., and Kullerstrand, L. J. (1988). Prostaglandin F2-alpha-1-isopropyl ester lowers intraocular pressure without decreasing aqueous humor flow, *Am. J. Ophthalmol.*, 105:30.
38. Larsen, J. D., Bundgaard, H., and Lee, V. H. L. (1988). Prodrug forms for the sulfonamide group. II. Water-soluble amino acid derivatives of N-methylsulfonamides as possible prodrugs, *Int. J. Pharm.*, 47:103.
39. Ahmed, I., and Patton, T. F. (1985). Importance of the noncorneal absorption route in topical ophthalmic drug delivery, *Invest. Ophthalmol. Vis. Sci.*, 26:584.
40. Maren, T. H., and Jankowska, L. (1985). Ocular pharmacology of sulfonamides: The cornea as barrier and depot, *Curr. Eye Res.*, 4:399.
41. Ahmed, I., Gokhale, R. D., Shah, M. V., and Patton, T. F. (1987). Physicochemical determinants of drug diffusion across the conjunctiva, sclera, and cornea, *J. Pharm. Sci.*, 76:583.
42. Chien, D. S., Homsy, J. J., Gluchowski, C., and Tang-liu, D. D. S. (1990). Corneal and conjunctival/scleral penetration of p-aminoclonidine, AGN 190342, and clonidine, *Curr. Eye Res.*, 9:1051.

43. Hitoshi, S., Bundgaard, H., and Lee, V. H. L. (1989). Design of prodrugs to selectively reduce timolol absorption on the basis of the differential lipophilic characteristics of the cornea and the conjunctiva. *Invest. Ophthalmol. Vis. Sci.*, 30(Suppl.):25.
44. 66. Rao, C. S., and Schoenwald, R. D. (1992). Biopharmaceutical evaluation of ibufenac, ibuprofen, and their hydroxyethoxy analogs in the rabbit eye, *J. Pharmacokinet. Biopharm.*, (in press.).
45. Apt, L., Henrick, A., and Silverman, L. M. (1979). Patient compliance with use of topical ophthalmic corticosteroids, *Am. J. Ophthalmol.*, 87:210.
46. Ponticello, G. S., Freedman, M. B., Habecker, C. N., Lyle, P. A., Schwam, H., Varga, S. L., Christy, M. E., Randall, W. C., and Baldwin, J. J. (1987). Thienothiopyran-2-sulfonamides: A novel class of water-soluble carbonic anhydrase inhibitors. *J. Med. Chem.*, 30:591.
47. Sugrue, M. F., Gautheron, P., Grove, J., Mallorga, P., Viader, M. P., Schwam, H., Baldwin, J. J., Christy, M. E., and Ponticello, G. S., (1990). MK-927: A topically active ocular hypotensive carbonic anhydrase inhibitor, *J. Ocul. Pharmacol.*, 6:9.
48. Sugrue, M. F., Mallorga, P., Schwam, H., Baldwin, J. J., and Ponticello, G. S. (1990). A comparison of L-671,152 and MK-927, two topically effective ocular hypotensive carbonic anhydrase inhibitors, in experimental animals, *Curr. Eye Res.*, 9:607.
49. Pfeiffer, N., Hennekes, R., Lippa, E. A., Grehn, F., Garus, H., and Brunner-Ferber, F. L. (1990). A single dose of the topical carbonic anhydrase inhibitor MK-927 decreases IOP in patients, *Br. J. Ophthalmol.*, 74:405.
50. Sugrue, M. F., Gautheron, P., Mallorga, P., Nolan, T. E., Graham, S. L., Schwam, H., Shepard, K. L., and Smith, R. L. (1990). L-662,583 is a topically effective ocular hypotensive carbonic anhydrase inhibitor in experimental animals, *Br. J. Pharmacol.*, 99:59.
51. Eller, M. G., Schoenwald, R. D., Dixson, J. A., Segarra, T., and Barfknecht, C. F. (1985). Topical carbonic anhydrase inhibitors IV: Relationship between excised corneal permeability and pharmacokinetic factors, *J. Pharm. Sci.*, 74:525.
52. Hansch, C., and Leo, A. (1983). *Log P and Parameter Database*. Comtex Scientific Corp., New York.
53. Michelson, S. R., Schwam, H., Baldwin, J. J., Mallorga, G. S., Ponticello, R. L., Smith, R. L., and Sugrue, M. F. (1989). Topically instilled MK-927: Lack of correlation between corneal penetration rate constant and ocular hypotensive activity in rabbits. *Invest. Ophthalmol. Vis. Sci.*, 30(Suppl.):24.
54. Lewis, R. A., Schoenwald, R. D., Eller, M. G., Barfknecht, C. F., and Phelps, C. D. (1984). Ethoxzolamide analogue gel. A topical carbonic anhydrase inhibitor, *Arch. Ophthalmol.*, 102:1821.
55. Lewis, R. A., Schoenwald, R. D., Barfknecht, C. F., and Phelps, C. D. (1986). Aminozolamide gel. A trial of a topical carbonic anhydrase inhibitor in ocular hypertension, *Arch. Ophthalmol.*, 104:842.
56. Lewis, R. A., Schoenwald, R. D., and Barfknecht, C. F. (1988). Aminozolamide suspension: The role of the vehicle in a topical carbonic anhydrase inhibitor, *J. Ocul. Pharmacol.*, 4:215.
57. Putnam, M. L., Schoenwald, R. D., Duffel, M. W., Barfknecht, C. F., Segarra, T. M., and Campbell, D. A. (1987). Ocular disposition of aminozolamide in the rabbit eye. *Invest. Ophthalmol. Vis. Sci.*, 28:1373.
58. Bar-Ilan, A., Pessah, N. I., and Maren, T. H. (1989). Ocular hypotensive activity and disposition of the topical carbonic anhydrase inhibitor 6-hydroxy-benzo[b]thiophene-2-sulfonamide, L-650,719, in the rabbit, *J. Ocul. Pharmacol.*, 5:99.
59. Edelhauser, H. F., and Maren, T. H. (1988). Permeability of human cornea and sclera to sulfonamide carbonic anhydrase inhibitors. *Arch. Ophthalmol.*, 106:1110.
60. Lee, V. H. L., Chang, S. C., Oshiro, C. M., and Smith, R. E. (1985). Ocular esterase composition in albino and pigmented rabbits: Possible implications in ocular prodrug design and evaluation. *Curr. Eye Res.*, 4:1117.

61. Bergamini, M. V. W. (1984). The metabolic mechanisms affecting drug actions in the eye. *In*: *Glaucoma: Applied Pharmacology in Medical Treatment* (S. M. Drance and A. H. Neufeld, eds.). Grune & Stratton, Orlando, Florida, pp. 151–184.

62. Lee, V. H. L., Chien, D. S., and Sasaki, H. (1988). Ocular ketone reductase distribution and its role in the metabolism of ocularly applied levobunolol in the pigmented rabbit, *J. Pharm. Exp. Ther.*, 246:871.

63. Shimada, S., Mishima, H., Kitamura, S., and Tatsumi, K. (1988). Metabolism of drugs in the eye. Drug-reducing activity of preparations from bovine ciliary body, *Curr. Eye Res.*, 7:1069.

64. Lee, V. H. L., Morimoto, K. M., and Stratford, Jr., R. E. (1982). Esterase distribution in the rabbit cornea and its implications in ocular drug bioavailability, *Biopharm. Drug Dispos.*, 3:291.

65. Bodar, N., and Varga, M. (1990). Effect of a novel soft steroid on the wound healing of rabbit cornea, *Exp. Eye Res.*, 50:183.

66. Bodar, N., and Prokai, L. (1990). Site- and stereospecific ocular drug delivery by sequential enzymatic bioactivation, *Pharm. Res.*, 7:723.

67. Bodar, N., El-Koussi, A. A., Kano, M., and Khalifa, M. (1988). Soft drugs. 7. Soft beta-blockers for systemic and ophthalmic use, *J. Med. Chem.*, 31:1651.

68. Wu, W. M., Hammer, R. H., and Bodor, N. (1988). Short-acting soft mydriatic agents. *Pharm. Res.*, 5(Suppl.):S99.

69. Wu, W. M., Hammer, R. H., and Bodor, N. (1988). Short-acting soft mydriatic agents. *Pharm. Res.*, 5(Suppl.):S99.

70. Havener, W. H. (1983). Ocular pharmacology. *In*: *Autonomic Drugs*, 5th ed. Mosby, St. Louis, pp. 379–390.

71. Duffel, M. W., Ing, I. S., Segarra, T. M., Dixson, J. A., Barfknecht, C. F., and Schoenwald, R. D. (1986). N-Substituted sulfonamide carbonic anhydrase inhibitors with topical effects on intra-ocular pressure, *J. Med. Chem.*, 29:1488.

72. Schoenwald, R. D., and Houseman, J. A. (1982). Disposition of cyclophosphamide in the rabbit and human cornea, *Biopharm. Drug Dispos.*, 3:231.

73. Qiu, Y. H., and Schoenwald, R. D., unpublished data.

74. Schoenwald, R. D. (1990). Ocular drug delivery. Pharmacokinetic considerations, *Clin. Pharmacokinet.*, 18:255.

75. Baldwin, J. J., Ponticello, G. S., Anderson, P. S., Christy, M. E., Murcko, M. A., Randall, W. C., Schwam, H., Sugrue, M. F., Springer, J. P., Gautheron, P., Grove, J., Mallorga, P., Viader, M.-P., Mckeever, B. M., and Navia, M. A. (1989). Thienothiopyran-2-sulfonamides: Novel topically active carbonic anhydrase inhibitors for the treatment of glaucoma, *J. Med. Chem.*, 32:2510.

16
Ocular Iontophoresis

**James M. Hill, Richard J. O'Callaghan, and
Jeffery A. Hobden** *Louisiana State University Medical Center
School of Medicine, New Orleans, Louisiana*

I. GENERAL PRINCIPLES OF IONTOPHORESIS

Iontophoresis (Greek *iontos* = ion; *phoresis* = to bear) is the process in which a direct current drives ions into cells or tissues. According to electrical principles, opposite charges attract one another and like charges repel. Therefore, cations (positive ions) are attracted to the cathode (negative electrode) and repelled by the anode (positive electrode). Similarly, anions (negative ions) are attracted to the anode and repelled by the cathode. When iontophoresis is used for drug delivery, the ions of importance are charged molecules of drug. If the drug molecules carry a positive charge, they are driven into the tissues at the anode; if negatively charged, at the cathode.

The basic design of an iontophoresis unit is a battery-operated device with a mA (milliampere) meter to measure the current, a rheostat to control the amount of current flowing through the system, and two electrodes. Platinum is the best material for the electrodes, since it releases almost no ions, undergoes degradation at a very slow rate, and is nontoxic.

Iontophoresis requires a complete electrical circuit in the body, with direct current passing from the anode to the cathode and from the cathode back to the anode. The two electrodes are placed as close to each other anatomically as possible; the current follows the path of least resistance through the body, which is an excellent conductor of electricity. Active processes occur where the electrodes are attached; ions (drugs) that enter cells or tissue near the electrode usually remain in those tissues until they are transported or altered by physiological processes. Figure 1 shows a diagram of ocular iontophoresis of a positively charged drug in a rabbit.

The solution or preparation to be iontophoresed should have a minimum of extraneous ions. The molecule to be delivered by iontophoresis should have a strong net charge (anionic or cationic). The salt form of a drug is usually used for iontophoresis, since the dissociated salt is highly soluble and has a high charge density. In general, the concentration of the ionized drug in solution can range from 0.01 to 5.0%. Other physicochemical

OCULAR IONTOPHORESIS

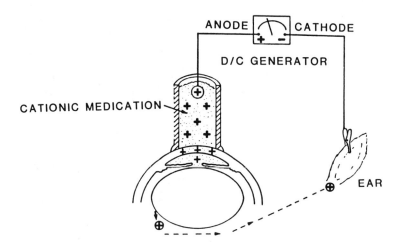

Figure 1. Ocular iontophoresis in the rabbit. The drug is placed in a cylindrical eye cup with a central diameter of 9–12 mm; the inner circumference of the eye cup fits within the corneoscleral limbus. The current is controlled by a rheostat on the direct current transformer. In general, the current should not exceed 2.0 mA and the time no longer than 10 min. In the case illustrated here, the drug molecules (cations) have a positive charge. Therefore, the platinum electrode connected to the anode (the positively charged pole) is placed in contact with the solution. The other electrode (cathode) is connected to the ear or front leg of the rabbit to complete the circuit. The positively charged anode drives the positively charged drug molecules from the solution into the eye at a greater rate than would be observed with simple diffusion.

characteristics, such as pH, conductivity, and ionic strength of the solution, often have to be determined for the specific drug or ion to be iontophoresed.

A. Electrical Laws

For ocular iontophoresis, only a few laws of physics and chemistry are important. One is Ohm's law:

$$V = IR$$

where V is the electromotive force in volts, I is the current in mA, and R is the resistance in ohms. At constant voltage, any change in resistance results in a change in the current. With ocular iontophoresis and most other iontophoretic applications, resistance decreases during the procedure. The result is that the current (mA) increases and must be reduced by adjustment of the rheostat. Any iontophoretic device that has a constant current compensator has an advantage over one that does not.

Another physical law important for ocular iontophoresis is Coulomb's law:

$$Q = IT$$

where Q is the quantity of electricity, I is the current in mA, and T is time in minutes. Thus, Q, which is the total current dosage, can be expressed as mA-minutes. Specific conditions for ocular iontophoresis can be expressed as a minimum, maximum, or range of mA-minutes.

Finally, a third important physical principle is Faraday's law:

$$D = \frac{IT}{IZIF}$$

where D is the drug delivered in gram-equivalents, I is the current in mA, T is time in minutes, IZI is the valence of the drug, and F is Faraday's constant. Faraday's constant is the electrical charge carried by 1 gram-equivalent of a substance. The importance of this relationship is that if more current is applied, more drug enters the ocular tissues.

II. HISTORICAL ASPECTS OF IONTOPHORESIS

Aetius, an ancient Greek physician, described the use of the shock of the torpedo ray, an electric fish, for the treatment of gout (1). The concept of applying a direct electric current to increase the penetration of charged particles into tissues for therapy was reportedly first described by Veratti in 1747. The first controlled studies of iontophoresis were conducted in 1901 by Leduc (2,3), who demonstrated the iontophoresis of strychnine sulfate and potassium cyanide in a classic rabbit experiment.

Sir Stewart Duke-Elder, in the 1962 edition of his classic work, *System of Ophthalmology* (4), reviewed the use of iontophoresis in ophthalmology from 1908 to 1956, citing more than 30 publications. The earliest description of ocular iontophoresis cited by Duke-Elder was published by Wirtz in 1908; he performed iontophoresis of zinc salts for the treatment of corneal ulcers. The most recent cited study was published in 1956 by Witzel (5) on the use of iontophoresis of antibiotics for the treatment of ocular infections. From 1936 to 1954, two prominent ophthalmologists, von Sallman (6–8) and Erlanger (9–11), were among the leading proponents of the clinical use of ocular iontophoresis.

Over the past 30 years, iontophoresis has been adapted for use in a variety of medical specialties, including dermatology, dentistry, and ophthalmology. Table 1 provides a list of selected reviews on iontophoresis (4,12–17) describing early and recent devices, as well as ocular and general medical applications, for this procedure.

Table 1. Iontophoresis Reviews

Topic	Author(s)	Year	Reference
Ocular therapy	Duke-Elder	1962	4
General aspects	Harris	1967	12
Dermatology	Sloan and Soltani	1986	13
Dentistry	Gangarosa	1983	14
Devices	Tyle	1986	15
Peptides and proteins	Banga and Chien	1988	16
Ocular drug delivery	Shofner et al.	1989	17

III. MEDICAL APPLICATIONS OF IONTOPHORESIS

A. Iontophoresis in General Medicine and Dentistry

1. Diagnosis of Cystic Fibrosis

Iontophoretic application of pilocarpine is a diagnostic test for cystic fibrosis (18,19) that is approved by the U.S. Food and Drug Administration. In this test, the iontophoresed pilocarpine induces sweating; high concentrations of sodium and chloride ions in the sweat are considered pathognomonic for the disease. This procedure, which has been widely employed since 1959, is particularly useful in children less than 1 year old, because it is essentially painless and takes only 3–5 min to complete.

2. Treatment of Hyperhidrosis

One of the most successful applications of iontophoresis is in the treatment of the dermatological disorder hyperhidrosis (13). Hyperhidrosis is a clinical condition resulting in extremely excessive sweating in various parts of the body; iontophoresis of tap water inhibits this sweating in localized areas. Although palmar and plantar hyperhidrosis have been treated very successfully with iontophoresis, the treatment of axillary hyperhidrosis has not been as successful.

3. Treatment of Hypersensitive Teeth and Oral Ulcers

Iontophoresis of sodium fluoride to teeth that are exquisitely sensitive to thermal stimuli has been a useful and successful therapy in dentistry (14). For example, teeth previously shown to be hypersensitive to cold lose their sensitivity to heat and cold immediately after iontophoresis of sodium fluoride and the effects are long lasting. The mechanisms by which teeth become hypersensitive and by which iontophoresis alleviates the condition are not fully understood. One possibility is that exposed dentin allows fluid movement through microtubules which stretch from the exposed surface to the pulp. Alternatively, the nerves near the pulp may become unusually excitable owing to exposure and constant stimulation. The mechanism of the reversal of hypersensitivity is probably related to one of these causal mechanisms; i.e., tubular blockage or reduction of nerve impulse generation.

Two common types of oral ulcers have been treated by iontophoresis of an antiviral or anti-inflammatory agent (14). Herpes orolabialis can be treated by idoxuridine or vidarabine monophosphate (Ara-AMP) iontophoresis (14). Aphthous lesions, which have no known etiology, are treated by methyl prednisolone sodium succinate iontophoresis (14).

B. Iontophoresis in Ophthalmology

Table 2 provides a list of the drugs, dyes, and other charged molecules reviewed below. The cations (positive ions) are used in anodal (positive electrode) iontophoresis; they include four antibiotics, one antifungal, one anesthetic agent, one adrenergic agonist (epinephrine), one adrenergic antagonist (timolol maleate), and two agents that act to inhibit the adrenergic metabolic pathway. The anions (negative ions) are used in cathodal (negative electrode) iontophoresis; they include three antivirals, two antibiotics, one steroid, one staining (dye) agent, and one antiproliferative agent.

Table 2. Ions Used in Ocular Iontophoresis

Ion	Potential clinical application
Cations used for anodal iontophoresis	
Gentamicin	T_x *Pseudomonas* keratitis
Tobramycin	T_x *Pseudomonas* keratitis
Ciprofloxacin	T_x *Pseudomonas* keratitis
Vancomycin	T_x *Pseudomonas* keratitis
Ketoconazole	T_x Fungal infection
Lidocaine	Anesthesia
Epinephrine	HSV-1 shedding
Timolol maleate	HSV-1 shedding
α-Methylparatyrosine	T_x glaucoma
6-Hydroxydopamine	T_x glaucoma
Anions used for cathodal iontophoresis	
Ara-AMP	T_x Herpes keratitis; stromal disease
Idoxuridine	T_x Herpes keratitis
Acyclovir	T_x Herpes stromal disease
Cefazolin	T_x Endophthalmitis
Ticarcillin	T_x Endophthalmitis
Dexamethasone	T_x Inflammation
Fluorescein	Study aqueous humor dynamics
5-Fluorouracil (5-FU)	Enhance glaucoma surgery, T_x ocular tumors

1. Glaucoma

a. Fluorescein for Studies of Aqueous Humor Dynamics

In 1966, Jones and Maurice (20) published a new method for measuring the rate of flow of the aqueous humor in patients using iontophoresis of fluorescein and a slit-lamp fluorophotometer. The iontophoresis solution (10% sodium fluorescein in 2% agar with 0.1% methylhydroxybenzylate as a preservative) was applied for 10–15 s with a current of 0.2 mA. No side effects were observed. Although their specific findings are not relevant to the purposes of this chapter, many of the procedures they developed are still used today by investigators studying aqueous humor or fluid dynamics of the anterior chamber. Other early investigators included Starr (21), who reported results similar to those of Jones and Maurice (20) using iontophoresis of fluorescein at 0.2 mA for 30–60 s, and Holm (22), who observed pupillary flow of fluorescein after saturating the anterior chamber by ionto-phoresis (0.5 mA for 4 min) through a cotton-wick electrode.

Tonjum and Green (23) quantified the effects of variable amounts of current and length of application on fluorescein iontophoresis through rabbit globes in an in vitro system. They used platinum electrodes, current ranging from 0.5 to 4.0 mA, and application times between 10 s and 4 min. They found that within this range, the amount of current was unimportant provided it was applied for at least 10 s.

In a 1982 review, Brubaker (24) described the procedures and techniques used to study the flow of aqueous humor in the human eye. He noted that these methods were essentially similar to those described in 1966 by Jones and Maurice (20). First, topical anesthesia was applied. Then a gel 5 mm in diameter, containing 2% agar and 10% fluorescein, was placed on the central cornea. The agar contained nonconducting salt other than sodium fluorescein and had significantly limited conductivity. A 45-V battery was used to apply the current. The agar gel constituted the negative electrode; to complete the circuit, the patient held the positive electrode in his hand. The current (0.2 mA) was applied for 5–7 s. The current was stopped before the agar and fluorescein were removed from the cornea to minimize the chance of producing a focal area of high current density. In more than 2500 iontophoretic applications of fluorescein, essentially no side effects of the iontophoretic procedure were observed.

b. Adrenergic Agents for Treatment of Glaucoma

In the early to mid-1970s, a number of investigators (25–29) conducted studies on ocular iontophoresis of 6-hydroxydopamine and α-methylparatyrosine, two pharmacological agents that block the synthesis of norepinephrine. 6-Hydroxydopamine, a congener of norepinephrine, causes the reversible destruction of nerve terminals in the anterior segment. The theory behind the treatment involved the depletion of ocular norepinephrine, which would result in an increased sensitivity to glaucoma drugs such as epinephrine.

Iontophoretic studies were done in rabbits, normal volunteers, and glaucoma patients with primary open-angle glaucoma. Kitazawa et al. (25,26) were the first to report the results of iontophoresis of 6-hydroxydopamine (1.0%, 0.75 mA, 3 min) in rabbit and human eyes. High concentrations of radiolabeled 6-hydroxydopamine were achieved in ocular tissues in rabbit eyes and intraocular pressure was reduced in normal human eyes. The results of a later study of patients with primary open-angle glaucoma treated by iontophoresis of 6-hydroxydopamine combined with topical epinephrine led Kitazawa et al. (27) to conclude that this regimen had some clinical value in the management of open-angle glaucoma.

Watanabe et al. (28) studied the iontophoresis of 6-hydroxydopamine in 137 eyes in 100 patients, 77 of which had primary open-angle glaucoma. In 49 patients with sufficient data for analysis, this procedure was therapeutically effective in 41%, questionable in 31%, and ineffective in 28%.

Colasanti and Trotter (29) iontophoresed rabbit eyes with α-methylparatyrosine (4.0%, 3 mA, 5 min). This drug, which is similar to 6-hydroxydopamine, produced a significant decrease in the concentration of norepinephrine in rabbit ocular tissues. No clinical studies with α-methylparatyrosine were done in normal human subjects or in patients with primary open-angle glaucoma.

All of the investigators (25–29) noted that iontophoresis was the most practical method for the administration of 6-hydroxydopamine to sensitize the eye to glaucoma drugs and that this procedure had some clinical value in the management of this disease. However, since long-acting antiglaucoma agents such as timolol, levobunolol, and betaxolol became available in the late 1970s, iontophoresis of 6-hydroxydopamine for the therapy of glaucoma has become superfluous.

c. 5-Fluorouracil for Control of Cellular Proliferation After Glaucoma Surgery

Kondo and Araie (30) published the first report describing transscleral iontophoresis of 5-fluorouracil (5.0%, 0.5 mA, 30 s) in the rabbit eye. An electrode 7 mm in diameter was placed on the bulbar conjunctiva 4 mm posterior to the limbus in the superior temporal quadrant. In addition to 5% 5-fluorouracil, the iontophoresis solution also contained 8.47% tris(hydroxymethyl)aminomethane (pH = 8.4, 865 mOsm).

5-Fluorouracil acts as an antiproliferative agent to prevent cellular replication. The concentration of 5-fluorouracil required for 50% inhibition of rabbit conjunctival fibroblasts in culture is 0.2–0.5 µg/mL; the iontophoretic concentration for human dermal fibroblasts in culture is 0.3 µg/mL. Thirty minutes after iontophoresis, the concentration of 5-fluorouracil in the conjunctiva was 50 µg/g of tissue and in the sclera 21 µg/g of tissue. Over the next 10 h, the amount of 5-fluorouracil decreased to 0.6 µg/g in the conjunctiva and 1.2 µg/g in the sclera. These concentrations were still high enough to produce more than a 50% inhibition of cellular proliferation.

Delivery of 5-fluorouracil by transscleral iontophoresis would eliminate the need for subconjunctival injections, which carry the risk of bleeding, infections, scarring, and undesired drug penetration into other ocular tissues. This approach offers a simple and effective way to introduce this antiproliferative agent into the conjunctiva and sclera, possibly improving the efficacy of antiglaucoma surgery by interfering with healing and thereby maintaining patency of the drainage openings. Other uses include reducing the recurrence of pterygia and treatment of localized malignancies of the cornea or conjunctival surface (30). To date, however, no studies have been done in experimental models of disease or in human eyes.

2. Ocular Anesthesia

Sisler (31) reported iontophoresis of lidocaine to the tarsal conjunctiva prior to surgical excision of conjunctivolithiasis plaques and other intra- and subconjunctival lesions.

The anesthetic solutions used were either 4% lidocaine plus 1:1,000 epinephrine or 2% lidocaine plus 1:2,000 epinephrine. A current of 0.5 mA was applied for 10 min. Twenty-seven patients with lesions of the tarsus and tarsal conjunctiva were treated. Since the blepharoconjunctiva adheres tightly to the tarsal plate, the injection of local anesthesia is not feasible. None of the patients with papillomas, superficial chalazions, or conjunctivolithiasis reported any discomfort in the eyelids or the arm to which the negative electrode was attached; only a mild sensation to touch was described. Three patients who reported pain had chalazions of the deeper portion of the tarsus and required injection of local anesthesia. This is the only report in the literature of iontophoresis of an anesthetic agent to adnexal areas for pain prevention.

Meyer et al. (32) reported iontophoresis (2 mA, 12 min) of 4% lidocaine to eyelids of patients for anesthesia prior to blepharoplasty or ptosis repair. Also, pain sensations after anesthesia by iontophoretic or topical application of 4% lidocaine were compared in 10 normal volunteers. Both surgical patients and volunteers reported significantly less pain after iontophoresis of the anesthetic, and no side effects of the process were observed.

3. Antibiotics and an Antifungal Agent for Treatment of Ocular Infections

Transcorneal iontophoresis of an antibiotic results in high and sustained concentrations of drug in the cornea and aqueous humor, with the potential for treating bacterial keratitis and anterior segment infections. With the crystalline lens in place, however, virtually no drug reaches the vitreous via this route of administration. Transscleral iontophoresis can bypass the lens and deliver drug to the vitreous in sufficient amounts to be therapeutic in the management of posterior segment infections, such as endophthalmitis.

a. Transcorneal Iontophoresis

Hughes and Maurice (33) found that transcorneal iontophoresis of gentamicin in the rabbit eye increased permeability to the antibiotic more than 100-fold, compared to topical exposure under the same conditions with no current applied. Suggestions for clinical use included the use of a gel wick or a soft contact lens presoaked in the drug solution as applicators.

Fishman et al. (34) described transcorneal iontophoresis of gentamicin to uninfected, aphakic rabbit eyes. Gentamicin iontophoresis (50 mg/mL at 0.75 mA for 10 min) yielded peak corneal (71 μg/g) and aqueous humor (78 μg/mL) concentrations 30 min after treatment. The peak vitreous concentration (10.4 μg/mL) was observed 16 h after treatment. Therapeutic concentrations of gentamicin were still present in the vitreous 24 h after iontophoresis. This study suggests that even transcorneal iontophoresis has the potential to deliver high concentrations of gentamicin to the posterior segment in aphakic eyes; since many patients with endophthalmitis are aphakic, either transcorneal or transscleral iontophoresis may provide effective routes of administration for antibiotic therapy of this disease in properly selected patients.

Grossman et al. (35) applied 10% gentamicin in 2% agar iontophoretically to rabbit corneas. This form of iontophoresis resulted in significantly higher and longer-lasting gentamicin concentrations in the cornea compared to a 20-mg subconjunctival injection. In a summary table, these authors describe all of the published reports of ocular iontophoresis of gentamicin that predate their own paper, specifically noting the details of the various conditions employed and the drug levels obtained in the cornea, aqueous humor, and vitreous humor.

Studies from our laboratories have examined the use of transcorneal iontophoresis of various antibiotics, including tobramycin and ciprofloxacin (36–40). Rootman et al. (36) were the first to demonstrate the efficacy of transcorneal iontophoresis of the aminoglycoside, tobramycin, for the treatment of experimental *Pseudomonas* keratitis in the rabbit. Iontophoresis (0.8 mA for 10 min) of 2.5% tobramycin to corneas infected with 10^3 colony-forming units of *Pseudomonas aeruginosa* was performed 22 and 27 h after injection. The result was an average 6-log reduction in colony-forming units in the cornea relative to untreated corneas. Five hours after the last treatment (32 h after inoculation), 67% of the corneas had no viable bacteria; that is, were sterile. No other routes of administration, including topical drops or subconjunctival injection, resulted in corneas free of viable *Pseudomonas*.

In another study, the safety (no toxicity to corneal epithelium) and pharmacokinetics of transcorneal iontophoresis of tobramycin in uninfected rabbit eyes were demonstrated (37). Tobramycin iontophoresis resulted in very high and sustained antibiotic concentrations in the corneal epithelium, corneal stroma, and aqueous humor. Furthermore, scanning electron microscopy following transcorneal iontophoresis showed only a limited disruption of the corneal epithelium and slit-lamp examination revealed no visible abnormalities. Light microscopy of a cornea treated with iontophoresis for 5 min showed normal stroma and endothelium and minimal epithelial disruption (Fig. 2). After 10 min of iontophoresis, the epithelium showed focal edema and disruption of the epithelial cell layers (Fig. 2). Histologically, specimens obtained 8 and 16 h after iontophoresis showed no defects in the corneal epithelium.

We (38) also described the pharmacokinetics of 2.5% tobramycin applied iontophoretically to uninfected, mock-infected, and *Pseudomonas aeruginosa*–infected rabbit corneas. The results showed high concentrations of antibiotic in all corneas (600–800 μg/g of tissue). Iontophoresis delivered five times more drug than bathing the cornea with the same concentration of tobramycin in an eye cup and 20 times more than applying 1.36% tobramycin as fortified drops.

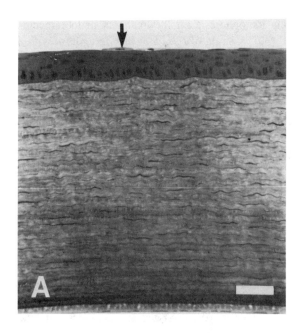

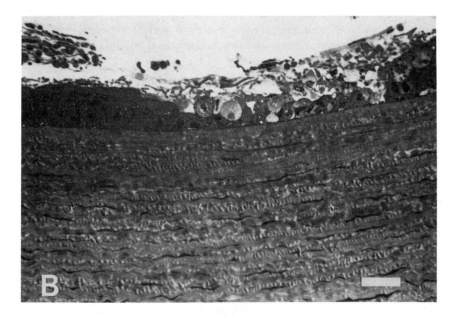

Figure 2. (A) Light microscopic section of cornea treated by transcorneal iontophoresis of tobramycin for 5 min. The stroma and endothelium appear normal. There is minimal disruption (arrow) of the surface epithelial cells. (Bar = 50 μm) (B) Light microscopic section of cornea treated in the same way for 10 min. The stroma looks normal, but focal disruption of the layers of the epithelium can be seen. (Bar = 25 μm) (From Ref. 37.)

Similarly, the power of tobramycin iontophoresis for the treatment of tobramycin-resistant *Pseudomonas* was determined (39). A strain of *Pseudomonas aeruginosa* with a minimum inhibitory concentration (MIC) for tobramycin of 31 µg/mL was injected into the corneal stroma in rabbit eyes. Iontophoresis of 2.5% tobramycin yielded a 3-log reduction in the number of bacteria. These results show that iontophoresis can deliver concentrations of antibiotic sufficient to combat a clinically resistant strain of bacteria in the cornea.

In one of our most recent studies (40), transcorneal iontophoresis was used to deliver the fluoroquinolone ciprofloxacin to rabbit corneas infected with an aminoglycoside-resistant strain of *Pseudomonas*. Iontophoresis of 1 or 2.5% ciprofloxacin reduced the numbers of colony-forming units by more than 5 logs relative to untreated controls and was significantly more effective than topical application of 0.75% ciprofloxacin drops or bathing the cornea with an eye cup containing 2.5% ciprofloxacin for 10 min. The concentrations of ciprofloxacin in the aqueous humor were 84, 30, and 25 µg/mL after iontophoresis, drops, and eye cup bathing, respectively. This was the first report of iontophoresis of a fluoroquinolone for therapy of experimental *Pseudomonas* keratitis.

Choi and Lee (41) were the first to demonstrate that vancomycin, a high molecular weight (1448 D), complex glycopolypeptide, can be applied to the eye by corneal iontophoresis. The antibiotic was prepared as a 5% solution. The area of contact between the drug solution and the cornea was 30 mm^2. Current (0.5 mA) was applied for 5 min. The peak concentration of vancomycin in the cornea was 10.8 µg/g of tissue 30 min after ocular iontophoresis. The peak concentration in the aqueous humor was 12.4 µg/mL 2 h after iontophoresis. Concentrations in the aqueous humor after iontophoresis were essentially equivalent to those achieved by a 25-mg subconjunctival injection (12.4 vs. 14.7 µg/mL, respectively). This study showed that a high molecular weight antibiotic could be administered by iontophoresis as an alternative to subconjunctival injection.

b. Transscleral Iontophoresis

Barza et al. (42) reported that transscleral iontophoresis delivered therapeutic concentrations of three antibiotics (cefazolin, ticarcillin, or gentamicin) to the vitreous humor of uninfected rabbit eyes. Two specific modifications of standard corneal procedures were used. First, the reservoir holding the drug was placed over the pars plana, thus bypassing the lens-iris barrier, and second, the contact area of the fluid that delivered both the antibiotic and the current was kept small (approximately 1 mm in diameter). The result was antibiotic concentrations in the range of 94–207 µg/mL in the vitreous humor. The significance of this study was that high concentrations of antibiotics were achieved in the vitreous by direct delivery not involving intraocular injection.

Another study from the same laboratory (43) showed transscleral iontophoresis of gentamicin to be a clinically useful supplement to intravitreal injections for endophthalmitis caused by *Pseudomonas aeruginosa*. At each treatment interval, the bacteria count was lower and the rate of sterilization was higher in rabbit eyes that received both intravitreal gentamicin and transscleral iontophoresis of gentamicin compared to rabbits that received gentamicin only by a single, 100-µg intravitreal injection. These results support the potential use of iontophoresis as a supplement for the treatment of bacterial endophthalmitis.

The same research group was the first to report the use of a nonhuman primate (cynomolgus monkey) to study the pharmacokinetics of transscleral iontophoresis of gentamicin (44) (Fig. 3). The procedure produced high and sustained concentrations of

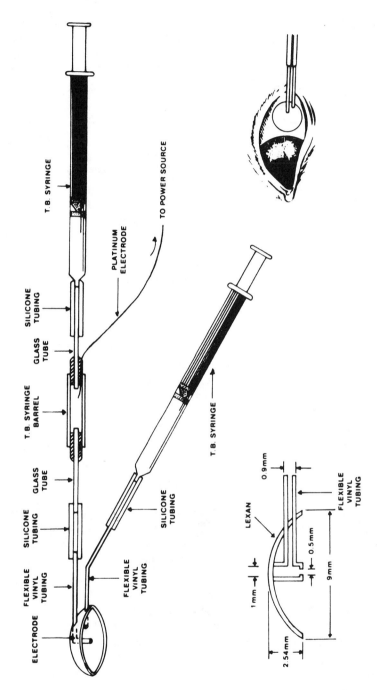

Figure 3. Diagram of apparatus used for transscleral iontophoresis in cynomolgus monkeys (44). The device is a modification of the device used previously by this research group in rabbit eyes (42). (From Ref. 44.)

antibiotic in the vitreous, with very few side effects. Indirect ophthalmoscopy showed that four of the six eyes had small retinal burns, approximately 2.5 mm in diameter, in the area of the pars plana over which the electrode was applied. All electroretinograms were normal. The results indicate that transscleral iontophoresis is a safe and effective noninvasive technique that can deliver therapeutic concentrations of antibiotic to the vitreous and is well tolerated in the primate eye. The preliminary success demonstrated in this study suggests that investigations in human eyes may be warranted.

Other studies in rabbit eyes have shown variable results. Burstein et al. (45) found that transscleral iontophoresis of gentamicin to uninfected rabbit eyes yielded antibiotic concentrations in the vitreous in the range of 10–20 μg/mL, which is one-fifth to one-tenth the concentrations reported by Barza et al. in the primate eye (44). In their rabbit study, Burstein et al. used a small silicone rubber tube with an internal diameter of 2.4 mm; they applied a solution of ^{125}I-labeled gentamicin (50 mg/mL) by means of a 2-mA current to four perilimbal sites for 3 min each. A biological assay was used to determine the concentration of gentamicin in the vitreous. These investigators found that the total surface area of the electrode was inversely proportional to the amount of antibiotic delivered. A 4.5-mm^2 applicator delivered approximately 20 times more drug to the vitreous than a 28-mm^2 applicator. As was also seen in the studies by Barza et al. (42–44) described above, a small area of contact in iontophoresis results in a higher concentration of drug in the eye.

The results of transscleral iontophoresis of 10% gentamicin in 2% agar reported by Grossman et al. (35) were similar to their findings with transcorneal iontophoresis described above. With a current of 2 mA for 10 min and a contact area 2 mm in diameter, significant concentrations of gentamicin were delivered to the vitreous humor. Peak vitreous concentrations (53.4 μg/mL) were achieved 16 h after iontophoresis; concentrations remained at inhibitory levels for 24 h. No damage to the retina or sclera was seen, in contrast to the slight damage reported by Barza et al. (44) in monkey eyes using gentamicin in a liquid solution. The absence of side effects with the agar-based drug applicator is significant and could facilitate the use of transscleral iontophoresis for the treatment of patients with bacterial endophthalmitis or other clinical conditions that require high concentrations of antibiotics in the vitreous.

In conjunction with their transcorneal studies described above, Choi and Lee (41) also investigated transscleral iontophoresis for delivery of vancomycin to the vitreous humor. A current of 3.5 mA was applied to a 5% vancomycin solution for 10 min; the contact area was approximately 25–30 mm^2 of the temporal sclera overlying the pars plana. Peak concentration (13.4 μg/mL) in the vitreous was reached 2 h after iontophoresis; 16 h after iontophoresis, the concentration of vancomycin in the vitreous was still nearly 3 μg/mL. Bactericidal concentrations for gram-positive organisms isolated from patients with endophthalmitis have been reported as equal to or less than 4 μg/mL (41). Therefore, antibiotic levels produced by transscleral iontophoresis in this study were, for the most part, at or near the required therapeutic concentrations. This is the first report of a high molecular weight glycopolypeptide antibiotic delivered to the vitreous humor by transscleral iontophoresis.

Grossman and Lee (46) attempted to administer an antifungal agent, ketoconazole, to the vitreous by transscleral iontophoresis. Ketoconazole was prepared as a 0.5 mg/mL solution in distilled water adjusted to pH 2.7 with HCl. The inner diameter of the applicator was 3 mm; the contact area was 7.1 mm^2. The current used was 5 mA for 15 min. However, the peak concentration, achieved 1–2 h after treatment, was only 0.1 µg/mL, which is not sufficient for therapeutic fungicidal activity. These results suggest that compounds that are not water soluble between pH 4.5 and 8.0 may not be good candidates for administration by iontophoresis.

4. Steroids for Treatment of Ocular Inflammation

Lachaud (47) delivered steroids to both rabbit and human eyes by iontophoresis. Hydrocortisone acetate (0.1%, 3 mA, 10 min) was used in the rabbit studies. Iontophoresis produced higher concentrations of steroid compared to frequent topical drops (0.5%) or subconjunctival injection (0.1 mL, 2.5%). In human studies, dexamethasone acetate (7 mg%, 1–2 mA, 20 min) was used to treat a variety of clinical conditions, including idiopathic uveitis. Lachaud (47) concluded that iontophoresis resulted in therapeutic concentrations of the steroid in the rabbit eye and that a significant proportion of the patients with uveitis benefitted in terms of more rapid recovery and/or increased comfort. However, it should be noted that the clinical study did not involve comparisons with eyes receiving other therapies or with untreated control eyes.

Lam et al. (48) performed transscleral iontophoresis of dexamethasone (30%, 1.6 mA, 25 min) into rabbit eyes. The diameter of the cylinder holding the drug solution in contact with the sclera was 0.7 mm. Peak steroid concentrations in the choroid-retinal tissue following iontophoresis, subconjunctival injection (1 mg), or retrobulbar injection (1 mg) were 122, 18.1 and 6.6 µg/g tissue, respectively, and in the vitreous humor, 140, 0.2, and 0.3 µg/mL, respectively. Even 24 h after iontophoresis, significant therapeutic levels of dexamethasone remained: 3.3 µg/mL in the vitreous and 3.9 µg/g in the choroid-retina. These results show that transscleral iontophoresis can produce high-peak and long-lasting therapeutic concentrations of this anti-inflammatory drug in the rabbit eye.

5. Antivirals and Adrenergic Agents in the Treatment and Study of Ocular Herpes Simplex Virus Infection

a. Antivirals for Treatment of Epithelial Keratitis

In 1977, Hill et al. (49) demonstrated that the antiviral agents idoxuridine (IDU), phosphonoacetic acid (PAA), and vidarabine monophosphate (Ara-AMP) could be iontophoresed into the murine epidermis and that high and sustained concentrations of these drugs could be achieved.

A year later, Hill et al. (50) were the first to describe the pharmacokinetics of Ara-AMP after iontophoresis in uninfected rabbit eyes. Tritium-labeled Ara-AMP was applied topically or by transcorneal iontophoresis (0.5 mAmp for 4 min using the cathode in contact with the drug solution). The amounts of radiolabeled drug in the cornea, aqueous humor, and iris were 3 to 12 times higher after iontophoresis than after topical application. Scanning electron micrographs of the corneal epithelium obtained 4 min after iontophoresis showed limited damage to a few superficial cells; specimens obtained 60 min after treatment showed no changes. These results revealed that iontophoresis of an antiviral agent could provide superior penetration of the cornea compared to topical drops, and that iontophoresis was safe in terms of the absence of damage to the corneal epithelium.

Shortly thereafter, this group (51) was also the first to demonstrate the antiviral activity of iontophoretically applied Ara-AMP in the treatment of experimental herpes simplex virus (HSV) keratitis. Ara-AMP was used because the parent compound, vidarabine, was shown to be effective in the treatment of HSV-1 infection after topical or systemic administration. Ara-AMP is the phosphorylated form of vidarabine; the molecule is highly charged and is, therefore, an ideal candidate for iontophoresis.

Epithelial herpetic keratitis was induced in rabbit eyes by inoculation of HSV-1 McKrae strain. Transcorneal iontophoresis of Ara-AMP (0.3 M, 3.4%) was initiated 24 h after infection and was done once daily in both eyes for 3 consecutive days. Iontophoresis of 0.9% sodium chloride was done in another group of infected rabbits on the same schedule. Three additional groups of rabbits received topical 10% Ara-AMP, 0.5% idoxuridine, or 0.9% sodium chloride five times daily for 4 days. All eyes underwent slit-lamp biomicroscopy by masked observers, who scored the severity of disease daily for 10 consecutive days after treatment was begun. Mean epithelial lesion scores and mean total anterior segment lesion scores were calculated. The means for the eyes treated by iontophoresis of Ara-AMP were significantly lower (i.e., less severe disease of shorter duration) compared to the scores of eyes treated with iontophoresis of sodium chloride or topically with Ara-AMP, idoxuridine, or sodium chloride.

b.   Antivirals for Treatment of Stromal Disease

Subsequently, Hill et al (52) compared the efficacy of ocular iontophoresis and intravenous administration of acyclovir and Ara-AMP for the treatment of HSV-1 stromal infection in the rabbit eye. Disease was induced by means of an intrastromal injection of purified HSV-1 McKrae strain; treatment was begun 24 h later. Three groups received iontophoresis (0.5 mA for 4 min) once daily for 5 consecutive days: either 3.4% (0.2 M) Ara-AMP, 5% (0.22 M) acyclovir; or sodium chloride (0.14 M). Two groups received intravenous infusion twice daily for 8 consecutive days: either 50 mg/kg acyclovir or 20 mg/kg sodium chloride. Two ophthalmologists performed masked evaluation of the disease severity by slit-lamp biomicroscopy for up to 22 days after viral inoculation.

Iontophoresis of acyclovir or Ara-AMP significantly reduced the course of the disease compared to iontophoresis of sodium chloride. Intravenous administration of acyclovir significantly reduced disease compared to intravenous sodium chloride. Acyclovir was equally effective regardless of route of administration; iontophoretically applied Ara-AMP was as effective as acyclovir. However, the amount of acyclovir given intravenously, in terms of the total dose per animal, was significantly higher than the amount given by iontophoresis, which achieved the same therapeutic effect. These results suggested that iontophoresis of acyclovir or Ara-AMP, either alone or in combination with intravenous administration of acyclovir, could be of value in the treatment of patients with HSV-1 stromal keratitis.

c.   Adrenergic Agents for Experimental Induction of Viral Shedding in the
     Study of Ocular Herpetic Disease

Attempts to study recurrent ocular HSV-1 infection required a reliable in vivo model of viral reactivation. The relationship between stress and recurrent disease suggested a role for epinephrine in this process, and various investigators had shown that topically applied or intramuscularly injected epinephrine could, in fact, lead to the reactivation of herpes in rabbits.

Iontophoresis seemed to be an ideal procedure for ensuring the penetration of large amounts of epinephrine into the cornea. In the early 1980s, Kwon et al. (53) were the first to report the induction of viral shedding by transcorneal iontophoresis of this adrenergic agent in rabbits harboring latent HSV-1. Epinephrine iontophoresis (0.01% at 0.8 mA for 8 min) was performed once daily for 3 consecutive days. Viral shedding was determined by culturing tear film in cell culture followed by antigenic or nucleic acid analysis to confirm the identity of the viral isolate. The results showed that unilateral iontophoresis 60 days after viral inoculation resulted in HSV-1 shedding in all treated eyes. Over the past 10 years, this reliable and highly efficient means of inducing viral shedding has been the basis for the development of animal models for studying the kinetics of HSV-1 ocular shedding and induction of clinical corneal epithelial herpetic disease in animals. In particular, these studies have examined reactivation of virus latent in the trigeminal ganglia, pharmacologic aspects of treatment, and the virology of HSV-1 latency, reactivation, and recurrence of clinical disease.

In 1982, Kwon et al. (54) further characterized ocular HSV-1 shedding induced by epinephrine iontophoresis by determining the titers and kinetics of the virus in the rabbit tear film. All treated rabbits shed virus; the HSV-1 titers rose, peaked, and fell with time after iontophoresis. These results provided additional evidence for the reliability of this animal model in the study of ocular reactivation of herpes.

Two later studies from this research group (55,56) used ocular iontophoresis of epinephrine to characterize the appearance of infectious virus in the nerves and ganglia after reactivation from the latent state. Hill et al. (55) showed that infectious virus could be detected more rapidly from cultured neuronal tissue extirpated from rabbits that had undergone iontophoresis of epinephrine compared to tissue from rabbits that had not been exposed to iontophoresis of this adrenergic agent. Also, Shimomura et al. (56) quantified infectious virus in the ganglia after reactivation by ocular epinephrine iontophoresis.

In all of the early studies described above (53–56), HSV-1 strain McKrae was used to infect the New Zealand white rabbit. Willey et al. (57) described for the first time reactivation of latent virus by epinephrine iontophoresis in a mouse model. BALB/c mice were infected with HSV-1 strain McKrae following corneal scarification. Epinephrine (0.01%) was applied by transcorneal iontophoresis 28 days postinoculation. Ocular shedding of HSV-1 occurred in 16 of 23 (70%) treated mice. Spontaneous viral shedding (no epinephrine iontophoresis) occurred in 3 of 97 (3%) untreated mice.

A major disadvantage of epinephrine iontophoresis is that the animals must be anesthetized once a day for 3 consecutive days. Another disadvantage is the time involved for 3 consecutive days of epinephrine iontophoresis. Shimomura et al. (58) developed a method of inducing ocular shedding that involves a single iontophoresis of 6-hydroxydopamine followed by topical application of epinephrine over several days. This approach was based on earlier procedures developed by investigators who were attempting to use iontophoresis of adrenergic agents in the treatment of glaucoma (25–29). As described above, 6-hydroxydopamine causes a selective and reversible degeneration of sympathetic nerve terminals in the anterior segment, after which the innervated structures of the eye are exquisitely sensitive to extremely dilute solutions of epinephrine.

To induce virus shedding in the rabbit using this new method, 1% 6-hydroxydopamine was administered by iontophoresis under various conditions: 0.75 mA for 3 min; 0.5 mA for 8 min; or 0.5 mA for 4 min. Iontophoresis was performed only once. Chemical sympathectomy was considered to be successful when pupillary dilatation did not occur 30 min after topical instillation of 1% hydroxyamphetamine. Two drops of 2% epinephrine were applied topically 6 h after iontophoresis and twice daily for the next 4 days. All treated eyes (17/17; 100%) shed HSV-1, regardless of the iontophoretic conditions.

In the mouse model (59), 6-hydroxydopamine iontophoresis followed by topical drops of 0.1% epinephrine plus 1% prednisolone resulted in the highest numbers of HSV-1–positive eyes, mice, and total shedding days compared to topical steroid or 6-hydroxydopamine iontophoresis plus topical epinephrine alone. Also, in the mouse, latent HSV-1 strain W yielded higher rates of reactivation than latent strain McKrae.

All previous studies of epinephrine iontophoresis used the levo(-) form of epinephrine. In a dose-response experiment using separate rabbits for each dose (60), levo(-)epinephrine was, in fact, shown to be significantly more potent than dextro(+)epinephrine for inducing HSV-1 ocular shedding. The data suggested that the mechanism of induction of HSV-1 ocular shedding by epinephrine is perhaps correlated with the receptor potency of levo(-)epinephrine.

Hill et al. (61) were the first to report the quantification of plaque-forming units of HSV-1 shed into the tear film after sensitizing rabbit eyes by iontophoresis of 6-hydroxydopamine followed by topical instillation of 2% epinephrine. Titers ranged up to nearly 10^5 plaque-forming units/eye.

A subsequent study (62) showed that dipivefrin hydrochloride could be used in place of epinephrine in this reactivation model. Dipivefrin hydrochloride is a prodrug of epinephrine, which is converted enzymatically within the cornea. Because penetration of the prodrug is greatly enhanced, compared to penetration of epinephrine, less drug can be given; in clinical studies, 0.1% dipivefrin hydrochloride was as effective as topical 1 or 2% epinephrine. Using iontophoresis of 6-hydroxydopamine with topical application of 0.1% dipivefrin hydrochloride, Hill et al. (62) demonstrated a positive correlation between HSV-1 ocular shedding and recurrent HSV-1 corneal epithelial lesions. This was the first report showing that an adrenergic drug could induce both HSV-1 ocular shedding (reactivation) and HSV-1 corneal epithelial lesions (recurrence) in rabbits harboring latent virus.

Virtually all of the studies demonstrating iontophoretic induction of herpesvirus reactivation have involved HSV-1 strain McKrae. There are, however, many different HSV strains, and the patterns of corneal pathology produced by these strains show specific and reproducible differences (63–66). In a study of reactivation of 10 HSV-1 strains by iontophoresis of an adrenergic agent, Hill et al. (67) found a wide divergence in rates of shedding. Herpes simplex virus strain McKrae produced the most consistent results, with reactivation occurring in 75–100% of treated eyes. Strain Syn[+] 17 could be reactivated in more than 70% of the eyes, whereas strains McIntyre, KOS, F, and CGA-3 could not be reactivated at all. However, all of these viral strains yielded the same high percentage (75–100%) of latency in the trigeminal ganglia of infected rabbits. These results indicate that latency in the trigeminal or superior cervical ganglia is only one component necessary for ocular reactivation, and biological differences among the strains may play an important, if not as yet clearly defined, role.

The relationship between the ganglionic and neural structures and viral latency and reactivation were also investigated using the iontophoretic model. Zhang et al. (68) studied the effect of surgical sympathectomy on the ability of rabbits harboring latent HSV-1 to shed virus after iontophoresis of 6-hydroxydopamine and topical epinephrine. The results showed that rabbits that underwent bilateral removal of the superior cervical ganglia had the same ability to shed virus as sham-operated rabbits. Thus, iontophoresis of adrenergic agents induces HSV-1 shedding in the outer eye from sources other than, or in addition to, the superior cervical ganglia.

Rivera et al. (69) were the first to show a temporal relationship between ocular viral reactivation and the presence of viral particles in corneal nerves after epinephrine iontophoresis. Transmission electron microscopy revealed viral particles in unmyelinated axons but in low frequency. No enveloped virions were found. This study suggests that corneal iontophoresis of epinephrine reactivates HSV-1 in the ganglia and that the virus is translocated from the ganglia to the cornea by axonal transport mechanisms. This report was also the first evidence of anterograde intra-axonal transport of viral particles in response to ocular epinephrine iontophoresis.

Penetrating keratoplasty was used to demonstrate that induction of viral shedding by iontophoresis of epinephrine in the rabbit eye is not possible unless the corneal nerves are intact (70). After penetrating keratoplasty, the area of the transplant is effectively denervated for up to 90 days. Two weeks after surgery, iontophoresis of 0.1% epinephrine was performed at 0.8 mA for 8 min, once daily for 3 consecutive days, using an eye cup smaller in diameter than the transplant. Only one of 12 (8%) of the eyes that underwent penetrating keratoplasty shed virus, whereas 8 of 12 (67%) of the unoperated contralateral eyes showed cultures positive for HSV-1. Successful induction of shedding after penetrating keratoplasty (71) by systemic administration of cyclophosphamide and dexamethasone showed that surgical denervation of the transplant does not interfere with the appearance of virus in the cornea but apparently does, in some way, interfere with the iontophoretic signal for reactivation.

One mechanism of ocular reactivation by epinephrine might be correlated with receptor potency of levo(-)epinephrine (60). Epinephrine is known to activate both alpha- and beta-adrenergic receptors in the eye. If viral reactivation were induced exclusively by activation of a beta-adrenergic receptor, the epinephrine response should be inhibited by a beta-adrenergic receptor antagonist. Studies from our (72–74) and other (68,75) laboratories assessed the effect of topically applied timolol maleate, a nonspecific $beta_1, beta_2$-adrenergic receptor blocking agent, on ocular HSV-1 reactivation after iontophoresis of 6-hydroxydopamine. Zhang et al. (68) reported that HSV-1 ocular shedding was reduced when 0.5% timolol was used in place of epinephrine in rabbit eyes supersensitized to adrenergic agents by ocular iontophoresis of 6-hydroxydopamine. Other investigators, however, did not observe this effect (72–75).

In fact, timolol produced another, seemingly contradictory effect. Studies in rabbits (73) and mice (75) showed that direct transcorneal iontophoresis of timolol induced ocular HSV-1 shedding. Furthermore, iontophoresis of timolol once daily for three consecutive days could induce a corneal epithelial lesion in the rabbit eye (72). In the first report of a beta-adrenergic receptor antagonist causing HSV-1 ocular shedding in a nonhuman primate, Rootman et al. (76) used iontophoresis of timolol to induce HSV-1 ocular shedding in the squirrel monkey (*Saimiri sciureus*).

The results of these studies demonstrated that the receptor potency of epinephrine alone is not an exclusive reactivator of ocular herpes. The data suggested that both timolol (a beta-adrenergic receptor antagonist) and epinephrine (an alpha- and beta-adrenergic receptor agonist) could induce ocular shedding. The finding that these two agents could influence the same event had been previously reported by Cyrlin et al. (77), who described the additive effect of topically applied epinephrine and timolol in the reduction of intra-ocular pressure. The in vivo mechanism that produced this paradoxical effect could not be explained, and neither, at this time, can we explain the observation that iontophoretic delivery of these two theoretically opposing adrenergic agents induces viral reactivation in animals that harbor latent HSV-1 strain McKrae.

Iontophoresis of adrenergic agents to rabbits harboring latent virus has been used in ocular reactivation studies involving mutants of HSV-1. Caudill et al. (78) used iontophoresis of 1% 6-hydroxydopamine followed by topical 2% epinephrine to determine the efficacy of viral reactivation of HSV-1 mutants that did not express the viral enzyme thymidine kinase (TK). The viral strain was NIH 11124; the viral thymidine kinase activity of cells infected with this strain was 0%. This study from Gordon's group (78) showed for the first time that HSV-1 thymidine kinase negative mutants could establish latency in the rabbit, be reactivated by iontophoretically applied adrenergic stimulation, and be shed in the preocular tear film, much like their TK-positive counterparts.

Hill et al. (79), using a mutant (X10-13) which could not produce a latently associated ribonucleic acid (RNA) transcript (LAT negative) and a genetically engineered positive mutant XC-20 (LAT positive), were able to demonstrate that the LAT-positive strain, which was similar to the parent HSV-1 strain Syn$^+$ 17, could be reactivated by iontophoresis with high efficiency in rabbits. However, the LAT-negative strain (X10-13) had very limited reactivation. The results of this study suggested that the latently associated transcript may play a role in viral reactivation. Data on ganglionic latency showed that the establishment and maintenance of latency was accomplished regardless of whether the LAT transcript was present (XC-20) or absent (X10-13). Similar results were found in mice using mutants X10-13 and XC-20 (80).

A variety of studies in addition to those discussed above have used iontophoresis of epinephrine to study experimental viral reactivation, as well as the treatment and prevention of recurrent herpetic disease (81–89). In all, these studies have validated the precision and reproducibility of the iontophoretic model of viral reactivation and the utility of this model in the search for therapeutic answers to one of the most common infectious causes of blinding eye disease.

IV. COMMERCIAL DEVICES FOR IONTOPHORESIS

Table 3 provides a list of companies that produce iontophoresis devices, their addresses and phone numbers, as well as a brief description of one specific model manufactured by each company.

V. CONCLUSIONS

Ocular iontophoresis offers a drug delivery system that is fast, painless, safe, and, in most cases, results in the delivery of a high concentration of the drug to a specific site. Experimentally, iontophoresis has proven extremely useful as a reliable system for inducing reactivation of herpes in various models of this ocular disease. Clinically, however, aside from ocular iontophoresis of fluorescein in patients to study anterior segment fluid dynamics, few studies have been done in humans. One reason is that most ocular drugs can be effectively delivered without the use of iontophoresis. However, the increased incidence of bacterial keratitis, frequently resulting in corneal scarring, offers a clinical condition that may benefit from drug delivery by iontophoresis. Iontophoretic application of antibiotics may enhance their bactericidal activity and reduce the severity of disease; similar application of other types of drugs, such as anti-inflammatory agents, could prevent or reduce vision-threatening side effects. At this time, however, a role for iontophoresis in clinical ophthalmology remains to be identified.

Table 3. Commercially Available Iontophoresis Equipment

Company	Model number/description
Life-Tech, Inc. 10920 Kinghurst Houston, TX 77099 (713) 495-9411 (800) 231-9841 Fax (713) 495-7960	Iontophor-PM model number 6110 PM. This model provides a painless, safe, and effective method of delivering high concentrations of drug into a localized skin area. This unit is battery operated, compact, and portable. It is an excellent unit for maintaining constant current.
IOMED, Inc. 1290 West 2320 South, Suite A Salt Lake City, UT 84119 (801) 975-1191 (800) 621-3347 Fax (801) 975-7366	Phoresor II model number PM 700. This model provides an effective, safe, and easy to use system mostly for iontophoretic drug application to the skin. The unit is battery operated, compact, and portable.
Wescor, Inc. 459 South Main Street Logan, UT 84321 (801) 752-6011 (800) 453-2725 Fax (801) 752-4127	Macroduct model 3700. This model is used for sweat testing (pilocarpine iontophoresis). It is accurate and easy to operate.
Dagan Corporation 2855 Park Avenue Minneapolis, MN 55407 (612) 827-5959 Fax (612) 827-6535	Dagan model 6400. Iontophoresis current generator. AC to transformer for DC. Current 0–0.2 mA.
MedTherm Corporation 2604 Newby Road Huntsville, AL 35805 (205) 837-2000	Electro-Medicator Model A1. This model is used for dental research and clinical practice. It is easy to operate and has AC charging or direct use of AC.
MedTronic, Inc. 7000 Central Avenue, NE Minneapolis, MN 55432 (612) 574-4000 (800) 328-2518 Fax (612) 574-4879	Model 9820. This iontophoretic device is part of complete system (Model 9800) for sweat analysis after pilocarpine iontophoresis.
Parkell 155 Schmitt Boulevard Farmingdale, NY 11735 (516) 249-1134 (800) 243-7446 Fax (516) 249-1242	Desensitron II Stock No. D6423D. This model is used for treatment of hypersensitive teeth by iontophoresis of fluoride ions.
Fischer Co., Inc. 517 Commercial Street Glendale, CA 91203 (213) 245-2746 Fax (213) 245-2748	Fischer Galvanic Unit, Model MD-1. This iontophoresis unit can be used to treat large areas (hyperhidrosis patients) and can deliver up to 50 mA of current.
Farrall Instruments, Inc. 3724 Arch Avenue Grand Island, NE 68803 (308) 384-1530 Fax (308) 384-2667	Model IPS-25. This unit is battery operated with a current-limiting regulator. It has a current control range of 0–5 mA DC. Farrall Instruments was the first company (in 1958) to manufacture an iontophoresis unit for commercial distribution.

ACKNOWLEDGMENTS

Louis P. Gangarosa, D.D.S., Ph.D., is acknowledged as the person who introduced iontophoresis to one of the authors (JMH). Dr. Gangarosa's optimism, advice, and encouragement are greatly appreciated. Specific research from the laboratories of JMH described in this review was funded in part by U.S. Public Health Service grants EY06311, EY08771, EY02580, and EY02377 from the National Eye Institute and AI06246 from the National Institute of Allergy and Infectious Diseases, National Institutes of Health, Bethesda, MD. The authors wish to acknowledge the secretarial assistance of Ms. Ada Rivera. None of the authors have any financial or proprietary interest in any agents or devices mentioned in this review.

REFERENCES

1. Shriber, W. J. (1975). The direct current and ion transfer. *In: A Manual of Electrotherapy* (W. J. Shriber, ed.). Lea & Febiger, Philadelphia, p. 124.
2. Leduc, S. (1901). Introduction des substances medicamenteuses dans la profondeur des tissus par le courant electrique, *Rev. Med.*, 10:147.
3. Leduc, S. (1908). *Electric Ions and Their Use in Medicine.* Rebman, London.
4. Duke-Elder, S. (1962). Iontophoresis. *In: System of Ophthalmology*, Vol. VII: *The Foundations of Ophthalmology* (S. Duke-Elder, ed.). Mosby, St. Louis, p. 507.
5. Witzel, S. H., Fielding, I. Z., and Ormsby, H. L. (1956). Ocular penetration of antibiotics by iontophoresis, *Am. J. Ophthalmol.*, 42:89.
6. von Sallmann, L. (1944). Penicillin and sulfadiazine in the treatment of experimental intraocular infections with *Staphylococcus aureus* and *Clostridium welchii, Arch. Ophthalmol.*, 31:54.
7. von Sallmann, L. (1945). Penetration of penicillin into the eye, *Arch. Ophthalmol.*, 34:195.
8. von Sallmann, L., and Meyer, K. (1944). Penetration of penicillin into the eye, *Arch. Ophthalmol.*, 31:1.
9. Erlanger, G. (1936). On the scientific and practical value of ionization in ophthalmology. Recent advances and researchers, *Br. J. Ophthalmol.*, 20:213.
10. Erlanger, G. (1939). Iontophoretic medication in ophthalmology. Theoretic and practical aspects, *Arch. Phys. Ther.*, 20:16.
11. Erlanger, G. (1954). Iontophoresis, a scientific and practical tool in ophthalmology, *Ophthalmologica*, 128:232.
12. Harris, R. (1967). Iontophoresis. *In: Therapeutic Electricity and Ultraviolet Radiation*, 2nd ed. (S. Licht, ed.). Waverly Press, Baltimore, p. 156.
13. Sloan, J. B., and Soltani, K. (1986). Iontophoresis in dermatology: A review, *J. Am. Acad. Dermatol.*, 15:671.
14. Gangarosa, L. P., Sr. (1983). *Iontophoresis in Dental Practice.* Quintessence, Chicago, p. 1.
15. Tyle, P. (1986). Iontophoretic devices for drug delivery. Review, *Pharm. Res.*, 3:318.
16. Banga, A. K., and Chien, Y. W. (1988). Iontophoretic delivery of drugs: Fundamentals, developments and biomedical applications, *J. Controlled Rel.*, 7:1.
17. Shofner, R. S., Kaufman, H. E., and Hill, J. M. (1989). New horizons in ocular drug delivery, *Ophthalmol. Clin. N. Am.*, 2:15.
18. Gibson, L. E., and Cooke, R. E. (1959). A test for concentration of electrolytes in sweat in cystic fibrosis of the pancreas utilizing pilocarpine by iontophoresis, *Pediatrics*, 23:545.
19. Carter, E. P., Barrett, A. D., Heeley, A. F., and Kuzemko, J. A. (1984). Improved sweat test method for the diagnosis of cystic fibrosis, *Arch. Dis. Child.*, 59:919.
20. Jones, R. F., and Maurice, D. M. (1966). New methods of measuring the rate of aqueous flow in man with fluorescein, *Exp. Eye Res.*, 5:208.

21. Starr, P. A. J. (1966). Changes in aqueous flow determined by fluorophotometry, *Trans. Ophthalmol. Soc. U.K.*, 86:639.

22. Holm, O. (1968). A photogrammetric method for estimation of the pupillary aqueous flow in the living human eye, I, *Acta Ophthalmol.*, 46:254.

23. Tonjum, A. M., and Green, K. (1971). Quantitative study of fluorescein iontophoresis through the cornea, *Am. J. Ophthalmol.*, 71:1328.

24. Brubaker, R. F. (1982). The flow of aqueous humor in the human eye, *Trans. Am. Ophthalmol. Soc.*, 80:391.

25. Kitazawa, Y., and Horie, T. (1974). Denervation supersensitivity induced by chemical sympathectomy with 6-hydroxydopamine, *Jpn. J. Ophthalmol.*, 18:109.

26. Kitazawa, Y., Nose, H., and Horie, T. (1973). The effects of chemical sympathectomy on intraocular pressure of the normal human subjects, *Acta Soc. Ophthalmol. Jpn.*, 77:1901.

27. Kitazawa, Y., Nose, H., and Horie, T. (1975). Chemical sympathectomy with 6-hydroxydopamine in the treatment of primary open-angle glaucoma, *Am. J. Ophthalmol.*, 79:98.

28. Watanabe, H., Levene, R. Z., and Bernstein, M. R. (1977). 6-Hydroxydopamine therapy in glaucoma, *Trans. Am. Acad. Ophthalmol. Otolaryngol.*, 83:69.

29. Colasanti, B. K., and Trotter, R. R. (1977). Enhanced ocular penetration of the methyl ester of alpha-methyl-para-tyrosine after iontophoresis, *Arch. Int. Pharmacodyn. Ther.*, 228:171.

30. Kondo, M., and Araie, M. (1989). Iontophoresis of 5-fluororacil into the conjunctiva and sclera, *Invest. Ophthalmol. Vis. Sci.*, 30:583.

31. Sisler, H. A. (1978). Iontophoretic local anesthesia for conjunctival surgery, *Ann. Ophthalmol.*, 10:597.

32. Meyer, D. R., Linberg, J. V., and Vasquez, R. J. (1990). Iontophoresis for eyelid anesthesia, *Ophthalmic Surg.*, 21:845.

33. Hughes, L., and Maurice, D. (1984). A fresh look at iontophoresis, *Arch. Ophthalmol.*, 102:1825.

34. Fishman, P. H., Jay, W. M., Hill, J. M., Rissing, J. P., and Shockley, R. K. (1984). Iontophoresis of gentamicin into aphakic rabbit eyes: sustained vitreal levels, *Invest. Ophthalmol. Vis. Sci.*, 25:343.

35. Grossman, R. E., Chu, D. F., and Lee, D. A. (1990). Regional ocular gentamicin levels after transcorneal and transscleral iontophoresis, *Invest. Ophthalmol. Vis. Sci.*, 31:909.

36. Rootman, D. S., Hobden, J. A., Jantzen, J. A., Gonzalez, V. R., O'Callaghan, R. J., and Hill, J. M. (1988). Iontophoresis of tobramycin for the treatment of experimental *Pseudomonas* keratitis in the rabbit, *Arch. Ophthalmol.*, 106:262.

37. Rootman, D. S., Jantzen, J. A., Gonzalez, J. R., Fischer, M., Beuerman, R., and Hill, J. M. (1988). Pharmacokinetics and safety of transcorneal iontophoresis of tobramycin in the rabbit, *Invest. Ophthalmol. Vis. Sci.*, 29:1397.

38. Hobden, J. A., Rootman, D. S., O'Callaghan, R. J., and Hill, J. M. (1988). Iontophoretic application of tobramycin to uninfected and *Pseudomonas aeruginosa*–infected rabbit corneas, *Antimicrob. Agent Chemother.*, 32:978.

39. Hobden, J. A., O'Callaghan, R. J. Hill, J. M., Reidy, J. J., Rootman, D. S., and Thompson, H. W. (1989). Tobramycin iontophoresis into corneas infected with drug-resistant *Pseudomonas aeruginosa, Curr. Eye Res.*, 8:1163.

40. Hobden, J. A., Reidy, J. J., O'Callaghan, R. J., and Hill, J. M. (1990). Ciprofloxacin iontophoresis for aminoglycoside-resistant pseudomonal keratitis, *Invest. Ophthalmol. Vis. Sci.*, 31:1940.

41. Choi, T. B., and Lee, D. A. (1988). Transscleral and transcorneal iontophoresis of vancomycin in rabbit eyes, *J. Ocul. Pharmacol.*, 4:153.

42. Barza, M., Peckman, C., and Baum, J. (1986). Transscleral iontophoresis of cefazolin, ticarcillin, and gentamicin in the rabbit, *Ophthalmology*, 93:133.

43. Barza, M., Peckman, C., and Baum, J. (1987). Transscleral iontophoresis as an adjunctive treatment for experimental endophthalmitis, *Arch. Ophthalmol.*, 105:1418.

44. Barza, M., Peckman, C., and Baum, J. (1987). Transscleral iontophoresis of gentamicin in monkeys, *Invest. Ophthalmol. Vis. Sci.*, 28:1033.

45. Burstein, N. L., Leopold, I. H., and Bernacchi, D. B. (1985). Trans-scleral iontophoresis of gentamicin, *J. Ocul. Pharmacol.*, 1:363.
46. Grossman, R., and Lee, D. A. (1989). Transscleral and transcorneal iontophoresis of ketoconazole in the rabbit eye, *Ophthalmology*, 96:724.
47. Lachaud, J. P. (1965). Considerations on the use of corticoids by ionization in certain ocular diseases, *Bull. Soc. D'Ophtalmol. France*, 65:84 [French].
48. Lam, T. T., Edward, D. P., Zhu, X., and Tso, M. O. M. (1989). Transscleral iontophoresis of dexamethasone, *Arch. Ophthalmol.*, 107:1368.
49. Hill, J. M., Gangarosa, L. P., and Park, N. H. (1977). Iontophoretic application of antiviral chemotherapeutic agents, *Ann. N.Y. Acad. Sci.*, 284:604.
50. Hill, J. M., Park, N. H., Gangarosa, L. P., Hull, D. S., Tuggle, C. L., Bowman, K., and Green, K. (1978). Iontophoretic application of vidarabine monophosphate into rabbit eyes, *Invest. Ophthalmol. Vis. Sci.*, 17:473.
51. Kwon, B. S., Gangarosa, L. P., Park, N. H., Hull, D. S., Fineberg, E., Wiggins, C., and Hill, J. M. (1979). Effects of iontophoretic and topical application of antiviral agents in treatment of experimental HSV-1 keratitis in rabbits, *Invest. Ophthalmol. Vis. Sci.*, 18:984.
52. Hill, J. M., Kwon, B. S., Burch, K. D., deBack, J., Whang, I., Jones, G. T., Luke, B., Andrews, P., Harp, R., Shimomura, Y., Hull, D. S., and Gangarosa, L. P. (1982). Acyclovir and vidarabine monophosphate: A comparison of iontophoretic and intravenous administration for the treatment of HSV-1 stromal keratitis, *Am. J. Med.*, 73:300.
53. Kwon, B. S., Gangarosa, L. P., Burch, K. D., deBack, J., and Hill, J. M. (1981). Induction of ocular herpes simplex virus shedding by iontophoresis of epinephrine into rabbit cornea, *Invest. Ophthalmol. Vis. Sci.*, 21:442.
54. Kwon, B. S., Gangarosa, L. P., Green, K., and Hill, J. M. (1982). Kinetics of ocular herpes simplex virus shedding induced by epinephrine iontophoresis, *Invest. Ophthalmol. Vis. Sci.*, 22:818.
55. Hill, J. M., Kwon, B. S., Shimomura, Y., Colborn, G. L., Yaghmai, F., and Gangarosa, L. P. (1983). Herpes simplex virus recovery in neural tissues after ocular HSV shedding induced by epinephrine iontophoresis to the rabbit cornea, *Invest. Ophthalmol. Vis. Sci.*, 24:243.
56. Shimomura, Y., Dudley, J. B., Gangarosa, L. P., and Hill, J. M. (1985). HSV-1 quantitation from rabbit neural tissues after reactivation induced by ocular epinephrine iontophoresis, *Invest. Ophthalmol. Vis. Sci.*, 26:121.
57. Willey, D. E., Trousdale, M. D., and Nesburn, A. B. (1984). Reactivation of murine latent HSV infection by epinephrine iontophoresis, *Invest. Ophthalmol. Vis. Sci.*, 25:945.
58. Shimomura, Y., Gangarosa, Sr., L. P., Kataoka, M., and Hill, J. M. (1983). HSV-1 shedding by iontophoresis of 6-hydroxydopamine followed by topical epinephrine, *Invest. Ophthalmol. Vis. Sci.*, 24:1588.
59. Gordon, Y. J., Araullo-Cruz, T. P., Romanowski, E., Ruziczka, L., Balouris, C., Oren, J., Cheng, K. P., and Kim, S. (1986). The development of an improved murine iontophoresis reactivation model for the study of HSV-1 latency, *Invest. Ophthalmol. Vis. Sci.*, 27:1230.
60. Hill, J. M., Shimomura, Y., Kwon, B. S., and Gangarosa, L. P. (1985). Iontophoresis of epinephrine isomers to rabbit eyes induced HSV-1 ocular shedding, *Invest. Ophthalmol. Vis. Sci.*, 26:1299.
61. Hill, J. M., Dudley, J. B., Shimomura, Y., and Kaufman, H. E. (1986). Quantitation and kinetics of induced HSV-1 ocular shedding, *Curr. Eye Res.*, 5:241.
62. Hill, J. M., Haruta, Y., and Rootman, D. S. (1987). Adrenergically induced recurrent HSV-1 corneal epithelial lesions, *Curr. Eye Res.*, 6:1065.
63. Wander, A. H., Centifanto, Y. M., and Kaufman, H. E. (1980). Strain specificity of clinical isolates of herpes simplex virus, *Arch. Ophthalmol.*, 98:1458.
64. Centifanto-Fitzgerald, Y. M., Yamaguchi, T., Kaufman, H. E., Tognon, M., and Roizman, B. (1982). Ocular disease pattern induced by herpes simplex virus is genetically determined by a specific region of viral DNA, *J. Exp. Med.*, 155:475.
65. Oh, J. O., Moschini, G. B., Okumoto, M., and Stevens, T. (1972). Ocular pathogenicity of types 1 and 2 herpesvirus hominis in rabbits, *Infect. Immun.*, 5:412.

66. Oh, J. O., and Stevens, T. R. (1973). A comparison of types 1 and 2 herpesvirus hominis infection of rabbit eyes. I. Clinical manifestations, *Arch. Ophthalmol.*, 90:473.

67. Hill, J. M., Rayfield, M. A., and Haruta, Y. (1987). Strain specificity of spontaneous and adrenergically induced HSV-1 ocular reactivation in latently infected rabbits, *Curr. Eye Res.*, 6:91.

68. Zhang, W. H., Briones, O., and Dawson, C. R. (1986). Effect of autonomic mediators in recurrent shedding of herpes simplex in the rabbit eye, *Curr. Eye Res.*, 5:79.

69. Rivera, L., Beuerman, R. W., and Hill, J. M. (1988). Corneal nerves contain intra-axonal HSV-1 after virus reactivation by epinephrine iontophoresis, *Curr. Eye Res.*, 7:1001.

70. Rootman, D. S., Haruta, Y., Hill, J. M., and Kaufman, H. E. (1988). Corneal nerves are necessary for adrenergic reactivation of ocular herpes, *Invest. Ophthalmol. Vis. Sci.*, 29:351.

71. Haruta, Y., Rootman, D. S., Xie, L., Kiritoshi, A., and Hill, J. M. (1989). Recurrent HSV-1 corneal lesions in rabbits induced by cyclophosphamide and dexamethasone, *Invest. Ophthalmol. Vis. Sci.*, 30:371.

72. Haruta, Y., Rootman, D. S., and Hill, J. M. (1988). Recurrent HSV-1 corneal epithelial lesions induced by timolol iontophoresis in latently infected rabbits, *Invest. Ophthalmol. Vis. Sci.*, 29:387.

73. Hill, J. M., Shimomura, Y., Dudley, J. B., Berman, E., Haruta, Y., Kwon, B. S., and Maguire, L. J. (1987). Timolol induces HSV-1 ocular shedding in the latently infected rabbit, *Invest. Ophthalmol. Vis. Sci.*, 28:585.

74. Rootman, D. S., Haruta, Y., Hill, J. M., and Kaufman, H. E. (1989). Trifluridine decreases ocular HSV-1 recovery, not recurrent HSV-1 lesions following timolol iontophoresis in the rabbit, *Invest. Ophthalmol. Vis. Sci.*, 30:678.

75. Harwick, J., Romanowski, E., Araullo-Cruz, T., and Gordon, Y. J. (1987). Timolol promotes reactivation of latent HSV-1 in the mouse iontophoresis model, *Invest. Ophthalmol. Vis. Sci.*, 28:580.

76. Rootman, D. S., Haruta, Y., and Hill, J. M. (1990). Reactivation of HSV-1 in primates by transcorneal iontophoresis of adrenergic agents, *Invest. Ophthalmol. Vis. Sci.*, 31:597.

77. Cyrlin, M. N., Thomas, J. F., and Epstein, D. L. (1982). Additive effect of epinephrine to timolol therapy in primary open angle glaucoma, *Arch. Ophthalmol.*, 100:414.

78. Caudill, J. W., Romanowski, E., Araullo-Cruz, T., and Gordon, Y. J. (1986). Recovery of a latent HSV-1 thymidine kinase negative strain following iontophoresis and co-cultivation in the ocularly infected rabbit model, *Curr. Eye Res.*, 5:41.

79. Hill, J. M., Sedarati, F., Javier, R. T., Wagner, E. K., and Stevens, J. G. (1990). Herpes simplex virus latent phase transcription facilitates *in vivo* reactivation, *Virology*, 174:117.

80. Cook, S. D., Paveloff, M. J., Doucet, J. J., Cottingham, A. J., Sedarati, F., and Hill, J. M. (1991). Ocular herpes simplex virus reactivation in mice latently infected with latency-associated transcript mutants, *Invest. Ophthalmol. Vis. Sci.*, 32:1558.

81. Hill, J. M., Haruta, Y., Yamamoto, Y., Jones, M. D., Wingate, H. L., and Jemison, M. T. (1987). Lack of efficacy of adenosine-5'-monophosphate against HSV-1 ocular shedding in rabbits, *J. Ocul. Pharmacol.*, 3:31.

82. Demangone, M., Hill, J. M., and Kwon, B. S. (1987). Effects of ACV therapy during simultaneous reactivation of latent HSV-1 in the New Zealand albino rabbit, *Antiviral Res.*, 7:237.

83. Dunkel, E. C., and Pavan-Langston, D. (1987). HSV-induced reactivation: Contributions of epinephrine after corneal iontophoresis, *Curr. Eye Res.*, 6:75.

84. Gordon, Y. J., Caudill, J. W., Romanowski, E., and Araullo-Cruz, T. (1987). HSV-1 latency: Thymidine kinase requirements and the round-trip theory, *Curr. Eye Res.*, 6:611.

85. Mayers, M., Matli, M., Okumoto, M., Samy, M., and Smolin, G. (1985). Recombinant human interferon alpha-D in HSV-1 recurrence in the rabbit, *Invest. Ophthalmol. Vis. Sci.*, 26:237.

86. Nesburn, A. B., Willey, D. E., and Trousdale, M. D. (1983). Effect of intensive acyclovir therapy during artificial reactivation of latent herpes simplex virus, *Proc. Soc. Exp. Biol. Med.*, 172:316.

87. Smolin, G., Matli, M., Okumoto, M., Mayers, M., and Samy, M. (1984). Use of recombinant interferon to prevent recurrent herpes virus shedding, *Curr. Eye Res.*, 3:1069.
88. Trousdale, M. D., Gordon, Y. J., Peters, A. C. B., Gropen, T. I., Nelson, E., and Nesburn, A. B. (1984). Evaluation of lithium as an inhibitory agent of herpes simplex virus in cell cultures and during reactivation of latent infection in rabbits, *Antimicrob. Agents Chemother.*, 25:522.
89. Trousdale, M. D., Robin, J. B., Willey, D. E., and De Clerq, E. (1987). Intentional reactivation of latent ocular herpes infection during BVDU therapy, *Curr. Eye Res.*, 6:1471.

17

A New Ophthalmic Delivery System

Mark C. Richardson and Peter H. Bentley *Smith & Nephew Research Ltd., York University, Science Park, England*

I. INTRODUCTION

The formulation of drugs for ocular delivery has occupied the attention of a large number of workers over many years. The most common dosage forms have been, and remain, solutions, suspensions and ointments. The relative advantages/disadvantages of these systems has been described elsewhere in this book but the primary problem is the short precorneal residence time due to tear turnover, solution drainage, and nonproductive absorption.

There have been many approaches to improve the precorneal residence time, and thereby increase corneal penetration. These have included increasing the viscosity of solutions with polymers such as polyvinylalcohol (PVA) or hydroxypropylmethyl cellulose, the use of nonerodible inserts with rate-limiting membranes, pH or ionic sensitive gels, erodible inserts, and mucoadhesive polymers. These approaches have been well reviewed elsewhere (1–3).

A primary consideration in the development of any ocular delivery system is its ease of use and comfort to the patient. Inserts have suffered in the past owing to their difficult and unreliable application resulting in poor patient acceptance and compliance. Other workers (3) have taken the view that patient compliance with inserts was so poor that the only way to improve ocular drug delivery was to take existing solution dosage forms and modify them to sustain drug release.

The new ophthalmic delivery system (NODS) (4) is a method for presenting drugs to the eye within a water-soluble, drug-loaded film. It provides for accurate, reproducible dosing in an easily administered, preservative-free form. It overcomes many of the problems found previously with inserts and in addition offers significant improvements in bioavailability over drops (5).

II. DEVELOPMENT

Figure 1 shows in diagrammatic form the appearance and dimension of a NODS device. Essentially the device consists of a water-soluble drug-loaded flag approximately 4 mm

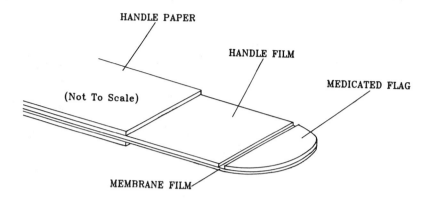

Figure 1. NODS: Diagram of appearance.

long and 6 mm wide with an area of 21 mm^2 and weight of approximately 500 μg which is attached to a water-soluble handle film via a soluble membrane approximately 0.7 mm in length. All three regions of the device are made from the same grade of water-soluble polyvinyl alcohol (PVA), varying only in thickness (handle 30 μ, membrane 3–4 μ and flag 20 μ). To make handling the device easier, the handle film is covered with a paper backing on both sides. The whole device is sealed as an individual unit into a moisture-proof package and sterilized by gamma-irradiation.

For administration, the flag is placed into the conjunctival sac and on contact with the tear fluid, the membrane rapidly dissolves, releasing the flag. The handle is then withdrawn and discarded. The flag, once in the sac, begins to hydrate and soften and release the drug.

The choice of the water-soluble polymer, PVA, was based upon the requirement for a polymer which formed robust but flexible films without plasticizer and which had a history of safe use in the eye. A number of polymers were studied but PVA had the advantage of widescale current use in ophthalmic solutions as a viscolizer, and the ability to be plasticized by water.

Experimentation in volunteers using blank NODS was used to select the ideal shape and dimensions of the device for easy patient or clinical administration.

III. FORMULATION

The inclusion of drugs into the NODS system offers several formulation advantages:

1. The essentially anhydrous nature of the system means that for drugs with poor aqueous stability, which cannot easily be formulated into drops, NODS offers a stable formulation route.
2. The pH of the flag can be adjusted (and buffers added if needed) for the optimum drug activity and corneal penetration even if the drug is poorly stable at this pH in solution.
3. The system is unit dose and, therefore, preservatives can be excluded, reducing the risk of sensitivity reactions.
4. Dosage is accurate, the flag containing a precisely controlled amount of drug, and therefore the risk of side effects due to overdosing can be minimized for certain drugs.

5. The system offers improved bioavailability, owing to prolonged ocular residence time, compared with drops and ointments and this will be discussed in detail later. This feature allows the use of lower total doses and hence reduced side effects compared with drops.
6. Both soluble and insoluble drugs can be formulated.

The advantages with respect to stability are illustrated with the drug pilocarpine nitrate. Normally, pilocarpine is formulated at pH 4.5 in solution. This is the optimum for stability but not for absorption. At pH 7, the drug exists as its base form to the extent of 50% and it is this form which is believed to have enhanced corneal penetration. However, at pH 7, significant decomposition would be expected over a few days in solution (6). When formulated into NODS at neutral pH, stability in excess of 1 year at 20°C can be demonstrated, whereas a corresponding solution lost 50% within 4 weeks' duration.

One aspect of the manufacture and processing of NODS which needs to be considered during formulation is the stability of the drugs to γ-irradiation during terminal sterilization (25 kGy in the United Kingdom). Drugs for ophthalmic use have not traditionally been sterilized by γ-irradiation and, therefore, an important activity in assessing whether a drug can be formulated into NODS is to assess any degradation which occurs. This has important toxicological implications, since the degradation products will not necessarily be the same as the aqueous products and toxicology studies on final NODS will need to reflect this fact.

IV. OCULAR CLEARANCE RATES

As mentioned earlier, one advantage of delivering drugs in a water-soluble film is to prolong the ocular residence time. This can intuitively be predicted by considering the likely differences in time taken for aqueous drop drainage and that for an anhydrous film to hydrate, soften, and dissolve. The residence time for any given dose of drug in the eye is likely to be greater with NODS than with a drop and hence bioavailability will be improved for similar doses. The ocular residence time for NODS was compared in human volunteers with a solution using the technique of γ-scintigraphy and employing a gamma camera. This was facilitated by the incorporation first of an insoluble marker, technecium-99m (^{99m}Tc)–labeled sulfur colloid, which will give an estimate of the residence time of the PVA film vehicle (and that of a poorly soluble drug within the vehicle). Second, a soluble marker was used, diethylenetriaminepentacetic acid (^{99m}Tc-DTPA), which will give an estimate of the residence time of a soluble compound in the eye when carried in the PVA film vehicle. Detailed methodology has been well described elsewhere by Wilson (7).

A. Scintigraphic Clearance Using ^{99m}Tc–Sulfur Colloid

Films were prepared on the day of the trial and were cut into sections (25 mm^2), each weighing 1.0 ± 0.2 mg and containing 2.0 ± 0.6 MBq of activity. Ten subjects were used and each was acclimatized to the room conditions for 30 min prior to the study. Each subject was positioned 5 cm from the collimator on the camera with their head supported and instructed to remain in this position throughout the period. The square of PVA was placed under the lower eyelid and a series of dynamic images of 15-s duration acquired for 15.5 min.

Three regions of interest (ROIs) were discriminated; i.e., the cornea, the inner canthus, and the lacrimal duct (Fig. 2). The counts in each region were corrected for background and

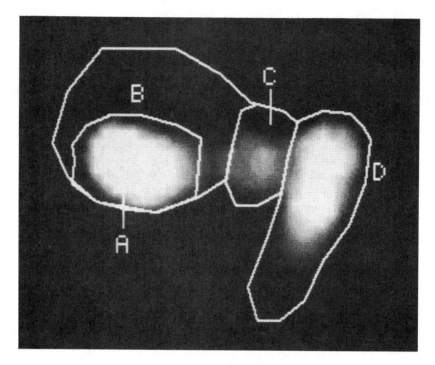

Figure 2. Summed gamma camera image of a human eye showing regions of interest (ROIs) after administration of a NODS radiolabeled with ^{99m}Tc DTPA. A: NODS (i.e. area of administration); B: corneal surface; C: inner canthus; D: nasolacrimal duct.

radioactive decay. Data were then normalized and curves of the mean corneal clearance were constructed.

The PVA film was observed to soften within the first minute and by 2 min released activity outlined the lower tear margin and lacrimal sac. By 6 min, considerable dissolution had taken place and lacrimal duct is clearly host to a large amount of marker. In the last frame at 13 min, the film had completely dissipated. Figure 3 shows the mean data (±SEM) for the clearance of the marker, and hence the film, from the corneal ROI. The mean curve showed a monoexponential clearance with a mean half-life of 8 min. The anticipated value for a solution is a few seconds and other workers have shown that greater than 75% of the dose is eliminated within the first minute (8). Individuals showed marked differences in rate of clearance with half-lifes between 2 and 24 min (9).

B. Scintigraphic Clearance Using ^{99m}Tc–Diethylenetriaminepentacetic Acid (^{99m}Tc-DTPA)

The basic methodology for this study was as described above but using the soluble marker incorporated into the PVA and a total of 12 volunteers. In addition, a pH 7 solution containing the marker was used and compared with the film on a separate occasion in each volunteer. Figure 4 shows the mean data (±SEM) for the clearance of the marker, and therefore a soluble drug, from the corneal ROI when added to an aqueous solution and a

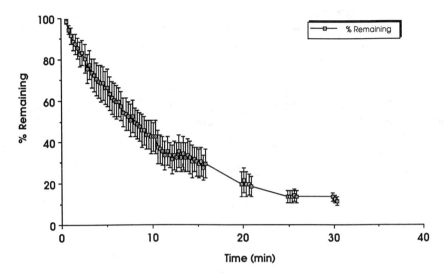

Figure 3. Loss of ^{99m}Tc-labeled sulfur colloid from corneal area of interest with time following administration in NODS film to human volunteers (n = 10). Mean data are shown (±SEM).

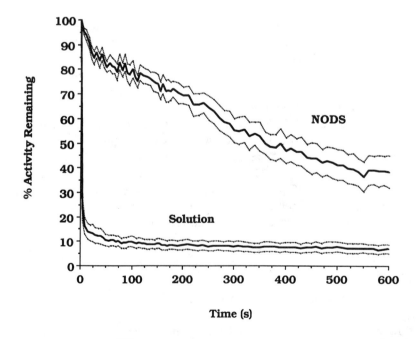

Figure 4. Loss of ^{99m}Tc-labeled DTPA from corneal area of interest with time following administration in NODS film or in solution to human volunteers (n = 12). Mean data are shown (±SEM).

PVA film. The mean half-life of the drop was approximately 3.0 s whereas that for the film was 6.8 min. As previously, volunteers showed marked differences in clearance rate between 2.5 and 14.0 min (10).

C. Conclusions

As mentioned earlier, it is clear that the primary determinant of the efficacy of an ophthalmic delivery system is the time which it allows the drug to remain in the precorneal film. Therefore, an increase in ocular residence time is likely to improve the drug bioavailability to the eye. As shown above, an aqueous solution of a water-soluble drug is likely to have a half-life ($t_{1/2}$) of only 3 s, whereas the NODS system has been shown to have a $t_{1/2}$ for the PVA film itself of approximately 8 min and for a water-soluble drug incorporated into the film a $t_{1/2}$ of approximately 7 min. A poorly soluble drug incorporated into the film is likely to have a $t_{1/2}$ equivalent to that of the film above.

The above prolonged ocular residence times combined with the ability to formulate an ionic drug at the optimum pH for absorption are, therefore, likely to lead to a significantly improved bioavailability for drugs in NODS compared with other delivery systems.

V. HUMAN EFFICACY AND BIOAVAILABILITY STUDIES

The NODSs have been studied in humans for both ease of administration/comfort and efficacy with a range of placebo NODSs and drug-loaded NODSs. Some of the key studies are summarized below.

A. Tropicamide

Tropicamide is a drug widely used for mydriasis and is generally administered as a 0.5% solution. A study was carried out in 12 human volunteers to compare the effects produced by a 125-μg tropicamide-NODS and one drop of a 0.5% solution (containing 125 μg drug) in contralateral eyes. The effects evaluated were mydriasis (using a pupillometer to measure pupil diameter), abolition of light reflex (determined using a slit-lamp), and cycloplegia (determined using a near-point ruler).

The mydriasis results are shown in Figure 5. The peak effect for both formulations occurred between 30 and 45 min. However, NODS gave a statistically significant ($p < 0.05$) greater mean pupil diameter up to 7 h. The results for light reflex (Fig. 6) and cycloplegia (Fig. 7) also show an enhanced effect for NODS compared with a solution at equivalent doses. The NODS-tropicamide (125 μg) is considered to be a satisfactory mydriatic/cycloplegic, whereas a tropicamide solution (0.5%w/v) was only an adequate mydriatic. The data therefore show, as anticipated, an improved bioavailability of NODS compared with solutions (11).

B. Chloramphenicol

The increase in tear concentrations following administration of NODS was revealed in the following trial (12).

A study in 12 human volunteers was carried out in which NODS containing a mean dose of 122.8 μg chloramphenicol was applied to the outer canthus and compared with Minims (trademark of Smith & Nephew) (0.5%, 25 μl ≡ 125 μg) drops and with

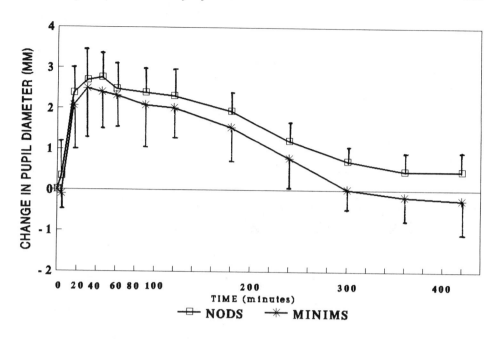

Figure 5. Tropicamide-NODS—Mydriasis. Mean change in pupil diameter (±SD) in comparison with solution.

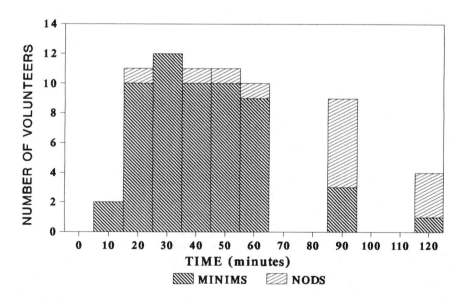

Figure 6. Tropicamide-NODS—Number of volunteers showing abolition of light reflex in comparison with solution.

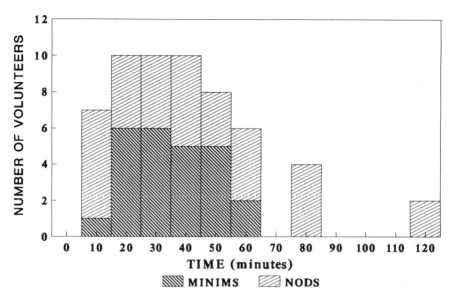

Figure 7. Tropicamide-NODS—Number of volunteers showing cycloplegia (accommodation <2 diopters) in comparison with solution.

Chloromycetin (trademark of Parke-Davis) ointment (1%, 12.5 mg = 125 μg), both applied to the lower conjunctival sac. Separate randomized groups allowed tears to be collected using a micropipette at six time points up to 64 min postadministration. Concentrations of the drug were measured by HPLC with a detection limit of 0.5 ng/sample. The tear concentration-time curves are presented in Figure 8 and the area under the curves (AVCs) and relative bioavailabilities are given in Table 1. It is evident that following administration of the drop, tear concentrations fall rapidly to below 10 μg/ml at 16 min. Levels generated by NODS or the ointment remain fairly constant between 2 and 8 min with levels from NODS being two- to threefold higher than from ointment, after which they decline. Levels at 1 h in either case are in excess of the minimum inhibitory concentrations (2 μg/mL) for the majority of bacteria sensitive to this drug. In terms of AUC, NODSs are 2.1-fold and 13.9-fold more effective than the ointment or drops, respectively.

C. Pilocarpine

The increase in bioavailability using NODS in comparison to drops has also been demonstrated by measuring the miotic effects of pilocarpine nitrate (13). In this study in healthy volunteers (n = 8, age 19–36 years), Minims eye drops (2%, 1 drop delivering 518 μg) were compared in one eye with NODS containing either 40, 80, or 170 μg of pilocarpine nitrate adjusted to pH 7 with potassium hydroxide. The other eye served as control in all cases. Drug effects on pupil diameter and light reflex amplitude up to 24 h postadministration were calculated as differences in measured values between treated and untreated eyes.

Figure 9 shows the mean miosis plotted against time for the four treatments and Table 2 provides the values for the peak miosis, AUC, and light reflex inhibition (%), calculated as follows:

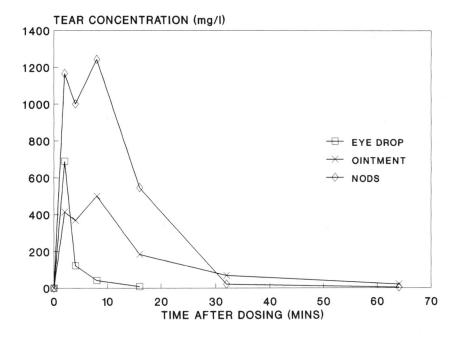

Figure 8. Chloramphenicol-NODS: Tear concentrations at different times following administration of NODS, 1% ointment, or 0.5% drop to human volunteers (n = 12). Mean data are shown.

$$LRI\ (\%)\ =\ \frac{(RAU_t - RAT_t) - (RAU_o - RAT_o)}{RAU_t}\ \times 100$$

where RAT = reflex amplitude (treated eye) in mm, RAU = reflex amplitude (untreated eye) in mm, each at time (t) or at time t = 0

It is evident that in terms of peak responses, AUC, or light reflex inhibition (LRI) the ranking is NODS 170 µg > NODS 80 µg > 2% drop > NODS 40 µg. As indicated in Table 2, it is possible to calculate from these data the NODS dose equivalent to the 2% eye drop to be about 67 µg, indicating a relative bioavailability of 578 ÷ 67 = 7.7.

In a more recent study (10) referred to earlier, NODS film incorporating both pilocarpine nitrate (63 µg, neutralized to pH 7) and a soluble ^{99m}Tc-labeled derivative was studied in healthy volunteers in comparison to a corresponding drop formulation. The miosis

Table 1. Chloramphenicol: NODS (Dose, AUC [from Tear Concentration-Time Curves] and Relative Bioavailability [RB] Values Following Administration of Chloramphenicol to Human Volunteers as NODS, Ointment, or Drops)

Formulation	Dose (µg)	AUC (g/L/min)	RB
NODS	123	18.75	13.9
1% Ointment	125	8.70	6.5
0.5% Drop	125	1.34	1.0

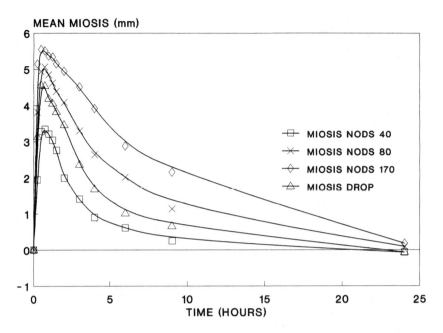

Figure 9. Pilocarpine NODS: Miosis at different times following administration of NODS (containing 40, 80, or 170 µg) or as 2% drop to human volunteers (n = 8). Mean data are shown.

time-curve confirmed the earlier study in that the AUC (to 5 h postadministration) for both treatments were not statistically different (i.e., 63 µg in the NODS ≡ 1 drop of 2%). However, the maximal pupil constriction arising from NODS administration was statistically greater than that from the drop (Table 3). In addition, the NODS produced a significant lowering of intraocular pressure (IOP) compared to the control which was not statistically different from IOP lowering by the drop formulation.

Similarly, the maximal changes in IOP were not significantly different.

Table 2. Pilocarpine: NODS (Peak Miosis, Miosis AUCs [From Miosis Time-Curve, Fig. 9] and Light Reflex Inhibition [LRI] Values Following Administration of Pilocarpine Nitrate to Human Volunteers, as NODS and Drops)

Formulation	Miosis peak (mm)	Miosis AUC (mm h)	LRI (%)
NODS 40 µg	3.42	12.23	60.3
NODS 80 µg	5.07	33.78	88.2
NODS 170 µg	5.67	50.70	95.0
Drops 2%	4.65	22.07	78.4
NODS equiv (µg)	67.1	65.6	68.5

Source: Adapted from Ref. 13.

Table 3. Pilocarpine: NODS (Peak Miosis, Miosis AUC (from Diameter Time-Curves), IOP Lowering AUC (from IOP Time-Curves) and Maximal IOP Lowering Following Administration to Human Volunteers as NODS [67 µg] or as 2% Drops)

	Units	NODS (63 µg)	Solution (2%)
Miosis peak	mm ±s.d	2.87 ± 0.89	1.8 ± 0.95
Pupil diameter	mm.h ±s.d.	17.0 ± 3.9	19.6 ± 4.8
IOP AUC_{0-5}	mm Hg.h ±s.d.	50.8 ± 8.7	56.2 ± 13
Max. IOP Lowering	mm Hg ±s.d.	3.29 ± 1.68	2.67 ± 1.57

VI. USER ACCEPTABILITY

A. Patient Acceptance

A new formulation for ophthalmic administration must address the ease of self-administration, often by elderly patients with poor eyesight, for chronic conditions such as glaucoma.

In a trial in healthy volunteers (n = 201, ages 18+ years), who were not regular drop users, unmedicated NODS carrying approximately 1.5 µg of fluorescein to enable the clear flag to be visualized, were self-administered to each eye twice a day for 7 days. The volunteers had been given instructions as to use both verbally and in writing. Expert assessment on days 1 and 7, together with an analysis of completed reports, indicated that 94% of the volunteers were inserting NODS successfully on day 7 and 76% had learned to do this by day 2. There was no significant difference between sexes or age groups in this respect. The majority preferred to use a mirror when using NODS, and experienced a slight foreign body sensation following release of the flag to the eye. Eighty-one percent of the volunteers believed this lasted less than 2 min but was only slightly uncomfortable. The NODS were considered well tolerated, easy to use, and convenient.

In a further trial, patients (n = 38) with primary open-angle glaucoma, all experienced drop users, applied NODS-fluorescein to one eye and artificial tear drops to the other twice a day for 7 days. Again, there was expert assessment on days 1 and 7 and patients completed a report. Analysis revealed that 68% of patients successfully inserted NODS on day 7 and 71% indicated that they preferred NODS to drops or found them equally acceptable. The majority of these patients preferred to use a mirror to aid the insertion.

B. Physician Acceptance

To assess ease of use and acceptability in outpatient clinics, a total of 174 patients at three U.K. centers with a mean age of 62 years, range 18–93 years, received NODS-tropicamide containing 125 µg in one eye or both eyes (279 eyes). The NODSs were administered by 14 nurses and 3 ophthalmologists, who found the NODSs quick and easy to apply and acceptable for routine use. The majority of patients recorded some initial discomfort as a transient stinging sensation on initial insertion.

In these and other trials in humans, NODSs have been well tolerated and safe to use.

VII. TOXICITY

Chronic administration of unmedicated NODS to the eyes of rabbits caused no observable toxic effects when the eyes were viewed macroscopically or microscopically or following examination histologically.

Aqueous solutions of PVA up to concentrations of 3–4% are approved for use in humans by direct instillation into the eye. An exposure of 1000–2000 μg of PVA per drop would be expected, which is two to four times the amount contained in the NODS flag.

No significant additional symptoms have been seen with medicated NODSs to date that were considered NODS related and above those expected from the particular drug itself. When medicated NODSs were compared with ointments or drops in rabbits, any irritancy effects normally associated with the drug are often considerably less pronounced with the NODS formulation when a bioequivalent dose is used.

VIII. CONCLUSIONS

These studies have shown that NODSs provide easily administered unit-dose formulations without the need for preservatives. Drug dose may be lowered by factors of 3–13 on account of increased bioavailability compared to other conventional formulations. They have been well received by both patients and physicians in terms of ease of administration, comfort, and effectiveness.

REFERENCES

1. Lee, V. H. L., and Robinson, J. R. (1986). Review: Topical ocular drug delivery: Recent developments and future challenges, *J. Ocul. Pharmacol.*, 2:67.
2. Lee, V. H. L. (1990). Review: New directions in the Optimization of ocular drug delivery, *J. Ocul. Pharmacol.*, 6:157.
3. Robinson, J. R. (1990). Mucoadhesive ocular drug delivery systems. *In*: Bioadhesion—Possibilities and Future Trends (R. Gurny and H. E. Junginger, eds.). Wiss Verl-Ges., Stuttgart.
4. Lloyd, R. (Smith & Nephew Research, Ltd.) U.K. Patent 2097680 (1985).
5. Bentley, P. H. (April 1990). Essentially as presented at the 9th Pharmaceutical Technology Conference "A New Ophthalmic Delivery System (NODS)." Veldhoven, The Netherlands; Abstract Vol. 2, p. 7.
6. Nunes, M. A., and Brochmann-Hanssen, E. (1974). Hydrolysis and epimerisation kinetics of pilocarpine in aqueous solution, *J. Pharm. Sci.*, 63:717.
7. Wilson, C. G. (1987). Scintigraphic evaluation of polymeric formulations for ophthalmic use. *In*: Ophthalmic Drug Delivery (FIDIA Research Series Vol. II) (M. F. Saettone, M. Bucci, and P. Speiser, eds.). Springer-Verlag, Berlin.
8. Zaki, I., Fitzgerald, P., Hardy, J. G., and Wilson, C. G. (1986). A comparison of the effect of viscosity on the precorneal residence of solutions in rabbit and man, *J. Pharm. Pharmacol.*, 38:463.

9. Fitzgerald, P., Wilson, C. G., Greaves, J. L., Frier, M., Hollingsbee, D., Gilbert, D., and Richardson, M. (1992). Scintigraphic assessment of the precorneal residence of a new ophthalmic delivery system (NODS) in man, *Int. J. Pharmaceut.*, 83:177.
10. Greaves, J. L., Wilson, C. G., Birmingham, A. T., Bentley, P. H., and Richardson, M. C. (1992). Scintigraphic studies on the corneal residence of a New Ophthalmic Delivery System (NODS): Rate of clearance of a soluble marker in relation to duration of pharmacological action of pilocarpine, *Br. J. Clin. Pharmac.*, 33:603.
11. Richardson, M. C. (April 1990). Poster 17 at the 9th Pharmaceutical Technology Conference, "An Investigation of Tropicamide NODS compared with Tropicamide Solution in Human Volunteers." Veldhoven, The Netherlands, Abstract Vol. 2, p. 307.
12. Hollingsbee, D. A., Hughes, K., and Gilbert, D. (October 1986). Poster presented at the International Symposium on Ophthalmic Drug Delivery, "A Comparison of the Human Ocular Bioavailability of Chloramphenicol Administered as a Solution, an Ointment and a Water Soluble Polymeric Film Insert." Pisa, Italy.
13. Kelly, J. A., Molyneux, P. D., Smith, S. A., and Smith, S. E. (1989). Relative bioavailability of pilocarpine from a Novel Ophthalmic Delivery System and conventional eyedrop formulations, *Br. J. Ophthalmol.*, 73:360.

18
Ocular Penetration Enhancers

Jiahorng Liaw   *School of Pharmacy, Taipei Medical College, Taipei, Taiwan*

Joseph R. Robinson   *School of Pharmacy, University of Wisconsin, Madison, Wisconsin*

I. INTRODUCTION

Owing to its importance in the conversation of normal optics of the eye, the cornea is protected from noxious substances in the environment by a variety of mechanisms, most notably a high tear secretion rate flushing its surface, as well as an impermeable corneal surface epithelium. Unfortunately, from a therapeutic standpoint, these protective mechanisms make it difficult to assure an effective concentration of drug at the intended site. Thus, an understanding of these mechanisms is a prerequisite for development of effective delivery systems.

Topical ocular drug delivery, using conventional dosage forms such as solutions, suspensions, and ointments, is relatively inefficient, because less than 10% of an applied dose is absorbed across the cornea into the eye. This low drug absorption is caused by both the impermeable nature of the corneal epithelium, as well as various precorneal loss processes, which include binding of drugs to proteins in tears with subsequent loss through tear drainage, nonproductive absorption of drugs across the conjunctiva and into the systemic circulation, and rapid drainage of instilled aqueous solutions into the nasal passages (1,2).

Scientists who have attempted to improve the bioavailability of topical ocular drugs have sought to extend the time of ocular contact by using nanoparticles, liposomes, gels, inserts, latex systems, and bioadhesives (3–7). Others have sought to improve the permeability of the cornea to drugs by transiently modifying the integrity of the corneal epithelium through chelating agents and surfactants (8,9). Attempts have also been made to improve specific drug permeability using the prodrug approach by making simple, reversible, modifications to the drug's chemical structure (10). These approaches have yielded slight to moderate improvements in the bioavailability of ocular drugs (2). In contrast, the ocular bioavailability of topically applied peptides and proteins is expected to be lower or at least no better than the ocular bioavailability of small drug molecules. The difficulty that peptides and proteins encounter in crossing the corneal epithelium arises from their

369

unfavorable molecular size, charge, and hydrophilicity, as well as their susceptibility to degradation by peptidases in the eye. Over the years, attempts have been made to improve ocular bioavailability of peptides and proteins, most notably through the use of penetration enhancers, such as actin filament inhibitors, surfactants, bile salts, chelators, and organic compounds (11,12).

Although some of these enhancers have been shown to be effective, they normally create multiple effects on the tissues and oftentimes cause problems associated with tissue irritation and damage. Undoubtedly, one of the major factors contributing to the limited success of this approach is the lack of information on basic transport mechanisms of drugs and how such mechanisms can be regulated. Therefore, this chapter will concentrate on mechanisms/methods of enhancing such delivery.

II. KINETIC MODEL OF PRECORNEAL DRUG DISPOSITION

As a prelude to discussion of corneal penetration enhancers, in order to appreciate the magnitude of enhancement that is required, it is helpful to describe the kinetics of drug movement in the front of the eye from an applied dose. A simple model of precorneal drug movement will suffice to demonstrate the principle.

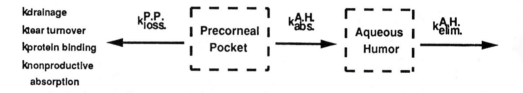

Scheme I.

Scheme I depicts an elementary kinetic model to account for drug movement in the front of the eye.

Inspection of scheme I suggests that if the left-hand portion, representing the loss components from the front of the eye, were not present, the drug concentration versus time profile in the aqueous humor would look identical to a comparable blood serum versus time profile for orally administered drug. In effect there would be an ascending and descending part of the curve such as is depicted in Figure 1.

Depending on the magnitude of the $k_{abs.}^{AH}$ and $k_{elim.}^{AH}$ would determine the assignment of rate constants to the right (descending) or left (ascending) part of the curve. For many drugs, pilocarpine can be used as an example, the true $k_{abs.}^{AH} \approx 0.003$ min^{-1} and the $k_{elim.}^{AH} \approx 0.02$ min^{-1}. Thus, since $k_{abs.}^{AH} \ll k_{elim.}^{AH}$, it fits the classic "flip-flop" model and hence the right-hand portion of the curve in Figure 1 corresponds to $k_{abs.}^{AH}$ and the left-hand curve corresponds to $k_{elim.}^{AH}$. Recall that this analysis was with the assumption that no loss from the precorneal pocket occurred; i.e., all of the rate constants on the left hand side of scheme 1 equal zero. In reality, all of these terms are not zero and indeed are rather large. A typical combined k_{loss}^{PP} constants (they are all first-order and can therefore be summed) are $k_{loss}^{PP} = 0.45$–0.65 min^{-1}. This gives rise to a kinetic scheme referred to as a "parallel elimination" process, as depicted in scheme II.

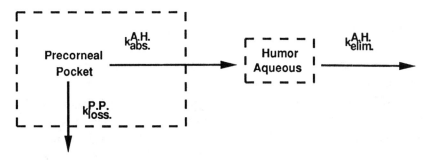

Scheme II.

The dotted box indicates the "parallel elimination" aspect of the descriptive term. One of the characteristics of this process is that the apparent $k_{abs.}^{AH}$ is actually the sum of the true $k_{abs.}^{AH}$ in the aqueous humor and the k_{loss}^{PP} in the precorneal pocket, thus

apparent $k_{abs.}^{AH}$ = true $k_{abs.}^{AH}$ + k_{loss}^{PP}

apparent $k_{abs.}^{AH}$ = 0.003 + 0.55 = 0.533

hence, the new kinetic scheme is

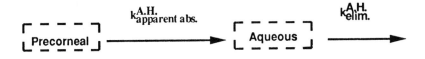

Scheme III.

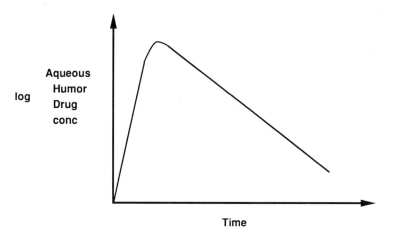

Figure 1.

Note that there is no longer a "flip-flop" model and the kinetic scheme is "well-behaved."

Inspection of the magnitudes of the two rate constants k_{loss}^{PP} and $k_{abs.}^{AH}$ provides a sense of the magnitude changes that are necessary to improve ocular bioavailability. Thus, $k_{abs.}^{AH}$ = 0.003 min^{-1} and k_{loss}^{PP} = 0.5 min^{-1}. To significantly improve the bioavailability of topically applied drugs, it is necessary to very substantially reduce k_{loss} through dosage form manipulation or substantially increase $k_{abs.}^{AH}$; i.e., corneal permeability through permeability enhancers. An additional perspective of the relative impermeability of the cornea is shown in Table 1, in which the permeability constants for a few drugs in the cornea and other tissues are compared. Recognizing the potential difficulties of broad generalization, inspection of Table 1 suggests that the cornea has a permeability to small organic molecules that is somewhere between that of the skin and the buccal area, both of which are considered relatively impermeable tissues.

III. TRANSPORT CHARACTERISTIC OF EPITHELIAL TISSUE

Transport across epithelia occurs via two pathways: transcellular and paracellular. The former involves cell/tissue partitioning/diffusion, channel diffusion, and carrier-mediated transport. In contrast, the latter represents diffusive and convective transport occurring through intercellular spaces and tight junctions. Diffusive transport is a dissipative process

Table 1. Comparative Permeability Coefficients (in cm/s) of Several Drugs Between the Cornea and Other Tissues

Permeant	MW	Rabbit/dog buccal	Rabbit cornea	Human skin
Water	18	3.7×10^{-5} (rabbit) 2.6×10^{-5} (dog)	1.5×10^{-4}	1.4×10^{-7}
Glycerol	92	6.0×10^{-7}	4.5×10^{-6}	
Benzylamine	107	1.4×10^{-5}	1.76×10^{-5}	
Octanol	130	2.2×10^{-5}		1.4×10^{-5}
Amphetamine	135	1.5×10^{-5}		3.9×10^{-9}
Salicyclic acid	138	9.3×10^{-7}	7.4×10^{-6}	
Estradiol	272	6.6×10^{-6}		1.1×10^{-6}
Progesterone	314	8.9×10^{-6}	1.8×10^{-5}	4.2×10^{-7}
Ouabain	584	6.5×10^{-6}		1.1×10^{-9}

Source: Modified from Ref. 47.

that depends upon the difference in solute concentration and the permeability-surface area properties of the membrane. In contrast, convective transport is dominated by a balance of hydrostatic and osmotic gradients, solute concentration, and hydraulic and reflection coefficients of the restrictive barrier. As a first approximation, the epithelia can be depicted as a simple electrical circuit consisting of resistors (aqueous shunt paths) and capacitors (membrane lipid matrix). Resistance depends on the molecular dimension of the aqueous transport pathway, and the charge lining it, whereas the capacitance depends on dielectric constant of the insulating medium and geometry of the membrane; i.e., surface area and thickness.

The transport barrier of the epithelia has two basic properties: the "permeability," which can be quantified by the electrical resistance measurement, and the "permselectivity," which is a measure of the ability of the membrane to discriminate or show preference for transport of molecules of different charges. Based on the resistive and other transporting properties of the membrane, i.e., the transmembrane potential, epithelia can be classified as leaky or tight (13). Generally, epithelia with resistance in the range of 10–100 Ω cm^2 are considerably leaky, whereas those with resistance ranging from 300 to 10,000 Ω cm^2 are "tight" tissues. The cornea is general classified as a moderately tight or moderately leaky tissue (400–1000 Ω cm^2), as shown in Table 2 (14). Typical relative permselectivities for cations and anions in the corneal epithelia shown cation selectivity. This has been explained by the nature of the paracellular pathway, which is lined with negative charges that discriminate against passive movement of anions through the hydrated channel.

Barrier permselectivity is a complex phenomenon which combines not only a passive contribution from electrostatic shunt activity, probably due to membrane fixed charges, but also an active contribution from cell membrane activity. The latter is generally a reflection of carriers and pumps residing in the membrane. Since they are interrelated, i.e., the active potential can enhance or retard passive permeation depending on the polarity and

Table 2. Electrical Resistances and Permselectivities of Various Epithelia

Tissue	Species	Resistance (Ω cm^2)	P_K:	P_{NA}:	P_{Cl}
Proximal renal tube	Dog	6–7	1.10	1.00	0.72
Gallbladder	Rabbit	20	2.30	1.00	0.23
Small intestine					
duodenum	Rat	98			
jejunum	Rat	51	1.60	1.00	0.20
ileum	Rabbit	100	1.14	1.00	0.20
Colon	Rabbit	385	1.00	1.00	
Gastric mucosa					
antrum	Necturus	1,730	1.00		0.86
fundus	Necturus	2,230			
Urinary bladder	Toad	3,755	1.40	1.00	0.72
Amphibian skin	Toad	763		1.00	0.53
	Frog	8,700	1.33	1.00	4.46
Cornea	Rabbit	989	0.12	1.00	0.1
Free solution			1.47	1.00	1.52

magnitude of the potential, interpretation of permselectivity data is normally difficult unless the two contributions can be separated. In the cornea, more is known about active permselectivity owing to its importance in conservation of corneal transparency and maintenance of its metabolic function.

The primary role of transport phenomena across the cornea is related to the preservation of hydration and transparency of this tissue. The basic process consists of ionic pumps located in the boundary cellular layers that limit the amount of water in the stroma. At low degree of hydration, the cornea is transparent but becomes opaque when water is accumulated in the tissue. Through membrane active transport systems, the cornea generates a transepithelial potential which is negative on the epithelial side and positive on the endothelial side (15). Transepithelial sodium transport is dependent on its ability to cross the apical and basolateral membranes. In rabbit cornea, transepithelial sodium transport from the tears into the epithelium can be accounted for simply in terms of passive diffusion along its electrochemical gradient. This passive movement is the rate-limiting step in the active absorption of sodium into the stroma, as demonstrated by the direct correlation between apical membrane cation conductance. The extrusion of sodium from the cells into the stroma occurs in opposition to an electrochemical gradient, a process that requires an active transport mechanism in the basolateral membrane. The addition of ouabain, a sodium pump inhibitor, to the bathing solution has been shown to reduce transepithelial potential. This action by ouabain indicates that Na-K-ATPase and the associated pump are involved in ion transport in the corneal tissue. Accumulated evidence indicates that this process is only specific to certain ions; i.e., in rabbit cornea, where the majority of data have been obtained, the active potential arises from an inward sodium transport from tears to aqueous humor (15) and an outward chloride transport in the reverse direction (16).

In corneal and some epithelial cells, such as those involved in absorbing nutrients from the gut, carrier proteins are distributed asymmetrically in the plasma membrane/ epithelial layers and thereby contribute to the transcellular transport of absorbed solutes (17–19,48). As shown in Figure 2, this transcellular sodium transport depends on two sets of membrane-bound carrier proteins: One is confined to the apical surface and an active pump delivers selected molecules into the epithelial cell from the lumen of the gut; the other, sodium-independent transport proteins, which are confined to the basolateral surface, allows the same molecules to leave the cell by facilitated diffusion into the extracellular fluid on the other side. Directional pumping is maintained by a tight junction. Thus, the apical set of carrier proteins must not be allowed to migrate to the basolateral surface. Furthermore, the spaces between the epithelial cells must be sealed so that the transported molecules cannot diffuse back down into the lumen through the intercellular space. The Na-K-ATPase that maintains the sodium gradient across the plasma membrane of these cells is located in the basolateral domain. Also in this laboratory, we have shown evidence of lysine-sodium cotransport, and a corresponding energy-dependent system in the rabbit cornea (20). By decreasing the concentration of sodium and incubation with the sodium pump suppressor substance, ouabain, at the epithelial side, ^{14}C-lysine permeability from the epithelial to endothelial side decreased under both conditions. Cooperstein (18) also indicated that aminoisobutyric acid is ouabain-sensitive and dependent upon the presence of extracellular sodium at the corneal epithelial cells of the toad.

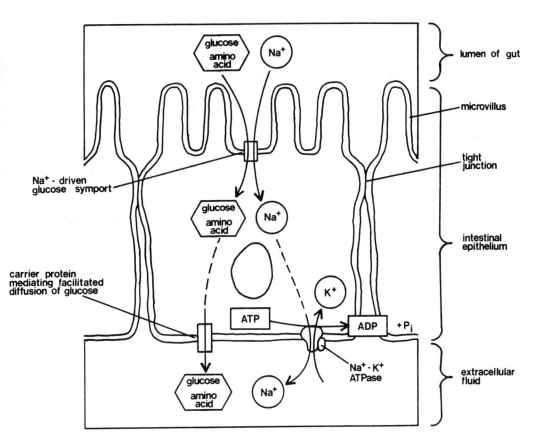

Figure 2. Transport proteins are confined to different regions of the plasma membrane in epithelial cells of the small intestinal or corneal tissues.

IV. MECHANISMS OF ACTION OF PENETRATION ENHANCERS

The precise mechanisms by which penetration enhancers improve corneal drug absorption are beginning to gain attention. It has been proposed that penetration enhancers improve corneal drug transport by two methods. The first method is an expanded paracellular pathway; i.e., 1) compounds that change the cell cytoskeleton, 2) alter tight junctions by promoting the transport of glucose or amino acids with sodium transport, and 3) choosing cationic molecules. The second approach is to enhance transcellular transport through 1) interaction with lipid membrane, and 2) interaction with the protein component of the cell membrane.

A. Expanded Paracellular Pathway

The permeability barrier of the cornea to hydrophilic molecules is thought to reside largely with the superficial surface of the epithelium; i.e., top two layers. Klyce et al. (21) showed that the apical surface of the corneal epithelium alone contributes over half of the total electrical resistance of the entire cornea. This is due to the presence of annular tight junctions or zonulae occludentes, which completely surround the superficial cells of the epithelium, thus effectively sealing the epithelium to all but the smallest hydrophilic molecules: Grass and Robinson have shown that the aqueous channel of the cornea has a size cutoff of around 90 D. Thus, for water, methanol, ethanol, and propanol, there appears to be aqueous channels to accommodate transcorneal movement for these compounds. Tight junctions are also present in the corneal endothelium but, unlike those at the epithelial surface, these do not extend around the cells as complete occluding belts. This is reflected by the size cutoff of permeant molecules through the corneal endothelium of around 20 nm, which means that it is readily permeable to colloidal tracers (23,24). Likewise, the basal and wing cells of the epithelium and the stroma are relatively unimportant as barriers to permeation. An elegant demonstration of the role of cell-cell junctional spaces in drug movement is to monitor horseradish peroxidase (HRP) (40 kD) movement through the cornea. Injection of HRP into the aqueous humor and monitoring its progress through the cornea using immunocytochemical staining reveals that HRP readily penetrates the corneal endothelium and stroma as well as the bottom three to four layers of the corneal epithelium. Two to three cell layers from the corneal surface HRP diffusion stops due to tight cell-cell junctions (25).

1. Cytoskeletal Modulation of Corneal Permeability

While tight junctions of the corneal epithelium have not been exclusively studied, much is known about tight junctions in general from work in other tissues and in cell monolayers (26,27). Tight junction are bandlike regions in which the membranes of adjacent epithelial cells appear to contact one another, and these bands completely encircle the superficial epithelial cells. Over the years, studies have shown that the cytoskeleton participates in regulation of epithelial permeability in a variety of conditions (28). Ultrastructural evidence also indicate that microfilaments and microtubules exhibit a close association with cellular junctions (29). Cereijido et al. (30) demonstrated that actin microfilaments of cultured epithelial cells form a complete ring at the lateral borders of the cells, where tight junctions are located. Disruption of these filaments, e.g., by treatment with specific cytoskeleton-active agents such as cytochalasin B and by removal of extracellular calcium, results in an increase in tight junction permeability (31). The exact mechanism for the regulation of tight junctions is unclear at present, but probably involves specific interactions between microfilaments and certain tight junction proteins. Indeed, a number of specific junctional proteins, such as ZO-1 (32) and cingulin (33) have been recently identified in various epithelia, including the colon, kidney, testes, and cornea.

Additional experiments performed in this laboratory further explored the potential of cytoskeletal modulators as corneal penetration enhancers (11). The data showed that an increase in corneal permeability indicates changes in the integrity of junctional expansion, which in turn results in a parallel drop in the electrical resistance by cytochalasin B treatment or EDTA–calcium chelator–treated tissues. The electrical resistance is primarily a measure of ionic conductance through shunt or paracellular pathways, consisting of tight junctions and intercellular spaces in series. In addition to monitoring the change in electrical resistance, experimental modulation of tight junctions in the cornea by cytochalasin B and EDTA was also examined morphologically by means of confocal fluorescence microscopy. Treatment with EDTA and deoxycholate allowed significant ingress of propidium iodide, a nuclear stain, into the surface epithelial cells, indicating permeabilization of the cell membranes and thus potential tissue damage; cytochalasin B, on the other hand, appeared to induce only minimal cell permeabilization. It thus appears that cytochalasin B acts via a paracellular pathway rather than by permeabilizing the individual epithelial cells. Indeed, cytochalasin B is an actin microfilament inhibitor. This may prove to be a preferable mode of action for penetration enhancers, particularly in the case of tight junction–controlled epithelia such as the cornea.

2. Alter Tight Junctions by Promoting Glucose or Amino Acid with Sodium Cotransport

Pappenheimer and Reiss (34) demonstrated that in the presence of 25 mM glucose, alanine, or leucine, fluid flow from the jejunum and upper ileum of the rat was doubled, as was clearance of creatinine (MW 113,3.2Å), PEG 4000 (MW 4000, 12.4Å), and inulin (MW 5,500, 14Å). Moreover, Pappenheimer showed that there was a two- to threefold decrease in resistance with a simultaneous increase of membrane surface (capacitance) and width of the intercellular junctions and lateral spaces (lower resistance) (49). The equivalent pore radius was estimated to be 50 Å. This response was dependent on oxygen tension, suggesting the involvement of some energy-dependent contractile process.

According to this mechanism, active transport of glucose or amino acids, which is coupled to sodium transport, across the intestinal mucosa into the intercellular lateral spaces creates an osmotic force for fluid flow. This in turn triggers contraction of the perijunctional actomyosin ring, resulting in increased paracellular permeability (35). Martinez-Palomo et al. (36) showed that solutions made hypertonic with lysine induce a reversible opening of the tight junction of the toad urinary bladder without gross deformation of the junction compared with hypertonic solutions of urea or sucrose. By measuring transepithelial membrane resistance, increasing concentration of lysine (50 mM) in the apical solution decreased the transepithelial resistance and was reversed when an isotonic solution was replaced on the apical side of the epithelium. When urea or sucrose is used, the minimal increases in osmolarity that produced a drop in transepithelial resistance corresponded to concentrations of 150 mM for urea and 300 mM for sucrose. Also, in this laboratory, we have shown that transcorneal movement of lysine is a sodium-dependent and ouabain-sensitive transcorneal movement from the epithelial to endothelial side (20). Thus, this could be a possible reversible mode for penetration enhancement.

Involvement of actin filaments in this process is indicated by a gradual increase in paracellular permeability upon exposure to cytochalasins, drugs that disrupt actin filaments (35) which are known to interact directly with the zonula occludens (ZO) or indirectly through disruption of the more extensive actin filament interaction with the zonula adherens (ZA). Phorbol esters, through stimulating protein kinase C (a calcium/phospholipid–dependent enzyme), induced opening of tight junctions, as judged from increased paracellular permeability of the LLC-PK1 cell monolayers to D-mannitol and PEG 4000 (37). A positive correlation between transepithelial resistance of cultured intestinal epithelia, their transepithelial mannitol fluxes, and number of strands in their occluding junctions has been established (38).

3. Charge Type and Charge Density Effect on Transcorneal Absorption

In addition to the general permeability barrier, transepithelial delivery of peptides and proteins via the paracellular route may also depend on the type and degree of charge selectivity of the epithelia. This is due to the fact that drugs are generally charged and the epithelia are known to possess permselective properties; i.e., the ability to discriminate or show preference to passage of certain charged molecules. Barrier permselectivity is a complex phenomenon which combines not only a passive contribution from electrostatic shunt activity, probably due to membrane fixed charges, but also an active potential contribution from cell membrane activity. With regard to passive permselectivity, recent studies by Rojanasakul and Robinson (39) have indicated that the cornea contains both positively and negatively charged groups whose magnitude and polarity depends on the degree of protonation. At pHs above the isoelectric point, pI = 3.2, the cornea carries a net negative charge and is selective to positively charged molecules. Below the pI, the reverse is valid. Based on these findings, a study of the in vitro flux of lysine (MW 146, positive charge) and glutamic acid (MW 147, negative charge) was conducted (40). Results from these experiments indicated an approximately two- to threefold difference in the permeability of the two compounds, with lysine being more absorptive. Also, Zadunaisky et al. (41) showed that epinephrine ($pK_a=8.50$), assuming just a pH difference of one log unit, yields a fivefold increase in drug concentration on the more acidic side.

B. Enhanced Transcellular Transport

Enhancers that increase transcellular permeability to drugs probably do so by affecting membrane lipids and proteins components. For instance, by using Fourier transform infrared spectroscopy (FT-IR) method (42), Potts et al. have indicated that oleic acid exerts a significant effect on the stratum corneum (SC) lipids by lowering the lipid transition temperature in addition to increasing the conformational freedom or flexibility of the endogenous lipid alkyl chains above their transition temperature. The enhanced transport of molecules across the SC was through the formation of permeable interfacial defects within the SC lipid layers which effectively decrease either the diffusional path length or the resistance. Tomita et al. (43) indicated that caprylate interacted mainly with proteins, whereas caprate interacted with both proteins and lipids. Using one or more of the above techniques, fatty acids and their derivatives have been found to act primarily on the phospholipid component of membranes thereby creating disorder and resulting in increased permeability (12).

The extraction of cholesterol out of the epithelial membrane was postulated to be the mechanism by which medium chain monoglycerides glyceryl-1-monooctanoate, glyceryl-1-monodecanoate, and glyceryl-1-monododecanoate promoted rectal cefoxitin absorption. Some fatty acids, however, act on the protein component in membranes. This is certainly the case for caprylate (12). Salicylates also act on the protein component of plasma membranes as indicated by their effect on fluorescence polarization of sodium 8-anilino-1-naphthalenesulfonate (ANS) incorporated in the brush border membrane vesicles of the rat small intestine. Additional evidence is that the enhancers released entrapped carboxyfluorescein from brush border membrane vesicles but not from liposomes made of phosphatidylcholine:cholesterol 1:1 and phosphatidylcholine:cholesterol:phosphatidic acid 1:1:0.1 (44).

Nonprotein thiols are yet another membrane component where certain enhancers act. In most tissues, the nonprotein thiols are composed almost entirely of glutathione. Boyd et al. (45) reported that glutathione comprised as high as 95% of nonprotein thiols in the rat glandular stomach. The good correlation between reduced nonprotein thiols and enhanced transport of hydrophilic compounds suggests an important role for nonprotein thiols in preventing the transport of hydrophilic compounds (12). Compounds known to affect nonprotein thiols include diethyl maleate (46) and salicylates. For example, Nishihata et al.

(50) showed that depletion of these nonprotein thiols by treatment with SH-modifying agents like diethyl maleate, diethyl ethoxymethylenemalonate, ethanol, or salicylates enhanced the mucosal to serosol transport of many hydrophilic compound including cefoxitin and phenol red in rat intestinal tissue.

V. CONCLUSIONS

In conclusion, it can be seen that one of the principal problems in ocular delivery of drugs is relatively low permeability of these drugs across ocular tissues. While an obvious solution to this problem would appear to be the use of penetration enhancers, this avenue has not been extensively studied to date. This chapter outlines an alternative approach to an empirical search for ocular penetration enhancers; i.e., to identify enhancers based on a detailed knowledge of the permeation pathway. It appears that the cytoskeletal modulator, cytochalasin B, as well as enhancing sodium cotransport with amino acids or glucose and perhaps selecting charge type of molecules will be able to increase the corneal intercellular permeability, but with substantially less membrane damage. Results to date suggest that these methods may be acting on a paracellular permeation pathway, indicting that it may yet be possible to develop penetration enhancers with highly specific foci of action, good reversibility, and minimal toxicity for ocular delivery.

REFERENCES

1. Sieg, J. W., and Robinson, J. R. (1976). Mechanistic studies on transcorneal permeation of pilocarpine, *J. Pharm. Sci.*, 65:1816.
2. Lee, V. H. L., and Robinson, J. R. (1986). Topical drug delivery: recent developments and future challenges, *J. Ocular Pharmacol.*, 2:67.
3. Wood, R. W., and Robinson, J. R., et al. (1985). Ocular disposition of poly-hexyl-2-cyano acrylate nanoparticles in the albino rabbit, *Int. J. Pharm.*, 23:175.
4. Lee, V. H. L., and Urrea, P. T., et al. (1985). Ocular drug bioavailability from topically applied liposomes, *Surv. Ophthalmol.*, 29:335.
5. March, W. F., and Stewart, R. M., et al. (1982). Duration of effect of pilocarpine gel, *Am. J. Ophthalmol.*, 100:1270.
6. Salminen, L., and Urtti, H., et al. (1983). Prolonged pulse-entry of pilocarpine with a soluble drug insert, *Graefes Arch. Clin. Exp. Ophthalmol.*, 221:96.
7. Hui, H. W., and Robinson, J. R. (1985). Ocular drug delivery of progesterone using a bioadhesive polymer, *Int. J. Pharm.*, 26:203.
8. Grass, G. M., and Robinson, J. R. (1985). Effects of calcium chelating agents on corneal permeability, *Invest. Ophthalmol. Vis. Sci.*, 26:110.
9. Burstein, N. L. (1984). Preservative alteration of corneal permeability in humans and rabbits, *Invest. Ophthalmol. Vis. Sci.*, 25:1453–1459.
10. Chang, S. C., et al. Improved corneal penetration of timolol by prodrugs as a means of to reduce systemic frog load, *Invest. Ophthalmol. Vis. Sci.*, in press.
11. Rojanasakul, Y., Liaw, J., and Robinson, J. R. (1990). Mechanisms of action of some penetration enhancears in the cornea: Laser scanning confocal microscopic and electrophysiology studies, *Int. J. Pharm.*, 66:133.
12. Lee, V. H. L. (ed.). (1990). *Peptides and Proteins Drug Delivery*. Marcel Dekker, New York.
13. Fromter, E., and Diamond, J. (1972). Route of passive ion permeation in epithelia, *Nature New Biol.*, 235:9–13.
14. Rojanasakul, Y. (1989). "Mechanistic Studies of Ocular Peptide Absorption and Its Enhancement by Various Penetration Enhancers." Ph.D. Thesis, University of Wisconsin–Madison.

15. Donn, A., Maurice, D. M., et al. (1959). Studies on the living cornea in vitro I: Method and physiologic measurement, *Arch. Ophthalmol.*, 62:741–747.

16. Klyce, S. D., and Neufeld, D. (1973). The activation of chloride transport by epinephrine and DB C-AMP in the cornea of rabbit, *Invest. Ophthalmol.*, 12:127–139.

17. Riley, M. V., Linz, D. H., et al. (1973). Entry of amino acid into the rabbit cornea, *Exp. Eye Res.*, 15:677–681.

18. Cooperstein, D. F. (1985). Amino acid transport by corneal epithelial cells from the toad, bufo marinus, *Comp. Biochem. Facial.*, 81:427–430.

19. Alberts, B., Watson, J. D., et al. (1989). *Molecular Biology of the Cell*, 2 ed. Garland, pp. 310–311.

20. Liaw, J., and Robinson, J. R. (1991). The effect of amino acid charge type and density on corneal transport, *Controlled Release Soc.*, in press.

21. Klyce, S. D. (1972). Electrical profiles in the corneal epithelium, *J. Facial. (Lond.)*, 226:407–429.

22. Grass, G. M., and Robinson, J. R. (1988). Mechanisms of corneal drug penetration 1: In vivo and in vitro kinetics, *J. Pharm. Sci.*, 77:3–14.

23. Hirsch, M., and Renard, G. (1977). Study of the ultrastructure of the rabbit corneal endothelium by the freeze-fracture technique: Apical and lateral junctions, *Exp. Eye Res.*, 25:277–288.

24. Burstein, N. L. (1979). Corneal endothelial permeability to electron opaque tracers demonstrated by modified propane jet cryofixation, *J. Cell Biol.*, 83(suppl.):300.

25. Tonjum, A. M. (1974). Permeability of horseradish peroxidase in the rabbit corneal epithelium, *Acta Ophthalmol.*, 52:650–658.

26. Meza, I., and Martinez-Palomo, A. (1980). Occluding junction and cytoskeletal components in a cultured transporting epithelium, *J. Cell Biol.*, 87:746–754.

27. Cereijido, M., Meza, I., and Martinez-Palomo, A. (1981). Occluding junctions in cultured epithelial monolayers, *Am. J. Physiol. Facial.*, 240:C96–C102.

28. Frederiksen, O., and Leyssac, P. P. (1977). Effects of cytochalasin B and dimethylsulfoxide on isoosmotic fluid transport by rabbit gall-bladder in vitro, *J. Facial (Lund.)*, 265:103–118.

29. Craig, W. S., and Prado, J. V. (1979). Alpha-actinin localization in the junction complex of the intestinal epithelial cells, *J. Cell Biol.*, 80:203–210.

30. Cereijido, M., et al. (1980). Structural and functional membrane polarity in cultured monolayers of MDCK cells, *J. Membr. Biol.*, 52:147–149.

31. Cohen, E., et al. (1985). Formation of tight junctions in the epithelial cells, *Exp. Cell Res.*, 156:103–116.

32. Stevenson, B. R., et al. (1986). Identification of ZO-1: a high molecular weight polypeptide associated with the tight junction in a variety of epithelia, *J. Cell Biol.*, 103:755–766.

33. Citi, S., et al. (1988). Cingulin, a new peripheral component of tight junctions, *Nature*, 333: 272–276.

34. Pappenheimer, J. R., and Reiss, K. Z. (1987). Contribution of solvent drag through intercellular junctions to absorption of nutrients by small intestine of the rat, *J. Membr. Biol.* 100:123.

35. Madara, J. L., et al. (1986). Effects of cytochalasin D on occluding junctions of intestinal absorptive cells: Further evidence that the cytoskeleton may influence paracellular permeability and junctional charge selectivity, *J. Cell Biol.*, 102:2125.

36. Martinez-Palomo, A. (1975). Structure of tight junctions in epithelia with different permeability, *Proc. Natl. Acad. Sci. U.S.A.*, 72:4487–4491.

37. Mullin, J. M., and O'Brien, T. (1986). Effect of tumor promoters on LLC-PK1, *Am. J. Physiol.*, 251:C597.

38. Madara, J. L., and Dharmsataphorn, K. (1985). Occluding junction structure-function relationships in a cultured epithelial monolayer, *J. Cell Biol.*, 101:2124.

39. Rojanasakul, Y., and Robinson, J. R. (1989). Transport mechanisms of the cornea: Characterization of barrier permselectivity, *Int. J. Pharm.*, 55:237–246.

40. Liaw, J., Rojanasakul, Y., and Robinson, J. R. (1989). Effect of drug charge type and density on corneal drug transport, *Pharm. Res.*, 6:s90.

41. Zadunaisky, J. A., and Spinowitz, B. (1976). Drugs and ocular tissues, 57–78.

42. Ongpipattanakul, B., et al. (1991). Evidence that oleic acid exists in a separate phase within stratum corneum lipids, *Pharm. Res.*, 8:350–354.

43. Tomita, M., et al. (1988). Enhancement of colonic drug absorption by the transcellular permeation route, *Pharm. Res.*, 5:786.

44. Kajii, H., et al. (1986). Effect of salicylic acid on the permeability of the plasma membrane of the small intestine of the rat: a fluorescence spectroscopic approach to elucidate the mechanism of promoted drug absorption, *J. Pharm. Sci.*, 75:475.

45. Boyd, S. C., et al. (1979). High concentrations of glutathione in glandular stomach: Possible implications for carcinogenesis, *Science*, 205–209, 1979.

46. Nishihata, T., et al. (1986). The effect of salicylates concentration on the uptake of salicylates and cefmetazole into rat isolated small intestinal epithelial cells, *Pharm. Res.*, 3:345.

47. Harris, D., and Robinson, J. R. (1990). Bioadhesive polymers in peptide drug delivery, *Biomaterials*, 11:652–658.

48. Cooperstein, D. F. (1983). Na-K-ATPase activity and transport processes in toad corneal epithelium, *Comp. Biochem. Facial.*, 87:1119–1121.

49. Madara, J. L., and Pappenheimer, J. R. (1987). Structural basis for physiological regulation of paracellular pathways in intestinal epithelia, *J. Membr. Biol.*, 100:149.

50. Murakami, M., et al. (1988). Intestinal absorption enhanced by unsaturated fatty acids: Inhibitory effect of sulfhydryl modifiers, *Biochim. Biophys. Acta*, 293:238.

19
Intracameral, Intravitreal, and Retinal Drug Delivery

Joel A. Schulman   *Louisiana State University School of Medicine,*
Shreveport, Louisiana

Gholam A. Peyman   *Louisiana State University Medical Center*
School of Medicine, New Orleans, Louisiana

I. INTRODUCTION

The treatment of many ocular disorders is hampered by poor penetration into the eye of many systemically administered drugs. The tight junctional complexes (zonulae occludens) of the retinal pigment epithelium (RPE) and retinal capillaries are the site of the blood-ocular barrier. This barrier inhibits penetration of substances, including antibiotics, into the vitreous. To circumvent the barrier, different routes of intraocular drug delivery along with different methods of prolonging the therapeutic effect of a drug have been investigated.

II. ENDOPHTHALMITIS

Endophthalmitis occurs when replicating microorganisms invade the internal structures of the eye, resulting in intraocular inflammation (1). Endophthalmitis may be of either exogenous or endogenous origin and be caused by bacterial, fungal, or parasitic invasion of the eye. Exogenous endophthalmitis is three times more common than the endogenous type.

When the infection involves the sclera and extraocular orbital structures, it is termed a panophthalmitis. Endophthalmitis occurs most frequently as a complication of intraocular surgery (2).

A. Clinical Diagnosis

Endophthalmitis represents a disease state that may present at one extreme as an acute fulminant vision-threatening ocular emergency and at the other as a vision-decreasing chronic low-grade inflammation. Endophthalmitis caused by virulent microorganisms typically presents with a destructive, painful, and hyperacute course (3). In contrast, the organisms in chronic endophthalmitis are usually either fungal or anaerobic bacteria (4,5). Unlike the acute form, indolent endophthalmitis usually has an insidious onset with an indolent course. Patients with chronic endophthalmitis may show an initial transient response when treated with steroids but eventually the inflammation becomes refractory to steroids (4).

The ocular findings in acute and chronic endophthalmitis and visual prognosis for the eye are influenced by a variety of factors, including host resistance, occurrence and extent of trauma, virulence of the microorganism, time between onset of disease and initiation of therapy, exogenous versus endogenous infection, and the length and modification of therapy (6).

B. Causes

Endophthalmitis is a complication of ocular surgery, penetrating ocular trauma, or metastatic ocular involvement. The spectrum of pathogenic organisms varies significantly among these subgroups of endophthalmitis, influencing the selection of antimicrobial agents. Knowledge of the microbiology associated with each subgroup of endophthalmitis is important when choosing drugs for initial treatment (7). Furthermore, treatment modalities will vary depending upon whether the offending organism is bacterial or fungal.

Endophthalmitis most frequently occurs following intraocular surgery (8). In a large series (9) involving 81 cases of endophthalmitis treated with vitrectomy, the most common clinical setting followed intraocular surgery (65%). Perforating trauma was the clinical setting in 20% of cases, whereas the remainder of the cases (15%) were endogenous in origin. Fifty-four percent of cases followed cataract surgery. In a second series (10) involving 36 cases of infectious endophthalmitis, 66.6% of cases developed after intraocular surgery, with cataract extraction accounting for 47.2% of the total cases. A third series (11) involved 76 patients referred with the diagnosis of endophthalmitis; 63% of the 54 culture-positive cases followed previous intraocular surgery, 22% had sustained penetrating ocular trauma, and 15% resulted from a metastatic infection.

The treatment of endophthalmitis remains controversial. Results of clinically randomized studies to determine the most appropriate therapy do not exist. For instance, studies comparing the results in eyes treated with or without vitrectomy are usually biased, since the more severe cases undergo vitrectomy (12). Treatment of endophthalmitis is determined by a variety of factors, including the pathogenic organisms, the extent of intraocular involvement, and the course of the infection.

The results of treatment of endophthalmitis before the use of antibiotics were uniformly poor (13–16). Even after the introduction of potent antibiotics, treatment of endophthalmitis was associated with significant visual loss in the majority of eyes (17). Achieving adequate concentrations of antibiotics in the infected tissue and maintaining the drug levels for a prolonged period of time are crucial considerations when evaluating different routes of administration of antibiotics used to treat endophthalmitis. Routine and conventional methods of systemic, topical, and subconjunctival administration of antibiotics have yielded poor results (13,15,18,19). Seventy-three percent of patients were found by Leopold to retain less than finger-counting vision in a review of 103 cases of endophthalmitis from 1944 to 1960 (20).

Penetration of topically applied medication into the anterior chamber is generally poor. The action of the eyelids along with the flow of tears which dilutes the eye drops rapidly removes the medication from the corneal surface. These actions minimize contact of the medication with the cornea, usually resulting in limited corneal penetration and low drug levels in the anterior chamber (21,22).

Collagen shields are composed of non–cross-linked porcine collagen with average dissolution times of 12, 24, and 72 h. These lenses act as a drug reservoir when soaked in antibiotics or steroids. The proteolytic action of tears and the mechanical action of the eyelids result in biodegradation of these lenses, which mold to the surface of the cornea. Medication is released with degradation of the shields, with resulting aqueous levels at least equivalent or higher when compared to frequent topical administration (23–28). The shields eliminate the need for frequent topical application of medication and problems associated with poor patient compliance (23–25). Yet vitreous levels of gentamicin following collagen shield delivery were found to be negligible (26).

Subconjunctival administration of antibiotics is used prophylactically after surgery to prevent endophthalmitis (29). This method of administration usually fails to produce high intravitreal drug levels (with the exception of a few of the newer antibiotics [29,30]) but generally results in bactericidal concentrations of many antimicrobial agents in the anterior chamber (31–33). Following parenteral administration, many antibiotics penetrate the anterior chamber, achieving therapeutic concentrations against many pathogenic organisms (32–39).

With the exception of some of the newer antibiotics (40–42), most antimicrobial agents administered parenterally fail to achieve sufficient intravitreal levels to be effective against many common organisms causing endophthalmitis (43–50). One experimental study has demonstrated that multiple, regularly repeated parenteral injections may result in therapeutic vitreous drug levels in inflamed eyes (51). Additionally, well-documented systemic side effects limit the use of several antimicrobial agents in the treatment of endophthalmitis (50).

Most studies (52,53) indicate that a single intravenous injection of an antimicrobial agent produces very low or undetectable drug levels; a few agents, including imipenem (40) and lipid-soluble drugs such as chloramphenicol and tetracycline, achieve therapeutic drug levels (54). Although the levels of antibiotics administered intravenously have been shown to vary significantly in the presence of both intraocular inflammation and different pathological states (54,55) such as proliferative vitreoretinopathy and rubeosis irides, the intraocular penetration is considered inadequate to treat endophthalmitis with the possible exception of a blood-retinal barrier compromised by infection (51).

Poor penetration into the vitreous can be explained in part by the tight junctional complexes (zonulae occludens) that interconnect cells of the retinal pigment epithelium and also tightly bind together the endothelial cells forming the walls of the retinal capillaries. These surfaces, which prohibit intercellular passage of fluids between cells, form the so-called blood-retinal barrier (56). This barrier inhibits bulk flow of materials, including exogenous antibiotics, into the vitreous. This may explain why the necessary intravitreal bactericidal concentration of antibiotics cannot be achieved by systemic administration. By the time the intravitreal infection breaks down this barrier, the retina has been irreversibly damaged.

The most logical means of bypassing physiological and anatomical barriers that might prevent rapid attainment of high vitreous drug concentrations appears to be through intravitreal injection. Intravitreal injection of antibiotics was first studied by von Sallmann and associates (57–59), who successfully treated early experimental staphylococcal endophthalmitis in rabbits with intravitreal injection of nontoxic doses of penicillin. Leopold (60) also found that the intravitreal injection of penicillin in rabbits favorably influenced the course of experimental endophthalmitis. These data led von Sallmann and others to attempt this method of treating clinically diagnosed endophthalmitis (58,59,61,62). A few cases were apparently cured; that is, the eyes were saved, although recovery of vision was rarely, if ever, achieved (58–62). In one instance, a patient with good visual results had no documented evidence of pyogenic organisms before treatment. Actually, the description of the case was more consistent with intense iridocyclitis after extracapsular cataract extraction than with endophthalmitis (63).

Intravitreal injection of antibiotics was abandoned for almost 2 decades, largely because the clinical results of intravitreal treatment of endophthalmitis with penicillin were discouraging. The usual course inevitably resulted in phthisis and useful vision was rarely maintained. In addition, because penicillin G given subconjunctivally achieved bactericidal concentrations in the vitreous (64), intravitreal injection was considered unnecessary. However, since a high percentage of infected eyes were still being lost and because direct intravitreal injections of antibiotics provides a high intraocular level of antibiotics, this method of drug delivery was again explored.

In a series of experiments, Peyman and associates (65–81) attempted 1) to determine the toxic level of various intravitreal antibiotics by clinical observation, histologic study, and electroretinography, 2) to measure the clearance of nontoxic doses of various antibiotics from the intraocular fluids after intravitreal injection, and 3) to compare intravitreal administration with combined systemic and subconjunctival administration in treating experimentally induced and human endophthalmitis. Intravitreal injections were given slowly into the anterior part of the vitreous, with the needle bent and directed away from the retina to avoid retinotoxicity. A nontoxic dose can become toxic if the site of injection is too close to the retina or if the injection is too rapid or forceful.

At this time other investigators also determined the clearance of various antibiotics (44,45,47,56–64,66,82–93). Nontoxic amounts were injected into the vitreous cavity, and the animals were killed at various intervals. Using in many instances the disk-sensitivity techniques of Kirby, the intravitreal concentrations were obtained at different intervals following intravitreal injection.

Several antibiotics were tested to determine a safe nontoxic dose that could be added to vitrectomy infusion fluid (94). Retinal toxicity was evaluated with ERG recordings and histopathological examination.

Experimental endophthalmitis (82) was produced by injecting various organisms into rabbit eyes. Endophthalmitis was treated by intravitreal injection of antibiotics at various time intervals. Other animals were treated with combined intravitreal injection of antibiotics and vitrectomy or conventional techniques of parenteral and subconjunctival injection of antibiotics. Significantly better results were apparent in animals receiving intravitreal antibiotics than in the conventional-treatment groups. Experimental data demonstrated no significant differences between animals treated with either intravitreal antibiotics alone or intravitreal antibiotics and vitrectomy. The only advantages of vitrectomy were to obtain clearer media and more rapid resolution of infection.

The volume of the vitreous in rabbit eyes is 1.5 mm, compared with 4 mm in humans. This size differential appears significant. Clinically, Peyman and associates determined the prognosis is better in severely infected eyes using intravitreal antibiotic injection and vitrectomy than with intravitreal injection alone.

The results of animal experiments form the bases for clinical trials in humans. The first large-scale investigation involved 26 eyes in 25 patients with endophthalmitis treated with either intravitreal injection alone or intravitreal injection in conjunction with vitrectomy

(82). The investigators found that 77% of patients retained their eye and 46 percent of patients had visual acuities better than 20/100; 27% of patients had vision ranging from light perception to 20/300, and 4% of patients had no light perception. Both aqueous and vitreous taps were recommended to obtain specimens appropriate for immediate microscopic examination and culture. When the vitreous was severely involved or fungal endophthalmitis suspected, primary vitrectomy was performed with the addition of selected antimicrobial agents in the intravitreal infusion fluids (96).

Two factors influenced results in this series. The majority of eyes that had visual acuities of 20/100 or better were treated within 36 h after the onset of symptoms. Eyes infected with organisms elaborating significant exotoxins and proteolytic enzymes did poorer than did the other eyes. Another series reported by Vastine and coworkers (97) confirmed that the visual prognosis in eyes with endophthalmitis treated with intravitreal antibiotics is related to these same factors: 1) interval between onset of symptoms and administration of intravitreal antibiotics, and 2) exotoxin and proteolytic activity of the organisms isolated from the eye.

III. GENERAL RESULTS OF EXPERIMENTATION

Animal experimentation using intravitreal injections was performed by different investigators (98–105) to determine the retinal toxicity of many commonly used antibiotics. Animal eyes injected with intravitreal antibiotics underwent electroretinography (ERG) and histopathological studies at various intervals.

Recent studies have involved electron microscopy (99–105), since the incipient toxicity of an injected antibiotic may be manifested solely by electron microscopic changes and only at higher, more toxic doses do gross light microscopic alterations become evident. Previous studies employing only light microscopic examination may not have been adequately sensitive (102) (Table 1).

The recommended intravitreal doses of many antibiotics were calculated to produce concentrations below the level toxic to the rabbit or primate eye. Unfortunately, little information is available on the dose-response relationship involving different antimicrobials for pathogenic agents in the vitreous; this information would be helpful in selecting the most effective concentration for intravitreal injection and avoiding underdosing or overdosing patients with endophthalmitis (106).

Experimental studies have demonstrated that following intravitreal injection, immediate high vitreous concentrations can be achieved and usually sustained for a prolonged period without retinal toxicity (107). Based on both the experimental data and clinical results, intravitreal injection of antimicrobial agents is now an established component in the treatment of infectious endophthalmitis.

IV. DRUG LEVELS IN THE VITREOUS

Talley and associates (108) divided aphakic rabbits with experimental endophthalmitis into three groups treated with either intravitreal antibiotics alone, intravitreal antibiotics with vitrectomy, or vitrectomy. The study demonstrated vitrectomy enhanced treatment results when used in conjunction with intravitreal antibiotics. A study by Ficker and associates (109) involving 17 patients with coagulase-negative *Staphylococcus aureus* endophthalmitis treated with vitrectomy, intraocular antibiotics, systemic antibiotics, and steroids also

Table 1. Ocular Anti-Infectives

Drug	Systemic dose (adult)	Topical (%)	Subconjunctival dose (mg)	Aqueous conc. from subconj. (µg/mL)	Intravitreal dose (mg)	Vitreous half-life (h)	Infusion solution conc. (µg/mL)
PENICILLINS							
Ampicillin	150–200 mg/kg/day IV		100		5	6	
Aziocillin	Up to 350 mg/kg/day IV		100	12			
Carbenicillin	400–600 mg/kg/day IV	10	100		0.5–2.0	10–20	
Dicloxacillin	0.125–0.5 g q6h PO/IM						
Methicillin	1–2 g q4h IV/IM	10	100		2	3–5	20
Nafcillin	1–2 g q4h IV/IM						
Oxacillin	1–2 g q4h IV/IM	6.6	100		0.5		10
Penicillin G	2–4 million U q4–6h IV	0.1	50,000–1 million U		0.2–0.3	3	10
Piperacillin	200–500 mg/kg/day IV/IM	5–10			1.5		
Ticarcillin	250–300 mg/kg/day IV/IM	5–10	100–150		3		

CEPHALOSPORINS							
Cefamandole	0.5 g q6h–2 g q4h IM/IV		12.5				
Cefazolin	0.25 g q8h–2 g q4h IM/IV	5–10	50–100		0.5–2.0	7	
Cefotaxime	1 g q8h–2 g q4h IM/IV	5–10	100	5	0.4		
Cefsulodin	1–1.5 g q6h IV		100				
Ceftazidime	1–2 g q8–12 h IV/IM		125	8	2	16	
Ceftriaxone	1–2 g q12–24 h IM/IV		100		2	12	
Cephalothin	0.5 g q6h–2 g q4h IM/IV	5	50–125		2		
Moxalactam	1 g q8h–2 g q4h IM/IV	10	100		1.25	20	
AMINOGLYCOSIDES							
Amikacin	15 mg/kg/day divided q8–12 h IM/IV	0.5–1.5	25	4	0.4	24	10
Gentamicin	3–5 mg/kg/day divided q8h IM/IV	0.3–1.5	10–40	4	0.2	12–35	8
Netilmicin	4.0–6.5 mg/kg/day divided q8h IM/IV				0.25	24	

Table 1. (Continued)

Drug	Systemic dose (adult)	Topical (%)	Subconjunctival dose (mg)	Aqueous conc. from subconj. (µg/mL)	Intravitreal dose (mg)	Vitreous half-life (h)	Infusion solution conc. (µg/mL)
Tobramycin	3–5 mg/kg/day divided q8h IM/IV	0.3–1.5	20–40		0.2	16	10
Neomycin		0.3–3.3					
MISCELLANEOUS							
Aztreonam	1 g q8h–2 g q6h IV				0.1	7.5	
Bacitracin		10,000 u/mL	10,000 U				
Ciprofloxacin	250–750 mg q12h PO				0.1 mg		
Clindamycin	150–450 mg q6h PO 150–900 mg q8h IV/IM	1–5	150		1	7–8	9
Chloramphenicol	0.25–0.75 g q6h PO 50 mg/kg/day IM/IV		50–100		2	10	10
Cotrimoxazole	2.5–5.0 mg/kg q6h IV	TMP 16 SMZ 80			1.6 (TMP)		
Fusidic Acid	500 mg tid PO/IV		Not recommended				
Imipenem	0.5–1.0 g q6h IV/IM				0.5		16

Drug	Dosage						
Metronidazole	7.5 mg/kg q6h IV						8
Teicoplanin	200 mg/day IV/IM	5	67	18	0.75		
Vancomycin	1 g q12h IV		25		1	30	
ANTIFUNGALS							
Amphotericin B	0.25 mg/kg, increase 0.5 mg/kg daily IV	0.1–5.0	0.750		0.005–0.010		
Clotrimazole	60–100 mg/kg/day PO	1	5–10				
Econazole	30 mg/kg/day IV/200 mg tid PO	1					
Fluconazole	50–400 mg/day PO/IV				0.1		
Flucytosine	50–150 mg/kg/day PO	1			0.1		
Itraconazole	50–400 unit/day PO				0.01		
Ketoconazole	200–1200 mg/day PO	1			0.54		
Miconazole	600 mg q12h IV	1	5–10	3–4	0.025–0.05		
Natamycin		5					
Oxiconazole					0.1		

Table 1. (Continued)

Drug	Systemic dose (adult)	Topical (%)	Subconjunctival dose (mg)	Aqueous conc. from subconj. (μg/mL)	Intravitreal dose (mg)	Vitreous half-life (h)	Infusion solution conc. (μg/mL)
Terconazole			5		0.01		
ANTIVIRALS							
Acyclovir	5–15 mg/kg q8h IV/200–600 5×/day PO	3 (oint)	2.5–25.0	23–309	0.24		40
Ethyldeoxyuridine					0.02		20
Investigational foscarnet	60 mg/kg Q 80 × 14 days				1		
Ganciclovir	Induction: 5 mg/kg q12h IV Maintenance: 6 mg/kg Q day				0.2–0.4		
Idoxuridine							
Trifluridine		10			0.02		60
Vidarabine	5–15 mg/kg/day in q12 h doses IV				20–30 μg/ 0.1 mL		32

For further information on systemic dosing suggest American Hospital Formulary.

Some dosing information has been extrapolated from animal studies. Extensive clinical data may be lacking. These doses are only guidelines. Clinical judgment is essential, especially in patients with intraocular gas, oil, among other substances.

concluded vitrectomy is effective when combined with intraocular antibiotics and systemic steroids when the clinician is confronted with moderate to severe endophthalmitis.

Talamo and associates (110) experimentally demonstrated the threshold toxic dose for aminoglycosides administered intravitreally was not altered by the surgical status of the eye. However, the data must be further evaluated.

Inflammation in experimental studies has been found to increase the penetration of some of the newer antimicrobial agents, including cefazolin, following intravenous administration into the vitreous cavity, allowing greater drug penetration across the blood-retinal barrier (51). Inflammation has a dual effect on elimination of some drugs from the vitreous. Experimental evidence demonstrated inflammation prolongs the half-life of cefazolin, β-lactam antibiotics, and penicillins. These antibiotics are removed by a retinal pump mechanism which is damaged by inflammation (51,111–113). In contrast, lipid-insoluble aminoglycosides are eliminated by an anterior route through the anterior chamber which involves aqueous circulation (113), increasing drug clearance (114,115).

Studies which have reported very low to nondetectable intravitreal drug levels following a single intravenous dose have usually been performed in noninflamed phakic eyes (51). Vitreous levels of cefazolin following a single intravenous injection were low in two studies (55,116). Martin and associates (51), using an experimental model of endophthalmitis, found repeated intravenous doses of cefazolin administered on a regular schedule in animals with inflamed eyes resulted in an incremental increase in vitreous drug concentration. Forty-nine hours after injection, the vitreous drug concentration was well above the minimum inhibitory concentration for organisms susceptible to cefazolin. This experimental design resembled clinical usage where repeated intravenous injections are administered on a regular schedule over a 2- to 3-day period, since drug levels following intravitreal injection which are initially high but decline in many (111,117) instances by 48 h to levels inadequate to provide significant coverage. Repeated intravitreal drug injections may cause retinotoxicity (118); regularly repeated intravenous administration of a drug which by 48 h produces a cumulative rise in achieved therapeutic vitreous levels may be useful as adjunct therapy for endophthalmitis.

V. GENERAL THERAPEUTIC PRINCIPLES GOVERNING THE TREATMENT OF ENDOPHTHALMITIS

Pathophysiological differences between exogenous (occurring as a complication of intraocular surgery, ocular trauma, or from an infectious corneal ulcer extending into the eye) and endogenous or bloodborne endophthalmitis influence the treatment of these two types of endophthalmitis (119).

Lesions that develop in endogenous endophthalmitis begin in the blood vessels of the choroid and retina. The blood-retinal barrier is disrupted, and then foci of infection extend to areas close to the chorioretinal blood vessels and spread to the vitreous (120). Because of damage to the blood-retinal barrier, parenterally administered antibiotics may reach therapeutic concentrations in the retina and vitreous at the site of infection (121).

Systemic administration of antimicrobial agents without recourse to intravitreal antibiotics has been successful in treating many cases of endogenous endophthalmitis (119).

Greenwald (119) has noted intravitreal antibiotics are usually not required in treating metastatic bacterial endophthalmitis with just involvement of the anterior segment or demonstrating vitreous involvement with just one or two discrete foci of inflammation.

Prompt treatment with intense intravenous administration of antibiotics using the initial and repeat doses based on the treatment recommended for meningitis and other severe infections appears to be the most important factor in treatment of these eyes. Treatment must be continued until the systemic infection is eradicated; antibiotic usage is modified when necessary to conform to culture and sensitivity test results.

Cases with mild vitreous involvement usually respond to systemic antibiotics. Vitrectomy and intravitreal antibiotics may be necessary in endogenous endophthalmitis with extensive vitreous involvement, since the outcome may be influenced by the physical state of the vitreous (122).

Incomplete vitreous detachment as a response to intraocular inflammation may result in both tangential and anterior-posterior vitreous traction resulting in macular pucker, traction retinal detachment, and retinal tears which may cause rhegmatogenous retinal detachment. Vitrectomy is usually not indicated in the presence of total vitreous detachment, since traction on the retina should not exist (122).

Exogenous endophthalmitis begins following inoculation of organisms into the vitreous (119).

Limited ocular penetration into the vitreous of most antimicrobial agents after parenteral administration due to low permeability during ocular circulation through the capillary endothelium has been noted. Intravitreal injection is advocated to overcome anatomical barriers and achieve therapeutic drug concentrations in the vitreous. Vitrectomy may also be required to remove active nodes of infection and prevent secondary vitreous changes (123).

VI. METHODS TO INCREASE INTRAOCULAR THERAPEUTIC EFFECTS WHILE REDUCING DRUG TOXICITY

The treatment of many posterior segment disorders, including endophthalmitis, viral retinitis, proliferative vitreoretinopathy, and intraocular inflammation after intravitreal surgery or uveitis, requires therapeutic levels of drugs in the vitreous cavity.

As previously noted in the treatment of endophthalmitis, the concentration levels achieved by topical, subconjunctival, or systemic administration of drugs have not usually been sufficient to be effective (124), since the blood-retinal barrier prevents the transport of most systemically administered drugs into the vitreous cavity. To achieve therapeutic concentrations of drugs in this compartment, intravitreal injections are often necessary.

Intravitreal injections, however, must be repeated in many clinical situations to maintain adequate therapeutic levels, and may be associated with ocular complications such as lens damage, retinal injury, infection, or bleeding in an already compromised eye. Moreover, the initial peak levels achieved by some drugs immediately after injection may result in ocular toxicity, further complicating the disease process (124–129).

Several methods have been designed to prolong the therapeutic effect of a drug and to reduce its toxicity. The first reported was that of Michelson et al. (130) in 1979, using a rabbit model of endophthalmitis to compare the efficacy of administering gentamicin using an osmotic minipump with that of administration by a standard intravitreal injection. A similar pump device was used later by Eliason and Maurice (131) for continuous long-term delivery of substances into the various compartments of the eye. The behavior of the system was evaluated by measuring the fluorescein turnover rate in the anterior chamber.

A method for prolonged drug infusion into the vitreous cavity was developed by Miki et al. in experimental animals (132). A cannula was inserted into the vitreous cavity and a silicone plate was used to control the location of the tip of the cannula. Fluorescein was administered to demonstrate the patency of the system.

None of these methods has achieved widespread use in clinical practice.

VII. LIPOSOME-ENCAPSULATED DRUGS

Liposomes are membranelike vesicles used to encapsulate drugs. Liposomes are made from phospholipids, such as lecithin, phosphatidylglycerol, and phosphatidylserine. Sterols (cholesterol and ergosterol), when incorporated into liposomes, increase the rigidity and stability of this macromolecule. Additional substances, including glycolipids, organic bases or acids, artificial polymers, or membrane proteins, may be added to influence the chemical, physical, and biological properties (133–136).

Liposomal intercalation before intravitreal injection has been used to enhance a drug's therapeutic index by primarily confining the drug's action to the local site of injection, increasing the amount of drug delivered to the target tissues, serving as a sustained-release depot extending the drug's half-life, and decreasing or minimizing intraocular side effects through a controlled-release effect (133).

Several types of liposomes are currently available as drug carriers. Large multilaminar liposomes consist of a series of lipid bilayers alternating with aqueous compartments. These structures are reasonably stable and are several microns in diameter. Multilaminar liposomes are formed when phospholipids are dispersed in an aqueous layer. Unilaminar liposomes are single-compartment vesicles containing a large internal aqueous space surrounded by a single bilipid membrane. Several methods are available to produce these unilaminar vesicles, including sonication of multilaminar liposomes, rapid injection of alcoholic lipid solutions into the aqueous phase, ether evaporation, and reverse-phase evaporation. These unilaminar liposomes vary in size depending on the methods used in their preparation (136).

The multivesicular liposome, a third type of liposome, consists of a cluster of numerous monolayered vesicles (thousands) surrounded by an outer lipid monolayer. An aqueous droplet is entrapped within each vesicle. Each liposome is large, ranging in diameter from 10 to 100 μm and can be visualized without magnification (137).

Incorporation of drugs into liposomes depends not only on the type of liposome (133) but also on the physical properties of the drug. Nonpolar drugs bind to the lipid membrane of the vesicle, whereas polar drugs are encapsulated in the aqueous compartment of liposomes (136).

The reticuloendothelial system (RES) plays a significant role in removing liposomes following parenteral administration (136). The mechanism by which liposomes are removed from the vitreous is unknown (137,138). Drugs entrapped within liposomes and administered parenterally have been successfully used in animal models to treat several infections and malignant diseases and for delivery of chemotherapeutic agents, steroids, enzymes, and chelating agents to tissues composing part of the RES (133). Depositing liposome-encapsulated drugs into specific sites has proved effective in selective disorders. This approach has been used in the treatment of experimental arthritis and tumors by injecting agents directly into involved joints or organs harboring malignancies (133).

Liposome-encapsulated antimicrobial agents improve the ocular delivery of drugs following topical and subconjunctival administration. Schaeffer et al. reported that liposome encapsulation enhanced the corneal penetration of topically applied penicillin and indoxole (139). Smolin and associates treated acute and chronic herpetic keratitis in albino rabbits and found that idoxuridine was more effective entrapped in liposomes than a comparable regimen of free drug (140). Dharma and colleagues reported that the corneal penetration of liposomal idoxuridine was significantly increased over the regular form of the drug for 6 h (141). After a single topical application for up to 3 h, liposome-bound triamcinolone acetate produced significantly higher drug concentrations in various ocular tissues, including the cornea, sclera, and aqueous humor than the suspension (142). Barza and coworkers demonstrated that subconjunctival injections of encapsulated gentamicin improved corneal concentrations (143).

Recent studies have demonstrated the vitreal concentration profiles for several antimicrobial agents have been increased by liposomal binding prior to intravitreal injection (144). Tremblay and associates (144) reported intravitreal injection of liposome-bound amphotericin B in doses ranging from 5 to 20 µg produced no retinal toxicity, whereas concentrations ranging from 4 to 10 µg/mL were present in the vitreous 5 weeks after administration. In contrast, retinal toxicity was observed by ophthalmological examination and histological studies 5 weeks after intravitreal injection of the free drug in doses as low as 5 µg.

Barza (145) found that liposomal intercalation reduced retinal toxicity of amphotericin B by at least fourfold and elevated the threshold damage for permanent retinal toxicity after a single intravitreal injection. Fishman and associates (146) demonstrated that the duration of therapeutic levels in the vitreous cavity was significantly increased when gentamicin was entrapped within liposomes. Effective inhibitory concentrations of liposome-encapsulated clindamycin were present compared to undetectable levels of the free drug 48 h after intravitreal injection in the rabbit (147).

Similarly, Alghadyan et al. (148) demonstrated liposome encapsulation decreases the toxicity of intravitreally administered penicillin G and prolongs the half-life in the vitreous by a factor of 10.

Two studies (129,149) have demonstrated experimentally induced endophthalmitis can be treated with encapsulated antimicrobial agents. Intravitreal liposome-encapsulated penicillin G (4000 units 0.1) was more efficacious than the free form of this antimicrobial in treating experimentally induced streptococcal endophthalmitis. A second study showed intravitreally administered clindamycin in two different concentrations (1 and 2 mg/0.1 mL) was effective in the treatment of *Staphylococcus aureus* endophthalmitis. Infection was halted in the 13 treated eyes, whereas one eye (treated with 1 mg/0.1 mL) continued to show signs of endophthalmitis. The six control eyes which received drug-free liposomes and three eyes not treated were lost to infection (129).

In a preliminary human study (150), a single intravitreal injection of liposome-encapsulated chemotherapeutic agent was effective in treating patients with acute toxoplasmosis retinochoroiditis, presumed *Propionibacterium acnes* endophthalmitis after cataract surgery, and presumed cytomegaloviral retinitis associated with acquired immunodeficiency syndrome (AIDS).

Different methods are available to target liposomes either to promote the interaction between specific cells or tissues and the encapsulated drug or release the contents of liposomes at specific sites (151). One approach involves temperature-sensitive liposomes which are formulated to release their contents in response to hyperthermia (152).

Khoobehi and associates (152), using rabbits, evaluated the feasibility of increasing the concentration of drugs in the anterior chamber of the eye using microwaves as an external triggering mechanism to release carboxyfluorescein (CF) and cytosine arabinoside (an antimetabolite) from temperature-sensitive liposomes. After intravenous injection of liposome-encapsulated CF, its concentration in the anterior chamber of eyes where the ciliary body's temperature was selectively increased by microwaves was eight times greater than in the control eyes. The same procedure done with liposome-encapsulated cytosine arabinoside yielded a 4.1 times greater concentration than in the control eye. These results suggested temperature-sensitive liposomes may be potentially useful as a new method for targeting the delivery of drugs and dye to specific sites inside the eye.

A similar liposome dye method was also used to measure retinal blood velocity and flow rate in primates (153). Argon laser was used to release a bolus of dye in the retina following systemic injection of liposome-encapsulated fluorescent dye. The volumetric flow rate and the distance traveled by the dye in retinal vessels of different diameters were calculated by measuring the distance traveled by the dye in a specific vein over a set time interval.

The laser beam was also used to release cytosine arabinoside from temperature-sensitive liposomes in vitro. Dynamic studies of the release of the drug from liposomes, diluted in blood flowing in a capillary tube at 40 μm/min, were conducted using an argon dye laser operating either in the blue-green mode (488/514 nm) or in the dye mode (577 nm). A radiolabeled marker was used to monitor the drug release. The results showed that the drug could indeed be released from liposomes that did not contain dye at energy levels that are not likely to be harmful to the tissue. At identical power levels, the release of the drug was greater at 577 nm than at 488/514 nm, probably owing to the greater light absorbance of hemoglobin at the longer wavelength. The results indicate the potential for the site-specific release of a variety of molecules in the ocular vasculature.

The externally controlled delivery of the drug using lasers has certain advantages over other systems. It appears likely that laser light could be used to release drugs at levels that are not toxic to the adjacent tissue and to release various drugs that can treat, destroy, or control the growth of the tissue in a specific area. Because liposomes persist in the circulation longer than many drugs administered intravenously, it may be possible to increase drug delivery to the targeted area in the retina (154).

Other investigators (155) used a similar method of dye delivery in primates by encapsulating the fluorescent dye carboxyfluorescein which was released by a short laser burst delivered to a retinal artery. This technique, which was repeatable as many as 100 times in 1 h, allowed visualization of the dye front throughout the retinal vasculature. The choroidal background, which can obscure retinal capillary details present in fluorescein angiograms, was eliminated and this technique was repeatable in contrast to fluorescein angiography, which usually is limited to a single injection. The technique appears to be safe and may be clinically useful in retinal vascular diseases which can cause damage to the retinal capillary network.

VIII. IONTOPHORESIS

Iontophoresis is a method of drug delivery which utilizes an electric current to drive a polar drug across a semipermeable membrane (156–178). In otolaryngology, the tympanic membrane and inner ear canal have been anesthetized by local anesthesia delivered by this technique (160). Transtympanic iontophoresis has been demonstrated to increase dexamethasone sodium phosphate levels in intratympanic fluid (161). Dentists have used iontophoresis to anesthetize teeth and to achieve local anesthesia of the oral mucosa (162) and deliver fluoride for hypersensitive dentin (162–164). The sweat test used by pediatricians and other physicians to diagnose cystic fibrosis involves transcutaneous delivery of pilocarpine hydrochloride by iontophoresis (174). Lidocaine iontophoresis has been demonstrated to be effective in achieving short-term safe anesthesia of eyelid skin (165).

Iontophoresis was first used by Von Sallmann in the early 1940s to treat experimental ocular disorders (166–168). Investigators have demonstrated the passage of some drugs crossing the cornea; penetration into the anterior chamber is increased sometimes 10- to 200-fold (159,161) by iontophoresis.

Corneal iontophoresis of gentamicin, tobramycin (169,172), and ciprofloxacin (170) has been effective in treating experimental pseudomonas keratitis (157).

Fishman and associates (158), using aphakic rabbits, demonstrated that iontophoresis was an effective means of delivering therapeutic levels of gentamicin in a noninvasive way across the cornea into ocular tissues, including the vitreous. An earlier report had demonstrated that this technique in phakic rabbits delivered high antibiotic concentrations to the cornea and anterior chamber but not to the vitreous. Removing the lens in rabbit eyes simulated the anatomical condition of pseudophakic endophthalmitis.

Transscleral iontophoresis has been shown experimentally to be an effective method to achieve and maintain therapeutic intravitreal levels of ionizable drugs, whereas avoiding complications of direct intravitreal drug injection, which include retinal toxicity from the drug or a small risk of retinal damage or endophthalmitis from the technique. The ora serrata appears best suited for transscleral iontophoresis because of a limited vascular circulation and the negligible effect on vision should any retinal damage occur (172).

Among the factors affecting intravitreal drug levels are the magnitude and duration of the applied current, the ionic charge on the drug molecule, which dictates the polarity of the electricity to allow the drug to be carried by the current, and the design of the application electrode. Discomfort limits the current to less than approximately 2 sec. To increase the drug crossing the sclera, the area of contact with the outside globe must be minimized, which may be achieved by using a narrow tube to hold the drug. This tube is placed in contact with the eyeball at the ora serrata (171).

Experimental intravitreal delivery by iontophoresis of a variety of drugs in therapeutic concentrations has been documented. These drugs include dexamethasone (156), cefazolin (172), ticarcillin (172), gentamicin (172,173,176), vancomycin (177), and ketoconazole (173).

In comparing corneal to transscleral iontophoresis, the latter technique is not only usually superior in facilitating drug penetration into the vitreous but the former method is ineffective in circumventing the lens diaphragm barrier in phakic eyes and will not deliver drugs into the vitreous in these eyes (172).

Transscleral iontophoresis in monkeys using gentamicin administered six times over a 2-week period demonstrated gentamicin levels comparable to levels produced by direct intravitreal injection of 100–200 µg the human eyes. With the exception of small retinal burns over the area where the electrode was applied, indirect ophthalmoscopy and electroretinography failed to demonstrate any pathology (176). Barza and associates (172) experimentally demonstrated intravitreal drug penetration following transscleral ionto-phoresis correlated with the duration of iontophoresis and the strength of the current but not with the drug solution concentration (172). The penetration of antibiotics was similar in both uninflamed eyes and eyes with endophthalmitis (172).

Barza and associates (178), using an animal model of infective endophthalmitis, demonstrated intravitreal injection of gentamicin was markedly less effective than the combined use of intravitreal injection followed by transscleral iontophoresis of gentamicin in reducing bacterial colony counts.

Experimental studies suggest iontophoresis is well tolerated, aside from some discom-fort and the possibility of small areas of retinal destruction not extending beyond the small area of placement of the external tube containing both the electrode and drug (172,175). Only limited studies involving iontophoresis on humans have been performed (59,179). Based on available data, iontophoresis shows some promise as an adjunct procedure in the treatment of endophthalmitis.

IX. MICROSPHERES

The established use of polymers based on lactic and glycolic acid in general surgery has made them suitable for experimental drug delivery systems (180,181). These systems may delay the clearance of the drug and reduce the need for repeated injections, thereby lowering the risk of complications.

Moritera et al. (182) reported the use of polymer microspheres containing 5-fluoro-uracil as a controlled drug delivery system in the vitreous cavity. Khoobehi et al. (183) used sodium fluorescein (NaF) entrapped in microspheres of lactide and lactide/glycolide (L/G) polymers for noninvasive quantitation of the clearance of the drug after intravitreal injection.

The intravitreal injection of drugs entrapped in microspheres is another potential means of prolonging therapeutic drug concentrations in the vitreous cavity.

Polymer microspheres based on copolymers of different substances, most commonly lactic and glycolic acid, have achieved wide usage in general surgery and are being evaluated as drug carriers (184). Investigation of the potential of polylactic acid (L-lactic acid) and DL-lactide was first reported by Kulkarni et al. (184,185).

Other materials subject to investigation include peptide polymers. Peptide/protein biopolymers have been developed to deliver drugs or hormones in the treatment of various diseases. These biopolymers are inactive by gastrointestinal administration, but have gained increasing recognition for transdermal controlled delivery of drugs (186–192).

Additional experiments demonstrated that the clearance of Na-fluorescein entrapped in microspheres made of polymers of lactic and glycolic acid is delayed when compared with the administration of free NaF (183). The methods of entrapment can be modified to improve the efficiency of the system, thereby increasing the efficiency of the drug. If drugs such as antibiotics or steroids can be adequately encapsulated into polymer microspheres, a sustained release of the drug is expected to continue as long as the microspheres remain in the eye. These delivery systems may prolong the therapeutic effects of drugs and avoid the initial high peak levels associated with free drug injection. Whether polymer microspheres present a better method of prolonging the therapeutic efficiency of drugs in the eye than other systems must be determined in future studies. Microspheres appear to be easier to prepare and store than liposomes.

X. VIRAL RETINITIS

Cytomegalovirus is the most frequently implicated cause of viral retinitis. Less common pathogens include two other members of the herpes virus family, herpes simplex and virus varicella-zoster virus. Cytomegaloviral and herpes simplex infections of the retina are almost always found in patients with immunological deficiencies (193).

Viral retinitis has assumed an increasingly prominent role in ophthalmological diseases as the incidence of ocular infections has significantly increased in recent years with the widespread use of parenteral corticosteroids and immunosuppressive agents (194). Also, the number of immunocompromised patients associated with acquired immunodeficiency syndrome (AIDS) is reaching epidemic proportions (195), because the total number of cases continues to double approximately every 11 months (196). Occasionally, viral retinitis may also occur in individuals with cancer or other debilitating diseases in which the patient has a lowered resistance to infection (197). Reports rarely describe viral retinitis (with the exception of acute retinal necrosis) in immunologically competent adults (198).

XI. CYTOMEGALOVIRAL RETINITIS

Retinitis produced by cytomegalovirus (CMV) occurs almost exclusively in newborns with cytomegalic inclusion disease or in immunosuppressed hosts, including individuals with cancer or AIDS and those receiving immunosuppressive drugs for organ transplantation (199–201). Improving immunity by decreasing or discontinuing immunosuppressive medication has been demonstrated to cause regression and healing of CMV retinitis in non-AIDS patients (197,201–203). To date, restoration of immunity has been impossible in patients with AIDS (204); consequently, treatment of CMV retinitis remains difficult.

Cytomegalovirus is the most common opportunistic ocular infection associated with retinitis in patients with AIDS. Often bilateral, the retinitis has been estimated to occur in 15–40% of patients with this immunodeficiency disorder (205).

Although the natural history of CMV retinitis not well understood, a large body of evidence now suggests the prognosis for eyes with retinitis from cytomegalovirus is poor, because the natural course of the infection is relentlessly progressive, eventually leading to blindness in many instances (205).

Though the rate of progression of CMV retinitis varies in individuals with AIDS, prolonged stabilization or regression of this retinitis has not been reported in this group of patients (206). In one series, CMV retinitis was the initial AIDS-defining opportunistic infection in 3% of individuals (207). In another series of patients, CMV retinitis was either the initial manifestation of AIDS alone or presented simultaneously with another opportunistic infection, providing the ophthalmologist the opportunity to make the diagnosis of AIDS in these patients (208).

Ganciclovir and foscarnet are the two approved antiviral agents used in treating CMV retinitis in AIDS patients. Each drug is administered initially in high doses during induction treatment, followed by a lower dose continuous maintenance regimen.

Ganciclovir was the first antiviral agent demonstrating therapeutic activity against CMV retinitis in patients with AIDS. A nucleoside analog of acyclovir, ganciclovir differs only by the addition of a 3' carbon and hydroxy group to the acyclic side chain. At low concentrations nontoxic to uninfected cells, both antiviral drugs are potent inhibitors of herpes simplex types 1 and 2 and varicella-zoster. In vitro tests have demonstrated that ganciclovir possesses 10 to 100 times greater activity against various laboratory and clinical isolates of cytomegalovirus than acyclovir (209,210).

Several case series without controlled observation have documented the usefulness of intravenously administered ganciclovir in the management of cytomegaloviral retinitis by delaying or reducing vision loss in AIDS patients (201,205,211–217). Based on clinical evidence (204,217) and verified by histopathological examinations (203,218) of retinal tissue from patients with AIDS and cytomegaloviral retinitis receiving ganciclovir therapy at the time of death or tissue biopsy, ganciclovir has been determined to act as a virustatic agent rather than completely eliminating the virus from the retina.

At least 80% of patients responded to an induction therapy which involves administration of 10 mg/kg per day in two divided doses over a 2-week period (216). Discontinuation of this parenterally administered agent invites relapse (213). The likelihood of recurrence of the retinitis is diminished by placing patients on a low-dose maintenance regimen. Maintenance therapy consists of either daily administration of 5 mg/kg intravenously or 6 mg/kg administered as a 1-h intravenous infusion 5 days a week (219).

Despite the use of preventive therapy, one series reported reactivation of the virus has been documented in 40 to 50% (207) of patients continuously receiving a maintenance dosage for longer than 3 weeks (201). However, ganciclovir appears to prevent CMV retinitis from developing in the second eye if not involved with this disease; the majority of patients with unilateral retinitis develop retinitis in the opposite eye if not treated parenterally with ganciclovir (206,207,220).

Ganciclovir has a relatively small margin of safety. Complications following parenteral administration in humans include leukopenia, fever, anorexia, itching associated with hives, thrombocytopenia, progressive neuropathy, diarrhea, psychosis, hallucinations, and phlebitis, which may limit the tolerance of some patients scheduled for a therapeutic course with this antiviral agent (203,217). Holland et al. evaluated complications associated with ganciclovir treatment for CMV retinitis in 20 patients with AIDS (201). Reversible neutropenia requiring temporary termination of therapy for variable periods of time developed in 25% of the 20 patients placed on initial treatment and 36% (live patients) of the 14 patients who received maintenance therapy with ganciclovir. Ussery et al. reported that thrombocytopenia or neutropenia may develop in up to 70% of patients receiving intravenous ganciclovir, necessitating temporary termination of drug use (221). Other side effects reported include inhibition of spermatogenesis, gastrointestinal mucosal atrophy and necrosis, rash, and phlebitis at the injection site (222).

Laboratory testing during induction consists of a complete blood count, including differential and platelet counts, performed two to three times weekly and then weekly while maintenance treatment is administered. Monthly serum creatine levels must be obtained. Ganciclovir dosages must be decreased when creatinine clearance is below 80 mL/min (219).

In one AIDS patient with CMV retinitis treated with ganciclovir, the development of thrombocytopenia preceded bilateral vitreous hemorrhage (223). Life-long parenteral therapy with ganciclovir may be burdensome for patients with AIDS. Possible deterrents that may affect the quality of life include the expense of therapy, complications associated with indwelling catheters (such as sepsis), inconvenience of frequent drug administration, and frequent hospital or clinic visits if maintenance therapy is not provided at home (125,217,224).

Retinal detachment was reported in 29% of eyes in a series of 17 patients (34 eyes) whose CMV retinitis had resolved with ganciclovir treatment. Multiple breaks in thin, peripheral atrophic retina caused the retinal detachments. Proliferative vitreoretinopathy complicated several eyes with retinal detachments before surgical repair could be undertaken. Endoretinal biopsy specimens obtained from two eyes during vitrectomy for retinal detachment repair revealed cytomegalovirus in retinal tissue, despite ongoing treatment with ganciclovir that appeared clinically effective (225).

The administration of zidovudine, a drug licensed by the U.S. Food and Drug Administration (FDA) which is effective against HIV, has been proven beneficial in prolonging life in patients with AIDS (204,221).

The causative agent of AIDS, the human immunodeficiency virus (HIV), has been isolated from most ocular tissue, including the retina (226). Recent evidence suggests HIV infection of the retina may enhance the probability of developing CMV retinitis. The HIV but not the CMV has been implicated in the development of retinal microangiopathy (227,228) and the virus has been isolated from the vascular endothelium. This damage to the vascular endothelium may increase the propensity of CMV to invade the retina (227,228).

Experiments have shown coinfection with both CMV and HIV enhances the replication of both viruses and dual infections of the retina with HIV and CMV have been reported which would present direct viral interactions (229). Additional evidence also suggests CMV coinfection accelerates the progression of HIV disease (230).

The role of zidovudine in treating CMV retinitis in patients with AIDS has not been established (207). Zidovudine appears generally ineffective in treating this infection (207,231) but in some individuals a beneficial effect has been documented (231–234), probably due to zidovudine's enhancing effect on the immune system (235).

Zidovudine does not have any direct antiviral effect on CMV (231,232) but may act by diminishing HIV enhancement of CMV infection or improving the immune status (229–231). The combined use of zidovudine and foscarnet may be additive in treating CMV retinitis. Foscarnet also inhibits HIV replication and one report suggests a secondary function of improving the host's general condition when both drugs were given concurrently to patients with AIDS and CMV retinitis (236).

Jabs and associates (207) reported CMV retinitis developing in six patients being treated with zidovudine for AIDS. The lesions continued to progress in five patients, whereas the sixth individual demonstrated complete resolution. D'Amico et al. (233) also described a single patient with AIDS whose CMV retinitis responds to zidovudine.

Zidovudine is frequently associated with marked bone marrow suppression (204,221) and usually is incompatible with ganciclovir. This places the physician in a dilemma when treating AIDS patients with CMV retinitis, since both drugs are associated with dose-limiting granulocytopenia. This toxicity usually limits concomitant therapy with both agents.

Multiple opportunistic infections are also associated with this complex disorder. Amphotericin B and trimethoprim-sulfa are among the therapeutic agents which, despite being myelosuppressive, may be required to treat life-threatening opportunistic infections.

The myelosuppression caused by ganciclovir may be worsened by concurrent administration with these other agents, necessitating discontinuation or severely limiting the use of ganciclovir (221).

Testosterone levels in males and the neutrophil count are evaluated when concomitant therapy is considered in an AIDS patient with CMV retinitis. Approximately 15–20% of homosexual men with AIDS demonstrated primary hypogonadism. The administration of testosterone results in correction of the gonadal dysfunction and improvement in bone marrow reserves. Utilizing careful modifications in zidovudine, both drugs may be used together with the zidovudine dose adjusted or stopped, depending on fluctuations of the absolute granulocyte count (235).

Foscarnet has been efficacious in treating CMV retinitis associated with AIDS (237–239) and other causes of immunosuppression (240) and nonocular tissue infections in immunocompromised patients (241,242). Foscarnet is an antiviral agent which acts at concentrations not toxic to host cell DNA polymerases by inhibiting many viral ribonucleic acid (RNA) and deoxyribonucleic acid (DNA) polymerases (236). Approximately 30% of patients receiving foscarnet develop renal toxicity, but this virostatic antiviral agent can be administered concurrently with antiretroviral therapy (237).

The second most serious complication is hypocalcemia, which has produced severe and at times fatal complications when foscarnet was administered to patients also receiving pentamidine (219). Seizures and arrhythmias may be due to resultant hypocalcemia when foscarnet is administered too rapidly or an overdose of the drug given. Changes in mental status (243) have been associated with hypocalcemia (219). Additional side effects reported that usually are minor include thrombophlebitis and local irritation at the infusion site (242,244).

While receiving foscarnet induction therapy, serum levels of calcium, creatinine, magnesium hemoglobin values, and potassium should be obtained two to three times weekly and during maintenance treatment at weekly intervals (219). Coadministration of other nephrotoxic drugs should be avoided (242). Adjustment of drug dosage while on maintenance therapy based on patient weight and creatine clearance should be done at weekly intervals and two to three times weekly during induction treatment (245).

A study demonstrated 29 of 30 eyes with CMV retinitis complicating AIDS responded to a 3-week course of induction therapy with foscarnet (236). All eyes not placed on maintenance therapy demonstrated a relapse within 3 weeks after induction treatment was terminated and three of the six patients on maintenance demonstrated a relapse within the first 5 weeks on this regimen. This very preliminary data suggested a higher rate of relapse occurring in patients receiving maintenance therapy with foscarnet compared to ganciclovir (236). Other studies show a similar relapse rate for patients with CMV retinitis on maintenance treatment with either ganciclovir or foscarnet (219). Unlike ganciclovir, foscarnet does not produce bone marrow toxicity, allowing concurrent use of this antiviral agent with zidovudine (246). The main toxicity caused by foscarnet is nephrotoxicity. Additional toxic effects include neurotoxicity, anemia, and hypocalcemia which tends to occur with a too rapid drug infusion or overdose and may cause cardiac arrhythmias (236). The drug irreversibly binds to bone which may contribute to changes in serum calcium and phosphorus levels noted in some individuals while receiving foscarnet (236).

Synergistic or additive effects have been demonstrated in vitro when a combination of ganciclovir and foscarnet was used. The data suggest coadministration could reduce the dose of each drug or the drugs administered could be alternated. Both therapeutic regimens would reduce side effects (219,247,248).

Placement of a central line is needed for most patients starting therapy with ganciclovir or foscarnet, since administration of either drug is usually for the duration of the patient's life. The anatomical location of the CMV retinitis determines when therapy must be started, with sight-threatening lesions near the fovea or optic nerve requiring immediate treatment. In contrast, lesions involving the peripheral retina which are not sight threatening or inactive lesions in the more central retina may be observed (219). An open randomized study demonstrated ganciclovir and foscarnet have similar efficacy against CMV retinitis (246).

A preliminary study (249) is presently being conducted with AIDS patients with CMV retinitis receiving 1000 mg of oral ganciclovir three times a day. This multiple dosing study, involving AIDS patients with stable retinitis or with no retinitis but who are instead shedding CMV, had no terminations among the first 11 patients enrolled.

Recent data also indicate some of the newer experimental antivirals, including dideoxycytodine (ddc) and dideoxyinosine (ddl) do not produce hematological complications. These agents may be possibly used to replace zidovudine in treating AIDS patients with CMV retinitis (210,214,215) placed on combination therapy with ganciclovir rather than discontinuing zidovudine (235).

Ganciclovir therapy is most frequently interrupted due to neutropenia; a decreased dosage of ganciclovir is less effective than the full-dose therapy (219). The properties of recombinant human granulocyte-macrophage colony-stimulating factor (rHUGM-CSF) which make it attractive as an adjunct in myelosuppressive therapy are increased survival time of neutrophils and eosinophils, stimulation of the differentiation and proliferation of macrophages and granulocytes, and enhancement of neutrophil chemotaxis and of phagocytic and cytocidal activity against yeasts and bacteria (250–252). Preliminary results involving 16 patients who became neutropenic while on ganciclovir demonstrated that all patients following rHUGM-CSF therapy were able to resume ganciclovir treatment at 5–10 mg/day for up to 8 months. The rHUGM-CSF is administered subcutaneously and the dose is incrementally increased in patients depending on the neutrophil response (253).

A preliminary study involving 36 patients demonstrated both drugs are well tolerated when administered together; the side effects associated with rHUGM-CSF include eosinophilia and myalgia. The rHUGM-CSF combined with ganciclovir (21 patients) compared to the ganciclovir-alone group demonstrated a trend showing both a decreased number and duration of neutropenic episodes and shortening of the interval when ganciclovir treatment had to be interrupted owing to neutropenia.

None of the five patients in part B of this study who received concomitant zidovudine treatment in addition to ganciclovir and rHUGM-CSF has developed significant neutropenia. In contrast, three of four patients receiving concomitant treatment with ganciclovir and zidovudine have developed neutropenia. Administration of rHUGM-CSF to these patients has reversed the neutropenia (254).

Before the introduction of ganciclovir and foscarnet, no satisfactory agents existed for the treatment of CMV retinitis in patients with AIDS. Unfortunately, both antiviral agents require maintenance therapy and parenteral administration and produce side effects that may restrict their use in some individuals. Efforts to control CMV retinitis failed using tolerable doses of antiviral agents and lymphokines, including acyclovir (255–260) with and without interferon (259), vidarabine (256–258,260,261) (adenine arabinoside), and interferon (259,262). Additionally, argon laser has failed to slow the spread of CMV retinitis (263).

In addition, transfer factor (264), vidarabine (260), and idoxuridine (265) have been ineffective against CMV retinitis in individuals immunocompromised from causes other than AIDS. Laboratory studies have demonstrated that parenteral use of steroids accelerates systemic cytomegaloviral infection in mice (266).

Other possible therapeutic regimens for the treatment of CMV retinitis are being investigated. Intravitreal injection of different antimicrobial agents that overcome anatomical barriers to achieve therapeutic but nontoxic drug concentrations in the vitreous body, whereas avoiding systemic toxicity associated with parenteral drug administration, has become a part of the standard treatment of endophthalmitis. This has prompted the evaluation of various intravitreally injected antiviral drugs to determine ocular toxicity levels and vitreous concentration time profile (124).

Studies (209,267) using a rabbit model demonstrated intravitreal ganciclovir injections up to 400 µg were nontoxic based on clinical examinations, histopathological studies, and electroretinography. Pharmacological data showed that intravitreal ganciclovir levels above the mean inhibitory dose for CMV were maintained for 60 h following a single intravitreal injection of this antiviral agent in rabbit eyes (210) and serial injections of 200 µg in one human eye (126). A more recent study demonstrated multiple intravitreal doses as low as 25 µg given weekly over a 5-week period can cause retinal toxicity, which may temper some of the initial enthusiasm over intravitreal use of this antiviral agent (268).

A small number of individuals with CMV retinitis associated with AIDS have been treated with intravitreal ganciclovir (126,221,269,270).

Heinemann (270) used intravitreal ganciclovir in seven patients with CMV retinitis associated with AIDS. Systemic therapy with ganciclovir was discontinued in six patients owing to myelosuppression and in the remaining individual because of hepatotoxicity. Induction therapy involving six injections consisting of 200 µg of ganciclovir over an 18-day period produced a favorable response in all patients. Relapse occurred in two eyes while on maintenance therapy with weekly intravitreal ganciclovir injections with the dose unchanged. Owing to their debilitated course, neither patient could tolerate a repeated period of induction therapy; therefore, weekly intravitreal injections were increased to 300 µg/0.1 mL, with one eye responding favorably, whereas the disease continued to progress in the second eye. *Staphylococcus epidermidis* endophthalmitis developed in one eye and a retinal detachment considered unrelated to the intravitreal injections developed from a break located at a distance from the injection site at the junction between normal and necrotic retina.

Ussery et al. treated 14 eyes of 11 patients with intravitreal injections of ganciclovir, either administered alone or as an adjunct to intravenous therapy with this antiviral agent (221). These 11 individuals with CMV retinitis and AIDS either had severe myelosuppression that precluded additional intravenous ganciclovir treatment or demonstrated progressive CMV retinitis involving the macula or optic nerve despite maximum tolerable intravenous therapy. The study lacked a matched control group. Suppression of the retinitis was demonstrated in 11 eyes, whereas three eyes demonstrated no improvement. The only significant complication was a retinal detachment occurring during injection.

Henry et al. (126) reported a 28-year-old man with AIDS and bilateral CMV retinitis who was ineligible for intravenous ganciclovir treatment because of hematological abnormalities. Twenty-eight intravitreal injections (200 μg/0.1 mL) were administered to his left eye, which over a 3-month period maintained useful vision with no evidence of intraocular toxicity. Following a single injection, the intravitreal ganciclovir remained above the ID_{50} for cytomegalovirus for approximately 62 h.

Schulman et al. demonstrated that an intravitreal ganciclovir injection up to 400 mg/0.02 mL was nontoxic to the retina (210). The intravitreal levels of this antiviral agent at 60 h were above the ID_{50} for several strains of human cytomegalovirus.

Peyman et al. (271) experimentally demonstrated a prolonged vitreous body drug level, without intraocular toxicity, that was within the range of the ID_{50} for different clinical and laboratory strains of viruses belonging to the herpes simplex family (including cytomegalovirus). The therapeutic levels were maintained up to 28 days following a single intravitreal injections (100 μg/0.1 mL or 200 μg/0.1 mL) of this liposome-encapsulated antiviral agent.

Peyman et al. used liposomes to capture a mixture of trifluridine (100 μg/0.1 mL) and ganciclovir (94 μg/0.1 mL) to determine if this method could achieve prolonged, nontoxic levels following injection (0.1 mL of suspension) into the vitreous of healthy albino rabbits (272). The concentrations of both drugs when injected together in liposomes were higher after 7 days for trifluridine and 14 days for ganciclovir than the ID_{50} for different viral isolates belonging to the herpes simplex family (including cytomegalovirus and varicella-zoster virus [VSV]). Trifluridine drug levels at 14 days postinjection were within the ID_{50} range for these same viral strains. No toxic effects were observed for up to 28 days after a single injection. Further study is needed to determine the full potential of this combination.

The first use of intravitreally administered liposome-encapsulated drugs in humans was reported by Peyman et al. (150). Individuals with cytomegaloviral retinitis, toxoplasmosis, retinochoroiditis, and chronic postoperative inflammation (probably secondary to *Propionibacterium acnes* infection) were successfully treated with intravitreal injections of antimicrobial agents bound to liposomes. This method of drug delivery produced no evidence of ocular toxicity and eliminated the need for multiple repeated drug injections, which enhances the chances of lens and retinal injury.

Interest has developed in the combination of different chemotherapeutic drugs (273,274) or a single antiviral agent with immunoregulatory agents, such as interferon (275), to treat viral infections. This strategy has worked in the treatment of bacterial endophthalmitis (124). Combined chemotherapy may be synergistic and may attack the pathogen at different metabolic or reproductive sites. These properties exhibited with certain antiviral combinations may prevent the emergence of drug-resistant organisms during antiviral therapy and allow agents to be administered in doses nontoxic to humans (204,273). Additionally, combination antiviral therapy may be required to treat retinitis caused by more than one virus. A recent report documented concurrent CMV and HSV retinitis and encephalitis in a patient with AIDS. Despite treatment with intravenous acyclovir, the patient died (276).

Small et al. tested four antiviral agents in various combinations for retinal toxicity after intravitreal injection and infusion in vitrectomy solutions (277). Each agent's individual nontoxic concentration in these routes of administration has been described previously in the literature. The study demonstrated that a concentration of 200 μg/0.1 mL of trifluorothymidine, 400 μg/0.1 mL of ganciclovir, 200 μg/0.1 mL of acyclovir, and 30 μg/0.1 mL of vidarabine could be combined for intravitreal injection without retinal toxicity. Also, 60 μg/mL of trifluorothymidine, 20 μg/mL of ganciclovir, 40 μg/mL of acyclovir, and

8 µg/mL of vidarabine could be combined in vitrectomy infusion solutions without producing retinal damage (277).

Cytomegalovirus is very sensitive to trifluorothymidine. When injected intravitreally, 42.9 µg of liposome-encapsulated trifluorothymidine prolonged the vitreal drug level within the range of ID_{50} for many strains of herpes virus and human cytomegalovirus 28 days after injection. This drug concentration produced no intraocular toxicity (138).

Different reports have suggested that herpes zoster plays a major role in the development of acute retinal necrosis (216,278–280). This association has significant implications regarding therapy of acute retinal necrosis (278). Viral retinitis caused by herpes simplex or herpes zoster and the infectious component of acute retinal necrosis have responded favorably to treatment with acyclovir (278,281), whereas this agent has been ineffective in treating CMV retinitis (206,216).

The intravitreal administration of antiviral agents, either individually or in combination, and the use of liposomal antimicrobial encapsulation represent two therapeutic approaches that may eventually prove beneficial in the primary or adjunct treatment of viral retinal infections, including cytomegaloviral retinitis in patients with AIDS.

XII. INTRAVITREAL CHEMOTHERAPEUTIC AGENTS AND PROLIFERATIVE VITREORETINOPATHY

Proliferative vitreoretinopathy (282) is an abnormality in which rhegmatogenous retinal detachment is complicated by proliferation of membranes on both surfaces of the detached retina and on the posterior surface of the detached vitreous gel. The clinical features of proliferative vitreoretinopathy (PVR) have been reported with rhegmatogenous retinal detachment since 1869 (283). It was not clear until Gonin [1904,1934] (284,285) that periretinal membrane formation was a complication and not the cause of retinal detachment.

Proliferative vitreoretinopathy accounts for the majority of failures following rhegmatogenous retinal detachment surgery (286). Contraction of the membranes creates tractional forces that can distort or detach the retina (282). Although successful retinal reattachment is possible in more patients with PVR because of improved surgical techniques, a significant number of cases fail owing to reproliferation and contraction of membranes (287).

Recent research has been centered on finding a pharmacological solution to the problem. A variety of pharmacological agents have been identified that act to inhibit the vitreoretinal scarring response (288–290). These agents attack different stages of PVR formation and some of them act on more than one stage.

XIII. INTRAVITREAL ANTINEOPLASTIC DRUGS IN PVR

Drugs such as steroids and nonsteroidal anti-inflammatory agents reduce the breakdown of the blood-ocular barrier and are particularly effective, since they act early in the pathway of the disease process (291).

Corticosteroids are the first pharmacological agents reported to modify vitreoretinal fibrosis in an experimental animal model (292). Although the initial basis for their selection was their perceived ability to inhibit fibroblastic proliferation, it is now generally accepted that one of their primary effects is the reduction of the inflammatory response in the eye, moderating the breakdown of the blood-ocular barrier (291). A single intravitreal injection of a high dose (1 mg) of slowly soluble corticosteroids, dexamethasone alcohol, and triamcinolone acetonide reduced retinal detachment from 57 and 84% to 24 and 20%, respectively, in a rabbit model of PVR (292,293).

Proliferative vitreoretinopathy is recognized as the major cause of failure in retinal detachment surgery (286,294). The cells characteristic of this disease create abnormal membranes which exert tangential traction on the retina and eventually lead to retinal detachment. The major cell components of these membranes are retinal pigment epithelial cells, myofibroblasts, and the glial cells. Although modern microsurgical techniques using vitrectomy instrumentation, membrane peeling, and the use of tamponading substances such as gas and silicone have improved the rate of success in these cases, regrowth of these cells has contributed to renewed failure of the surgery. Consequently, numerous investigators have chosen a pharmacological approach with intravitreal injection of antineoplastic drugs, such as 5-fluorouracil (5-FU), in the prevention of cell proliferation inside the eye (125,291,293–297).

A pharmacological approach to PVR, although effective in experimental animals, has not gained wide clinical application. The main disadvantage of this method is the rapid clearance of the drug from the eye and uncertainty about the nontoxic dose which has been recommended for intraocular injection. Although 5-FU appears to be least toxic (125,298) among the drugs studied, there has been controversy over the nontoxic dose (299). One explanation for the variable toxicity encountered in these studies might be the presence of freely diffusible free drug in the retinal tissue immediately after intravitreal injection. Another problem in treating PVR is that this disease process is slow, progressive, and requires long-term treatment with antineoplastic drugs over days and possibly weeks to be successful in inhibition of cell proliferation. To be effective, some concentration of this drug has to be maintained in the vitreous cavity for a long period of time. Free drug injected intravitreally in the vitrectomized eye has been shown to have a very fast clearance rate (300). Therefore, there is a need for a slow drug delivery system in the management of PVR.

Blumenkranz and associates (298) demonstrated that single intravitreal injection of 5-FU decreased the incidence of tractional retinal detachment in an animal model of PVR. Repeated subconjunctival injections of 5-FU enhanced the antiproliferative effect of intraocular 5-FU in rabbit eyes. Fishman et al. (301), using normal rabbit eyes, evaluated the clearance of intravitreal liposome-encapsulated 5-FU compared to the free compound and found the intravitreal levels of the encapsulated drug were six times the levels of free 5-FU 48 h after injection. Another study demonstrated in a phakic animal model of PVR that intravitreal liposome-encapsulated 5-FU resulted in a lower incidence of retinal detachment than free 5-FU (302).

Stern and associates (303) evaluated intraocular drug delivery in aphakic vitrectomized eyes to determine whether liposomes might cause retention of drugs for prolonged periods. These studies demonstrated liposomes are rapidly cleared from these eyes, making it unlikely that liposomes will improve the half-life of drugs in vitrectomized aphakic eyes. Instead, a small fraction of the liposomes directly bind to surfaces within the eye, including the internal limiting membrane of the retina and epiretinal membranes. Retinal toxicity is limited because liposomes are unable to gain access to the retina by penetrating the internal limiting membrane. Liposomes are endocytosized by cells in epiretinal membranes and then degraded intracellularly by lysosomes. This mechanism ensures selective delivery of liposome-intercalated drugs to membranes complicating PVR while minimizing retinal toxicity.

Joondeph et al. (302) investigated the use of liposome-encapsulated 5-FU in the treatment of PVR in an animal model. Doses of up to 1.6 mg administered intravitreally in rabbits demonstrated no retinal toxicity by histological or electroretinographic criteria. In an experimental animal model of PVR, intravitreal injection of homologous rabbit corneal fibroblasts caused tractional retinal detachments in 90% of eyes after 4 weeks. The addition of 1.6 mg of liposome-encapsulated 5-FU decreased the rate of detachment to 32% compared with 55% for 1 mg of free 5-FU.

Experiments were conducted with biodegradable microspheres containing anti-metabolites to assess the release of the drugs from the microspheres into the vitreous cavity of primates (304). Microspheres containing a mixture of radiolabeled and cold cytosine arabinoside (Ara-C) or 5-FU were prepared using a solvent evaporation process. A study evaluated the clearance of two antineoplastic drugs, 5-FU and Ara-C, bound to copolymers of lactic acid and glycolic acid after an intravitreal injection in primate eyes. A 0.1-mL aliquot of a suspension of the microspheres was then injected into one eye in each of eight African green monkeys. Half received 250 ± 10 µg of Ara-C and the others 375 ± 15 µg of 5-FU.

This study demonstrated that both 5-FU and Ara-C could be entrapped within this copolymer and therapeutic concentration could be maintained for up to 48 h after a single intravitreal injection of these drugs. Lower concentrations were maintained for up to 11 days.

Histological evaluation of the primate eyes injected with copolymer-drug combination demonstrated minimal inflammatory cell reaction in the vitreous cavity but otherwise normal retinal and lens structure. There is a continued interest in the development of an adjunct pharmacological therapy and a variety of agents have been evaluated thus, for only a small number of clinical studies (125,305,306) involving the effectiveness of chemotherapeutic agents in PVR have been performed (125,305–310). However, these will be difficult to design, considering the manifold manifestations of PVR and the different stages of retinal attachment in this disease process. Double-masked studies are needed to evaluate the concept of chemical inhibition of proliferating cells in the human eye.

XIV. INTRAVITREAL IMMUNOSUPPRESSIVE CYCLOSPORINE

Chronic endogenous uveitis and uveitis associated with Behçet's disease usually respond poorly to intensive treatment with steroids or cytotoxic drugs. The eventual outcome is usually blindness, which has necessitated the utilization of many other treatment modalities which have been unsuccessful (311–313).

Cyclosporine is a new immunomodulating drug which has been effective in treating experimental autoimmune (314) uveitis and clinically acute inflammation unresponsive to conventional treatment (315–318).

Cyclosporine is a highly stable, 11–amino acid, cyclical polypeptide that is almost totally insoluble in water. It is metabolized mostly in the liver and excreted in bile and has a plasma half-life of 19 h (319). Typical peak plasma concentration of 400–1200 ng/mL are reached in 3–4 h after oral administration. Typical trough levels are 100–400 ng/mL. In vitro activity of the drug has been shown at levels as low as 10 ng/mL (320). The drug's mechanism of action is believed to be through inhibition of synthesis of the lymphokine interleukin 2 by helper T cells. This lymphokine is involved in cytotoxic T-cell function. Topical effectiveness of cyclosporine has been shown by several researchers (321–323).

Systemic cyclosporine is not a benign drug. Approximately one-third of the patients in the above study developed renal toxicity. Systemic cyclosporine also has caused an increase incidence of viral infections, particularly the reactivation of infections caused by the Epstein-Barr virus (EBV) (319). Moreover, cyclosporine-treated patients have a greater incidence of lymphoma, which is thought to result from an unchecked proliferation of EBV-transformed B cells in immunosuppression (319). Gum hypertrophy, hirsutism, nausea, tremor, fluid retention, and allergic reactions can occur but are reversible reactions. Endomyocardial biopsy specimens of cardiac transplant recipients have shown diffuse interstitial fibrosis in all patients (319).

Considering the significant side effects from the systemically administered drug, an effective local mode of administration might avoid the toxic reactions. In addition, there might be increased efficacy with a greater drug concentration at the site of disease, which is possible only with local administration.

In a rabbit corneal allograft rejection model, it has been shown that topical (321,322), subconjunctival (323), and retrobulbar administration (324) of cyclosporine are effective in the prevention of graft rejection. None of these studies discovered significant side effects of the locally used cyclosporine. Considering the significant side effects of systemically administered cyclosporine, it is possible that a local mode of administration may be effective. In addition, one might find increased efficacy with the greater drug concentration at the site of disease.

Animal studies have shown that with the exception of eyes with serious uveitis, topical application of 2% cyclosporine A in olive oil resulted in nondetectable levels of the drug in all intraocular structures. Local applications of the drug in the severely inflamed eye resulted in significantly elevated cyclosporine levels only in the anterior segment structures (325,326).

BenEzra and associates (311) demonstrated no measurable levels of cyclosporine A in the aqueous and vitreous in human eyes with no ocular inflammation or mild uveitis following oral treatment with 5 mg/kg/day or topical application of 2% cyclosporine A eye drops. In eyes with severe uveitis, breakdown of the blood-retinal barrier resulted in significant levels of this drug in the aqueous and vitreous only when the drug was administered orally. Patients also had high blood level of cyclosporine A after oral administration.

Oh and associates (327) were able to suppress herpes simplex uveitis by a combination of systemic and intravitreal injections of cyclosporine. The half-life of free cyclosporine in the eye after intravitreal injection is expected to be short, because of its lipid solubility, which enhances it absorption via the retina surface, in addition to drainage via the trabecular meshwork.

Alghadyan et al. (328) demonstrated subconjunctival injection of 25 mg of either free or liposome-bound cyclosporine in albino rabbits gave reasonably high concentrations in the aqueous (1438 ng/mL and 1050 ng/mL, respectively) 4 days after the injection. Very low vitreous concentration (less than 30 ng) were obtained. The high aqueous concentration is important in the treatment of anterior uveitis and in prolonging the survival of the corneal graft.

Alghadyan and associates (328) demonstrated that intravitreal doses of less than 100 µg were nontoxic to the rabbit eye, whereas a second study by Grisolano and Peyman

(329) showed that intravitreal doses of 200 mg or more may cause patchy loss of outer segments of the retina. These same investigators (329) found no toxic effects in any animals treated with 100 μg or less of intravitreal cyclosporine. Because effective blood levels of cyclosporine are thought to be between a trough of 100 ng/mL and a peak of 1200 ng/mL, it is expected that a 100-μg dose in a 1.3-mL rabbit vitreous represents a very effective dose. If this dose were evenly distributed in the vitreous, the concentration would be 77 μg/mL.

Using liposomal encapsulation, normal ERG recordings and histological findings were present when up to 300 μg/mL was injected intravitreally in rabbit eyes (329).

The same investigators found the half-life of free cyclosporine compared to liposome-bound cyclosporine was approximately 6 h as opposed to 3 days after intravitreal injection of 100 μg of either free or liposome-bound cyclosporine (329).

Prolonging the presence of a therapeutic level of cyclosporine in the posterior part of the eye using liposomal encapsulation may be beneficial when treating severe posterior uveitis.

ACKNOWLEDGMENTS

Supported in part by U.S. Public Health Service grants EY07541 and EY02377 from the National Eye Institute, the National Institutes of Health, Bethesda, Maryland.

REFERENCES

1. Meredith, T. A. (1989). Clinical microbiology of infectious endophthalmitis. *In: Retina* (S. J. Ryan, ed.), Mosby, St. Louis, pp. 183–188.
2. Wilson, F. M., II (1987). Causes and prevention of endophthalmitis, *Int. Ophthalmol. Clin.*, 27:67–73.
3. Forster, R. K. (1978). Etiology and diagnosis of bacterial and postoperative endophthalmitis. *Ophthalmology*, 85:320–326.
4. Brady, S. E., Cohen, E. J., and Fischer, D. H. (1988). Diagnosis and treatment of chronic postoperative bacterial endophthalmitis. *Ophthalmic Surg.*, 19:580–584.
5. Nobe, J. R., Finegold, S. M., Hite, L. L., et al. (1987). Chronic anaerobic bacterial endophthalmitis in pseudophakic rabbit eyes. *Invest. Ophthalmol. Vis. Sci.*, 28:259–263.
6. Bohigian, G. M., and Olk, R. J. (1986). Factors associated with a poor visual result in endophthalmitis. *Am. J. Ophthalmol.*, 101:332–334.
7. Affeldt, J. C., Flynn, H. W., Jr., Forster, R. K., et al. (1987). Microbial endophthalmitis resulting from ocular trauma, *Ophthalmology*, 94:407–413.
8. Mandelbaum, S., and Forster, R. K. (1987). Postoperative endophthalmitis, *Int. Ophthalmol. Clin.*, 27:95–106.
9. Verbraeken, H., Geeroms, B., and Karemera, A. (1988). Treatment of endophthalmitis by pars plana vitrectomy, *Ophthalmologica*, 197:19–25.
10. Puliafito, C. A., Baker, A., Haaf, J., et al. (1982). Infectious endophthalmitis. Review of 36 cases, *Ophthalmology*, 89:921–929.
11. Rowsey, J. J., Newsom, D. L., Sexton, D. J., et al. (1982). Endophthalmitis. Current approaches, *Ophthalmology*, 89:1055–1066.
12. Stern, G. A., Engel, H. M., and Driebe, W. T., Jr. (1989). The treatment of postoperative endophthalmitis. Results of differing approaches to treatment, *Ophthalmology*, 96:62–67.
13. Neveu, M., and Elliot, A. J. (1959). Prophylaxis and treatment of endophthalmitis, *Am. J. Ophthalmol.*, 48:368–373.

14. Burns, R. P. (1959). Postoperative infections in an ophthalmologic hospital. With comments upon bacteriolophage typing of staphylococci as a preventative tool, *Am. J. Ophthalmol.*, 48:519.
15. Allan, H. F., and Mangiaracine, A. B. (1964). Bacterial endophthalmitis after cataract extraction. A study of 22 infections in 20,000 operations, *Arch. Ophthalmol.*, 72:454–462.
16. Hughes, W. F., Jr., and Owens, W. C. (1947). Postoperative complications of cataract extraction, *Arch. Ophthalmol.*, 38:577.
17. Peyman, G. A., and Schulman, J. A. (1989). Intravitreal drug therapy, *Jpn. J. Ophthalmol.*, 33:392–404.
18. Forster, R. K. (1974). Endophthalmitis. Diagnostic cultures and visual results, *Arch. Ophthalmol.*, 92:387–392.
19. Hattenhauer, J. M., and Lipsich, M. P. (1971). Late endophthalmitis after filtering surgery, *Am. J. Ophthalmol.*, 72:1097–1101.
20. Leopold, I. H. (1971). Doyne memorial lecture: Management of intra-ocular infection, *Trans. Ophthalmol. Soc. U.K.*, 91:575–610.
21. Maurice, D. M. (1980). Factors influencing the penetration of topically applied drugs, *Int. Ophthalmol. Clin.*, 20(3):21–32.
22. Alani, S. D. (1990). The ophthalmic rod. A new ophthalmic drug delivery system. *Graefes Arch. Clin. Exp. Ophthalmol.*, 228:297–301.
23. Phinney, R. B., Schwartz, S. D., Lee, D. A., and Mondino, B. J. (1988). Collagen-shield delivery of gentamicin and vancomycin, *Arch. Ophthalmol.*, 106:1599–1604.
24. Reidy, J. J., Limberg, M., and Kaufman, H. E. (1990). Delivery of fluorescein to the anterior chamber using the corneal collagen shield, *Ophthalmology*, 97:1201–1203.
25. Weissman, B. A., and Lee, D. A. (1988). Oxygen transmissibility, thickness, and water content of three types of collagen shields, *Arch. Ophthalmol.*, 106:1706–1708.
26. Unterman, S. R., Rootman, D. S., Hill, J. M., Parelman, J. J., Thompson, H. W., and Kaufman, H. E. (1988). Collagen shield drug delivery: Therapeutic concentrations of tobramycin in the rabbit cornea and aqueous humor. *J. Cataract Refract. Surg.*, 14:500–504.
27. Sawusch, M. R., O'Brien, T. P., and Updegraff, S. A. (1989). Collagen corneal shields enhance penetration of topical prednisolone acetate, *J. Cataract Refract. Surg.*, 15:625–628.
28. Reidy, J. J., Gebhardt, B. M., and Kaufman, H. E. (1990). The collagen shield. A new vehicle for delivery of cyclosporin A to the eye, *Cornea*, 9:196–199.
29. Jay, W. M., Shockley, R. K., Aziz, A. M., et al. (1984). Ocular pharmacokinetics of ceftriaxone following subconjunctival injection in rabbits, *Arch. Ophthalmol.*, 102:430–432.
30. Rubinstein, E., Triester, G., Avni, I., et al. (1987). The intravitreal penetration of cefotaxime in man following systemic and subconjunctival administrations, *Ophthalmology*, 94:30–34.
31. Orr, W. M., Jackson, W. B., and Colden, K. (1985). Intraocular penetration of netilmicin, *Can. J. Ophthalmol.*, 20:171–175.
32. Hillman, J. S., Jacobs, S. I., Garnett, A. J., et al. (1979). Gentamicin penetration and decay in the human aqueous, *Br. J. Ophthalmol.*, 63:794–796.
33. Barza, M., Kane, A., and Baum, J. (1980). Oxacillin for bacterial endophthalmitis. Subconjunctival, intravenous, both, or neither? *Invest. Ophthalmol. Vis. Sci.*, 19:1348–1354.
34. Busse, H., Seeger, K., and Wreesman, P. (1980). Concentrations of cefotaxime in the anterior chamber of the eye in rabbits and humans, *J. Antimicrob. Chemother.*, 6(Suppl. A):143–145.
35. Johnson, A. P., Scoper, S. V., Woo, F. L., et al. (1985). Azlocillin levels in human tears and aqueous humor, *Am. J. Ophthalmol.*, 99:469–472.
36. Mattila, J., Nerdrum, K., Rouhiainen, H., et al. (1983). Penetration of metronidazole and tinidazole into the aqueous humor in man, *Chemotherapy*, 29:188–191.
37. Quentin, C. D., and Ansorg, R. (1983). Penetration of cefotaxime into the aqueous humour of the human eye after intravenous application, *Graefes Arch. Clin. Exp. Ophthalmol.*, 220:245–247.

38. Axelrod, J. L., and Kochman, R. S. (1978). Cefamandole levels in primary aqueous humor in man, *Am. J. Ophthalmol.*, 85:342–348.

39. Axelrod, J. L., and Kochman, R. S. (1982). Moxalactam concentration in human aqueous humor after intravenous administration, *Arch. Ophthalmol.*, 100:1334–1336.

40. Axelrod, J. L., Newton, J. C., Klein, R. M., et al. (1987). Penetration of imipenem into human aqueous and vitreous humor, *Am. J. Ophthalmol.*, 104:649–653.

41. Axelrod, J. L., Klein, R. M., Bergen, R. L., et al. (1986). Human vitreous levels of cefamandole and moxalactam, *Am. J. Ophthalmol.*, 101:684–687.

42. Finlay, K. R., Carlson, C. L., and Chow, A. W. (1983). Ocular penetration of N-formimidoyl thienamycin (MK-787) and potentiation by dipeptidase inhibitor (MK-791), *Invest. Ophthalmol. Vis. Sci.*, 24:1147–1149.

43. Furgiuele, F. P. (1967). Ocular penetration and tolerance of gentamicin, *Am. J. Ophthalmol.*, 64:421–426.

44. Deur, H. A., and Maas, E. R. (1962). The penetration of several new penicillins into the tissues of the eye, *Ophthalmologica*, 144:316–322.

45. Furgiuele, F. P., Sery, T. W., and Leopold, I. H. (1960). New antibiotics. Their intraocular penetration, *Am. J. Ophthalmol.*, 50:614–622.

46. Leopold, I. H., and Nichols, A. (1946). Intraocular penetration of streptomycin following systemic and local administration, *Arch. Ophthalmol.*, 35:33–38.

47. Golden, B., and Coppel, S. P. (1970). Ocular tissue absorption of gentamicin, *Arch. Ophthalmol.*, 84:792–796.

48. Rubinstein, E., Goldfarb, J., Keren, G., et al. (1983). The penetration of gentamicin into the vitreous humor in man, *Invest. Ophthalmol. Vis. Sci.*, 24:637–639.

49. Peyman, G. A., May, D. R., Homer, P. I., et al. (1977). Penetration of gentamicin into the aphakic eye, *Ann. Ophthalmol.*, 9:871–880.

50. Doft, B. H. (1991). The endophthalmitis vitrectomy study (editorial), *Arch. Ophthalmol.*, 109:487–488.

51. Martin, D. F., Ficker, L. A., Aguilar, H. A., et al. (1990). Vitreous cefazolin levels after intravenous injection: Effects of inflammation, repeated antibiotic doses, and surgery, *Arch. Ophthalmol.*, 108:411–414.

52. Carney, M. D., and Peyman, G. A. (1987). Vitrectomy in endophthalmitis, *Int. Ophthalmol. Clin.*, 27:127–134.

53. Baum, J., Peyman, G. A., and Barza, M. (1982). Intravitreal administration of antibiotics in the treatment of bacterial endophthalmitis. III. Consensus, *Surv. Ophthalmol.*, 26:204–206.

54. Barza, M. (1979). Factors affecting the intraocular penetration of antibiotics. The influence of route, inflammation, animal species and tissue pigmentation, *Scand. J. Infect. Dis.*, 14(Suppl):151–159.

55. Axelrod, J. L., Klein, R. M., Bergen, R. L., et al. (1985). Human vitreous levels of selected antistaphylococcal antibiotics, *Am. J. Ophthalmol.*, 100:570–575.

56. Peyman, G. A., and Bok, D. (1972). Peroxidase diffusion in the normal and laser-coagulated primate retina, *Invest. Ophthalmol.*, 11:35–45.

57. Von Sallmann, L., Meyer, K., Di Grandi, J. (1944). Experimental study on penicillin treatment of ectogenous infection of vitreous, *Arch. Ophthalmol.*, 32:179–189.

58. Von Sallmann, L. (1945). Penicillin therapy of infections of the vitreous, *Arch. Ophthalmol.*, 33:455–462.

59. Von Sallmann, L. (1945). Penetration of penicillin into the eye: Further studies, *Arch. Ophthalmol.*, 34:195–201.

60. Leopold, I. H. (1945). Intravitreal penetration of penicillin and penicillin therapy of infections of the vitreous, *Arch. Ophthalmol.*, 33:211–216.

61. Rycroft, B. W. (1945). Penicillin and the control of deep intra-ocular infection, *Br. J. Ophthalmol.*, 29:57–87.

62. Schneider, J., and Frankel, S. S. (1947). Treatment of later postoperative intraocular infections with intraocular injection of penicillin, *Arch. Ophthalmol.*, 37:304.
63. Feigenbaum, A., and Kornbluth, W. (1945). Intravitreal injection of penicillin in a case of incipient abscess of the vitreous following extracapsular cataract extraction: Perfect cure, *Ophthalmologica*, 110:300.
64. Sorsby, A., and Ungar, J. (1948). Distribution of penicillin in the eye after injections of 1,000,000 units by the subconjunctival retrobulbar and intramuscular routes, *Br. J. Ophthalmol.*, 32:864.
65. Peyman, G. A., May, D. R., Ericson, E. S., et al. (1974). Intraocular injection of gentamicin: Toxic effects and clearance, *Arch. Ophthalmol.*, 92:42–47.
66. May, D. R., Ericson, E. S., Peyman, G. A., et al. (1974). Intraocular injection of gentamicin: Single injection therapy of experimental bacterial endophthalmitis, *Arch. Ophthalmol.*, 91: 487–489.
67. Axelrod, A. J., Peyman, G. A., and Apple, D. J. (1973). Toxicity of intravitreal injection of amphotericin B, *Am. J. Ophthalmol.*, 76:578–583.
68. Axelrod, A. J., and Peyman, G. A. (1973). Intravitreal amphotericin B treatment of experimental fungal endophthalmitis, *Am. J. Ophthalmol.*, 76:584–588.
69. Graham, R. O., and Peyman, G. A. (1974). Intravitreal injection of dexamethasone: Treatment of experimentally induced endophthalmitis, *Arch. Ophthalmol.*, 92:149–154.
70. Graham, R. O., Peyman, G. A., and Fishman, G. (1975). Intravitreal injection of cephaloridine in the treatment of endophthalmitis, *Arch. Ophthalmol.*, 93:56–61.
71. Koziol, J., and Peyman, G. (1974). Intraocular chloramphenicol and bacterial endophthalmitis, *Can. J. Ophthalmol.*, 9:316–321.
72. Peyman, G. A., Nelsen, P., and Bennett, T. O. (1974). Intravitreal injection of kanamycin in experimentally induced endophthalmitis, *Can. J. Ophthalmol.*, 9:322–327.
73. Nelsen, P., Peyman, G. A., and Bennett, T. O. (1974). BB-K8: A new aminoglycoside for intravitreal injection in bacterial endophthalmitis, *Am. J. Ophthalmol.*, 78:82–89.
74. Bennett, T. O., and Peyman, G. A. (1974). Use of tobramycin in eradicating experimental bacterial endophthalmitis, *Graefes Arch. Klin. Exp. Ophthalmol.*, 191:93–107.
75. Schenk, A. G., and Peyman, G. A. (1974). Lincomycin by direct intravitreal injection in the treatment of experimental bacterial endophthalmitis, *Graefes Arch. Klin. Exp. Ophthalmol.*, 190:281–291.
76. Bennett, T. O. and Peyman, G. A. (1974). Toxicity of intravitreal aminoglycosides in primates, *Can. J. Ophthalmol.*, 9:475–478.
77. Schenk, A. G., Peyman, G. A., and Paque, J. T. (1974). The intravitreal use of carbenicillin (Geopen) for treatment of *Pseudomonas* endophthalmitis, *Acta Ophthalmol.*, 52:707–717.
78. Paque, J. T., and Peyman, G. A. (1974). Intravitreal clindamycin phosphate in the treatment of vitreous infection, *Ophthalmic Surg.*, 5(3):34–39.
79. Daily, M. J., Peyman, G. A., and Fishman, G. (1973). Intravitreal injection of methicillin for treatment of endophthalmitis, *Am. J. Ophthalmol.*, 76:343–350.
80. Peyman, G. A., and Herbst, R. (1974). Bacterial endophthalmitis: Treatment with intraocular injection of gentamicin and dexamethasone, *Arch. Ophthalmol.*, 91:416–418.
81. Peyman, G. A., Vastine, D. W., Crouch, E. R., et al. (1974). Clinical use of intravitreal antibiotics to treat bacterial endophthalmitis, *Trans. Am. Acad. Ophthalmol. Otolaryngol.*, 78:OP862–OP875.
82. Peyman, G. A., Vastine, D. W., and Raichand, M. (1978). Symposium: Postoperative endophthalmitis: Experimental aspects and their clinical applications, *Ophthalmology*, 85:374–385.
83. Pincus, J., Deiter, P., and Sears, M. L. (1965). Experiences with five cases of postoperative endophthalmitis, *Am. J. Ophthalmol.*, 59:403–409.
84. Kanski, J. J. (1974). Treatment of late endophthalmitis associated with filtering blebs, *Arch. Ophthalmol.*, 91:339–343.
85. Sery, T. W., Paul, S. D., Leopold, I. H. (1957). Novobiocin, a new antibiotic. Ocular penetration and tolerance, *Arch. Ophthalmol.*, 57:100–109.

86. Furgiuele, F. P. (1964). New antibiotics. II. Their intraocular penetration, *Am. J. Ophthalmol.*, 58:443–447.

87. Faris, B. M., and Uwaydah, M. M. (1974). Intraocular penetration of semisynthetic penicillins: Methicillin, cloxacillin, ampicillin, and carbenicillin studies in experimental animals with a review of the literature, *Arch. Ophthalmol.*, 92:501–505.

88. Green, W. R., and Leopold, I. H. (1965). Intraocular penetration of methicillin. *Am. J. Ophthalmol.*, 60:800–804.

89. Records, R. E. (1966). The human intraocular penetration of methicillin, *Arch. Ophthalmol.*, 76:720–722.

90. Records, R. E., and Ellis, P. P. (1967). The intraocular penetration of ampicillin, methicillin, and oxacillin, *Am. J. Ophthalmol.*, 64:135–143.

91. Furgiuele, F. P. (1970). Penetration of gentamicin into the aqueous humor of human eyes, *Am. J. Ophthalmol.*, 69:481–483.

92. Coles, R. S., Boyle, G. L., Leopold, I. H., et al. (1971). Lincomycin levels in rabbit ocular fluids and serum, *Am. J. Ophthalmol.*, 72:464–467.

93. Boyle, G. L., Gwon, A. E., Zinn, K. M., et al. (1972). Intraocular penetration of carbenicillin after subconjunctival infection in man, *Am. J. Ophthalmol.*, 73:754–759.

94. Stainer, G. A., Peyman, G. A., Meisels, H., et al. (1977). Toxicity of selected antibiotics in vitreous replacement fluid, *Ann. Ophthalmol.*, 9:615–618.

95. Carney, M. and Peyman, G. A. (1987). Vitrectomy in endophthalmitis. *Int. Ophthalmol. Clin.*, 27(2):127–134.

96. Peyman, G. A., and Schulman, J. A. (1986). *Intravitreal Surgery: Principles and Practice.* Appleton-Century-Crofts, Norwalk, CT, pp. 410–413.

97. Vastine, D. W., Peyman, G. A., and Guth, S. B. (1979). Visual prognosis in bacterial endophthalmitis treated with intravitreal antibiotics, *Ophthalmic Surg.*, 10:76–83.

98. Semple, H. C., Liu, J. C., and Peyman, G. A. (1989). Intravitreal injection of piperacillin, *Ophthalmic Surg.*, 20:588–590.

99. Meschis, M., Grigoras, G., Ponakis, E., et al. (1990). ERG and electron microscopic findings after intravitreal use of aminoglycosides, *Ann. Ophthalmol.*, 22:255–262.

100. D'Amico, D. J., Caspers-Velu, L., Libert, J., et al. (1985). Comparative toxicity of intravitreal aminoglycoside antibiotics, *Am. J. Ophthalmol.*, 100:264–275.

101. D'Amico, D. J., Libert, J., Kenyon, K. R., et al. (1984). Retinal toxicity of intravitreal gentamicin. An electron microscopic study, *Invest. Ophthalmol.*, 25:564–572.

102. Ling, C. H., Peyman, G. A., and Raichand, M. (1985). Electron microscopic study of toxicity of intravitreal injections of gentamicin in primates, *Can. J. Ophthalmol.*, 20:179–183.

103. Philipp, W., Schmid, K., Steiner, H. J., et al. (1990). Toxicity and clearance of intravitreal cefotetan, *Graefes Arch. Clin. Exp. Ophthalmol.*, 228:475–480.

104. Carney, M., Kao, G., Peyman, G. A., et al. (1988). The intraocular penetration and retinal toxicity of teicoplanin. *Ophthalmic Surg.*, 19:119–123.

105. Heigle, T. J., and Peyman, G. A. (1990). Retinal toxicity of intravitreal ticarcillin, *Ophthalmic Surg.*, 21:563–565.

106. Davey, P. G., Barza, M., and Stuart, M. (1987). Dose response of experimental pseudomonas endophthalmitis to ciprofloxacin, gentamicin, and imipenem. Evidence for resistance to "late" treatment of infections, *J. Infect. Dis.*, 155:518–532.

107. Gardner, S. K. (1989). Treatment of bacterial endophthalmitis. Part I, *Ocular Ther. Rep.*, 2:1–4.

108. Talley, A. R., D'Amico, D. J., Talamo, J., et al. (1987). The role of vitrectomy in the treatment of postoperative bacterial endophthalmitis. An experimental study, *Arch. Ophthalmol.*, 105: 1699–1702.

109. Ficker, L. A., Meredith, T. A., Wilson, L. A., et al. (1988). Role of vitrectomy in staphylococcus epidermidis endophthalmitis, *Br. J. Ophthalmol.*, 72:386–389.

110. Talamo, J. H., D'Amico, D. J., Hanninen, L. A., et al. (1985). The influence of aphakia and vitrectomy on experimental retinal toxicity of aminoglycoside antibiotics, *Am. J. Ophthalmol.*, 100:840–847.

111. Barza, M., Kane, A., and Baum, J. (1983). Pharmacokinetics of intravitreal carbenicillin, cefazolin, and gentamicin in rhesus monkeys, *Invest. Ophthalmol. Vis. Sci.*, 24:1602–1606.

112. Barza, M., Kane, A., and Baum, J. (1982). The effects of infection and probenecid on the transport of carbenicillin from the rabbit vitreous humor, *Invest. Ophthalmol. Vis. Sci.*, 22:720–726.

113. Maurice, D. M., and Mishima, S. (1984). Ocular pharmacokinetics, *In: Pharmacology of the Eye. Handbook of Experimental Pharmacology*, Vol. 69 (M. Sears, ed.). Springer-Verlag, New York, p. 76.

114. Cobo, L. M., and Forster, R. K. (1981). The clearance of intravitreal gentamicin, *Am. J. Ophthalmol.*, 92:59–62.

115. Kane, A., Barza, M., and Baum, J. (1981). Intravitreal injection of gentamicin in rabbits. Effect of inflammation and pigmentation on half-life and ocular distribution, *Invest. Ophthalmol. Vis. Sci.*, 20:593–597.

116. Abel, R. Jr., Boyle, G. L., Furman, M., et al. (1974). Intraocular penetration of cefazolin sodium in rabbits, *Am. J. Ophthalmol.*, 78:779–787.

117. Ficker, L., Meredith, T. A., Gardner, S., et al. (1990). Cefazolin levels after intravitreal injection. Effects of inflammation and surgery, *Invest. Ophthalmol. Vis. Sci.*, 31:502–505.

118. Oum, B. S., D'Amico, D. J., and Wong, K. W. (1989). Intravitreal antibiotic therapy with vancomycin and aminoglycoside. An experimental study of combination and repetitive injections, *Arch. Ophthalmol.*, 107:1055–1060.

119. Greenwald, M. J., Wohl, L. G., and Sell, C. H. (1986). Metastatic bacterial endophthalmitis. A contemporary reappraisal, *Surv. Ophthalmol.*, 31:81–101.

120. Jones, D. B. (1980). Chemotherapy of experimental endogenous Candida albicans endophthalmitis, *Trans. Am. Ophthalmol. Soc.*, 78:846–855.

121. Cuhna-Vaz, J. (1979). The blood-ocular barriers, *Surv. Ophthalmol.*, 23:279–296.

122. Barrie, T. (1987). The place of elective vitrectomy in the management of patients with Candida endophthalmitis, *Graefes Arch. Clin. Exp. Ophthalmol.*, 225:107–113.

123. O'Day, D. M., Head, W. S., Robinson, R. D., et al. (1985). Intraocular penetration of systemically administered antifungal agents, *Curr. Eye Res.*, 4:131–134.

124. Peyman, G. A., and Schulman, J. A. (1986). *Intravitreal Surgery: Principles and Practice.* Appleton-Century-Crofts, New York, pp. 407–455.

125. Blumenkranz, M., Hernandez, E., Ophir, A., et al. (1984). 5-fluorouracil. New applications in complicated retinal detachment for an established antimetabolite, *Ophthalmology*, 91:122–130.

126. Henry, K., Cantrill, H., Fletcher, C., et al. (1987). Use of intravitreal ganciclovir (dihydroxypropoxymethyl guanine) for cytomegalovirus retinitis in a patient with AIDS, *Am. J. Ophthalmol.*, 103:17–23.

127. Jaffe, G. J., Whichter, J. P., Biswell, R., et al. (1986). *Propionibacterium acnes* endophthalmitis seven months after extracapsular cataract extraction and intraocular lens implantation, *Ophthalmic Surg.*, 17:791–793.

128. Meisler, D. M., Palestine, A. G., Vastine, D. W., et al. (1986). Propionibacterium endophthalmitis after extracapsular cataract extraction and intraocular lens implantation, *Am. J. Ophthalmol.*, 102:733–739.

129. Rao, V. S., Peyman, G. A., Khoobehi, B., et al. (1989). Evaluation of liposome-encapsulated clindamycin in staphylococcus aureus endophthalmitis, *Int. Ophthalmol.*, 13:181–185.

130. Michelson, J. B., and Nozik, R. A. (1979). Experimental endophthlamitis treated with an implantable osmotic minipump, *Arch. Ophthalmol.*, 97:1345–1346.

131. Eliason, J. A., and Maurice, D. M. (1980). An ocular perfusion system, *Invest. Ophthalmol. Vis. Sci.*, 19:102–105.

132. Miki, K., Ohkuma, H., and Ryan, S. J. (1984). A method for chronic drug infusion into the eye, *Jpn. J. Ophthalmol.*, 28:140–146.

133. Juliano, R. L., and Layton, D. (1980). Liposomes as a drug delivery system. *In: Drug Delivery Systems* (R. L. Juliano, ed.). Oxford University Press, New York, pp. 189–236.

134. Lee, V. H., Urrea, P. T., Smith, R. E., et al. (1985). Ocular drug bioavailability from topically applied liposomes, *Surv. Ophthalmol.*, 29:335–348.

135. Lopez-Berestein, G. (1987). Liposomes as carriers of antimicrobial agents, *Antimicrob. Agents. Chemother.*, 31:675–678.

136. Lopez-Berestein, G., Kasi, L., Rosenblum, M. G., et al. (1984). Clinical pharmacology of the ^{99m}Tc-labeled liposomes in patients with cancer, *Cancer Res.*, 44:375–378.

137. Liu, K. R., Peyman, G. A., Khoobehi, B., et al. (1987). Intravitreal liposome-encapsulated trifluorothymidine in a rabbit model, *Ophthalmology*, 94:1155–1159.

138. Assil, K. K., and Weinreb, R. N. (1987). Multivesicular liposomes. Sustained release of the antimetabolite cytarabine in the eye, *Arch. Ophthalmol.*, 105:400–403.

139. Schaeffer, H. E., and Krohn, D. L. (1982). Liposomes in topical drug delivery, *Invest. Ophthalmol. Vis. Sci.*, 22:220–227.

140. Smolin, G., Okumoto, M., Feiler, S., et al. (1981). Idoxuridine-liposome therapy for herpes simplex keratitis, *Am. J. Ophthalmol.*, 91:220–225.

141. Dharma, S. K., Fishman, P. H., and Peyman, G. A. (1986). A preliminary study of corneal penetration of ^{125}I-labeled idoxuridine liposome, *Acta Ophthalmol.*, 64:298–301.

142. Singh, K., and Meze, M. (1983). Liposomal ophthalmic drug delivery system. I. Triamcinolone acetate, *J. Pharmaceut.*, 16:339–344.

143. Barza, M., Baum, J., and Szoka, F., Jr. (1984). Pharmacokinetics of subconjunctival liposome-encapsulated gentamicin in normal rabbit eyes, *Invest. Ophthalmol. Vis. Sci.*, 25:486–490.

144. Tremblay, C., Barza, M., Szoka, F., et al. (1989). Reduced toxicity of liposome-associated amphotericin B injected intravitreally in rabbits, *Invest. Ophthalmol. Vis. Sci.*, 26:711–718.

145. Barza, M., Baum, J., Tremblay, C., et al. (1985). Ocular toxicity of intravitreally injected liposomal amphotericin B in rhesus monkeys, *Am. J. Ophthalmol.*, 100:259–263.

146. Fishman, P. H., Peyman, G. A., and Lesar, T. (1986). Intravitreal liposome-encapsulated gentamicin in a rabbit model. Prolonged therapeutic levels, *Invest. Ophthalmol. Vis. Sci.*, 27:1103–1106.

147. Fiscella, R., Peyman, G. A., and Fishman, P. H. (1987). Duration of therapeutic levels of intravitreally injected liposome-encapsulated clindamycin in the rabbit, *Can. J. Ophthalmol.*, 22:307–309.

148. Alghadyan, A. A., Peyman, G. A., Khoobehi, B., et al. (1988). Intravitreal injection of liposome-encapsulated penicillin. Toxicity and clearance, *Afro-Asian J. Ophthalmol.*, 7:40–42.

149. Alghadyan, A. A., Peyman, G. A., and Khoobehi, B. (1989). Intravitreal injection of liposome-encapsulated penicillin for the treatment of bacterial endophthalmitis, *Afro-Asian J. Ophthalmol.*, 7:43–45.

150. Peyman, G. A., Charles, H. C., Liu, K. R., et al. (1988). Intravitreal lipsome-encapsulated drugs: A preliminary human report, *Int. Ophthalmol.*, 12:175–182.

151. Alving, C. R., Steck, E. A., Hanson, W. L., et al. (1978). Improved therapy of experimental leishmaniasis by use of a liposome-encapsulated antimonial drug, *Life Sci.*, 22:1021–1026.

152. Khoobehi, B., Peyman, G. A., McTurnan, W. G., et al. (1988). Externally triggered release of dye and drugs from liposomes into the eye. An in vitro and in vivo study, *Ophthalmology*, 95:950–955.

153. Khoobehi, B., Peyman, G. A., Niesman, M. R., and Oncel, M. (1989). Measurement of retinal blood velocity and flow rate in primates using liposome-dye system, *Ophthalmology*, 96:905–912.

154. Khoobehi, B., Char, C. A., and Peyman, G. A. (1990). Assessment of laser induced release of drugs from liposomes. An in vitro study, *Laser Surg. Med.*, 10:60–65.

155. Zeimer, R. C., Guran, T., Shahidi, M., et al. (1990). Visualization of retinal microvasculature by targeted dye delivery, *Invest. Ophthalmol. Vis. Sci.*, 31:1459–1465.

156. Lam, T. T., Edward, D. P., Zhu, X. A., et al. (1989). Transscleral iontophoresis of dexamethasone, *Arch. Ophthalmol.*, 107:1368–1371.

157. Rootman, D. S., Hobden, J. A., Jantzen, J. A., et al. (1988). Iontophoresis of tobramycin for the treatment of experimental pseudomonas keratitis in the rabbit, *Arch. Ophthalmol.*, 106: 262–265.

158. Fishman, P. H., Jay, W. M., Rissing, J. P., et al. (1984). Iontophoresis of gentamicin into aphakic rabbit eyes. Sustained vitreal levels, *Invest. Opthalmol. Vis. Sci.*, 25:343–345.

159. Hughes, L., and Maurice, D. M. (1984). A fresh look at iontophoresis, *Arch. Ophthalmol.*, 102:1825–1829.

160. Bridger, M. M., Keene, M., Graham, J. M., et al. (1982). A device for iontophoretic anesthesia of the tympanic membrane, *J. Med. Eng. Technol.*, 6:62–64.

161. Sato, H., Takahashi, H., and Honjo, I. (1988). Transtympanic iontophoresis of dexamethasone and fosfomycin, *Arch. Otolaryngol. Head Neck Surg.*, 114:531–533.

162. Gangarosa, L. P. Sr. (1974). Iontophoresis for surface local anesthesia, *J. Am. Dent. Assoc.*, 88:125–128.

163. Gangarosa, L. P., and Park, N. H. (1978). Practical consideration in iontophoresis of fluoride for desensitizing dentin, *J. Prosthet. Dent.*, 19:173–178.

164. Gangarosa, L. P. (1982). How modern iontophoresis can improve your practice, *Quintessence Int.*, 10:1027–1038.

165. Meyer, D. R., Linberg, J. V., and Vasquez, R. J. (1990). Iontophoresis for eyelid anesthesia, *Ophthalmic Surg.*, 21:845–848.

166. Von Sallmann, L. (1944). Penicillin and sulfadiazine in the treatment of experimental intra-ocular infections with Staphylococcus aureus and Clostridium welchii, *Arch. Ophthalmol.*, 31:54–63.

167. Von Sallmann, L. (1944). Controversial points in ocular penicillin therapy, *Trans. Am. Ophthalmol. Soc.*, 83:1–67.

168. Von Sallmann, L. (1942). Sulfadiazine iontophoresis in pyocyaneus infection of rabbit cornea, *Am. J. Ophthalmol.*, 25:1292–1300.

169. Hobden, J. A., O'Callaghan, R. J., Hill, J. M., et al. (1989). Tobramycin iontophoresis into corneas infected with drug-resistant Pseudomonas aeruginosa, *Curr. Eye Res.*, 8: 1163–1169.

170. Hobden, J. A., Reidy, J. J., O'Callaghan, R. J., et al. (1990). Ciprofloxacin iontophoresis for aminoglycoside-resistant pseudomonal keratitis, *Invest. Ophthalmol. Vis. Sci.*, 31:1940–1944.

171. Maurice, D. M. (1986). Iontophoresis of fluorescein into the posterior segment of the rabbit eye, *Ophthalmology*, 93:128–132.

172. Barza, M., Peckman, C., and Baum, J. (1986). Transscleral iontophoresis of cefazolin, ticarcillin, and gentamicin in the rabbit, *Ophthalmology*, 93:133–139.

173. Burstein, N. L., Leopold, I. H., and Bernacchi, D. B. (1985). Transscleral iontophoresis of gentamicin, *J. Ocul. Pharmacol.*, 1:363–368.

174. Gibson, L. E., and Cooke, R. E. (1959). A test for concentration of electrolytes in sweat in cystic fibrosis of the pancreas utilizing pilocarpine by iontophoresis, *Pediatrics*, 23:545–549.

175. Hobden, J. A., Rootman, D. S., O'Callaghan, R. J., et al. (1988). Iontophoretic application of tobramycin to uninfected and Pseudomonas aeruginosa-infected rabbit corneas, *Antimicrob. Agents Chemother.*, 32:978–981.

176. Barza, M., Peckman, C., and Baum, J. (1987). Transscleral iontophoresis of gentamicin in monkeys, *Invest. Ophthalmol. Vis. Sci.*, 28:1033–1036.

177. Choi, T. B., and Lee, D. A. (1988). Transscleral and transcorneal iontophoresis of vancomycin in rabbit eyes, *J. Ocul. Pharmacol.*, 4:153–164.

178. Barza, M., Peckman, C., and Baum, J. (1987). Transscleral iontophoresis as an adjunctive treatment for experimental endophthalmitis, *Arch. Ophthalmol.*, 105:1418–1420.

179. Wright, R. E., and Stuart-Harris, C. H. (1945). Penetration of penicillin into the eye, *Br. J. Ophthalmol.*, 29:428–436.

180. Wood, D. (1980). Biodegradable drug delivery systems, *Int. J. Pharmaceut.*, 7:1–18.

181. Vert, M., Christel, P., Chabot, F., et al. (1984). Biodegradable plastic materials for bone surgery. In: *Macromolecular Biomaterials* (G. Hastings, P. Ducheyne, eds.), CRC Press, Boca Raton, FL, pp. 119–214.

182. Moritera, T., Ogura, Y., Arai, M., et al. (1989). Intravitreal drug delivery system using microspheres of biodegradable polymers, *Invest. Ophthalmol. Vis. Sci.*, 30(Suppl.):249.

183. Khoobehi, B., Stradtmann, M. O., Peyman, G. A., et al. (1991). Clearance of sodium fluorescein incorporated into microspheres from the vitreous after intravitreal injection, *Ophthalmic Surg.*, 22:175–180.

184. Kulkarni, R. K., Pani, K. C., Newman, C., et al. (1966). Polylactic acid for surgical implants, *Arch. Surg.*, 93:839–843.

185. Kulkarni, R. K., Moore, E. G., Hegyeli, A. F., et al. (1971). Biodegradable poly (lactic) acid polymers, *J. Biomed. Mater. Res.*, 5:169–181.

186. Chien, Y. W., Siddiqui, O., Sun, Y., et al. (1987). Transdermal iontophoretic delivery of therapeutic peptides/proteins. I. Insulin, *Ann. N.Y. Acad. Sci.*, 507:32–51.

187. Chien, Y. W. (1983). Logics of transdermal controlled drug administration, *Drug Dev. Indust. Pharm.*, 9:497–520.

188. Kligman, A. M. (1983). A biological brief on percutaneous absorption, *Drug Dev. Indust. Pharm.*, 9:521–560.

189. Chandrasekaran, S. K. (1983). Controlled release of scopolamine for prophylaxis of motion sickness, *Drug. Dev. Indust. Pharm.*, 9:627–646.

190. Higuchi, W. I., Gordon, N. A., Fox, J. L., et al. (1983). Transdermal delivery of prodrugs, *Drug Dev. Indust. Pharm.*, 9:691–706.

191. Breimer, D. D. (1984). Rationale for rate controlled drug delivery of cardiovascular drugs by the transdermal route, *Am. Heart J.*, 108:196–200.

192. Weber, M. A., and Drayer, J. I. M. (1984). Clinical experience with a rate-controlled delivery of antihypertensive therapy by a transdermal system, *Am. Heart J.*, 108:231–236.

193. Jabs, D. A., Schachat, A. P., Liss, R., et al. (1987). Presumed varicella zoster retinitis in immunocompromised patients, *Retina*, 7:9–13.

194. Sarkies, N. J. C., and Blach, R. K. (1985). Ocular disease in immunosuppressed patients, *Trans. Ophthalmol. Soc. UK.*, 104:243–247.

195. Freeman, W. R., and O'Connor, G. R. (1984). Acquired immune deficiency syndrome retinopathy, pneumocystis, and cotton-wool spots (Editorial), *Am. J. Ophthalmol.*, 98:235–237.

196. Centers for Disease Control (January 13, 1985). AIDS activity daily report.

197. Pollard, R. B., Egbert, P. R., Gallagher, J. G., et al. (1980). Cytomegalovirus retinitis in immunosuppressed hosts. I. Natural history and effects of treatment with adenine arabinoside, *Ann. Intern. Med.*, 93:655–664.

198. England, A. C., Miller, S. A., and Maki, D. G. (1982). Ocular findings of acute cytomegalovirus infection in an immunologically competent adult, *N. Engl. J. Med.*, 307:94–95.

199. Rungger-Brändle, E., Roux, L., and Leuenberger, P. M. (1984). Bilateral acute retinal necrosis (BARN). Identification of the presumed infectious agent, *Ophthalmology*, 91:1648–1658.

200. Sarkies, N., Gregor, Z., Forsey, T., et al. (1986). Antibodies to herpes simplex virus type I in intraocular fluids of patients with acute retinal necrosis, *Br. J. Ophthalmol.*, 70:81–84.

201. Holland, G. N., Sakamoto, M. J., Hardy, D., et al. (1986). Treatment of cytomegalovirus retinopathy in patients with acquired immunodeficiency syndrome. Use of the experimental drug 9-[2-hydroxy-1-(hydroxymethyl)ethoxymethy] guanine, *Arch. Ophthalmol.*, 104: 1794–1800.

202. Rosecan, L. R., Laskin, O. L., Kalman, C. M., et al. (1986). Antiviral therapy with ganciclovir for cytomegalovirus retinitis and bilateral exudative retinal detachments in an immunocompromised child, *Ophthalmology*, 93:1401–1407.

203. D'Amico, D. J., Talamo, J. H., Felsenstein, D., et al. (1986). Ophthalmoscopic and histologic findings in cytomegalovirus retinitis treated with BW-B759U, *Arch. Ophthalmol.*, 104: 1788–1793.

204. Hirsch, M. S., and Kaplan, J. C. (1987). Treatment of human immunodeficiency virus infections, *Antimicrob. Agents Chemother.*, 31:839–843.

205. Henderly, D. E., Freeman, W. R., Causey, D. M., et al. (1987). Cytomegalovirus retinitis and response to therapy with ganciclovir, *Ophthalmology*, 94:425–434.

206. Holland, G. N., Buhles, W. C. Jr., Mastre, B., et al. (1989). The UCLA CMV Retinopathy Study Group. A controlled retrospective study of ganciclovir treatment for cytomegalovirus retinopathy, *Arch. Ophthalmol.*, 107:1759–1766.

207. Jabs, D. A., Enger, C., and Bartlett, J. (1989). Cytomegalovirus retinitis and acquired immunodeficiency syndrome, *Arch. Ophthalmol.*, 107:75–80.

208. Henderly, D. E., Freeman, W. R., Smith, R. E., et al. (1987). Cytomegalovirus retinitis as the initial manifestation of acquired immunodeficiency syndrome, *Am. J. Ophthalmol.*, 103: 316–320.

209. Schulman, J., Peyman, G. A., Horton, M. B., et al. (1986). Intraocular penetration of new antiviral agent, hydroxyacyclovir (BW-B759U), *Jpn. J. Ophthalmol.*, 30:116–124.

210. Schulman, J., Peyman, G. A., Horton, M. B., et al. (1986). Intraocular 9-([2-hydroxy-1-(hydroxymethyl)ethoxy]methyl) guanine levels after intravitreal and subconjunctival administration, *Ophthalmic Surg.*, 17:429–432.

211. Felsenstein, D., D'Amico, D. J., Hirsh, M. S., et al. (1985). Treatment of cytomegalovirus retinitis with 9-[2-hydroxy-1-(hydroxymethyl) ethoxymethyl] guanine, *Ann. Intern. Med.*, 103:377–380.

212. Palestine, A. G., Stevens, G., Jr., Lane, H. C., et al. (1986). Treatment of cytomegalovirus retinitis with dihydroxy propoxymethyl guanine, *Am. J. Ophthalmol.*, 101:95–101.

213. Holland, G. N., Sidikaro, Y., Kreiger, A. E., et al. (1987). Treatment of cytomegalovirus retinopathy with ganciclovir, *Ophthalmology*, 94:815–823.

214. Collaborative DHPG Treatment Study Group. (1986). Treatment of serious cytomegalovirus infections with 9-(1,3-dihydroxy-2-propoxymethyl)guanine in patients with AIDS and other immunodeficiencies, *N. Engl. J. Med.*, 314:801–805.

215. Rosecan, L. R., Stahl-Bayliss, C. M., Kalman, C. M., et al. (1986). Antiviral therapy for cytomegalovirus retinitis in AIDS with dihydroxy propoxymethyl guanine, *Am. J. Ophthalmol.*, 101:405–418.

216. Jabs, D. A., Newman, C., De Bustros, S., et al. (1987). Treatment of cytomegalovirus retinitis with ganciclovir, *Ophthalmology*, 94:824–830.

217. Orellana, J., Teich, S. A., Friedman, A. H., et al. (1987). Combined short- and long-term therapy for the treatment of cytomegalovirus retinitis using ganciclovir (BW B759U), *Ophthalmology*, 94:831–838.

218. Pepose, J. S., Newman, C., Bach, M. C., et al. (1987). Pathologic features of cytomegalovirus retinopathy after treatment with the antiviral agent ganciclovir, *Ophthalmology*, 94: 414–424.

219. Jacobson, M. A., and O'Donnell, J. J. (1991). Approaches to the treatment of cytomegalovirus retinitis. Ganciclovir and foscarnet, *J. Acquir. Immune Def. Syndr.*, 4(Suppl. 1):S11–S15.

220. Freeman, W. R. (1989). Intraocular antiviral therapy (editorial), *Arch. Ophthalmol.*, 107: 1737–1739.

221. Ussery, F. M. III, Gibson, S. R., Conklin, R. H., et al. (1988). Intravitreal ganciclovir in the treatment of AIDS-associated cytomegalovirus retinitis, *Ophthalmology*, 95:640–648.

222. Hennis, H. L., Scott, A. A., and Apple, D. J. (1989). Cytomegalovirus retinitis, *Surv. Ophthalmol.*, 34:193–203.

223. Robinson, H. R., Teitelbaum, C., and Taylor-Findlay, C. (1989). Thrombocytopenia and vitreous hemorrhage complicating ganciclovir treatment (letter). *Am. J. Ophthalmol.*, 107:560–561.

224. Jacobson, M. A., de Miranda, P., Cederberg, D. M., et al. (1987). Human pharmacokinetics and tolerance of oral ganciclovir, *Antimicrob. Agents Chemother.*, 31:1251–1254.

225. Freeman, W. R., Henderly, D. E., Wan, W. L., et al. (1987). Prevalence, pathophysiology, and treatment of rhegmatogenous retinal detachment in treated cytomegalovirus retinitis, *Am. J Ophthalmol.*, 103:527–536.

226. Govig, B., Jackson, W. B., and Gilmore, N. (1988). Preventing transmission of human immuno-deficiency virus in ophthalmologic practice, *Can. J. Ophthalmol.*, 23:5–7.

227. Pomerantz, R. R., Kuritzkes, D. R., de la Monte, S. M., et al. (1987). Infection of the retina by human immunodeficiency virus type I, *N. Engl. J. Med.*, 317:1643–1647.

228. Cantrill, H., Henry, K., Jackson, B., et al. (1988). Recovery of human immunodeficiency virus from ocular tissues in patients with acquired immune deficiency syndrome, *Ophthalmology*, 95:1458–1462.

229. Skolnik, P. R., Kosloff, B. R., and Hirsch, M. S. (1988). Bidirectional interactions between human immunodeficiency virus type I and cytomegalovirus, *J. Infect. Dis.*, 157:508–514.

230. Webster, A. (1991). Cytomegalovirus as a possible cofactor in HIV disease progression, *J. Acquir. Immune Def. Syndr.*, 4(Suppl):547–552.

231. Skolnick, P. R., Pomerantz, R. J., de la Monte, S., et al. (1989). Dual infection of the retina with human immunodeficiency virus type I and cytomegalovirus, *Am. J. Ophthalmol.*, 107: 361–372.

232. Guyer, D. R., Jabs, D. A., Brent, A. M., et al. (1989). Regression of cytomegalovirus retinitis with zidovudine. A clinicopathologic correlation, *Arch. Ophthalmol.*, 107:868–874.

233. D'Amico, D. J., Skolnick, P. R., Kosloff, B. R., et al. (1988). Resolution of cytomegalovirus with zidovudine therapy, *Arch. Ophthalmol.*, 106:1168–1169.

234. Fay, M., Freeman, W., Wiley, C., et al. (1988). Atypical retinitis in the acquired immuno-deficiency syndrome, *Am. J. Ophthalmol.*, 105:483–490.

235. Causey, D. (1991). Concomitant ganciclovir and zidovudine treatment for cytomegalovirus retinitis in patients with HIV infection. An approach to treatment, *J. Acquir. Immune Def. Syndr.*, 4(Suppl 1):S16–S21.

236. Lehoang, P., Girard, B., Robinet, M., et al. (1989). Foscarnet in the treatment of cytomegalo-virus retinitis in acquired immune deficiency syndrome, *Ophthalmology*, 96: 865–874.

237. Holland, G. N. (1992). Acquired immunodeficiency syndrome and ophthalmology. The first decade, *Am. J. Ophthalmol.*, 114:86-95.

238. Le Hoang, P., Robinet, M., Materon, S., et al. (1987). Cytomegalovirus retinitis in the acquired immune deficiency syndrome (AIDS). Clinical, angiographic and pathologic aspects: Treatment with trisodium phosphonoformate (Foscarnet), *Int. Ophthalmol.*, 10:91.

239. Michon, C. P., Katlama, C., Le Hoang, P., et al. (1986). Foscarnet for cytomegalovirus (CMV) infection in AIDS. *In*: Program and Abstracts of the II International Conference on AIDS, Paris, France.

240. Chew, E., Walmsley, S., Fanning, M., et al. (1987). Treatment of CMV retinitis with trisodium phosphonoformate (foscarnet) (abstract), *Invest. Ophthalmol. Vis. Sci.*, 28(Suppl):394.

241. Studies of ocular complications of AIDS Research Group, in collaboration with the AIDS Clinical Trials Group (1992). Mortality in patients with the acquired immunodeficiency syndrome treated with either foscarnet or ganciclovir for cytomegalovirus retinitis, *N. Engl. J. Med.*, 326:213-220.

242. Farthing, C., Anderson, M. G., Ellis, M. E., et al. (1987). Treatment of cytomegalovirus pneumonitis with foscarnet (trisodium phosphonoformate) in patients with AIDS, *J. Med. Virol.*, 22:157–162.

243. Youle, M. S., Clarbour, J., Gazzard, B., et al. (1988). Severe hypocalcaemia in AIDS patients treated with foscarnet and pentamidine (letter), *Lancet*, 1:1455–1466.

244. Singer, D. R. J., Fallon, T. J., Schulenburg, W. E., et al. (1985). Foscarnet for cytomegalovirus retinitis (letter), *Ann. Intern. Med.*, 103:962.

245. Aweeka, F., Gambertogilio, J., Mills, J., et al. (1989). Pharmacokinetics of intermittently administered intravenous foscarnet in the treatment of acquired immunodeficiency syndrome patients with serious cytomegalovirus retinitis, *Antimicrob. Agents Chemother.*, 33: 742–745.

246. Graeme, M., Mathalone, B., and Gazzard, B. (1990). An Open Randomized Comparative Study of Foscarnet and Ganciclovir in the Treatment of CMV Retinitis. Abstract F.B. 95, presented at the 6th International Conference on AIDS, San Francisco.

247. Freitas, V. R., Fraser-Smith, E. B., and Matthews, T. R. (1989). Increased efficacy of ganci-clovir in combination with foscarnet against cytomegalovirus and herpes simplex virus type 2 in vitro and in vivo, *Antiviral Res.*, 12:205–212.

248. Manischewitz, J. F., Quinnan, G. V., Jr., Lane, H. C., et al. (1990). Synergistic effect of ganciclovir and foscarnet on cytomegalovirus replication in vitro, *Antimicrob. Agents Chemother.*, 34:373–375.

249. DeArmond, B. (1991). Future directions in the management of cytomegalovirus infections, *J. Acquir. Immune Def. Syndr.*, 4(Suppl. 1):S53–S60.

250. Metcalf, D., Begley, C. G., Johnson, G. R., et al. (1986). Biologic properties in vitro of a recombinant human granulocyte-macrophage colony-stimulating factor, *Blood*, 67:37–45.

251. Gasson, J. C., Weisbart, R. H., Kaufman, S. E., et al. (1984). Purified human granulocyte-macrophage colony-stimulating factor. Direct action on neutrophils, *Science*, 226:1339–1342.

252. Weisbart, R. H., Golde, D. W., Clark, S. C., et al. (1985). Human granulocyte-macrophage colony-stimulating factor is a neutrophil activator, *Nature*, 314:361–363.

253. Grossberg, H. S., Bonnem, E. M., and Buhles, W. C., Jr. (1989). GM-CSF with ganciclovir for the treatment of CMV retinitis in AIDS, *N. Engl. J. Med.*, 320:1560.

254. Hardy, W. D. (1991). Combined ganciclovir and recombinant human granulocyte-macrophage colony-stimulating factor in the treatment of cytomegalovirus retinitis in AIDS patients, *J. Acquir. Immune Defic. Syndr.*, 4(Suppl. 1):S22–S28.

255. Schulman, J. A., Peyman, G. A., Fiscella, R. G., et al. (1984). Parenterally administered acyclovir for viral retinitis associated with AIDS (letter), *Arch. Ophthalmol.*, 102:1750.

256. Friedman, A. H., Orellana, J., Freeman, W. R., et al. (1983). Cytomegalovirus retinitis. A manifestation of the acquired immune deficiency syndrome (AIDS), *Br. J. Ophthalmol.*, 67:372–380.

257. Bachman, D. M., Rodrigues, M. M., Chu, F. C., et al. (1982). Culture-proven cytomegalovirus retinitis in a homosexual man with the acquired immune deficiency syndrome, *Ophthalmology*, 89:797–804.

258. Neuwirth, J., Gutman, I., Hofeldt, A. J., et al. (1982). Cytomegalovirus retinitis in a young homosexual male with acquired immunodeficiency, *Ophthalmology*, 89:805–806.

259. Schuman, J. S., and Friedman, A. H. (1983). Retinal manifestations of the acquired immune deficiency syndrome (AIDS). Cytomegalovirus, Candida albicans, cryptococcus, toxoplasmosis and Pneumocystis carinii, *Trans. Ophthalmol. Soc. UK.*, 103:177–190.

260. Newman, N. M., Mandel, M. R., Gullett, J., et al. (1983). Clinical and histologic findings in opportunistic ocular infections. Part of a new syndrome of acquired immunodeficiency, *Arch. Ophthalmol.*, 101:396–401.

261. Holland, G. N., Pepose, J. S., Pettit, T. H., et al. (1983). Acquired immune deficiency syndrome. Ocular manifestations, *Ophthalmology*, 90:859–873.

262. Chou, S., Dylewski, J. S., Gaynon, M. W., et al. (1984). Alpha-interferon administration in cytomegalovirus retinitis, *Antimicrob. Agents Chemother.*, 25:25–28.

263. Stevens, G. Jr., Palestine, A. G., Rodrigues, M. M., et al. (1986). Failure of argon laser to halt cytomegalovirus retinitis, *Retina*, 6:119–122.

264. Rytel, M. W., Aaberg, T. M., Dee, T. H., et al. (1975). Therapy of cytomegalovirus retinitis with transfer factor, *Cell. Immunol.*, 19:8–21.

265. Cox, F., Meyer, D., and Hughes, W. T. (1975). Cytomegalovirus in tears from patients with normal eyes and with acute cytomegalovirus chorioretinitis, *Am. J. Ophthalmol.*, 80:817–824.

266. Henson, D., Smith, R. D., Gehrke, J., et al. (1967). Effect of cortisone on nonfatal mouse cytomegalovirus infection, *Am. J. Pathol.*, 51:1001–1012.

267. Pulido, J., Peyman, G. A., Lesar, T., et al. (1985). Intravitreal toxicity of hydroxyacyclovir (BW-8759U), a new antiviral agent, *Arch. Ophthalmol.*, 103:840–841.

268. Yoshizumi, M. D., Lee, D., Vinci, V., et al. (1990). Ocular toxicity of multiple intravitreal DHPG injections, *Graefes Arch. Clin. Exp. Ophthalmol.*, 228:350–355.

269. Heery, S., and Hollows, F. (1989). High-dose intravitreal gancyclovir for cytomegaloviral (CMV) retinitis, *Aust. N.Z. J. Ophthalmol.*, 17:405–408.

270. Heinemann, M. H. (1989). Staphylococcus epidermidis endophthalmitis complicating intravitreal antiviral therapy of cytomegalovirus retinitis (letter), *Arch. Ophthalmol.*, 107: 643–644.

271. Peyman, G. A., Khoobehi, B., Tawakol, M., et al. (1987). Intravitreal injection of liposome-encapsulated ganciclovir in a rabbit model, *Retina*, 7:227–229.

272. Peyman, G. A., Schulman, J. A., Khoobehi, B., et al. (1989). Toxicity and clearance of a combination of liposome-encapsulated ganciclovir and trifluridine, *Retina*, 9:232–236.

273. Smith, K. O., Galloway, K. S., Ogilvie, K. K., et al. (1982). Synergism among BIOLF-62, phosphonoformate and other antiherpetic compounds, *Antimicrob. Agents Chemother.*, 22:1026–1030.

274. Spector, S. A., Tyndall, M., and Kelley, E. (1982). "Effects of Acyclovir Combined with Other Antiviral Agents on Human Cytomegalovirus." Proceedings Symposium on Acyclovir, July 20, 1982, *Am. J. Med.*, 72(Suppl.):36–39.

275. deKoning, E. W. J., van Bijsterveld, P., and Cantell, K. (1983). Combination therapy for dendritic keratitis with acyclovir and α-interferon, *Arch. Ophthalmol.*, 101:1866–1868.

276. Pepose, J. S., Hilborne, L. H., Cancilla, P. A., et al. (1984). Concurrent herpes simplex and cytomegalovirus retinitis and encephalitis in the acquired immune deficiency syndrome (AIDS), *Ophthalmology*, 91:1669–1677.

277. Small, G. H., Peyman, G. A., Srinivasan, A., et al. (1987). Retinal toxicity of combination antiviral drugs in an animal model, *Can. J. Ophthalmol.*, 22:300–303.

278. Culbertson, W. W., Blumenkranz, M. S., Pepose, J. S., et al. (1986). Varicella zoster virus is a cause of the acute retinal necrosis syndrome, *Ophthalmology*, 93:559–569.

279. Browning, D. J., Blumenkranz, M. S., Culbertson, W. W., et al. (1987). Association of varicella zoster dermatitis with acute retinal necrosis syndrome, *Ophthalmology*, 94:602–606.

280. Yeo, J. H., Pepose J. S., Stewart, J. A., et al. (1986). Acute retinal necrosis syndrome following herpes zoster dermatitis, *Ophthalmology*, 93:1418–1422.

281. Peyman, G. A., Goldberg, M. F., Uninsky, E., et al. (1984). Vitrectomy and intravitreal antiviral drug therapy in acute retinal necrosis syndrome. Report of two cases, *Arch. Ophthalmol.*, 102:1618–1621.

282. The Retina Society Terminology Committee (1983). The classification of retinal detachment with proliferative vitreoretinopathy, *Ophthalmology*, 90:121–125.

283. Jaeger, E. V. (1869). Ophthalmoskopscher Atlas; Netzhautsrange, table XVI, figs. 73, 74, Deuticke, Leipzig, p. 121.

284. Gonin, J. (1904). La pathogenie du decollement spontane de la retina, *Ann. Ocul.*, 132:30.

285. Gonin, J. (1934). Le decollment de la retine, pathogenie, traitment, table XI. Payot, Lausanne.

286. Rachal, W. F., and Burton, T. C. (1979). Changing concepts of failures after retinal detachment surgery, *Arch. Ophthalmol.*, 97:480–483.

287. Machemer, R. (1988). Proliferative vitreoretinopathy (PVR). A personal account of its pathogenesis and treatment, *Invest. Ophthalmol. Vis. Sci.*, 29:1771–1783.

288. Peyman, G. A., and Schulman, J. (1985). Proliferative vitreoretinopathy and chemotherapeutic agents, *Surv. Ophthalmol.*, 29:434–442.

289. Wiedemann, P., and Heimann, K. (1986). Proliferative vitreoretinopathie. Pathogenese und moglichkeiten der behandlung mit zytostutiki, *Klin. Monatsbl. Augenheilkd.*, 188:559–564.

290. Barr, C. C., and Blumenkranz, M. S. (1989). New substances in the treatment of proliferative vitreoretinopathy, *Ophthalmol. Clin. North Am.*, 2:187–198.

291. Blumenkranz, M. S., and Hartzer, M. K. (1989). The mechanism of action of drugs for the treatment of vitreoretinal scarring. In: *Retina* (S. J. Ryan, B. M. Glaser, R. G. Michels, eds.). Mosby, St. Louis, pp. 401–411.

292. Tano, Y., Sugita, G., Abrams, G., et al. (1980). Inhibition of intraocular proliferations with intravitreal corticosteroids, *Am. J. Ophthalmol.*, 89:131–136.

293. Tano, Y., Chandler, D., and Machemer, R. (1980). Treatment of intraocular proliferation with intravitreal injection of triamcinolone acetonide, *Am. J. Ophthalmol.*, 90:810–816.

294. Machemer, R., Van Horn, D. L., and Aaberg, T. M. (1978). Pigment epithelial proliferation in human retinal detachment with massive periretinal proliferation, *Am. J. Ophthalmol.*, 85:181–191.

295. Fiscella, R., Peyman, G. A., Elvart, J., et al. (1985). In vitro evaluation of cellular inhibitory potential of various antineoplastic drugs and dexamethasone, *Ophthalmic. Surg.*, 16: 247–249.

296. Sunalp, M., Wiedemann, P., Sorgente, N., et al. (1984). Effects of cytotoxic drugs on proliferative vitreoretinopathy in the rabbit cell injection model, *Curr. Eye Res.*, 3:619–623.

297. Wiedemann, P., Sorgente, N., and Bekhar, C. (1985). Daunomycin in the treatment of experimental proliferative vitreoretinopathy, *Invest. Ophthalmol. Vis. Sci.*, 26:719–725.

298. Blumenkranz, M., Ophir, A., Clafin, A. J., et al. (1982). Fluorouracil for the treatment of massive periretinal proliferation, *Am. J. Ophthalmol.*, 94:458–467.

299. Kulnig, N., Binder, S., and Riss, B. (1984). Inhibition of experimental intraocular proliferation with intravitreal 5-fluorouracil: A transmission electron microscope study in rabbits, *Ophthalmologica*, 188:248–258.

300. Case, J. L., Peyman, G. A., Barrada, A., et al. (1985). Clearance in intravitreal ^{3}H-fluorouracil, *Ophthalmic Surg.*, 16:378–381.

301. Fishman, P. H., Peyman, G. A., and Hendricks, R. (1989). Liposome-encapsulated ^{3}H-5-FU in rabbits, *Invest. Ophthalmol. Vis. Sci.*, 13:361–365.

302. Joondeph, B. C., Peyman, G. A., Khoobehi, B., et al. (1988). Liposome-encapsulated 5-fluorouracil in the treatment of proliferative vitreoretinopathy, *Ophthalmic Surg.*, 19: 252–256.

303. Stern, W. H., Heath, T. D., Lewis, G. P., et al. (1987). Clearance and localization of intravitreal liposomes in aphakic vitrectomized eye, *Invest. Ophthalmol. Vis. Sci.*, 28:907–911.

304. Peyman, G. A., Conway, M., Khoobehi, B., et al. (1992). Clearance of microsphere-entrapped 5-fluorouracil and cytosine arabinoside from the vitreous of primates, *Int. Ophthalmol.*, 16:109–113.

305. Blankenship, G. W. (1989). Evaluation of a single intravitreal injection of 5-fluorouracil in vitrectomy cases, *Graefes Arch. Clin. Exp. Ophthalmol.*, 227:565–568.

306. Berman, D. H., and Gombos, G. M. (1989). Proliferative vitreoretinopathy. Does oral low-dose colchicine have an inhibitory effect? A controlled study in humans, *Ophthalmic Surg.*, 20: 268–272.

307. Wiedemann, P., Lemmen, K., Schmiedl, R., et al. (1987). Intraocular daunorubicin for the treatment and prophylaxis of traumatic proliferative vitreoretinopathy, *Am. J. Ophthalmol.*, 104:10–14.

308. Wiedemann, P., Evans, P. Y., Wiedemann, R., et al. (1989). A fluorescein angiographic study on patients with proliferative vitreoretinopathy treated by vitrectomy and intraocular daunomycin, *Int. Ophthalmol.*, 13:211–216.

309. Wiedemann, P., Lemmen, K. D., Wiedemann, R., et al. (1988). Eine randomisierte Studie zur Behandlung der proliferativen Vitreoretinopathie mit Daunomycin, *Fortschr. Ophthalmol.*, 85: 503–504.

310. Wiedemann, P., Leinung, C., Hilgers, R. D., et al. (1991). Daunomycin and silicone oil for the treatment of proliferative vitreoretinopathy, *Graefes Arch. Clin. Exp. Ophthalmol.*, 229: 150–152.

311. BenEzra, D., Maftzir, G., deCourten, C., et al. (1990). Ocular penetration of cyclosporin A. III: the human eye, *Br. J. Ophthalmol.*, 74:350–352.

312. Nussenblatt, R. B., Palestine, A. G., and Chan, C. C. (1983). Cyclosporin A therapy in the treatment of intraocular inflammatory disease resistant to systemic corticosteroids and cytotoxic agents, *Am. J. Ophthalmol.*, 96:275–282.

313. BenEzra, D., and Cohen, E. (1986). Treatment and visual prognosis in Behçet's disease, *Br. J. Ophthalmol.*, 70:589–592.

314. Nussenblatt, R. B., Salinas-Carmona, M. C., Gery, I., et al. (1982). Modulation of experimental autoimmune uveitis with cyclosporin A, *Arch. Ophthalmol.*, 110:1146–1149.
315. Graham, E. M., Sanders, M. D., James, D. G., et al. (1985). Cyclosporin A in the treatment of posterior uveitis, *Trans. Ophthalmol. Soc. UK.*, 104:146–151.
316. BenEzra, D., Cohen, E., Chajek, T., et al. (1988). Evaluation of conventional therapy versus cyclosporine A in Behçet's syndrome, *Transplant. Proc.*, 20(Suppl. 4):136–143.
317. BenEzra, D., Cohen, E., Rakotomalala, M., et al. (1988). Treatment of endogenous uveitis with cyclosporine A, *Transplant. Proc.*, 20(Suppl. 4):122–127.
318. Nussenblatt, R. B., Palestine, A. G., Chan, C. C., et al. (1983). Cyclosporin A therapy in the treatment of intraocular inflammatory disease resistant to systemic corticosteroids and cytotoxic agents, *Am. J. Ophthalmol.*, 96:275–282.
319. Abramowicz, M. (1983). Cyclosporine. A new immunosuppressive agent, *Med. Lett.*, 25: 77–78.
320. Lafferty, J. K., Borel, J. F., Hodgkin, P. (1983). Cyclosporin-A (CsA). Models for the mechanism of action, *Transplant. Proc.*, 15(Suppl. 4):2245.
321. Hunter, P. A., Garner, A. R., Wilhelmus, K. R., et al. (1982). Corneal graft rejection: A new rabbit model and cyclosporin-A, *Br. J. Ophthalmol.*, 66:292–302.
322. Mosteller, M. W., Gebhardt, B. M., Hamilton, A. M., et al. (1985). Penetration of topical cyclosporine into the rabbit cornea, aqueous humor, and serum, *Arch. Ophthalmol.*, 103: 101–102.
323. Kana, J. S., Hoffman, F., Buchen, R., et al. (1982). Rabbit corneal allograft survival following topical administration of cyclosporin A, *Invest. Ophthalmol. Vis. Sci.*, 22:686–690.
324. Salisbury, J. D., and Gebhardt, B. M. (1981). Suppression of corneal allograft rejection by cyclosporin A, *Arch. Ophthalmol.*, 99:1640–1643.
325. BenEzra, D., and Maftzir, G. (1990). Ocular penetration of cyclosporin A. The rabbit eye, *Invest. Ophthalmol. Vis. Sci.*, 31:1362–1366.
326. BenEzra, D., and Maftzir, G. (1990). Ocular penetration of cyclosporine A in the rat eye, *Arch. Ophthalmol.*, 108:584–587.
327. Oh, J. O., Minasi, P., Grabner, G., et al. (1985). Suppression of secondary herpes simplex uveitis by cyclosporine, *Invest. Ophthalmol. Vis. Sci.*, 26:494–500.
328. Alghadyan, A. A., Peyman, G. A., Khoobehi, B., et al. (1988). Liposome-bound cyclosporine. Retinal toxicity after intravitreal injection, *Int. Ophthalmol.*, 12:105–107.
329. Grisolano, J., and Peyman, G. A. (1986). Retinal toxicity study of intravitreal cyclosporin, *Ophthalmic Surg.*, 17:155–156.

20
Systemic Delivery of Drugs for Ophthalmic Diseases

Philip R. Mayer *Alcon Laboratories, Fort Worth, Texas*

I. INTRODUCTION

It is well-recognized that topical ophthalmic medications are not restricted to local effects in the eye but can be absorbed into the general circulation through nasolacrimal drainage, diffusion into conjunctival capillaries, or other mechanisms. Once present systemically, these drugs may provide both pharmacological and toxicological effects (1). It is just as apparent that systemic drugs may also distribute into ocular tissues. Certainly many systemic tissue distribution studies have demonstrated the presence of drug in ocular tissues and, in fact, several orally administered agents are marketed for ophthalmic indications. Three oral carbonic anhydrase inhibitors, acetazolamide, methazolamide, and dichlorphenamide, are routinely prescribed for lowering intraocular pressure. In addition, systemic doses of aldose reductase inhibitors may be utilized for treating diabetic retinopathy in the future. Other drugs are also capable of providing therapeutic concentrations in intraocular tissues following systemic administration. Therefore, while topical ophthalmic dosing provides the benefits of localized delivery with a decreased potential for systemic side effects, oral dosing may also be utilized in select cases for effective ocular therapy. The purpose of this chapter is to demonstrate this capability for certain systemic medications.

II. CARBONIC ANHYDRASE INHIBITORS

The carbonic anhydrase enzyme reversibly catalyzes the conversion between CO_2 and HCO_3-. Its presence is required in many tissues to provide a physiological equilibrium between these species. In the ciliary process of the eye, blocking the synthesis of HCO_3- slows the transport of Na^+ into aqueous humor, resulting in a concurrent decrease in aqueous humor formation and a lowering of intraocular pressure (2). This pharmacological effect and the potential for treating glaucoma were first recognized in 1954 (3).

Despite renewed interest in topically instilled carbonic anhydrase inhibitors (4), the only marketed drugs utilizing this mechanism of action are administered orally. The disadvantage of oral carbonic anhydrase inhibitors is the magnitude of systemic side effects that occur, including fatigue, depression, gastrointestinal upset, and others (5), which can be reduced with topical agents. Although all of the hurdles have not been overcome, newly synthesized, potent carbonic anhydrase inhibitors have solved the major problem with adapting these oral agents to topical dosing, low corneal permeability, and these topical agents show promise as effective intraocular pressure–lowering compounds (6,7). However, oral carbonic anhydrase inhibitors provide sufficient drug concentration in the ciliary process to control glaucoma, especially as adjunctive treatment.

It is somewhat unexpected that enough systemic drug can accumulate in the ciliary process to effectively block carbonic anhydrase there, since 99.9% of the enzyme must be inhibited (8). Because of the high enzyme turnover, drug must not only reach the active site, but also remain in high concentrations to have a sufficient duration of action. This is especially remarkable, since carbonic anhydrase inhibitors exhibit nonlinear, high-affinity binding to red blood cell carbonic anhydrase such that the large majority of an administered dose is present within the whole blood. Still, owing to the marked attraction of carbonic anhydrase inhibitors for their enzymatic active site, sufficient drug can accumulate and be retained in the ciliary process.

The disposition of methazolamide has been examined extensively by Bayne et al. (9). Methazolamide is sequestered in red blood cells and is released very slowly from enzyme-binding sites into the plasma prior to metabolism and eventual elimination. Although methazolamide has an intrinsic metabolic half-life of 7.5 h (9), this half-life would only be appropriate if there were no uptake and binding in red blood cells. Therefore, the apparent half-life is more appropriately hundreds of hours and may, in fact, be related to red blood cell turnover rate, known to be 3 months (10). Blood concentration versus time profiles show significant concentrations of methazolamide 6 weeks following the administration of a single 50-mg tablet (9).

With the avid binding to red blood cell carbonic anhydrase, inhibitor drug concentration is equivalent to carbonic anhydrase concentration (170 μM) (11). When saturation occurs, drug may effectively distribute to other tissue binding sites, most notably the ciliary process of the eye and the proximal tubule of the kidney. Indeed, this can be observed by the increase in methazolamide plasma concentrations above what would be expected on the basis of linear pharmacokinetic principles (9). This theory has been substantiated, both theoretically and by application in humans, by Maren et al. (11). Methazolamide plasma concentrations sufficient to result in the inhibition of carbonic anhydrase in the eye are obtained with multiple dosing, so that intraocular pressure is lowered. This led to a reduction in intraocular pressure to normal values in three out of four human subjects (11). Other studies documenting the therapeutic effectiveness of oral carbonic anhydrase inhibitors have been published (12,13).

Carbonic anhydrase inhibitors demonstrate the capacity of a systemic drug to distribute into the ciliary process of the eye and to provide a concentration suitable for inhibiting essentially all of the hydration of carbon dioxide and, therefore, decreasing the secretion of aqueous humor. Their retention at the carbonic anhydrase enzyme active site enables sufficient drug to accumulate intraocularly and block this enzyme effectively. They have become successful adjuncts to other antiglaucoma agents and assist in maintaining intraocular pressure control for 8–12 h.

III. ALDOSE REDUCTASE INHIBITORS

Owing to the anatomy of the eye, drug distribution to posterior ocular tissues is a difficult process. With topical ocular administration, only a small percentage of the dose penetrates the cornea to reach the aqueous humor. Then diffusion across the lens, iris-ciliary body, and vitreous humor must occur prior to any drug reaching the retina. However, retinal capillaries furnish oxygen, nutrients, and other biochemical substrates to the retina and surrounding tissue. The consistent delivery of drugs via this pathway surpasses the potential for drugs instilled into the cul-de-sac to reach the retina or other posterior eye tissues. Therefore, it is quite appropriate to consider systemic drug treatment as a first option for diabetic retinopathy or other anatomically related posterior eye diseases.

The aldose reductase enzyme has been implicated in the pathogenesis of complications which arise from long-term diabetes (14,15). These complications include neuropathy and nephropathy, purely systemic in origin, and retinopathy and cataracts, which are ophthalmic disorders. For these ocular disease states, cataracts will most likely be treated in topical ocular fashion by aldose reductase inhibitors. For example, one such agent, imirestat, shows higher lens concentrations after topical ocular dosing than can be achieved by intravenous administration of an equivalent dose (16). To achieve effective drug concentrations for almost any disease in this avascular ocular tissue, topical instillation will be required. However, the treatment of diabetic retinopathy will probably necessitate systemic drug therapy.

Diabetic retinopathy results from serious lesions present in retinal capillaries, basement membrane thickening though increasing in porosity, and the degeneration of intraocular pericytes. Clinically, the effects of retinopathy may result in blindness, such that it is the leading cause of new cases of blindness. Following from the hypothesis of aldose reductase inhibitor therapy for arresting diabetic complications, there have been extensive investigations to examine the benefits of these agents in preventing or reversing diabetic retinopathy. Significantly, all of these studies have utilized systemic administration of aldose reductase inhibitors.

The primary animal model used for studying retinopathy has been the rat, either rendered diabetic chemically or administered 30–50% galactose as part of their diet. The connection between aldose reductase–related retinopathy complications and the benefits of sorbinil, an aldose reductase inhibitor, were apparent in a one early study by Robison et al. (17). A year's treatment with 2 g/kg of oral sorbinil prevented the thickening of capillary basement membranes in galactosemic rat retinas.

Other aldose reductase inhibitors have provided evidence for the aldose reductase link in diabetic retinopathy and also for the ability of systemically administered drug, through the diet, to reach ocular tissues and prevent these histopathological changes. ONO 2235 mixed with a fructose-rich diet, maintained a normal microvascular basement membrane (18). Oral ADN-138 prevented electroretinogram abnormalities and polyol accumulation associated with diabetic hyperglycemic and galactosemic states in Sprague-Dawley rats (19). Over 2 years of oral tolrestat treatment in galactose-fed rats prevented basement membrane thickening, pericyte degeneration, microaneurysm formation, and other retinal changes observed with long-term galactosemia (20,21). Sorbinil has been shown in a recent study to alter various components of retinal capillary basement membrane thickening in the rat (22). In the galactosemic dog animal model, oral sorbinil and M79175 have prevented the formation of pericyte ghosts in retinal capillaries (23). Finally, in early human trials of sorbinil, the aldose reductase inhibitor has been shown to stabilize the blood-retinal barrier in a 6-month study (24).

Similarly to the carbonic anhydrase inhibitors, aldose reductase inhibitors are highly bound to their respective enzyme sites in ocular tissues in significant enough quantities to promote a specific therapeutic outcome. Histopathological and biochemical evidence indicates that oral aldose reductase inhibitors alter the vascular changes affected by diabetic retinopathy. Stabilizing retinal capillaries in animal models through oral administration demonstrates that systemic dosing of these agents results in the delivery of therapeutic concentrations of drug to active sites within the eye.

IV. OTHER SYSTEMIC DRUGS EFFECTIVELY DISTRIBUTING INTO OCULAR TISSUES

The general distributional behavior of a systemic drug dictates whether a compound penetrates ocular tissues. Since aqueous humor is formed from plasma by secretion processes, any relatively small molecular weight molecule may be present in aqueous humor. This may actually occur quite rapidly given the rate of aqueous formation. For example, upon the injection of pentobarbital or other agents for animal sacrifice, these drugs may be detected at relatively high concentrations in the aqueous humor in the short time between the intravenous bolus injection and the death of the animal.

Although it is conceivable that many systemic drugs could be utilized to treat ocular diseases, there are limited examples of this practice. Fluorescein is a widely used diagnostic aid for the study of blood-retinal and blood-aqueous barrier permeability. Though often instilled topically, it may be given as an oral or intravenous dose (25). Fluorescein is metabolized quickly to its glucuronide in the liver (26,27) but its fluorescent properties enable it to be quantitated in the eye noninvasively by fluorophotometry. Its rapid penetration into the aqueous and vitreous humors make this agent useful for the assessment of barrier function and other ocular disease states.

Various animal studies have demonstrated the ability of systemic antibiotics to reach infections in the eye in concentrations appropriate for treating various pathogens (28,29). Ciprofloxacin, a quinoline antibiotic, penetrates into the aqueous humor following oral administration. In a study of 101 human patients undergoing elective cataract lens removal, ciprofloxacin was dosed orally 1–4 h prior to surgery (30). Drug was measured in both serum and aqueous humor by high-performance liquid chromatography. Peak aqueous humor concentrations of 0.5–0.7 μg/mL were achieved 2–3 h after 1.0 or 1.5 g ciprofloxacin administration (Fig. 1). These levels in aqueous humor ranged from 3 to 15% of the corresponding serum drug level.

BCNU, an anticancer drug, was measured in rabbit aqueous and vitreous humor following intravenous injection (31). By comparing vitreous humor concentration-time profiles with those observed after topical ocular and subconjunctival administration, the authors suggested that intravenous injection of BCNU was the best route for treating choroidal and retinal tumors.

Although there is limited data available in the literature, it is likely that many other drugs, especially steroids and other anti-inflammatory agents, are administered orally to treat diseases localized in the eye. Owing to drug distribution properties, partition of sufficient drug into specific ocular tissues may result in a therapeutic concentration at the active site.

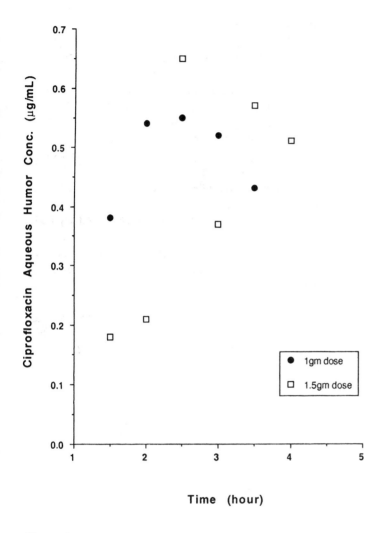

Figure 1.   Mean ciprofloxacin aqueous humor concentration versus time profiles ($n = 2$–5) following oral administration to humans undergoing cataract surgery. (Adapted from Ref. 29.)

V.   CONTRALATERAL EYE EFFECTS WITH TOPICAL OCULAR THERAPY

Because of the likelihood of systemic drugs to penetrate intraocular tissues, there is also the potential for drugs dosed in topical ocular fashion to reach the systemic circulation and to redistribute back into the eye. This phenomenon is not well recognized, but can be discerned as a crossover effect in a nontreated contralateral eye. The results can be seen as an additional benefit above one entirely due to an initial transit through the eye.

Initial screening of antiglaucoma agents has historically involved a monocular study design with the untreated eye serving as a control. However, a study with unilateral 0.5% timolol maleate treatment found a significant pressure drop in both the treated and untreated eyes (32). One-half of the subjects exhibited less than a 0.5 mmHg difference in the intraocular pressure reduction in both eyes. Timolol exhibits high-affinity binding to the β-adrenergic receptor in the ciliary process (33) and it is likely that uptake occurs in either the treated or untreated eye via the systemic circulation (34). Therefore, systemic absorption and redistribution to the eye can result in a more pronounced pharmacological effect.

The contralateral eye effects of the alpha-adrenergic antiglaucoma agent apraclonidine have been examined. A single 30-μL topical ocular dose of 1% apraclonidine was instilled in the right eye of New Zealand albino rabbits, with the left eye remaining untreated. Tissues were taken at periodic sampling times (n=3) through 6 h. Concentrations in various tissues of the dosed eye were approximately 10-fold greater than those achieved in the control eye. The apraclonidine aqueous humor concentration versus time profiles show that following peak concentrations achieved at 2 h, the undosed eye aqueous humor concentrations are 10% of the dosed eye (Fig. 2). For a vascularized eye tissue, iris-ciliary body concentrations in the undosed eye were 20% of the dosed eye. In the avascular cornea, only 3% of the dosed eye concentrations were present in the undosed eye. These data demonstrate the potential for systemic absorption and redistribution into ocular tissues, although contralateral eye concentrations 1 log scale lower than the dosed eye are unlikely to provide significant pharmacologic activity.

One is more likely to see a contralateral eye effect in a smaller laboratory animal. Brown Norway rats were utilized as the animal model for one study designed to correlate lens concentrations with biochemical inhibition of aldose reductase (35). AL01576, an aldose reductase inhibitor, was administered in the right eye only of rats either once, twice,

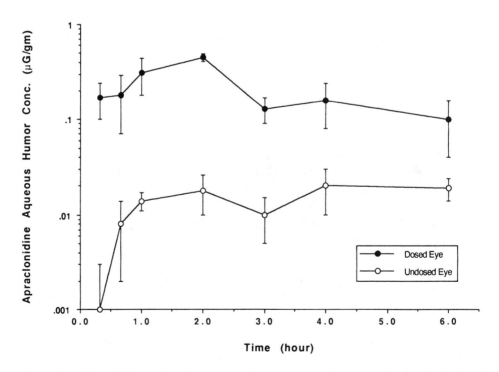

Figure 2. Mean (±SD) apraclonidine aqueous humor concentration versus time profiles in dosed and undosed rabbit eyes following unilateral instillation (*n* = 6).

or four times daily as a 0.1% suspension. After 6 weeks of treatment, the animals were sacrificed and drug concentrations were determined in both lenses by a bioassay technique. As shown in Figure 3, both the dosed and undosed eye lenses had similar concentrations, showing the predominant systemic contribution to ocular drug levels in this animal model. Other studies with the aldose reductase inhibitor imirestat (AL01576) have demonstrated the phenomena of drug crossover to an undosed contralateral eye (16). Following equivalent topical ocular and intravenous doses (50 µg) to New Zealand albino rabbits, ^{14}C-imirestat concentrations were remarkably similar in the undosed eye lens and aqueous and vitreous humor. Though drug concentrations were lower in the undosed eye when compared to the dosed eye, the data indicate that the uptake process into the lens, which is rich in aldose reductase, is a more long-term process leading to an eventual equilibrium with significant concentrations of imirestat in the undosed eye.

Systemic delivery of imirestat into ocular lens tissue has been investigated more extensively following multiple monocular doses. Thirty microliters of a 0.1% suspension was instilled twice daily into the right eye only of the New Zealand albino rabbit for 28

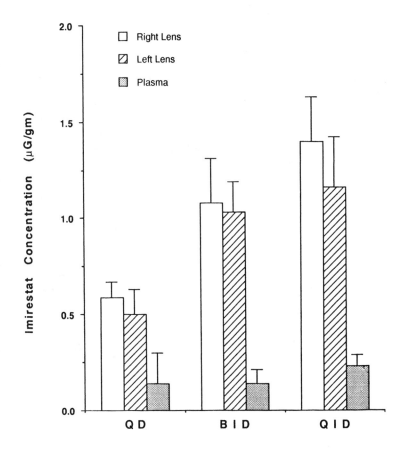

Figure 3. AL01576 concentrations (mean ±SD) in rat lenses and plasma following 42 days of 0.1% AL01576 treatment to the right eye only. Treatment regimens were once daily (QD), twice daily (BID), or four times daily (QID). (Adapted from Ref. 34.)

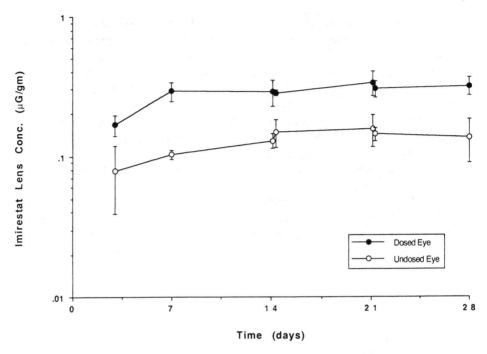

Figure 4. Mean (±SD) imirestat concentrations in the right (●) and left (○) rabbit lens following twice daily instillation of 0.1% imirestat ophthalmic suspension to the right eye only for 28 days.

days. Imirestat concentrations in the lens were measured by gas chromatography in three animals sacrificed at the end of a dosing interval on days 3, 7, 14, 21, and 28 of treatment; peak samples were also obtained on days 14 and 21. Steady-state conditions appear to have been achieved for lens concentrations after two weeks of dosing, with undosed eye imirestat concentrations approximately 40% of those observed in the dosed eye (Fig. 4). Therefore, even in the dosed eye, up to 40% of the concentration represents drug which has reached the general circulation and then redistributed into the eye to be taken up by the lens.

Cumulatively, these data indicate that a topical ocular drug may be absorbed systemically only to return to its site of action in the eye. This phenomena may more reasonably occur with a drug exhibiting a long systemic half-life or unique tissue-binding characteristics within the eye. Although not likely to provide a majority of the intended pharmacological effect, this systemic drug may be a substantial contributor to the compound's overall ophthalmic activity.

VI. SUMMARY

Topical ocular administration will always remain as the primary means of delivering drugs to treat ophthalmic diseases. However, systemic drugs may also partition into ocular tissues via active processes or passive diffusion. Based on this systemic-ocular equilibrium, sufficient drug may distribute to the eye, reach potential sites of pharmacological activity, and promote a therapeutic effect. Although most of the data demonstrating this route of delivery to the eye is based on smaller animal models, it is quite apparent that similar results may be observed in humans. It is important to recognize this potential for ocular drug treatment.

REFERENCES

1. Everitt, D. E., and Avorn, J. (1990). Systemic effects of medications used to treat glaucoma, *Ann. Intern. Med.*, 112:120.
2. Maren, T. H. (1987). Carbonic anhydrase: General perspectives and advances in glaucoma research, *Drug. Dev. Res.*, 10:255.
3. Becker, B. (1954). Decrease in intraocular pressure in man by a carbonic anhydrase inhibitor, Diamox. A preliminary report, *Am. J. Ophthalmol.*, 37:13.
4. Kass, M. A. (1989). Topical carbonic anhydrase inhibitors, *Am. J. Ophthalmol.*, 107:280.
5. Podos, S. M., and Serle, J. B. (1991). Topically active carbonic anhydrase inhibitors for glaucoma, *Arch. Ophthalmol.*, 109:38.
6. Higginbotham, E. J., Kass, M. A., et al. (1990). MK-927: A topical carbonic anhydrase inhibitor. Dose response and duration of action, *Arch. Ophthlamol.*, 108:65.
7. Lewis, R. A., Schoenwald, R. D., and Barfknecht, C. F. (1988). Aminozolamide suspension: The role of the vehicle in a topical carbonic anhydrase inhibitor, *J. Ocul. Pharmacol.*, 4:215.
8. Grant, W. M. (1970). Antiglaucoma drugs: Problems with carbonic anhydrase inhibitors. *In: Symposium on Ocular Therapy*, Vol. 6 (I. H. Leopold, ed.), Mosby, St. Louis, p. 19.
9. Bayne, W. F., Tao, F. T., et al. (1981). Time course and disposition of methazolamide in human plasma and red blood cells, *J. Pharm. Sci.*, 70:75.
10. Guyton, A. C. (1971). *Textbook of Medical Physiology*, Saunders, Philadelphia, p. 105.
11. Maren, T. H., Haywood, J. R., et al. (1977). The pharmacology of metazolamide in relation to the treatment of glaucoma, *Invest. Ophthalmol. Vis. Sci.*, 16:730.
12. Lehmann, B., Linner, E., and Wistrand, P. J. (1970). The pharmacokinetics of acetazolamide in relation to its use in the treatment of glaucoma and to its effects as an inhibitor of carbonic anhydrases, *Adv. Biosci.*, 5:197.
13. Stone, R. A., Zimmerman, T. J., et al. (1977). Low-dose methazolamide and intraocular pressure, *Am. J. Ophthalmol.*, 83:674.
14. Kinoshita, J. H. (1986). Aldose reductase in the diabetic eye, *Am. J. Ophthalmol.*, 102:685.
15. Kador, P. F., Robison, W. G., and Kinoshita, J. H. (1985). The pharmacology of aldose reductase inhibitors, *Ann. Rev. Pharmacol. Toxicol.*, 25:691.
16. Brazzell, R. K., Wooldridge, C. B., et al. (1990). Pharmacokinetics of the aldose reductase inhibitor imirestat following topical ocular administration, *Pharm. Res.*, 7:194.
17. Robison, W. G., Kador, P. F., and Kinoshita, J. H. (1983). Retinal capillaries: Basement membrane thickening by galactosemia prevented with aldose reductase inhibitor, *Science*, 221:1177.
18. Kojima, K., Matsubara, H., et al. (1985). Effects of aldose reductase inhibitor on retinal micro-angiopathy in streptozotocin-diabetic rats, *Jpn. J. Ophthalmol.*, 29:99.
19. Segawa, M., Hirata, Y., et al. (1988). The development of electroretinogram abnormalities and the possible role of polyol pathway activity in diabetic hyperglycemia and galactosemia, *Metabolism*, 37:454.
20. Robison, W. G., Nagata, M., et al. (1989). Aldose reductase and pericyte-endothelial cell contacts in retina and optic nerve, *Invest. Ophthalmol. Vis. Sci.*, 30:2293.
21. Robison, W. G., Tillis, T. N., et al. (1990). Diabetes-related histopathologics of the rat retina prevented with an aldose reductase inhibitor, *Exp. Eye Res.*, 50:355.
22. Das, A., Frank, R. N., et al. (1990). Increases in collagen type IV and laminin in galactose-induced retinal capillary basement membrane thickening-prevention by an aldose reductase inhibitor, *Exp. Eye Res.*, 50:269.

23. Kador, P. F., Akagi, Y., et al. (1988). Prevention of pericyte ghost formation in retinal capillaries of galactose-fed dogs by aldose reductase inhibitors, *Arch. Ophthalmol.*, 106:1099.

24. Cunha-vaz, J. G., Mota, C. C., et al. (1986). Effect of sorbinil on blood-retinal barrier in early diabetic retinopathy, *Diabetes*, 35:574.

25. Palestine, A. G., and Brubaker, R. F. (1981). Pharmacokinetics of fluorescein in the vitreous, *Invest. Ophthalmol. Vis. Sci.*, 21:542.

26. Chahal, P. S., Neal, M. J., and Kohner, E. M. (1985). Metabolism of fluorescein after intravenous administration, *Invest. Ophthalmol. Vis. Sci.*, 26:764.

27. Blair, N. P., Evans, M. A., et al. (1986). Fluorescein and fluorescein glucuronide pharmacokinetics after intravenous injection, *Invest. Ophthalmol. Vis. Sci.*, 27:1107.

28. Mester, U., Krasemann, C., and Werner, H. (1982). Cefsulodin concentrations in rabbit eyes after intravenous and subconjunctival administration, *Ophthalmic Res.*, 14:129.

29. Schechter, R. J. (1978). Systemic antibiotics for use in ocular infections-penicillin-resistant staphylococcus, *Ann. Ophthalmol.*, 10:422.

30. Sweeney, G., Fern, A. I., et al. (1990). Penetration of ciprofloxacin into the aqueous humor of the uninflamed human eye after oral administration, *J. Antimicrob. Chemother.*, 26:99.

31. Ueno, N., Refojo, M. F., and Liu, L. H. S. (1982). Pharmacokinetics of the antineoplastic agent 1,3-bis(2-chloroethyl)-1-nitrosourea (BCNU) in the aqueous and vitreous of rabbit, *Invest. Ophthalmol. Vis. Sci.*, 23:199.

32. Kwitko, G. M., Shin, D. H., et al. (1987). Bilateral effects of long-term monocular timolol therapy, *Am. J. Ophthalmol.*, 104:591.

33. Gregory, D. S., and Sears, M. L. (1980). Beta-adrenergic receptors in ciliary processes of the rabbit, *Invest. Ophthalmol. Vis. Sci.*, 19:203.

34. Urtti, A., and Salminen, L. (1985). A comparison between iris-ciliary body concentration and receptor affinity of timolol, *Acta Ophthalmol.*, 63:16.

35. Hockwin, O., Muller, P., et al. (1989). Determination of AL01576 concentration in rat lenses and plasma by bioassay for aldose reductase activity measurements, *Ophthalmic Res.*, 21:285.

21
Peptide and Protein Therapeutics in the Eye

Randall J. Erb *Clinical Research Foundation, Lenexa, Kansas*

I. INTRODUCTION

Proteins and peptides constitute critical molecules in the structure and function of biological systems. Their functions include (1):

Enzymatic catalysis
Transport and storage of small molecules
Coordinated motion via muscle contraction
Mechanical support from fibrous protein
Immune protection through antibodies
Generation and transmission of nerve impulses
Control of growth and differentiation via hormones

Proteins consists of amino acid building blocks, which differ in size, shape, charge, hydrogen-bonding capacity, and chemical reactivity (1). The combination of these parameters confer considerable latitude in peptide structure and function. The protein backbone is formed by joining the alpha-carboxyl group of an amino acid to the alpha-amino group of another amino acid with eventual loss of a molecule of water. Naturally occurring proteins exist primarily in the L-isomer configuration. The term *peptide* generally refers to an amino acid sequence with a relatively small number of amino acids.

Protein structure exhibits four levels of characteristics: primary, secondary, tertiary, and quaternary (1). Primary structure is described by the linear sequence of the amino acids in the backbone with disulfide locations. Secondary structure represents the spatial configuration of amino acids in close approximation to each other. In contrast, tertiary structure refers to the spatial configuration of amino acids that are greater distances from each other along the backbone. If a protein contains more than one polypeptide chain, it is said to consist of subunits. The spatial arrangement of these subunits confers the quaternary structure of a protein. Although this structural configuration imparts a high degree of functional flexibility to the biological system, the complexity creates significant problems in production and biological delivery for the pharmaceutical scientist, who is required to develop a stable and bioavailable peptide drug formulation.

A. Implications of Peptide Chemistry in Formulation and Delivery

The use of peptides as therapeutic agents presents challenges which are primarily associated with the peptide physiochemical properties. First, because of their molecular size, peptides are not likely to pass membrane barriers. Only if a peptide is sufficiently small or is actively transported is it apt cross membrane barriers. This implies that topical applications designed to penetrate ocular tissues may require absorption enhancers.

Second, peptides which rely on their secondary, tertiary, or quaternary structure for pharmacological activity will be inherently difficult to formulate into a viable pharmaceutical product.

B. Peptides and the Eye

The intact eye presents significant barriers to intraocular penetration of peptides proteins. The blood-retinal barrier diminishes ocular absorption of systemically delivered drugs, whereas the cornea and conjunctiva act as barriers for topically delivered drugs. Peptides are not generally able to penetrate these barriers without absorption enhancers. Consequently, the opportunity to use the ocular route for systemic administration of peptides is limited.

Peptides, having biological effects in the eye, will be categorized here as agents which are intended for use in ocular pathologies as well as those which directly or indirectly effect the eye via experimental or therapeutic administration by various nonocular routes.

1. Peptides Useful in Ocular Pathology

The number of peptides currently in use for ocular pathologies is generally limited to antibiotic preparations (bacitracin) to treat infections and enzymes (chymotrypsin) to promote wound healing. Topical application of cyclosporine has been used experimentally for the prevention of corneal allograft rejection (2). *Pseudomonas* elastase inhibitors have been evaluated for the management of corneal infections from *Pseudomonas aeruginosa* (3).

Capsaicin is a nonpeptide irritant, which causes pain in humans and experimental animals (4). Paradoxically, prolonged treatment with capsaicin causes insensitivity to painful stimuli through the local depletion of substance P (5), a neuropeptide associated with pain transmission (6). Gallar et al. (7) have shown that if capsaicin is administered to rabbit eyes for 3 weeks prior to producing an epithelial wound in the center of the cornea with n-heptanol, the healing time of the cornea is delayed. This observation supports the hypothesis that at least part of the tropic effects of sensory nerves on corneal epithelium are mediated by neuropeptides contained in peripheral nerve terminals (7). Such a phenomenon suggests that any condition or treatment, which modulates endogenous neuropeptide levels at corneal sensory nerve terminals in the eye, may well modify the rate of healing of the cornea.

a. Bacitracin

Bacitracin is an antibiotic polypeptide complex produced by *Bacillus subtilis* and *B. licheniformis* (4). Commercial bacitracin is a mixture of at least nine bacitracins, which is used for its antibacterial activity (4). The drug is applied topically to the eye for a variety of conditions, including eyelid burns, blepharitis, hordeolum, chalazion, and corneal superficial punctate keratitis (8). It is also used to treat optic neuritis (8). Bacitracin is not absorbed by ocular tissues. Its most frequent adverse reactions are localized hypersensitivity, including itching, swelling, and conjunctival erythema (9).

b. Chymotrypsin

Chymotrypsins are a group of proteolytic enzymes in pancreatic juice whose normal function is to hydrolyze peptide bonds during intestinal digestion (4). Chymotrypsin is a 25-kD enzyme, which consists of three polypeptide chains connected by two interchain disulfide bonds (1). Chymotrypsin is used clinically in the eye for enzymatic zonulysis for intracapsular lens extraction. Zonules are digested by a solution of chymotrypsin through irrigation of the posterior chamber through a corneoscleral incision (9). Reported adverse effects are transient increases in ocular pressure, moderate uveitis, corneal edema, and striation (9).

c. Cyclosporine

Cyclosporines are a group of biologically active metabolites produced by Fungi Imperfecti. The major components, cyclosporines A and C, are nonpolar cyclic oligopeptides, which have immunosuppressive, antifungal, and antiphogistic (inflammation-reducing) activity (4). Oral and intravenous cyclosporine is indicated for the prophylaxis of organ rejection in kidney, liver, and heart allogenic transplants (5).

Applied topically to the eye, cyclosporine may improve the prognosis for corneal allograft rejection (2). When cyclosporine A is administered by nonocular routes to rabbits and rats, it produces significant blood levels, but it can not be detected in ocular tissues (10,11). Administered to rabbits as eye drops, cyclosporine was bound to corneal and conjunctival epithelial cell membranes but was not found in significant levels in the conjunctiva, iris, lens, vitreous, or aqueous humor (10,12). Nevertheless, in spite of the apparent lack of penetration into eye structures, intramuscular cyclosporine can reactivate latent murine cytomegalovirus in mouse vitreous (13) and produce more severe stromal keratitis in herpes simplex viral infections in rabbits (14).

d. Pseudomonas Elastase Inhibitors

Although *Pseudomonas* elastase inhibitors are not commonly used clinically, such use represents an interesting therapeutic concept. When *Pseudomonas aeruginosa* infects the eye, it "melts" the cornea by elastase-mediated proteolysis. If left unchecked, proteolysis of ocular tissue can eventually cause corneal perforation. Since certain peptide derivatives inhibit elastase, they may be useful in the management of *Pseudomonas* infections. In 1983, Kessler et al. (3) demonstrated the feasibility of this approach when they treated *Pseudomonas*-infected rabbit eyes with three elastase inhibitors, benzyloxycarbonyl-L-leucyl-hydroxamate, phosphoryl-L-leucyl-L-phenylalanine, and 2-mercaptoacetyl-L-phenyl-alanyl-L-leucine (HSAc-Phe-Leu). HSAc-Phe-Leu, a known enkephalinase inhibitor (15), was found to be particularly effective. In fact, frequent topical application of HSAc-Phe-Leu completely prevented corneal melting (3).

2. Systemic Delivery of Peptides Through the Eye

The relatively impermeable barrier formed by the lipoidal corneal epithelium and conjunctiva prevents peptides from easily entering into the systemic circulation. Proteolytic enzymes, which can degrade a peptide before its absorption, are present in eye tissues and fluids and also provide a barrier to peptide absorption (16–19). To ameliorate these barriers, it is common to consider the use of absorption enhancers and peptidase inhibitors to increase peptide absorption.

Under normal circumstances, a portion of drug instilled into the conjunctival sac will be washed into the nasal lacrimal duct. Therefore, although a drug may be ocularly administered, some absorption may occur through ocular drainage apparatus into systemic circulation.

a. Enkephalins

Enkephalins are the 61st to 65th amino acid sequence of 91 amino acid beta-lipoprotein (20,21). Leucine enkephalin (Leu-E) and methionine enkephalin (Met-E) are the two naturally occurring opioid pentapeptides (20). Enkephalins are known to have neuro-transmitter and neuromodulator activities (22–24). These peptides are of particular interest to the medical community for possible therapeutic use as analgesics. Since enkephalins modulate dopamine release in the brain, these compounds may play significant role in behavior modification (25). Sandi et al. (26), for instance, have pointed out that rats treated with [D-Ala2-Met5] enkephalinamide have an altered propensity to drink alcohol. Finally, Met-E has been shown to be an immunostimulant, producing improvements in physio-logical symptoms in patients with AIDS (acquired immunodeficiency syndrome) related complex (ARC) (27).

Radiolabeled Leu-E administered topically to the eye without absorption enhancer has been shown to produce increasing (nearly linearly dependent) blood level radioactivity (Fig. 1) (28). This absorption was not efficient, however. Lee et al. have shown that less than 1% of the enkephalin dose applied to (rabbit) eyes becomes absorbed (17). An appreciable amount of enkephalin was metabolized by ocular proteases, which were not

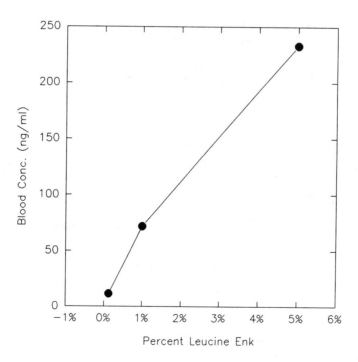

Figure 1. Plateau blood level of leucine enkephalin after ocular administration. (From Ref. 28.)

significantly inhibited by an aminopeptidase inhibitor, bestatin (17). The use of protease-resistant analogs of enkephalin may be a practical strategy to circumvent the metabolic barrier (17). This hypothesis was supported when [D-Ala2] metenkephalinamide, an aminopeptidase-resistant Met-E analog, was shown to produce significant (36%) systemic absorption (29).

Interestingly, there is some suggestion that while termination of chronic enkephalin dosing produces withdrawal, termination of enkephalinase inhibitors (which elevate endogenous enkephalins levels by catabolic inhibition) produces little withdrawal (30,31). This observation indicates that it may be better to administer protease inhibitors to produce therapeutic levels of endogenously generated enkephalins rather than to deliver enkephalins exogenously.

b. Glucagon

Glucagon is a 29–amino acid polypeptide unrelated to insulin which mediates conversion of liver glycogen to glucose. Glucagon is commercially available as a reconstitutible injection (IV, SC, or IM) for use in hypoglycemia (5). Although its molecule weight is significant (3483), glucagon (5%) was significantly absorbed through the eye (Figs. 2 and 3) (32). Since glucagon is currently administered by injection, in concept, ocular administration provides a potentially attractive alternative route of administration. Unfortunately, reconstituted glucagon for injection must be used shortly after reconstitution (5). This implies that glucagon is not stable in solution. This instability problem offers a significant challenge to pharmaceutical formulators trying to develop an ocular delivery system.

c. Insulin

Insulin consists of two polypeptide chains linked together with disulfide bonds. It aids glucose regulation in the body by promoting the entry of glucose into muscle and fat.

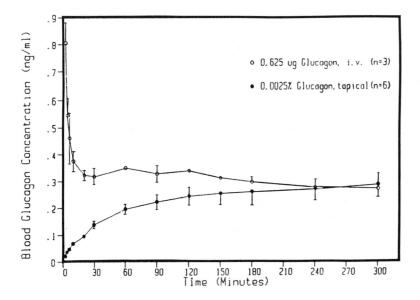

Figure 2. Comparison of blood glucagon concentration after IV injection and topical instillation of glucagon. Bars represent SEM. (Courtesy of Ref. 32.)

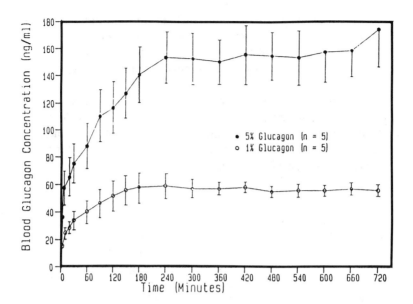

Figure 3. Absorption of glucagon into systemic circulation through eyes. Bars represent SEM. (Courtesy of Ref. 32.)

Insulin is used by diabetics to control blood glucose levels. The major disadvantage of insulin treatment, of course, is its need to be injected. So there is considerable interest in developing alternate routes of administration. One such possible route is topical ocular administration.

One study in rabbits suggests that insulin instilled into the eye was absorbed and can produce hypoglycemia (33). Insulin was administered with and without absorption promoters. With promoters, bioavailability ranged from 5% to about 12%; without promoter, insulin bioavailability from the eye was only about 1% (refer to discussion below on insulin pharmacokinetic information). The nasal mucosa was found to cause about four times more absorption of insulin than the conjunctival mucosa. The practicality of ocular insulin administration in humans will depend on whether absorption promoters will be required to produce therapeutic insulin levels; and whether these promoters lack chronic toxicity.

d. Luteinizing Hormone–Releasing Hormone

Luteinizing hormone–releasing hormone (LHRH) is a decapeptide neurohumoral hormone produced in the hypothalmus which stimulates the secretion of pituitary hormones (e.g., luteinizing hormone, LH) (34). Since LH is used therapeutically in humans for the treatment of infertility, LHRH may be useful as a prodrug.

Luteinizing hormone–releasing hormone instilled into the eye at concentrations of 0.0025% and 1 and 5% produced significant blood concentrations (Figs. 4 and 5) (32). Treatment of the eye with a peptidase inhibitor (Leu-Leu, 5mM) enhances ocular absorption of LHRH (Fig. 5). Intravenous therapeutic dosing maintains a blood concentration of about 0.3 ng/mL. Consequently, therapeutic blood levels appear to be achievable with topical ocular instillation of LHRH.

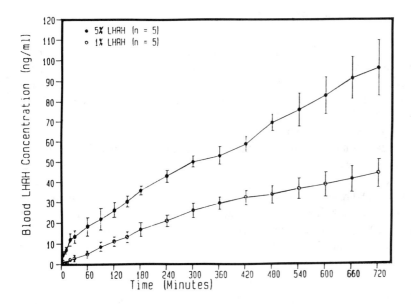

Figure 4. Absorption of LHRH into systemic circulation through eyes. Bars represent SEM. (Courtesy of Ref. 32.)

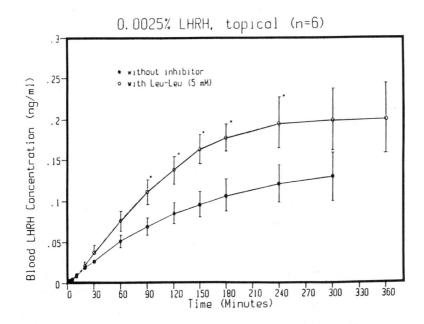

Figure 5. Enhancement of peptidase inhibitor (Leu-Leu, 5 mM) on systemic absorption of LHRH through eyes. Bars represent SEM. (Courtesy of Ref. 32.)

3. Peptides Which Affect the Eye by Miscellaneous Routes

a. Bradykinin

Bradykinin is an endogenous 9–amino acid tissue hormone belonging to a group of hypotensive peptides known as plasma kinins (35). It acts on smooth muscle, dilates peripheral vessels, increases capillary permeability, and is a potent pain-producing agent (4). Pharmacological, biochemical, and immunohistochemical studies have revealed that tachykinins (like bradykinin) are the most likely transmitters at peripheral as well as at central endings of primary sensory nerves (36).

Bradykinin evokes contraction in isolated rabbit iris sphincter muscle (37). Injection of bradykinin into the vitreous chamber of the rabbit eye caused miosis and disruption of the blood-aqueous barrier, which was manifested as aqueous flare (38). Substance P (SP) antagonists, [D-Pro2,D-Trp7,9]SP-11 and [Arg5,D-Trp7,9]SP-(5-11), block bradykinin contraction of the isolated rabbit sphincter pupillae muscle, which implies SP involvement (38). Bradykinin-induced contraction tachyphylaxis was demonstrated both in vitro and in vivo, whereas SP continued to produce contraction. This observation suggests that bradykinin depletes the neuronal pool of SP (38).

b. Cholecystokinin

Cholecystokinin (CCK) is a polypeptide hormone found in the mucosa of the upper intestine and in the peripheral and central nervous system (CNS) tissue (39). Peptide fragments of CCK cause acid secretion, gallbladder contraction, and pancreatic enzyme secretion. Intracameral injection of CCK in monkeys produced a direct effect on the pupillary sphincter mediated by type A CCK receptors on the muscle (40). Retinal release of acetylcholine was not affected by locally applied CCK sulfate (41).

c. Dynorphin(1-13)

Dynorphin is a potent 17–amino acid neuropeptide that contains leucine enkephalin as its amino-terminal sequence. Dynorphin(1-13) has been proposed as the specific endogenous ligand of the kappa opioid receptor (42).

Transmural electrical stimulation produced cholinergic and substance P–ergic responses in rabbit iris sphincter muscle (43). Effects of dynorphin(1-13) in this muscle suggest that it probably increases the presynaptic release of acetylcholine from the parasympathetic postganglionic nerves and reduces the kappa-type opioid receptor–mediated release of substance P from the trigeminal nerve (42).

d. Enkephalins

Although enkephalins and enkephalin-sensitive opiate receptors are endogenous to the eye (44–46), enkephalins apparently exert no tonic control over ocular function. On the other hand, exogenous opioids have long been known to produce pupillary effects in humans and animals (47–52). Erb et al. (53,54) have investigated the (rabbit) pupillary effect of intravenous methionine enkephalin (Met-E) and leucine enkephalin (Leu-E). Met-E infused at rates between 14 and 129 µg/min/kg produced a linear log dose pupillary response (Fig. 6) (54). At comparable infusion rates, less potent Leu-E produced a biphasic (miosis to mydriasis) response (53). This biphasic response appears to be the result of CNS-induced miosis at lower opioid dose levels, preempted by catecholamine-induced mydriasis at higher dose levels (48). Other pupillary observations in rabbits reveal that IV administration of peptides (N-carboxymethyl-phe-leucine and des-tyrosyl-leucine enkephalin), which inhibits enkephalinase, may increase endogenous enkephalins by preventing enkephalin degradation. This hypothesis stems from the observation that enkephalinase inhibitors

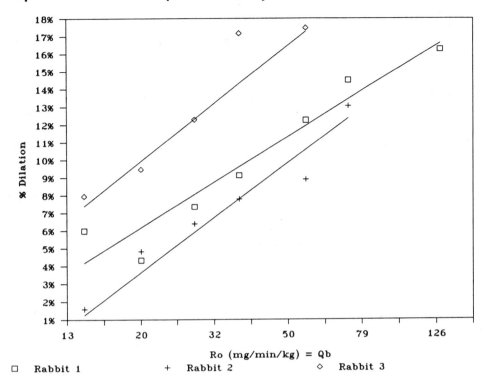

Figure 6. Dose-dependent pupillary response of methionine enkephalin in rabbits for the intra-venous steady-state condition. Each line represents the linear regression fit for one rabbit. (From Ref. 54.)

produce a mydriatic response, even though they have no intrinsic pharmacological activity of their own (53).

Cripps and Bennett investigated the effect of [D-Ala2] metenkephalinamide (DALA) on the peptidergic control of lacrimal duct function (55). DALA was previously shown to decrease intraocular pressure (56). Lacrimal peroxidase secretion was used to characterize DALA activity. DALA was able to inhibit basal activity by about 65%. The investigators concluded that DALA inhibits lacrimal adenyl cyclase via inhibitory, receptor-mediated, peptidergic regulation (55).

In a study designed to examine the effect of opiate peptides on the calcium-dependent release of [^{3}H]dopamine from the rabbit retina, it was found that enkephalin analogs inhibited the stimulation-evoked release of [^{3}H]dopamine through activation of stereo-selective presynaptic opiate receptors (57).

e. Neurotensin

Neurotensin is a tridecapeptide found in mammalian brain and gut tissues having a variety of hormonelike activities (4). Intracameral injection of 1–2 µg of neurotensin into the rabbit eye caused vasodilation in the anterior segment of the eye, a slight increase in aqueous humor concentration, and some decrease in intraocular pressure (58). It also caused miosis (59). Blockade of alpha- and beta-adrenoceptor subtypes, muscarinic receptors, or mu-opioid receptors did not affect neurotensin-induced miosis (59). Destruction of ocular dopamine nerve endings or blockade of D-2 dopamine receptors significantly inhibited the miotic response. Therefore, an intact dopamine pathway is probably required for the expression of neurotensin-induced miosis (59).

f. Penicillamine

Penicillamine (3-mercapto-D-valine) is a degradation product of β-lactam antibiotics. It is used therapeutically in the removal of excess copper in patients with Wilson's disease, cystinuria, or rheumatoid arthritis. The compound manifests its activity through chelation of metal ions. Because it is a single amino acid, it can be administered orally without degradation. Penicillamine can cause optic neuritis (5).

g. Somatostatin

Somatostatin is a tetradecapeptide which is a potent inhibitor in a number of systems, including central and peripheral neural, gastrointestinal, and vascular smooth muscle (4). It also inhibits the release of insulin and glucagon.

When somatostatin or an analog, cyclo(D-Trp-Lys-Thr-Phe-Pro-Phe), was intra-camerally injected or infused intra-arterially into normal eyes, no effect was observed on intraocular pressure, aqueous humor protein concentration, ocular blood flow, or pupil size (58). The agents did, however, attenuate the miotic response produced by a standard pain stimulus resulting from a topical application of 1% neutral formaldehyde. Somatostatin appeared to attenuate the miotic response to pain by preventing the release of substance P (58). Retinal release of acetylcholine was not affected by locally applied somatostatin, which did, however, reduce the amplitude of the b-wave of an electroretinogram (41).

h. Substance P

Substance P (SP) is an endogenous, 11–amino acid peptide belonging to a group of proteins, the tachykinins (60). It can cause pain or analgesia depending upon dose and animal responsiveness.

When capsaicin (a nonpeptide) was chronically administered to the eye, it depleted SP reserves and affected corneal healing time (5). In the rabbit eye, direct administration of SP produced miosis and a rise in the protein concentration in the aqueous humor by damaging the blood-aqueous barrier (61). Similar response in the eye was elicited by bradykinin, which apparently released local neuronal stores of SP (38). Retinal release of acetylcholine was not affected by locally applied substance P (41).

i.   Thyrotropin-Releasing Hormone

Thyrotropin-releasing hormone (TRH) is a tripeptide prohormone which stimulates the release and synthesis of thyrotropin. When TRH was injected intravitreally, intraocular pressure did not change (62). When the peptide was administered intravenously, however, intraocular pressure increased. The increased intraocular pressure coincided with plasma increases in epinephrine and norepinephrine. The conclusion was that TRH raised intra-ocular pressure through beta-adrenergic and muscarinic mechanisms (62).

j.   Vasoactive Intestinal Peptide

Vasoactive intestinal peptide (VIP) (porcine) is an endogenous 28 amino acid peptide (63) which is related to glucagon and secretin. It is believed to play an important role in neurotransmission. Its activities include relaxation of systemic and vascular smooth muscle and secretion of insulin.

When VIP was administered intracamerally, vasodilation occurred in the iris and ciliary body. It did not affect intraocular pressure, however (64). Vasoactive intestinal peptide had no apparent effect on pupil size or the blood-aqueous barrier. Although no arterial blood pressure changes were observed during intravenous administration, intra-ocular pressure rose and choroidal blood flow increased by 35%; anterior uvea blood flow was unaffected (64). The study indicated that VIP produced significant vasodilation in tissues at levels hardly affecting arterial blood pressure (64).

In another study in rabbits, no difference in the composition of lacrimal fluid was found between that stimulated by VIP as opposed to that stimulated by acetylcholine (65). The study concluded that different stimuli caused protein release either from the same secretory cells or from different populations of secretory cells containing the same secretory proteins (65).

II. PEPTIDE OCULAR PHARMACOKINETICS

Information on peptide ocular pharmacokinetics is limited. This is probably due to the paucity of peptides displaying significant transport into or across the globe. Pharmaco-kinetic studies on the precorneal administration of enkephalins, insulin, LHRH, and TRH are discussed below.

A. Enkephalins

Enkephalins are of potential interest for clinical use in pain therapy. Unfortunately, the two endogenous enkephalins, methionine enkephalin (Met-E) and leucine enkephalin (Leu-E), are not particularly well absorbed by the eye and are subject to degradation from a variety of ubiquitous proteases. In 1986, Lee et al. (17) demonstrated that only 1% of Met-E and 13% of Leu-E topical ocular doses were absorbed. To ameliorate this lack of absorption, absorption enhancers have been evaluated for their potential improvement of absorp-tion, and protease-resistant enkephalin analogs have been developed to reduce catabolism (17,19,29,66).

Without enhancer or surfactant, Leu-E 0.125% (31.25 µg/25 µL) topically admin-istered to the eye reached a plateau blood concentration of 11.5 ng/mL in 3–4 h and maintained relatively high levels for 8–9 h (28). Higher concentrations of 1% (0.25 mg/25 µL) and 5% (1.25 mg/25 µL) produced plateau blood concentrations of 72 ng/mL and 233 ng/mL, respectively (see Fig. 1). In contrast, when Leu-E was administered intra-venously, half-life was less than 30 min. The lowest point in the blood concentration following intravenous administration was 22 ng/mL at 5 h.

In homogenates of anterior segment tissues of rabbit eye, Met-E and Leu-E were found to be 90% hydrolyzed by aminopeptidases (18). This trend was paralleled in other absorp-tive mucosal tissues (nasal, rectal, vaginal, and buccal) (66). On the other hand, [D-Ala2] metenkephalinamide (YAGFM), which is resistant to aminopeptidase degradation, was primarily hydrolyzed by dipeptidyl carboxylpeptidase (18).

Ocularly applied YAGFM produced peak plasma concentrations in the rabbit within 20 min of instillation (29). The apparent YAGFM absorption rate was slower than the elimination rate, demonstrating "flip-flop" kinetics. Based upon the 120-min area under the curve, 36.1% ± 4.4% of YAGFM was absorbed. The conjunctival mucosa played as important a role as the nasal mucosa in the systemic absorption of YAGFM. Systemic absorption of YAGFM did not appear to be adversely affected by the presence of 5% polyvinyl alcohol.

B. Insulin

Ocular absorption of insulin was evaluated in the rabbit compared to intravenous and subcutaneous administration (Fig. 7) (33). Ocular insulin absorption was also evaluated in the presence of absorption promoters, polyoxyethylene-9-lauryl ether (PLE), sodium glycocholate (SG), sodium taurocholate (ST), and sodium deoxycholate (SD) (Fig. 8) (33). All promoters were used at concentrations of 1% w/v. Based upon the aqueous humor concentration time area under the curve, the bioavailability with PLE was 5.7 to 12.6%, with SG 4.9 to 7.9%, with ST 3.6 to 7.8%, and with SD 8.2 to 8.3%. Only 0.7 to 1.3% of the insulin was absorbed in the absence of absorption promoters. The absorption-promoting effect of SG was dose dependent over a range of 0.1–2%. At 1%, the promoting effect

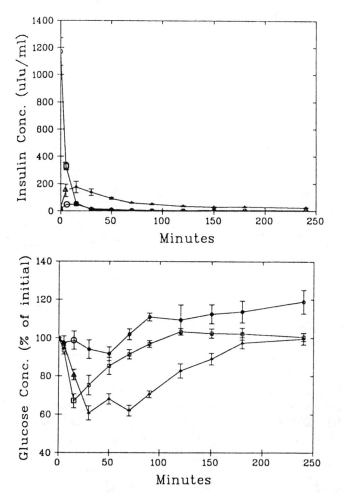

Figure 7.   Concentration-time profiles of insulin (upper plot) and glucose (lower plot) in plasma after IV (open square), SC (open triangle), and ocular (open circle) administration in albino rabbit. The insulin dose was 0.5 U for IV, 0.8 U for SC, and 10 U for ocular. The glucose concentration was expressed as percentage of value at time zero. Error bars represent SEM for four to six rabbits. (Courtesy of Ref. 33.)

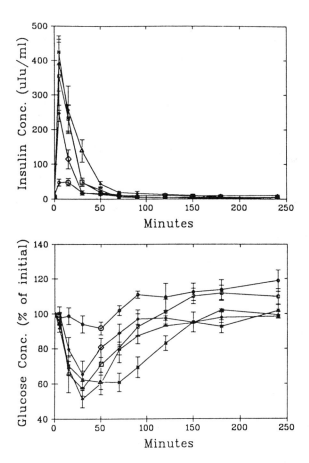

Figure 8. Concentration-time profiles of insulin (upper plot) and glucose (lower plot) in plasma after ocular administration of 10 U of insulin in the presence of 1% polyoxyethylene-9-lauryl ether (significantly different from ocular administration without absorption promoters, $P < 0.05$), 1% Na deoxycholate (open triangle), 1% Na glycocholate (open square), and 1% Na taurocholate (open diamond) compared with the control (open circle). The glucose concentration was expressed as percentage of value at time zero. Error bars represent SEM for four to six rabbits. (Courtesy of Ref. 33.)

lasted for about 5 min and disappeared by 15–30 min. Nasal mucosa was found to contribute about four times the absorption of that of the conjunctival mucosa (33).

C. Thyrotropin-Releasing Hormone and Luteinizing Hormone–Releasing Hormone

Precorneal application of 0.0025% TRH produced a plateau blood concentration of 0.05 ng/ml in 60 min (32). Levels remained high for at least 4 h. At 1%, a peak concentration of 26 ng/mL was reached in 2 h and remained there for 10 h (Fig. 9). At 5%, TRH peaked at 138 ng/mL in 60 min and gradually fell to a steady state of 60 ng/mL by 9 h after

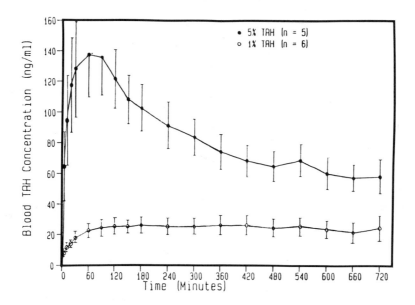

Figure 9. Absorption of TRH into systemic circulation through eyes. Bars represent SEM. (Courtesy of Ref. 32.)

the peak (Fig. 9). The dose-to-peak ratio was fairly constant over this range of doses, which signified linear kinetics. A therapeutic dose of TRH (15 µg/70 kg) administered intravenously maintained a blood concentration of 0.07 ng/mL. This was comparable to the blood levels produced by the 0.0025% ocular dose. The presence of peptidase inhibitors (Leu-Leu, 4mM; bestatin, 60 µM; and DL-thiorphan, 0.6 µM) did not affect TRH absorption (32).

After the instillation of 0.0025, 1, and 5 LHRH, blood levels increased steadily over a 12-h period without reaching a plateau (32). The highest concentrations for these doses were 0.13 ng/mL, 45 ng/mL, and 95 ng/mL, respectively. The decreasing amount of LHRH absorbed per dose administered indicated a saturation of the absorption process; the kinetics were dose-related, but were not linear. Intravenously administered LHRH (15 µg/70 kg) maintained blood levels at 0.25–0.3 ng/mL, which was slightly higher than the level reached with the 0.0025% ocular instillation. Leu-Leu (5 mM) was found to slightly (but significantly) increase LHRH absorption into systemic circulation (32).

Ocular administration appears to be a viable route of administration for TRH and LHRH.

III. CONCLUSIONS

Although the eye presents significant tissue and enzyme barriers, some peptide drugs can be delivered to systemic circulation via the ocular route of administration. In some cases, these barriers need to be ameliorated with absorption enhancers or enzyme inhibitors to produce significant bioavailability. In any case, for the foreseeable future, the ocular route of administration for peptides will probably be restricted to relatively small and relatively potent peptides, such as hormones and neuropeptides.

REFERENCES

1. Stryer, L. (1988). *Biochemistry*, 3rd ed. Freeman, New York, pp. 15–43.
2. Belin, M. W., Bouchard, C. S., and Phillips, T. M. (1990). Update on topical cyclosporin A. Background, immunology, and pharmacology, *Cornea* 9(3):184–195.
3. Kessler, E., Spierer, A., and Blumberg, S. (1983). Specific inhibition of Pseudomonas aeruginosa elastase injected intracorneally in rabbit eyes, *Invest. Ophthalmol. Vis. Sci.*, 24(8):1093–1097.
4. *The Merck Index*, 10th ed. (1983). Windholz, M. (ed.). Merck & Co., Inc., Rahway, New Jersey, p. 135.
5. *Physicians' Desk Reference*, 43rd ed. (1989). Medical Economics Company, Inc., Oradell, New Jersey, p. 1892.
6. Nawa, H., Hirose, T., Takashima, H., Inayama, S., and Nakanishi, S. (1983). Nucleotide sequences of cloned cDNAs for two types of bovine brain substance P precursor, *Nature*, 306:32–36.
7. Gallar, J., Pozo, M. A., Rebollo, I., and Belmonte, C. (1990). Effects of capsaicin on corneal wound healing, *Invest. Ophthalmol. Vis. Sci.*, 31(10):1968–1974.
8. *The Merck Manual*, 15th ed. R. Berkow (ed.). Merck & Co., Rahway, New Jersey, pp. 2213–2240.
9. *Physician's Desk Reference for Ophthalmology*, 15th ed. (1987), Medical Economics Company, Inc., Oradell, New Jersey, p. 65.
10. BenEzra, D., and Maftzir, G. (1990). Ocular penetration of cyclosporin A. The rabbit eye, *Invest. Ophthlamol. Vis. Sci.*, 31(7):1362–1366.
11. BenEzra, D., and Maftzir, G. (1990). Ocular penetration of cyclosporin A in the rat eye, *Arch. Ophthalmol.*, 108(4):584–587.
12. Stamer, L., Bohnke, M., Vogelberg, K., and Arndt, R. (1989). Tissue levels of locally applied cyclosporin A in the rabbit eye, *Fortschr. Ophthalmol.*, 86(5):540–542.
13. Rabinovitch, T., Oh, J. O., and Minasi, P. (1990). In vivo reactivation of latent murine cytomegalovirus in the eye by immunosuppressive treatment, *Invest. Ophthalmol. Vis. Sci.*, 31(4): 657–654.
14. Meyers-Elliott, R. H., Chitjian, P. A., and Billups, C. B. (1987). Effects of cyclosporin A on clinical and immunological parameters in herpes simplex keratitis, *Invest. Ophthalmol. Vis. Sci.*, 28(7): 1170–1178.
15. Alstein, M., Bachar, E., Vogel, Z., and Blumberg, S. (1983). Protection of enkephalins from enzymatic degradation utilizing selective metal-chelating inhibitors, *Eur. J. Pharmacol.*, 91: 353–361.
16. Lee, V. H. (1989). Peptidase activities in absorptive mucosa, *Biochem. Soc. Trans.*, 17(5): 937–940.
17. Lee, V. H., Carson, L. W., Kashi, S. D., and Stratford, R. E., Jr. (1986). Metabolic and permeation barriers to the ocular absorption of topically applied enkephalins in rabbits, *J. Ocul. Pharmacol.*, 2(4):345–352.
18. Kashi, S. D., and Lee, V. H. (1986). Hydrolysis of enkephalins in homogenates of anterior segment tissues of the albino rabbit eye, *Invest. Ophthalmol. Vis. Sci.*, 27(8):1300–1303.
19. Lee, V. H. (1988). Enzymatic barriers to peptide and protein absorption, *Crit. Rev. Ther. Drug Carrier Syst.*, 5(2):69–97.
20. Ronai, A. Z. (1982). Detection of endogenous ligands of opiate receptors. *In: Opioid Peptides*, Vol. III, *Opiate Receptors and Their Ligands*. CRC Press, Boca Raton, Florida, pp. 43–68.
21. Hughes, J., Smith, T. W., Kosterlitz, H. W., Fothergill, L. A., Morgan, B. A., and Morris, H. R. (1975). Identification of two related pentapeptides from the brain with potent opiate agonist activity, *Nature*, 258:577.

22. Frederickson, R. C. A. (1977). Enkephalin pentapeptides: A review of current evidence for a physiological role in vertebrate neurotransmission, *Life Sci.*, 21:23.

23. Kosterlitz, H. W., and Hughes, J. (1975). Some thoughts on the significance of enkephalin, the endogenous ligand, *Life Sci.*, 17:91.

24. Stewart, J. M., and Channabasavaiah, K. (1978). Evolutionary aspects of some neuropeptides, *Fed. Proc. Fed. Am. Soc. Exp. Biol.*, 38:2302.

25. Spanagel, R., Herz, A., and Shippenberg, T. S. (1990). The effects of opioid peptides on dopamine release in the nucleus accumbens: An in vivo microdialysis study, *J. Neurochem.*, 55(5): 1734–1740.

26. Sandi, C., Borrell, J., and Guaza, C. (1990). Enkephalins interfere with early phases of voluntary ethanol drinking, *Peptides*, 11(4):697–702.

27. Bhargava, N. H. (1990). Opioid peptide, receptors, and immune function, *NIDA Res. Monogr.*, 96:220–233.

28. Chiou, G. C., Chuang, C. Y., and Chang, M. S. (1988). Systemic delivery of enkephalin peptide through eyes, *Life Sci.*, 43(6):509–514.

29. Stratford, R. E., Jr., Carson, L. W., Dodda-Kashi, S., and Lee, V. H. (1988). Systemic absorption of ocularly administered enkephalinamide and inulin in albino rabbit: Extent, pathways, and vehicle effects, *J. Pharm. Sci.*, 77:838–842.

30. Maldonado, R., Feger, J., Fournie-Zaluski, M. C., and Roques, B. P. (1990). Differences in physical dependence induced by selective mu or delta opioid agonists and by endogenous enkephalins protected by peptidase inhibitors, *Brain Res.*, 520(1–2):247–254.

31. Schwartz, J.-C., Costen, J., and Lecomte, J.-M. (1985). Pharmacology of enkephalinase inhibitors. *In*: *Trends in Pharmacological Sciences*, Elsevier, Cambridge, 472–476.

32. Chiou, G. C., and Chuang, C. Y. (1988). Systemic delivery of polypeptides with molecular weights between 300 and 3500 through the eyes, *J. Ocular Pharmacol.*, 4(2):165–177.

33. Yamamoto, A., Luo, A. M., Dodda-Kashi, S., and Lee, V. H. (1990). The ocular route for systemic insulin delivery in the albino rabbit, *J. Pharmacol. Exp. Ther.*, 249(1):249–255.

34. Kalra, S. P., and Kalra, P. S. (1983). Neural regulation of luteinizing hormone secretion in the rat, *Endocrinol. Rev.*, 3:311.

35. Rocha e Silva, M. (1970). *Kinin Hormones.* Charles C Thomas, Springfield, Illinois.

36. Muramatsu, I. (1987). Peripheral transmission in primary sensory nerves, *Jpn. J. Pharmacol.*, 43/2:113–120.

37. Muramatsu, I., Ueda, N., and Fujiwara, M. (1987). Sensory tachykininergic response in the rabbit iris sphincter muscle, *Biomed. Res. (Jpn.)*, 8(Suppl.):59–63.

38. Bynke, G., Hakanson, R., Horig, J., and Leander, S. (1983). Bradykinin contracts the pupillary sphincter and evokes ocular inflammation through release of neuronal substance P, *Eur. J. Pharmacol.*, 91(4):469–475.

39. Dockray, G. J., Dimaline, R., Pauwels, S., and Varro, A. (1989). Gastrin and CCK-related peptides. *In*: *Peptide Hormones as Prohormones: Processing, Biological Activity, Pharmacology* (J. Martinez, ed.), Halsted Press, New York, pp. 244–284.

40. Bill, A., Anderson, S. E., and Almegard, B. (1990). Cholecystokinin causes contraction of the pupillary sphincter in monkeys but not in cats, rabbits, rats and guinea-pigs: Antagonism by loglumide, *Acta Physiol. Scand.*, 138(4):479–485.

41. Cunningham, J. R., and Neal, M. J. (1983). Effect of gamma-aminobutyric acid agonists, glycine, taurine and neuropeptides on acetylcholine release from rabbit retina, *J. Physiol. (Lond.)*, 336: 563–577.

42. Wuster, M., Schulz, R., and Herz, A. (1980). Highly specific opiate receptors for dynorphin-(1–13) in the mouse vas deferens, *Eur. J. Pharmacol.*, 62:235.

43. Ueda, N., Muramatsu, I., and Fujiwara, M. (1985). Dual effects of dynorphin(1–13) on cholinergic and substance P-ergic transmissions in the rabbit iris sphincter muscle, *J. Pharmacol. Exp. Ther.*, 232(2):545–550.

44. Tinsley, P. W., Fridland, G. H., Killmar, J. T., and Desiderio, D. M. (1988). Purification, characterization, and localization of neuropeptides in the cornea, *Peptides*, 9(6):1373–1379.
45. Drago, F., Gorgone, G., and Spina, F. (1980). Opiate receptors in the rabbit iris, *Nauyn-Schmiedebergs. Arch. Pharmacol.*, 315(1):1–4.
46. Slaughter, M. M., Mattler, J. A., and Gottlieb, D. I. (1985). Opiate binding sites in the chick, rabbit and goldfish retina, *Brain Res.*, 339(1):39–47.
47. Murray, R. B., Adler, M. W., and Korczyn (1983). Minireview: The pupillary effects of opioids, *Life Sci.*, 33:495–509.
48. Szekely, J. I. (1982). The role of endogenous opioids in the vegetative regulation. *In: Opioid Peptides*, Vol. II, *Pharmacology* (J. I. Szekely and A. Z. Ronai, eds.). CRC Press, Boca Raton, Florida, pp. 155–206.
49. Tallarida, R. J., Kramer, M. S., Roy, J. W., Kester, R. A., Murray, R. B., and Adler, M. W. (1977). Miosis and fluctuation in the rabbit pupil, *J. Pharmacol. Exp. Ther.*, 201:587.
50. Korczyn, A. D., Boyman, R., and Shifter, L. (1979). Morphine mydriasis in mice, *Life Sci.*, 24:1667.
51. Klemfuss, H., Tallirida, R. J., Adler, C. H., and Adler, M. W. (1979). Morphine-induced mydriasis and fluctuation in the rat: Time and dose relationships, *J. Pharmacol. Exp. Ther.*, 208:91.
52. Fanciullacci, M., Boccuni, M., Pietrini, U., and Sicuteri, F. (1980). The naloxone conjunctival test in morphine addiction, *Eur. J. Pharmacol.*, 61:319.
53. Erb, R. J. unpublished observation.
54. Erb, R. J., Her, L.-M., Abdallah, A., and Mitra, A. K. (1991). Pharmacodynamics and biophasic drug levels of methionine enkephalin, *Pharm. Res.*, in press.
55. Cripps, M. M., and Bennett, D. J. (1990). Peptide stimulation and inhibition of lacrimal gland adenyl cyclase, *Invest. Ophthalmol. Vis. Sci.*, 31(10):2145–2150.
56. Drago, F., Panissidi, G., and Bellomio, F. (1985). Effects of opiates and opioids on intraocular pressure of rabbits and humans, *Clin. Exp. Pharmacol. Physiol.*, 12(2):107–113.
57. Dubocovich, M. L., and Weiner, N. (1983). Enkephalins modulate (3H)dopamine release from rabbit retina in vitro, *J. Pharmacol. Exp. Ther.*, 224(3):634–639.
58. Stjernschantz, J., Sears, M. L., and Oksala, O. (1985). Effects of somastatin, a somastatin analog, neurotensin and met-enkephalin in the eye with special reference to the irritative response, *J. Ocul. Pharmacol.*, 1(1):59–70.
59. Hernandez, D. E., and Jennes, L. (1990). Inhibition of neurotensin-induced miosis by blockade of ocular dopamine pathways, *J. Ocul. Pharmacol.*, 6(1):31–36.
60. Euler, U. S., and Gaddum, J. H. (1931). An unidentified depressor substance in certain tissue extracts, *J. Physiol.*, 72:74–87.
61. Mandahl, A., and Bill, A. (1983). In the eye (D-Pro2, D-Trp7,9)-SP is a substance P agonist, which modifies the responses to substance P, prostaglandin E1 and antidromic trigeminal nerve stimulation, *Acta Physiol. Scand.*, 117(1):139–144.
62. Liu, J. H., Dacus, A. C., and Bartels, S. P. (1989). Thyrotropin releasing hormone increases intraocular pressure. Mechanism of action, *Invest. Ophthalmol. Vis. Sci.*, 30(10):2200–2208.
63. Tatemoto, K., and Mutt, V. (1980). Isolation of two novel candidate hormones using a chemical method for finding naturally occurring polypeptides, *Nature*, 285:517.
64. Nilson, S. F., and Bill, A. (1984). Vasoactive intestinal polypeptide (VIP); effects in the eye and on regional blood flow, *Acta Physiol. Scand.*, 121(4):385–392.
65. Dartt, D. A., Matkin, C., and Gray, K. (1988). Comparison of proteins in lacrimal fluid secreted in response to different stimuli, *Invest. Ophthalmol. Vis. Sci.*, 29(6):991–995.
66. Kashi, S. D., and Lee, V. H. (1986). Enkephalin hydrolysis in homogenates of various absorptive mucosae of the albina rabbit: Similarities in rates and involvement of aminopeptidases, *Life Sci.*, 38(22):2019–2028.

22
Ocular Delivery of Peptides and Proteins

Ramesh Krishnamoorthy and Ashim K. Mitra   *Purdue University, West Lafayette, Indiana*

I. INTRODUCTION

Recent advances in biotechnology have made possible the mass production of natural polypeptides and proteins for clinical use. Such advances in molecular biology have not only made large quantities of peptide and protein drugs available for clinical investigations but have also provided directions by which one could modify the peptide structure to enhance therapeutic potential. The application of peptide and protein-based drugs in the treatment of a variety of ailments has been well documented. Table 1 lists some of those therapeutic agents and their clinical use (1).

The barriers associated with the delivery of proteins as therapeutic agents are primarily associated with their physiochemical and pharmacokinetic properties (e.g., size, propensity to aggregate, adsorption characteristics, rapid systemic clearance). These factors cannot be considered trivial and research must be undertaken to gradually overcome or minimize them. Most of the protein compounds thus far have been delivered by invasive routes, such as parenteral injections. The disadvantages of repeated injections, particularly in the treatment of chronic ailments, deter many patients from undergoing intensive therapy. Parenteral administration is unsanitary unless sterile needles and syringes are used. It is associated with the risk of spreading acquired immunodeficiency syndrome (AIDS) and other infectious diseases. Phlebitis and tissue irritation are other complications of parenteral delivery. Numerous attempts have been made to utilize alternative noninvasive routes for peptide and protein administration (2–6). Approaches to overcome the barriers, i.e., low absorption and rapid metabolism of proteins at the site of administration, have been many (7,8). Although buccal (9), nasal (10–12), transdermal (13,14), tracheal (15), rectal (16), and vaginal (17) routes have been attempted, none has so far been found to be completely satisfactory. Following oral administration, peptides are rapidly degraded by luminal proteases and brush border and cytoplasmic aminopeptidases in the gastrointestinal tract and exhibit very low bioavailability (2,18,19).

In addition to these routes, the ocular route can be considered for the systemic delivery of proteins and peptides. This route is especially useful in delivering these agents for the local treatment of ailments that affect the anterior segment of the eye. Several peptides

Table 1. Examples of Some Proteins and Peptides and Their Possible Applications

Peptide/Protein	Indication
Growth Hormone	Increasing the height of children deficient in growth hormone
Insulin	Lowering blood glucose levels
Luteinizing hormone–releasing hormone (LHRH)	Inducing ovulation in women
Thyrotropin-releasing hormone (TRH)	Prolonging infertility and lactation in women
Gastrin antagonists	Reducing secretion of gastric acid
Somatostatin	Reducing bleeding of gastric ulcers
Neurotensin	Inhibition of gastric juice secretion
Nerve growth factor	Stimulating nerve growth and repair
β-Endorphin	Relieving pain
Enkephalins	Pain suppressor and reducing inflammation
Cholecystokinin	Suppressing appetite
Salmon calcitonin	Osteoporosis
Bradykinin	Improving peripheral circulation
Angiotensin antagonists	Lowering blood pressure
Tissue plasminogen factors	Dissolving blood clots
Cyclosporine	Inhibiting function of T lymphocytes
Interferon	Enhance activity of natural killer cells
Thymopoietin	Selective T-cell–differentiating hromone
Epidermal growth factor	Wound healing
Vasoactive intestinal peptide	Induce relaxation of smooth muscles
Substance P	Reducing inflammation, induce analgesia
Fibronectin	Helps in wound healing

whose roles in ocular pharmacology have been established have been shown to be able to traverse the cornea. Moreover, systemic delivery of polypeptide and protein drugs through the ocular route has several advantages:

1. Mode of delivery is convenient, i.e., eye drops.
2. Systemic absorption is extremely rapid.
3. The absorbed peptide can bypass the hepatic circulation and thus can avoid first-pass metabolism.
4. Formulations can be tailormade to prolong drug action and/or reduce drug concentrations to achieve consistent drug action with least side effects.
5. The dose size can be controlled accurately.

While this route is well accepted by patients, it yields low systemic bioavailability. The size, charge, and hydrophilic nature of proteins are the primary determinants of their extent of absorption. Because the systemic delivery of peptides depends on their transport and contact time with mucous membrane of the conjunctiva and the nasolacrimal system (20) the following factors need to be considered:

1. The eye drops used must be devoid of any local irritation and/or side effects.
2. Inclusion of permeation enhancers may be necessary when dealing with agents with molecular weight larger than 10,000.

3. The absolute quantity of polypeptide that can be placed in the eye cannot exceed 2.5 mg because the eye cannot endure more than 25 μL of a 10% (w/v) ophthalmic solution.

Some studies have pointed out that the systemic delivery of peptides via the ocular route may exert a local toxic response. Ocular peptide delivery is still in its infancy. This chapter will summarize the work done to date in this area and will review the experimental methods currently being employed.

II. MECHANISM OF PEPTIDE TRANSPORT

Protein transport across biological membranes depends upon a number of physical properties among which the size and polarity of the compound are most significant. From the changes in permeability coefficients under different experimental conditions, the major pathway of protein permeation can be hypothesized. The kinetic approach provides indirect evidence of the permeability characteristics and can be a powerful tool in deducing pathways.

Electrophysiological measurements and fluorescent confocal microscopy have been used to understand the mechanism of corneal drug permeation (21,22). The latter method provides a sensitive approach to monitoring flux across the corneal tissue and to characterize tissue damage. Confocal microscopy utilizes a laser computer system that permits visualization of a tissue specimen under light microscopy.

Insulin, polylysine, and thyrotropin-releasing hormone have been studied for their corneal permeability behavior using confocal microscopy (23). Based upon the results obtained, the movement of these peptides across the cornea appears to be governed by the following factors:

1. A paracellular route is favored irrespective of the charge or size of the peptide.
2. The outermost two cell layers of the corneal epithelium offer the maximum resistance; the intercellular spaces then widen, making the transport across the corneal layer easier.
3. Charge plays an important role in the transport of the small- to medium-sized peptides. The cornea offers greater resistance to negatively charged compounds than it does to positively charged ones.

Minor inflammation of the cornea and calcium chelation may cause a widening of the intercellular spaces, thereby allowing a substantial flux of the peptide compounds. If polypeptide absorption in therapeutic amounts across the cornea is to be achieved, it will be necessary to maintain prolonged contact of the peptide with the corneal surface and also to employ a proper penetration enhancer to potentiate flux across the intercellular spaces.

III. METHODS FOR ENHANCING PEPTIDE AND PROTEIN DELIVERY

Irrespective of the noninvasive route employed to deliver the peptide and protein drugs, some inherent delivery problems must be overcome. Table 2 lists some of the general methods that can be employed to negotiate such formulation difficulties.

Physical methods for increasing absorption such as iontophoresis and phonophoresis have both been examined extensively (24–27). Such methods of enhancement are quite complex and may lead to chemical and physical instability of the permeating protein (28–30). Erratic results may also be obtained due to different degrees of surface absorption.

Table 2. General Methods for Enhancing Protein Delivery

1. By increasing absorption through:
    (a) Application of physical methods like iontophoresis or phonophoresis
    (b) Coadministration with permeation enhancers
    (c) Incorporation into liposomes or other carriers
    (d) Chemical modification of primary structure and development of prodrugs

2. By minimizing metabolism through:
    (a) Covalent attachment to a polymer
    (b) Chemical modification of the primary structure
    (c) Targeting to specific tissues
    (d) Coadministration with an enzyme inhibitor

3. By prolonging blood levels through:
    (a) Use of bioadhesives
    (b) Protection using liposomes, polymers, or other carrier

Prolongation of the biological half-life of proteins and enhancement of their systemic bioavailability are also necessary. An attempt has been made by coadministering proteins with known enzyme inhibitors (31). The covalent attachment of polymers has also been shown to protect a number of proteins from enzymatic hydrolysis (32–36). Thus, azopolymers may be used to deliver proteins orally whereby the system could bypass the digestive enzymes of the small intestine; however, in the flora of the colon the polymer will release the protein. In any event, the problem of low bioavailability still exists and permeation enhancers may have to be used to overcome this obstacle.

The use of chemical permeation enhancers has been reviewed extensively relative to nasal, oral, and rectal absorption of proteins and peptides (7,18,37,38). Three major mechanisms of action are possible for these enhancers: perturbation of membrane integrity, expansion of the paracellular pathway, and increase in the thermodynamic activity of the permeating species.

The following section will briefly discuss the studies performed in other noninvasive routes of protein and peptide delivery, the findings of which may be useful in designing ocular peptide delivery systems.

A. Oral Route

The oral route, though the most convenient, is the least likely to be successful because of extensive degradation of proteins and peptides in the gut. Based on the concentration-dependent absorption of 1-desamino-8-D-arginine-vasopressin (dDAVP), Lundin et al. (39) suggested the process to be mediated by passive transport. Other investigators have shown that the permeability of peptides can be enhanced through prodrug modification designed to utilize the peptide transport system of the digestive tract (40–43). Coadministration of enzyme inhibitors may offer some protection in conjunction with a delivery system that can target the protein to the site of optimal absorption (7,44). The incorporation of absorption enhancers to improve the oral bioavailability of proteins has been well documented (45). Lundin et al. (46) showed that sodium taurodihydrofusidate (STDHF) enhanced both the in vitro and in vivo absorption of dDAVP. Schilling and Mitra (47) used the everted gas sac technique to evaluate the optimal site of insulin absorption. The addition of sodium glycocholate and linoleic acid enhanced insulin absorption in the duodenum and jejunum by eight- and threefold, respectively.

B. Nasal Route

The extensive network of blood capillaries underneath the nasal mucosa could provide effective systemic absorption of drugs. The nasal route is capable of providing a rapid absorption with a bioavailability relatively similar to that following subcutaneous injection. Nasal delivery of peptides and proteins has been reviewed (48,49). The polypeptides intended for delivery by this route should be readily soluble in a low mucosal irritant vehicle. It must also be absorbed in effective amounts to make this mode of administration both economical and acceptable (50). This route has been shown to be acceptable for peptides with 10 residues or less (51,52). When the number of amino acids in the peptide approaches 20 or more, satisfactory bioavailability is obtained only with a permeation enhancer (53). The nasal mucosa contains enzymes capable of hydrolyzing peptides such as leucine enkephalin. It appears that the human nasal passage contains a variety of peptidases with wide specificities. The enhancing effect of two enzyme inhibitors, amastatin and bestatin, a mucolytic agent, N-acetyl-L-cysteine, and the permeation enhancers palmitoyl-D,L-carnitine and L-α-lysophosphatidylcholine (LPC) on the nasal absorption of human growth hormone (hGH) was studied by O'Hagan et al. (54). The highest bioavailability relative to the subcutaneous injection was found with amastatin, followed by LPC and palmitoyl-D,L-carnitine. Tengamnuay and Mitra (55,56) found that mixed micelles of sodium glycocholate and fatty acids were more effective in enhancing the nasal delivery of peptides than the bile salt itself. Vadnere et al. (57) found that ethylenediaminetetraacetic acid (EDTA) and α-cyclodextrin were capable of increasing the bioavailability of leuprolide when given intranasally.

C. Buccal Route

Delivery of macromolecules through the buccal membrane has also received considerable attention in recent years (58–60). Both keratinized and nonkeratinized mucosae have been used in studying the in vitro rate of penetration of drugs through the buccal tissue. In vivo absorption of peptides/proteins from the buccal cavity is likely to be influenced by the presence of mucosal secretions and immunological reactions among other factors. Molecular size may not be the limiting factor in the buccal delivery of peptides (61). Gandhi and Robinson (62) described that amino acids penetrate the buccal membrane by an active process, whereas peptide drugs permeate passively. The buccal cavity exhibits greater proteolytic enzyme activity than the nasal or vaginal mucosa (63). The metabolic activity is shown to reside primarily in the epithelium (64). Aungst and Rogers (4,65) studied a variety of absorption enhancers to determine their effects on buccal absorption and showed that significant changes in the morphology of this mucosal barrier take place following exposure to the absorption enhancers.

D. Pulmonary

Delivery of protein and peptide drugs via the pulmonary route has also received significant attention in recent years. The walls of the alveoli are thinner than the epithelial/mucosal membrane; the surface area of the lung is much greater and the lungs receive the entire blood supply from the heart, all of which work in favor for the absorption of protein drugs more rapidly and to a greater extent. Of course, the lungs are rich in enzymes and overcoming this barrier is no easy task. Peptide hydrolases, peptidases, and a wide variety of proteinases are present in the lung cells (66). However, some proteinase inhibitors are also present at concentrations varying with the disease state which might work to prevent the destruction of administered peptides (67). Liposomal delivery of peptide and protein drugs through the pulmonary route have been attempted (68). Molecular modifications have also been undertaken to explore this route of protein and peptide delivery (69).

E. Ocular Route

Lee et al. recently reviewed the factors affecting corneal drug penetration (70). Rojanasakul showed that polylysine permeated through epithelial surface defects via an intracellular pathway when administered to the eye, whereas inulin predominates in the surface cells of the cornea (22). They noted that there was a significant amount of aminopeptidase activity present in the ocular fluids and tissues. Figure 1 summarizes the results of the metabolism of the topically applied enkephalins to the eye (71). Pretreatment with the peptidase inhibitor bestatin had a significant protease inhibitory effect albeit in the tears only.

Studies have been conducted with absorption enhancers to improve the delivery of peptides and proteins into the systemic circulation via the ocular route (72–74). Table 3 lists some of the penetration enhancers which have been used in the ocular delivery of some peptide like drugs. Ocular delivery of insulin to generate a therapeutic glucose lowering response requires a penetration enhancer (75). Yamamoto et al. (76) reported that the bioavailability of insulin could be improved in the following descending order by coadministration of the permeation enhancers: polyoxyethylene-9-lauryl ether> sodium deoxycholate> sodium glycocholate ~ sodium taurocholate.

IV. OCULAR DELIVERY OF PEPTIDE AND PROTEIN DRUGS

Instillation of a topical dose of a drug to the eye leads to absorption of the drug mainly through the conjunctival and corneal epithelia. The absorption into the systemic circulation may occur across the conjunctiva and sclera. However, for local absorption the cornea presents a significant barrier to the intraocular penetration of peptide drugs in view of their high molecular size and low lipophilicity. Lee (72) reported that the penetration of inulin through the cornea of the rabbit was probably occurring via a paracellular route rather than a transcellular route.

Systemic absorption of peptide and protein drugs following topical administration to the eye could occur through contact with the conjunctival and the nasal mucosae, the latter occurring as a result of the drainage through the nasolacrimal duct. When systemic effects are desired, absorption through the conjunctival and nasal mucosae needs to be maximized. One also needs to consider other competing processes present in the ocular tissues. Of these

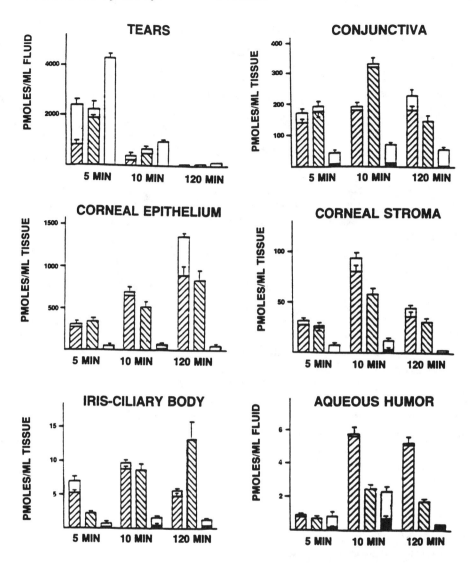

Figure 1. Concentration of intact (open bar) and degraded (marked bar) leucine enkephalin (/ / /), methionine enkephalin (\ \ \) or [D-Ala2]Met-enkephalinamide (filled bar) recovered in each part of the rabbit eye. (From Ref. 71.)

processes, absorption by the avascular cornea is an important one, since a large portion of the drug thus absorbed is distributed to adjacent ocular tissues.

Ahmed and Patton (77) also found that noncorneal (scleral) absorption accounted for about 80% absorption of inulin, a highly hydrophilic macromolecule, into the iris-ciliary body. This observation is important, since most therapeutic peptides act locally in the iris-ciliary body, which is contiguous with the sclera. Therefore macromolecular drug absorption would benefit from scleral absorption.

Besides the transport barrier, another factor severely limiting the ocular absorption of peptide drugs is metabolism by the ocular enzymes, specifically peptidases. The magnitude

Table 3. Penetration Enhancers Used to Improve Ocular Absorption

Enhancer	Effect
Azone	Threefold increase in cyclosporine absorption
Cetrimide, Cytochalasin B	Increased absorption of inulin
EDTA	Threefold increase in glycerol absorption
Taurocholate, Taurodeoxycholate	Increased permeation of insulin and FITC-dextran

of this enzymatic barrier is a significant one. Endopeptidases, like plasmin and collagenase, and exopeptidases, like aminopeptidases, are present in the ocular fluids and tissues. The endopeptidase levels are usually low unless the eye is inflamed (78,79) or injured (80) and are of little concern relative to the stability of topically applied doses. Lee (71) reported that within 5 min postinstillation of solution, about 90% of leucine enkephalin and almost 100% of methionine enkephalin (pentapeptides) were recovered in the corneal epithelium of the albino rabbit in a hydrolyzed form. Therefore, the aminopeptidases activity must be inhibited to facilitate ocular peptide absorption. Controlling these enzymes in the target tissues may not be practical given the fact that the same enzymes might be necessary for the homeostasis in the eye.

A more practical strategy for circumventing the enzymatic barrier would be to administer peptide analogs that are resistant to the principal peptidases but possess equivalent biological activity. Such conditions were met by [D-Ala^2]met-enkephalinamide, which resists aminopeptidase-mediated cleavage (71).

In addition, the presence of sites beyond the absorbing epithelia that are capable of degrading peptides and proteins, and the availability of multiple peptidases in a given site further decrease the absorption potential of such compounds. In general, there are insufficient data to assess accurately the magnitude of the enzymatic barrier in ocular tissues as compared to other alternative routes of delivery.

The future task then will be to optimize ocular peptide delivery by exploring one or a combination of the following approaches:

1. Enhanced residence time of the drug at the absorption site
2. Reduced enzymatic degradation of the drug both at the site of absorption as well as the site of action
3. Increased permeability of the drug across the ocular membranes
4. By utilizing absorption enhancers to improve corneal uptake

V. SYSTEMIC ADMINISTRATION OF PEPTIDES AND PROTEINS THROUGH THE OCULAR ROUTE

Systemic absorption of polypeptides and proteins primarily occur through contact with the conjunctival and nasal mucosae. Table 4 lists some of the peptides that could be administered through the ocular route (81). Almost all the studies involving the absorption of peptides and proteins in animal models have been carried out using labeled peptide samples (82–84). Apart from monitoring the blood concentrations for pharmacokinetic evaluation, pharmacodynamic studies have also been extensively pursued. Some of the biological response parameters include reduction in blood sugar by insulin, increase in

Table 4. Therapeutically Useful Peptides that Could Be Administered
Through the Ocular Route

Peptide	Application
ACTH	Antiallergic, decongestant anti-inflammatory
β-Endorphin	Analgesic
Calcitonin	Paget's disease, hypercalcemia
Glucagon	Hypoglycemic crisis
Insulin	Diabetes mellitus
Leu-enkephalin	Analgesic
Met-enkephalin	Immunostimulant
Oxytocin	Induce uterine contractions
Somatostatin	Attenuate miotic responses
TRH	Diagnosis of thyroid cancer
Vasopressin	Diabetes insipidus
VIP	Secretion of insulin

blood glucose by glucagon, analgesic effects by enkephalins, and increase in blood pressure by vasopressin.

Systemic peptide availability following ocular administration has been related to biological response. The study by Christie and Hanzal (85) showed that insulin instilled into the conjunctiva is absorbed rapidly, giving rise to a fairly constant and consistent lowering of blood sugar levels in rabbits. Another study with somatostatin and its analog revealed that there was an attenuation of the miotic response to noiceptive stimuli by these agents, whereas intracameral injection of 1–50 mg met-enkephalin had no effect on the miotic response (86).

Lee et al. (87) found that enkephalinamide and inulin are absorbed into the blood stream following topical ocular administration, the former to a greater extent than the latter. The authors proposed that depending on the molecular size, lipophilicity, and susceptibility to proteolysis, other peptides and proteins may also be absorbed to varying extents. Similarly, Chiou and Chuang (82) demonstrated the feasibility of effective systemic delivery of topically instilled peptides in the eye. Their findings suggest that systemic delivery of peptide drugs is a superior method than parenteral route, especially when the drug is potent and doses required are low. Enkephalin could effectively be absorbed systemically through the eye with the use of an absorption enhancer (83). This ocular route was found to be superior to administering the peptide by an intravenous route. Similar results have been obtained with other peptides like thyrotropin-releasing hormone (TRH), luteinizing hormone–releasing hormone (LHRH), glucagon, and insulin (82). Spantide, a tachykinin antagonist, is readily taken up into the rabbit eye following topical application. Measurable concentrations of the peptide were observed in the aqueous humor as well as in the general circulation. Similarly, insulin could be absorbed effectively into the systemic circulation through ocular instillation (88). The systemic absorption of 1% insulin through the eyes can be enhanced at least sevenfold when 1% of saponin, a surfactant, was added to the solution. This absorption enhancement was not affected by aminopeptidase inhibition. Recently, calcitonin, a polypeptide hormone, was found to be poorly absorbed into the systemic circulation through the ocular route (89). Inclusion of permeation enhancers like Brij-78 and BL-9 markedly improved its systemic absorption.

In summary, small polypeptides such as TRH (MW 300), enkephalins (MW ~600), LHRH (MW 1200), and glucagon (MW 3500) are absorbed to a significant extent through the eyes, almost to the extent of 99% (82). Polypeptides with larger molecular weight such as β-endorphin (MW ~5000) and insulin (MW ~6000) are also absorbed but to a much lesser extent. The absorption of such large molecular weight compounds can, however, be improved by simultaneous use of absorption enhancers (75).

VI. ENHANCED SYSTEMIC ABSORPTION WITH PERMEATION ENHANCERS

One of the major problems associated with the ocular delivery of peptide drugs is their poor systemic bioavailability. This may be overcome by using penetration enhancers. Most permeation enhancers need to be evaluated with caution, since most of these agents cause local irritation to the eye. Among them the most effective ones are Brij-78 and BL-9, because these compounds have been shown to enhance insulin absorption to a significant extent without causing any noticeable irritation (75). Table 5 lists the penetration enhancers that have been examined for enhancing insulin absorption by the ocular route and their relative performance (81). Saponin, fusidic acid, and Brij-99 possess high irritation potential and therefore cannot be used. As indicated earlier, the same surfactants are also capable of enhancing the absorption of calcitonin (89).

Table 5. Effects of Various Permeation Enhancers on Systemic Absorption of Insulin Following Ocular Administration

Permeation enhancer	Concentration of enhancer (%)	Insulin absorption enhanced (×)
Saponin	0.5	4.0
	1.0	7.0
Fusidic acid	0.25	2.3
	0.5	2.7
	1.0	3.9
	2.0	7.5
Polyethylene-9-laurylether (BL-9)	0.25	2.6
	0.5	4.5
	1.0	6.0
	2.0	7.6
Polyethylene-20-stearylether (Brij 78)	0.5	6.8
	1.0	6.3
Polyethylene-20-oleorylether (Brij 99)	0.5	4.0

The permeability barrier of the cornea to hydrophilic molecules is presumed to reside in the epithelial layer. The presence of tight junctions render the epithelium almost impermeable to all but the smallest molecules. Grass and Robinson have shown that the aqueous channel of the cornea has a cut-off of around 90 D (90). Other studies have suggested a close relationship between epithelial permeability (or tight junction integrity) and the cell cytoskeleton (91,92). Treatment with cytochalasins or removal of extracellular calcium ions cause opening of tight junctions and increase tight junction permeability (93,94). Cytoskeletal modulators have been explored as corneal penetration enhancers (95,96). The efficacy of EDTA, bile salts, and cytochalasin B (97) in enhancing the ocular permeability of hydrophilic compounds have been examined. Cytochalasin B has the ability to increase corneal permeability with minimum membrane damage, indicating its potential as an ocular penetration enhancer. Further development of novel penetration enhancers with highly specific foci of action, good reversibility, and minimal toxicity are needed for any realistic delivery of peptides and proteins by the ocular route.

VII. CONCLUSIONS

With the breakthrough in biotechnology, newer and more potent peptide and protein drugs are emerging in the market. The majority of these polypeptides require special delivery systems. However, since most of these compounds are very potent, require low doses, and are well absorbed from the mucous membrane, their delivery via the ocular route may be viable. However, one of the principal problems in the ocular delivery of peptide and protein drugs is that of relatively low bioavailability to the ocular tissues. This problem may be circumvented by the use of penetration enhancers. The conjunctival administration of this class of compounds to achieve therapeutic levels in the systemic circulation may well be possible in the near future. We hope that novel drug delivery systems would be developed to deliver potent polypeptide drugs through the ocular route.

REFERENCES

1. Lee, V. H. L. (1987). Ophthalmic delivery of peptides and proteins, *Pharm. Tech.*, 11:26.
2. Tobey, N., Heizer, W., Yeh, R., Huang, T. I., and Hoffner, C. (1985). Human intestinal brush border peptidases, *Gastroenterology*, 88:913.
3. Ziv, E., Lior, O., and Kidron, M. (1987). Absorption of protein via the intestinal wall, *Biochem. Pharmacol.*, 36:1035.
4. Aungst, B. J., Rogers, N. J., and Shefter, E. (1988). Comparison of nasal, rectal, buccal, sublingual and intramuscular insulin efficacy and the effects of bile salt absorption promoter, *J. Pharmacol. Exp. Ther.*, 244:23.
5. Aungst, B. J., and Rogers, N. J. (1988). Site dependence of absorption promoting actions of laureth-9, Na salicylate, Na_2EDTA, and apoprotinin on rectal, nasal and buccal insulin delivery, *Pharm. Res.*, 5:305.
6. Moore, J. A., Pletcher, S. A., and Ross, M. J. (1986). Absorption enhancement of growth hormone from the gastrointestinal tract of rats, *Int. J. Pharm.*, 34:35.
7. Lee, V. H. L. (1990). Protease inhibitors and penetration enhancers as approaches to modify peptide absorption, *J. Controlled Rel.*, 13:213.
8. Lee, V. H. L. (1988). Enzymatic barriers to peptide and protein absorption, *Crit. Rev. Ther. Drug. Carrier Syst.*, 5:69.
9. Anders, R., Merkle, H. P., Schurr, W., and Ziegler, R. (1983). Buccal absorption of protirelin: An effective way to stimulate thyrotropin and prolactin, *J. Pharm. Sci.*, 72:1481.

10. Salzman, R., Manson, J. E., Griffing, G. T., Kimmerle, R., and Ruderman, N. (1985). Intranasal aerosolized insulin: Mixed meal studies and long term use in Type I diabetes, *N. Engl. J. Med.*, 312:1078.
11. Moses, A. C., Gordon, G. S., Carey, M. C., and Flier, J. S. (1983). Insulin administration intranasally as an insulin-bile salt aerosol, effectiveness and reproducibility in normal and diabetic subjects, *Diabetes*, 32:1040.
12. Hirai, S., Ikenaga, T., and Matsuwaza, T. (1978). Nasal absorption of insulin in dogs, *Diabetes*, 27:296.
13. Siddiqui, O., Sun, Y., Liu, J. C., and Chien, Y. W. (1987). Facilitated transdermal transport of insulin, *J. Pharm. Sci.*, 76:341.
14. Kari, B. (1986). Control of blood glucose levels in alloxan-diabetic rabbits by iontophoresis of insulin, *Diabetes*, 35:217.
15. Wigley, F. M., Londono, J. H., Wood, S. H., and Shipp, J. C. (1971). Insulin across respiratory mucosae by aerosol delivery, *Diabetes*, 20:552.
16. Yamasaki, Y., Shichiri, M., Kawamori, R., Kikuchi, M., and Yagi, T. (1981). The effectiveness of rectal administration of insulin suppository on normal and diabetic subjects, *Diabetes Care*, 4:454.
17. Fisher, N. F. (1923). The absorption of insulin from the intestine, vagina and scrotal sac, *Am. J. Physiol.*, 67:65.
18. Lee, V. H. L., and Yamamoto, A. (1990). Penetration and enzymatic barriers to peptide and protein absorption, *Adv. Drug Deliv. Rev.*, 4:171.
19. Lee, V. H. L. (ed.) (1991). *Peptide and Protein Drug Delivery*, Marcel Dekker, New York.
20. Fraunfelder, F. T., and Meyer, S. M. (1987). Systemic side effects from ophthalmic timolol and their prevention, *J. Ocul. Pharmacol.*, 3:177.
21. Robinson, J. R. (1989). Ocular drug delivery. Mechanism(s) of corneal drug transport and mucoadhesive systems, *S.T.P. Pharma.*, 5:839.
22. Rojanasakul, Y., Paddock, S. W., and Robinson, J. R. (1990). Confocal laser scanning microscopic examination of transport pathways and barriers of some peptides across the cornea, *Int. J. Pharm.*, 61:163.
23. Harris, D., and Robinson, J. R. (1990). Bioadhesive polymers in peptide drug delivery, *Biomaterials*, 11:652.
24. Green, P., Hinz, R., Cullander, C., Yamane, G., and Guy, R. H. (1989). Iontophoretic delivery of amino acids and analogs, *Pharm. Res.*, 6:S148.
25. Miller, L., Kolaskie, C. J., Smith, G. A., and Riviere, J. (1990). Transdermal iontophoresis of gonadotrophin releasing hormone (LHRH) and two analogues, *J. Pharm. Sci.*, 79:490.
26. Sun, Y., Xue, H., and Liu, J. C. (1990). A unique iontophoresis system designed for transdermal protein drug delivery, *Pharm. Res.*, 7:S113.
27. Chien, Y. W., Lelawong, P., Siddiqui, O., Sun, Y., and Shi, W. M. (1990). Facilitated transdermal delivery of therapeutic peptides and proteins by iontophoretic delivery devices, *J. Controlled Rel.*, 7:1.
28. Dill, K. A. (1990). Dominant forces in protein folding, *Biochemistry*, 29:7133.
29. Creighton, T. E. (1990). Protein folding, *Biochem. J.*, 270:1.
30. Horbett, T. A., and Brash, J. L. (1987). Proteins at interfaces: Current issues and future prospects. *In: Proteins at Interfaces: Physicochemical and Biochemical Studies*. (T. A. Horbett and J. L. Brash, eds.). American Chemical Society, Washington, D.C., Chap. 1.
31. Okumura, K., Kiyohara, Y., Komada, F., Mishima, Y., and Fuwa, T. (1990). Protease inhibitor potentiates the healing effect of epidermal growth factor in wounded or burned skin, *J. Controlled Rel.*, 13:310.
32. Katre, N. V., Knauf, M. J., and Laird, W. J. (1987). Chemical modification of recombinant interleukin 2 by polyethylene glycol increases its potency in the murine Meth A sarcoma model, *Proc. Natl. Acad. Sci. U.S.A.*, 84:1487.

33. Yoshihiro, I., Casolaro, M., Kono, K., and Imanishi, Y. (1989). An insulin releasing system that is responsive to glucose, *J. Controlled Rel.*, 10:195.
34. Hori, R., Komada, F., Iwakawa, S., Seino, Y., and Okumura, K. (1989). Enhanced bioavailability of subcutaneously injected insulin coadministered with collagen in rats and humans, *Pharm. Res.*, 6:813.
35. Fuertges, F., and Abuchowski, A. (1990). The clinical efficacy of poly(ethylene glycol)-modified proteins, *J. Controlled Rel.*, 11:139.
36. Saffran, M., Kumar, G. S., Neckers, D. C., Pena, J., Jones, R. H., and Field, J. (1990). Biodegradable copolymer coating for oral delivery of peptide drugs, *Biochem. Soc. Trans.*, 18:752.
37. De Boer, A. G., Van Hoogdalem, E. J., Heijligers-Feigen, C. D., Verhoef, J. C., and Breimer, D. D. (1990). Rectal absorption enhancement of peptide drugs, *J. Controlled Rel.*, 13:241.
38. Pontiroli, A. E. (1990). Intranasal administration of calcitonin and of other peptides: Studies with different promoters, *J. Controlled Rel.*, 13:247.
39. Lundin, S., and Artursson, P. (1990). Absorption of vasopressin analogue, 1-desamino-8-D-arginine-vasopressin (dDAVP), in human intestinal epithelial cell line, CaCO-2, *Int. J. Pharm.*, 64:181.
40. Amidon, G. L., Sinko, P. J., Hu, M., and Leesman, G. D. (1989). Absorption of difficult drug molecules: Carrier mediated transport of peptides and peptide analogues. *In: Novel Drug Delivery and Therapeutic Application* (L. F. Presscot and W. S. Ninmo, eds.). Wiley, New York, Chap. 5.
41. Sinko, P. J., Hu, M., and Amidon, G. L. (1987). Carrier mediated transport of amino acids, small peptides and their drug analogs, *J. Controlled Rel.*, 6:115.
42. Hu, M., Subramaniam, P., Mosberg, H. I., and Amidon, G. L. (1989). Use of the peptide carrier system to improve the intestinal absorption of L-α-methyldopa: Carrier kinetics, intestinal permeabilities and in vitro hydrolysis of dipeptidyl derivatives of L-α-methyldopa, *Pharm. Res.*, 6:66.
43. Friedman, D. I., and Amidon, G. L. (1990). Characterization of the intestinal transport parameters for small peptide drugs, *J. Controlled Rel.*, 13:141.
44. Ungell, A., and Andreasson, A. (1990). The effect of enzymatic inhibition versus increased paracellular transport of vasopressin peptides, *J. Controlled Rel.*, 13:313.
45. Drewe, J., Vonderscher, J., Hornung, K., Munzer, J., Reinhardt, J., Kissel, T., and Beglinger, C. (1990). Enhancement of oral absorption of somatostatin analog Sandostatin in man, *J. Controlled Rel.*, 13:315.
46. Lundin, S., Pantzar, N., Hedin, I., and Westron, B. R. (1990). Intestinal absorption by sodium taurodihydrofusidate of a peptide hormone analogue (dDAVP) and a macromolecule (BSA) in vitro and in vivo, *Int. J. Pharm.*, 59:263.
47. Schilling, R. J., and Mitra, A. K. (1990). Intestinal mucosal transport of insulin, *Int. J. Pharm.*, 62:53.
48. Su, K. S. E. (1991). Nasal route delivery of peptide and protein drug delivery. *In: Peptide and Protein Drug Delivery* (V. H. L. Lee, ed.). Marcel Dekker, New York, Chap. 13.
49. Harris, A. S. (1986). Biopharmaceutical aspects of the intranasal administration of peptides. *In: Delivery Systems for Peptide Drugs*, (S. S. David, L. Illum, and E. Tomlinson, eds.). Plenum Press, New York, p. 191.
50. Sandow, J., and Petri, W. (1985). Intranasal administration of peptides, biological activity and therapeutic efficacy. *In: Transnasal Systemic Medications.* (Y. W. Chien, ed.). Elsevier, New York, Chap. 7.
51. Solbach, H. G., and Wiegelmann, W. (1973). Intranasal application of luteinizing hormone releasing hormone, *Lancet*, 1:1259.
52. Dashe, A. M., Kleeman, C. R., Czarczkes, J. W., Rubinoff, H., and Spears, I. (1964). Synthetic vasopressin nasal spray in the treatment of diabetes insipidus, *JAMA*, 190:113.
53. Flier, J. S., Moses, A. C., Gordon, G. S., and Silver, R. S. (1985). Intranasal administration of insulin efficacy and mechanism. *In: Transnasal Systemic Medications*, (Y. W. Chien, ed.). Elsevier, New York, Chap. 9.

54. O'Hagan, D. T., Critchley, H., Farraj, N. F., Fisher, A. N., Hohansen, B. R., David, S. S., and Illum, L. (1990). Nasal absorption enhancers for synthetic human growth hormone in rats, *Pharm. Res.*, 7:772.

55. Tengamnuay, P., and Mitra, A. K. (1990). Bile salt-fatty acid mixed micelles as nasal absorption promoters of peptides. I. Effects of ionic strength, adjuvant composition and lipid structure on the nasal absorption of [D-Arg^2]kyotrophin, *Pharm. Res.*, 7:127.

56. Tengamnuay, P., and Mitra, A. K. (1990). Bile salt-fatty acid mixed micelles as nasal absorption promoters of peptides. II. In vivo nasal absorption of insulin in rats and effects of mixed micelles on the morphological integrity of the nasal mucosa, *Pharm. Res.*, 7:370.

57. Vadnere, M., Adjei, A., Doyle, R., and Johnson, E. (1990). Evaluation of alternative routes for delivery of leuprolide, *J. Controlled Rel.*, 13:322.

58. Merkle, H. P., Anders, R., Sandow, J., and Schurr, W. (1985). Self adhesive patches for buccal delivery of peptides, *Proc. Int. Symp. Controlled Rel. Bioact. Mater.*, 12:85.

59. Squier, C. A., and Hall, B. K. (1985). The permeability of skin and oral mucosa to water and horseradish peroxidase as related to the thickness of the permeability barrier, *J. Invest. Dermatol.*, 84:176.

60. Yokosuka, T., Omori, Y., Hirata, Y., and Hirai, S. (1977). Nasal and sublingual administration of insulin in man, *J. Jpn. Diabetic Soc.*, 20:146.

61. Tolo, K., and Jonsen, J. (1975). In vitro penetration of tritiated dextrans through rabbit oral mucosa, *Arch. Oral Biol.*, 20:419.

62. Gandhi, R. B., and Robinson, J. R. (1990). Mechanism of transport of charged compounds across rabbit buccal mucosa, *Pharm. Res.*, 7:S116.

63. Dodda-Kashi, S. and Lee, V. H. L. (1986). Enkephalin hydrolysis in homogenates of various absorptive mucosae of the albino rabbit: Similarities in rate and involvement of aminopeptidases, *Life Sci.*, 38:2019.

64. Garren, K. W., and Repta, A. J. (1988). Buccal absorption. III. Simultaneous diffusion and metabolism of an aminopeptidase substrate in the hamster cheek pouch, *Pharm. Res.*, 6:966.

65. Aungst, B. J., and Rogers, N. J. (1989). Comparison of the effects of various transmucosal absorption promoters on buccal insulin delivery, *Int. J. Pharm.*, 53:277.

66. Crooks, P. (1990). Lung Peptidases and Their Activities. Presented at Respiratory Drug Delivery II, Keystone, Colorado.

67. Schankar, L. S., Mitchel, E. W., and Brown, R. A. (1986). Species comparison of drug absorption from the lung after aerosol inhalation or intratracheal injection, *Drug Metab. Dispos.*, 14:79.

68. Maruyama, K., Homberg, E., Kennel, S. J., Klibanov, A., Forchlin, V. P., and Huang, L. (1990). Characterization of in vivo immunoliposome targeting to pulmonary endothelium, *J. Pharm. Sci.*, 79:978.

69. O'Donnell, M. (1990). Novel Approaches to the Development of Peptide Bronchodilator Drugs. Presented at Respiratory Drug Delivery II, Keystone, Colorado.

70. Lee, V. H. L. (1990). Mechanisms and facilitations of corneal drug penetration, *J. Controlled Rel.*, 11:79.

71. Lee, V. H. L., Carson, L. W., Dodda-Kashi, S., and Stratford, R. E. (1986). Metabolic permeation barriers to the ocular absorption of topically applied enkephalins in albino rabbits, *J. Ocul. Physiol.*, 2:345.

72. Lee, V. H. L., Carson, L. W., and Takemoto, K. A. (1986). Macromolecular drug absorption in the albino rabbit eye, *Int. J. Pharm.*, 29:43.

73. Newton, C., Gebhardt, B. M., and Kaufman, H. E. (1988). Topically applied cyclosporine in azone prolongs corneal allograft survival, *Invest. Ophthalmol. Vis. Sci.*, 29:208.

74. Morimoto, K., Nakai, T., and Morisaka, K. (1987). Evaluation of permeability enhancement of hydrophilic compounds and macromolecular compounds by bile salts through rabbit corneas in vitro, *J. Pharm. Pharmacol.*, 39:124.

75. Chiou, G. C., and Ching, Y. C. (1989). Improvement of systemic absorption of insulin through the eyes with absorption enhancers, *J. Pharm. Sci.*, 78:815.

76. Yamamoto, A., Luo, A. M., Dodda-Kashi, S., and Lee, V. H. L. (1989). The ocular route for the systemic insulin delivery in the albino rabbit, *J. Pharm. Exp. Ther.*, 249:249.
77. Ahmed, I., and Patton, T. F. (1985). Importance of the noncorneal absorption route in topical ophthalmic drug delivery, *Invest. Ophthalmol. Vis. Sci.*, 26:584.
78. Pandolfi, M., Astedt, B., and Dyster-Aas, K. (1972). Release of fibrinolytic enzymes from the human cornea, *Acta. Ophthalmol.*, 50:199.
79. Berman, M., Manseau, E., Law, M., and Aiken, D. (1983). Ulceration is correlated with degradation of fibrin and fibronectin at the corneal surface, *Invest. Ophthalmol. Vis. Sci.*, 24:1358.
80. Hayasaka, S., and Hayasaka, I. (1979). Cathepsin B and collagenolytic cathepsin in the aqueous humor of patients with Bechet's disease, *Albrecht v. Graefes Arch. Klin. Exp. Ophthal.*, 206:103.
81. Chiou, G. C. (1991). Systemic delivery of polypeptide drugs through ocular route, *Ann. Rev. Pharmacol. Toxicol.*, 31:457.
82. Chiou, G. C., and Chuang, C. Y. (1988). Systemic delivery of polypeptides with molecular weights between 300 and 3500 through the eye, *J. Ocul. Pharmacol.*, 4:165.
83. Chiou, G. C., Chuang, C. Y., and Chang, M. S. (1988). Systemic delivery of enkephalin peptide through eyes, *Life Sci.*, 43:509.
84. Chiou, G. C., and Chuang, C. Y. (1988). Treatment of hypoglycemia with glucagon eye drops, *J. Ocul. Pharmacol.*, 4:179.
85. Christie, C. D., and Hanzal, R. F. (1931). Insulin absorptin by the conjunctival membranes in rabbits, *J. Clin. Invest.*, 10:787.
86. Stjernschantz, J., Sears, M. L., and Oksala, O. (1985). Effects of somatostatin, a somatostatin analog, neurotensin, and metenkephalin in the eye with special reference to the irritative response, *J. Ocul. Pharmacol.*, 1:59.
87. Lee, V. H. L., Carson, L. W., Dodda-Kashi, S. D., and Stratford, R. E. Jr. (1988). Systemic absorption of ocularly administered enkephalinamide and inulin in the albino rabbit: Extent, pathways and vehicle effects, *J. Pharm. Sci.*, 77:838.
88. Chiou, G. C., Chuang, C. Y., and Chang, M. S. (1989). Systemic delivery of insulin through eyes to lower the glucose concentration, *J. Ocul. Pharmacol.*, 5:81.
89. Li, B. H. P., and Chiou, G. C. Y. (1992). Systemic Administration of calcitonin through ocular route, *Life Sci.*, 50:349.
90. Grass, G. M., and Robinson, J. R. (1988). Mechanisms of corneal drug penetration I: In vivo and in vitro kinetics, *J. Pharm. Sci.*, 77:3.
91. Meza, I., Ibarra, G., Sabanero, M., and Cereijido, M. (1980). Occluding junctions and cytoskeletal components in cultures transporting epithelium, *J. Cell Biol.*, 87:746.
92. Madara, J. L., Barenberg, D., and Carlson, S. (1986). Effects of cytochalasin D on occluding junctions of intestinal absorptive cells: Further evidence that the cytoskeleton may influence paracellular permeability and junctional charge selectivity, *J. Cell Biol.*, 102:2125.
93. Bentzel, C. J., Hainau, B., Ho, S., Hui, S. W., Edelman, A., Anagnostopoulos, T., and Benedetti, E. L. (1980). Cytoplasmin regulation of tight junction permeability: effect of plant cytokinins, *Am. J. Physiol.*, 239:C75.
94. Martinez-Palomo, A., Meza, I., Beaty, G., and Cereijido, M. (1980). Experimental modulation of occluding junctions in a cultured epithelium, *J. Cell Biol.*, 87:736.
95. Aldridge, D. C., Armstrong, J. J., Speake, R. N., and Turner, W. B. (1967). The cytochalasins, a new class of biologically active mold metabolites, *Chem. Commun.*, 1:26.
96. Rothweiler, W., and Tamm, C. (1966). Isolation and structure of phomin, *Experientia*, 22:750.
97. Binder, M., and Tamm, C. (1973). The cytochalasins: A new class of biologically active microbial metabolites, *Agnew. Chem. Int. Edit.*, 12:370.

23
Regulatory Considerations

Robert E. Roehrs   *Alcon Laboratories, Fort Worth, Texas*

I. INTRODUCTION

The regulation of research and development of new ophthalmic drug delivery systems is based on laws enacted by the U.S. Congress* with implementing regulations promulgated and enforced by the U.S. Food and Drug Administration (FDA).[†]

If a drug delivery researcher is interested only in the in vitro performance of his or her system and/or its in vivo performance in laboratory research animals, then the FDA regulations can largely be ignored. However, if the delivery system is being designed and developed for use in human and/or veterinary medicine, then a knowledge of the regulations governing clinical testing and ultimately the application to market such a pharmaceutical dosage form will be essential.

II. BRIEF HISTORY OF DRUG REGULATIONS IN THE UNITED STATES

Federal legislation regulating the importation of adulterated articles dates back to the Import Drug Act of 1848. However, the first significant federal legislation regulating the interstate shipment of food and drugs was enacted in 1906 and was known as the Pure Food and Drug Act. It prohibited the interstate shipment of adulterated or misbranded foods or drugs. In 1912, it was amended by Congress to include false statements or fraudulent claims as part of the definition of a misbranded product (1).

A. Federal Food, Drug and Cosmetic Act of 1938

In 1938, a new law was passed as a result of the elixir of sulfanilamide disaster and the recognition that the 1906 Act and its amendments did not ban unsafe or toxic drugs. Sulfanilamide was one of the first synthetic anti-infective drugs and was widely used in powder form. The S. E. Massengill company recognized the usefulness of a liquid form for convenient oral use and discovered that diethylene glycol would dissolve the drug and provide a pharmaceutically elegant vehicle. It was not long after marketing the new dosage

---

*Federal Food, Drug and Cosmetic Act (FD&C).
[†]Code of Federal Regulations (CFR).

form that the poisonous nature of the vehicle was realized and over 100 deaths were attributed to its use (2).

The existing law did not require premarket testing for safety and the product could not be legally removed from the market because of its toxicity. The product was labeled as an "elixir" and therefore was judged to be misbranded in that it did not contain alcohol and because of this technical violation of the labeling provisions of the 1906 law the product was removed from the market.

The 1938 Act was passed to require drugs to be tested for safety and provide this proof to the FDA before marketing. It contained a "grandfather" clause which exempted certain drugs on the market the day prior to the effective date of the Act from new drug status. Some of these drugs are still on the market. It also added the regulation of cosmetics to FDA's responsibilities.

B. Kefauver-Harris Amendments of 1962

The Kefauver-Harris Amendments of 1962 were enacted largely in response to another therapeutic disaster, thalidomide. The drug was already marketed overseas without a prescription as a tranquilizer. It was under clinical investigation in the United States and a New Drug Application (NDA) was being reviewed by the FDA, who was withholding approval and insisting on further proof of safety. During the time FDA was reviewing the NDA, it was discovered in West Germany that thalidomide was associated with the severe birth defect of phocomelia. FDA seized the investigational supplies in the United States and only a small number of cases were reported in this country. This brought the entire drug development and government review of new medicinal agents under intense congressional and public scrutiny and debate (3).

The 1962 amendments are usually referred to as the drug efficacy amendments, since for the first time manufacturers were required to prove efficacy as well as safety. These amendments established the requirements for an Investigational New Drug application (IND) to be submitted to FDA before clinical research on human subjects can be initiated and requirements for NDAs to obtain FDA approval to market a new drug product. FDA completed rewriting these IND and NDA requirements in 1987 (4) and 1985 (5) respectively. We will review these current requirements in some detail in the next section as to their relevance to the regulation of ophthalmic drug delivery systems.

These amendments also established the important GMP, or Good Manufacturing Practice, regulations under which drugs may be removed from the market even if they are not "impure" but legally considered adulterated because they were not manufactured in accordance with the most current good manufacturing practices (21 CFR 210 & 211).

C. Environmental Regulations

The National Environmental Policy Act of 1974 requires FDA to assess the possible environmental effects when approving investigational research and market approval of new drug products. In 1985, FDA implemented new regulations requiring sponsors and applicants to provide a detailed environmental assessment in INDs and NDAs from which the agency would review and provide either a finding of no significant impact or request the preparation of a formal environmental impact statement (21 CFR 25).

D. Orphan Drug Act

The Orphan Drug Act of 1983 was passed to provide incentives for the research and development (R&D) leading to the market availability of drugs to treat rare diseases or conditions. Congress provided incentives in terms of research grants to conduct the necessary animal and clinical testing to obtain FDA approval, tax credits for R&D, and significant market exclusivity for the manufacturer who is the first to obtain approval. The exclusivity prohibits a second manufacturer from obtaining subsequent NDA approval for 7 years for the same drug and disease provided that an adequate supply of the drug to the market is maintained. More than one drug can be designated by FDA for the same rare disease and more than one sponsor may obtain designation using independent data for the same drug and disease or condition. A rare disease has been defined in the amended Act as one in which there are fewer than 200,000 patients with the disease in the United States or one in which the manufacturer cannot recover the R&D costs to bring the drug to the market. Congress is reviewing the success of the legislation and is likely to make some changes affecting the eligibility of a drug to be designated as an orphan drug as well as the market exclusivity incentive.

E. Drug Price Competition and Patent Restoration Act

The Waxman-Hatch Act was passed in 1984 and is officially known as the Drug Price Competition and Patent Restoration Act. The purpose of the legislation is to allow marketing of generic equivalents of pioneer NDA drugs approved since 1962 and thereby increase competition and lower drug prices. The procedure to obtain marketing approval is the Abbreviated New Drug Application (ANDA) and this has generated a large generic pharmaceutical industry. The ANDA applicant must demonstrate to FDA that their generic product is the "same as" the pioneer NDA product and in lieu of the costly NDA process demonstrate that it is bioequivalent to the pioneer. The ANDA is abbreviated in that the applicant does not have to repeat the expensive and time-consuming animal safety and human clinical studies to demonstrate efficacy and safety. However, the generic applicant is required to meet the same FDA requirements for chemistry, manufacturing, and quality control. Importantly, the Act also modified the patent law such that it is no longer an infringement of a patent to use a patented drug for all experimental purposes related to obtaining regulatory approval. Thus, the development of a generic equivalent can be accomplished at any time prior to patent expiration.

The second part of the Act provided incentives to the pioneer industry to continue the costly R&D into new therapeutic agents by extending, or in effect restoring, a limited portion of the patent term for new drugs. A U.S. patent has a term of 17 years, and by the time the product is eventually approved for marketing only a few years may actually remain on the patent before generic competition is made possible by the new law. The manufacturer who obtains the first NDA approval for a new molecular entity is entitled to apply for extension of the term of one unexpired patent by a formula which takes into account the time that it took to diligently pursue development during the clinical investigation phase and the time to obtain FDA approval of the marketing application. The patent term extension is subject to the limitations of a maximum of 5 years and a maximum total effective patent life with extension of 14 years. A subsequent NDA approval for a new salt, ester, dosage form, or use of the new molecular entity would not be eligible for patent term extension.

In addition to the possible patent term extension, a pioneer manufacturer can also obtain a period of market exclusivity against generic competition with the approval of an NDA or approval of a supplemental application for a new use. The market exclusivity provisions run concurrently with any patent term extension. In general, there is a 5-year period of market exclusivity for the first approval of a new chemical entity and a period of 3 years for all others when the criteria for clinical studies essential to approval are met.

The provisions of this Act do not cover antibiotic drugs. Antibiotics are regulated under Section 507 of the FD&C Act which provides for monographs to be issued by FDA at the time of NDA approval. These monographs then serve as the legal basis for approval of generic equivalents. Since the monograph system was already in place for generic antibiotic products, Congress did not see the need for additional incentives.

F. Drug Export Amendments Act of 1986

Prior to the passage of this Act, only drugs approved as safe and effective by FDA could be legally exported. This sometimes placed the U.S. pharmaceutical industry at a competitive disadvantage since new drugs are often first approved overseas and manufacturing plants had to be located outside of the United States to meet the need for drug substances and finished products in these markets. The new law allows export of unapproved new drugs to 21 countries which have premarket approval systems comparable to the United States. However, the export cannot occur until an application is approved by FDA. The drug must be approved in the importing country and the drug manufacturer must be actively pursuing marketing approval in the United States.

The new law does not affect the shipment of new drugs overseas for the sole purpose of clinical investigations. These supplies may be exported under a U.S.IND if the investigator is named in the IND or when approved by an alternate procedure when there is no IND (21 CFR 312.110).

III. REGULATORY REQUIREMENTS TO TEST AN OPHTHALMIC DRUG DELIVERY SYSTEM IN HUMANS

Before discussing the regulatory requirements for clinical testing of drugs in humans, we need to know what constitutes a drug for regulatory purposes, since the FD&C Act also regulates medical devices which could be delivery systems. The drug delivery researcher also needs to be aware of FDA's regulation of certain kinds of testing in animals.

A. Drug versus Device

A *drug* is legally defined as:

1. Articles recognized in the official *United States Pharmacopeia* (USP), official *Homeopathic Pharmacopeia of the United States*, or the *National Formulary* (NF) or any supplements to any of them
2. Articles intended for use in the diagnosis, cure, mitigation, treatment, or prevention of disease in man or other animals
3. Articles other than foods intended to affect the structure or any function of the body of man or other animals
4. Articles intended for use as a component of any article specified in the above three clauses

A *device* is defined as an instrument, apparatus, implement, machine, contrivance, implant, in vitro reagent, or other similar or related article, including any component, part, or accessory which is:

1. Recognized in the official NF or the USP or any supplements
2. Intended for use in the diagnosis of disease or other conditions, or in the cure, mitigation, treatment, or prevention of disease in man or other animals, or
3. Intended to affect the structure or any function of the body of man or other animals, and which does not achieve any of its principal intended purpose through chemical action within or on the body of man or other animals and which is not dependent upon being metabolized for the achievement of any of its principal intended purposes.

While there are some similarities in the two definitions, there are also important differences. The definition of a device lists specific types of articles that are covered and these are the articles that one typically would associate with a literal definition of a device. A device is also an accessory to one of these articles. For example, the contact lens care products which are often sterile solutions containing disinfectant chemicals or polymers which act as lubricants are regulated as devices since they are considered accessory products to the safe use of another device, a contact lens.

Another ophthalmic example is seen with the regulatory history of the Lacrisert®, which is a sterile rod-shaped solid consisting of a cellulosic polymer to be placed in the eye and slowly dissolve in the tears to provide lubrication for patients with painful dry eye diseases. FDA initially approved it as a device and then changed its mind and reclassified it as a drug (6). In doing so, FDA explained that the term *article* in the definition of a "drug" is a broad category in contrast with the specific types of articles listed in the "device" definition and that Lacrisert is not one of these specific articles. FDA also stated that a drug is a chemical or a combination of chemicals in liquid, paste, powder, or other drug dosage form that is ingested, injected, or instilled into body orifices, or rubbed or poured onto the body in order to achieve its intended medical purpose. Also note that the legal definition of a "drug" does not require it to achieve its intended purpose through chemical action or by being metabolized.

It is quite possible to have as a new ophthalmic drug delivery system a combination of a drug and a device. For example, the system could contain the drug in an aerosolized form which is associated with a novel apparatus to instill the drug directly into the eye in a manner which avoids the blink response. The delivery mechanism could be a universal applicator device to which various drugs are added in prepackaged form as cartridges. FDA has established a committee to initially review such applications and decide whether to conduct a primarily a drug review or a device review. In this example, the intended use as a drug would be the primary review.

We will be discussing the requirements for ophthalmic delivery systems in which a drug substance is incorporated for its pharmacological effects and as such is regulated as a "drug."

B. Human versus Animal Use

It is important to know that the investigational use of drugs in animals is also regulated by FDA. If the new drug is shipped interstate for the purpose of clinical investigation in animals, an exemption similar to a human IND is required and the label must bear the following statement (21 CFR 511.1b):

"Caution. Contains a new animal drug for use only in investigational animals in clinical trials. Not for use in humans. Edible products of investigational animals are not to be used for food unless authorization has been granted by the U.S. Food and Drug Administration or by the U.S. Department of Agriculture."

However, if the interstate shipment is intended solely for use in animals used only for laboratory research purposes, then it is exempted from the IND requirement if it is labeled as follows (21 CFR 511.1a):

"Caution. Contains a new animal drug for investigational use only in laboratory research animals or for tests in vitro. Not for use in humans."

Also, the exemption requires that due diligence be used to assure that the consignee is regularly engaged in conducting such tests and the shipment will actually be used as stated in the Caution. Records of the shipments must be kept for a period of 2 years after shipment and delivery and made available to an FDA inspector if requested.

C. Federal versus State Regulation

The FD&C Act regulates interstate shipments of drugs. However, FDA can also regulate the intrastate clinical testing of new drugs, since any component of the drug that is obtained through interstate commerce could bring the product within FDA's jurisdiction. Many states also have Drug laws which are identical to the federal law and it is possible to obtain permission from some states to conduct clinical investigation of new drugs much like the federal IND process.

D. IND Exemption for Clinical Testing in Humans

The FD&C Act Sections 505 and 507 requires the interstate shipment of new drugs to meet certain requirements, including prior FDA approval. If the shipment is for the purpose of clinical testing the drug in humans, then the law provides an exemption from some of the requirements. However, prior to the shipment of the drug, a notice claiming the exemption must be submitted to FDA. This notice is what is termed an Investigational New Drug application or IND (21 CFR 312). The clinical use of the drug cannot begin for 30 days from the date of the application or longer if so notified by FDA. Thus, if the application is acceptable to FDA, there is no formal approval issued other than a notice of receipt. FDA will during this 30-day period make an initial assessment of the clinical testing plans and the data provided to support the use in humans with particular emphasis on whether it is safe to conduct the testing. Beyond the initial 30-day review required by the regulation, FDA will conduct a more indepth review of the data submitted and may from time to time notify the sponsor regarding deficiencies in the application that must be corrected before additional clinical testing is undertaken.

The sponsor is required to submit an annual progress report of the clinical investigations and immediate reports of serious and unexpected adverse reactions in humans and certain findings in animal safety tests.

When is an IND required? An IND is always required for a *new drug*. A new drug is one that is not generally recognized among experts qualified by scientific training and experience as safe and effective for use under the conditions prescribed, recommended, or suggested in its labeling.* Certain drugs have been exempted from this definition if they were in use prior to enactment of the 1938 Act and if the labeling contains the same representations concerning the conditions of its use.

A new drug is not just a newly discovered chemical compound. This can best be illustrated by several examples of what legally constitutes a new drug:

1. The drug is a new derivative of a known molecule. For example, a prodrug of epinephrine such as dipivefrin.
2. A known drug which has been discovered to have a new therapeutic use. For example, a nonsteroidal anti-inflammatory agent to be used to inhibit miosis during cataract surgery.
3. A component of a drug is new for drug use. An EVA polymer film to control the rate of release of pilocarpine to the eye.
4. Two or more "old" drugs combined for drug use. For example, the combination of tobramycin and dexamethasone to form a new anti-infective–steroid combination.
5. A change in the route of administration; i.e., a topical ocular dosage form of acetazolamide for intraocular pressure (IOP) reduction.
6. A change in the dosage or strength of a drug.
7. A change in the intended patient population; i.e., use of an approved glaucoma drug to treat normotensive patients prior to laser surgery to prevent IOP spikes.
8. Add or delete an inactive component which changes the risk to benefit ratio for the drug.
9. The use of radiation sterilization for a drug product (21 CFR 200.30).

A new ophthalmic drug delivery system developed through chemical or pharmaceutical means is considered a new drug subject to FDA requirements for INDs to clinically evaluate its safety and effectiveness and NDAs to obtain approval to market.

E. The Content of an IND Application

FDA regulations specify the format and content requirements of an IND. This is shown in Table 1.

1. Clinical Testing

The first section of the IND informs FDA as to what drug is to be tested, the objectives of the clinical experiments, and the scientific rationale and existing knowledge. FDA uses this information to determine the adequacy of the technical data to support the proposed human experiments.

Clinical testing usually occurs in several phases and an IND can be filed for one or more of these phases (Table 2). Typically, an IND would be filed with specific protocol(s) for Phase 1 and a general outline of the plan for Phase 2. The IND can be amended as necessary to add additional protocols and a revised clinical plan included in the annual report. The clinical protocol is a critical element of the investigational phase for a new drug. FDA regulations establish requirements for the protocol (Table 3). The FDA medical officer reviewing the protocol will provide a critique as to its scientific and regulatory acceptability as well as the acceptability of the risk to human subjects. If the study is intended to be used as part of the NDA to establish safety and effectiveness, it would be important to know if FDA has any serious questions about the protocol before proceeding.

---

*FD&C Act Section 201(p).

Table 1. IND—Format and Content Outline*

Part 1   Form FDA 1571

Part 2   Table of Contents

Part 3   Introductory Statement—brief introductory statement to inclue:
  a. Name(s) of the drug
     Drug's pharmacological class
     Drug's structural formula
     Dosage form and formulation
     Route of administration
     Broad objectives and planned duration of the proposed clinical investigations
  b. Brief summary of previous human experience with the drug:
     Reference to other IND/NDAs, if pertinent
     Investigational or marketing experience in other countries that may be relevant to the
        safety of the proposed clinical investigation(s)
  c. Identification of countries where drug has been withdrawn from investigation or
     marketing for any reasons related to safety or effectiveness and reasons for
     withdrawal

Part 4   General Investigational Plan—brief description of the overall plan for investigating the
          drug product for the following year to include:
  a. Rationale for drug study
  b. Indication(s) to be studies
  c. General approach to be followed in evaluating the drug
  d. Kinds of clinical trials to be conducted in the first year (indicate if plans not developed
     for full year)
  e. Estimate number of patients to be given the drug
  f. Safety risks anticipated—any risks of particular severity or seriousness anticipated
     based on toxicology data or prior human experience with the drug or related
     drugs

Part 5   Investigator's Brochure—to contain the following information:
  a. Brief description of the drug (include structural formula) and the formulation
  b. Summary of the pharmacological and toxicological effects of the drug in animals and
     to the extent known, in man
  c. Summary of pharmacokinetics and biological disposition of the drug in animals and if
     known, in man
  d. Summary of information relating to safety and effectiveness in humans from prior
     clinical studies (can append reprints when pertinent and useful)
  e. Description of possible risks and side effects to be anticipated based on experience
     with the drug or with related drugs. Precautions or special monitoring to be done as
     part of the investigations.

Part 6   Clinical Investigation
  a. Protocol for each planned study
  b. Investigators
     Name and address and CV of each investigator
     Name of each subinvestigator
     Name and address of research facilities
     Name and address of IRB

Table 1. (Continued)

Part 6 (Continued)
  c. Monitor—name, title, and CV
  (*The* person responsible for monitoring the conduct and progress of the clinical investigations)
  Safety Monitor(s)—name, title and CV
  (The person or persons responsible for review and evaluation of information relevant to safety of the drug)
  d. Contract Research Organizations (CRO)
     i. Name and address of CRO used for any part of the clinical studies
     ii. Identify the studies and CRO monitor
     iii. List sponsor obligations transferred to CRO, if any
  e. Labeling for Clinical Supplies

Part 7 Chemistry, Manufacturing, and Controls Information
  a. Drug Substance
     1. Description of physical and chemical characteristics
     2. Name and address of manufacturer
     3. Method of preparation
     4. Reference Standard
     5. Specifications
     6. Methods of Analysis
     7. Stability
  b. Drug Product
     1. Components (reasonable alternatives)
        i. Inactive Components—Tests and Specifications
     2. Composition (reasonable variations)
     3. Name and Address of Manufacturer
     4. Manufacturing and Packaging Procedure
     5. Specifications
     6. Methods of Analysis
     7. Packaging
     8. Stability
     9. Labeling for Clinical Supplies
     10. Placebo—Composition, Manufacture and Control
     11. Environmental Analysis—Claim for Categorical Exclusion

Part 8 Pharmacology and Toxicology
  a. Pharmacology and Drug Disposition
     1. Section describing the pharmacologic effects and mechanism(s) of action of the drug in animals
     2. Section describing the ADME of the drug, if known
  b. Toxicology
     1. ID and qualifications of persons conducting and evaluating results of studies concluding reasonably safe to begin proposed investigations
     2. Statement where studies conducted and where records available for inspection
     3. Integrated summary of the toxicological effects of the drug in animals and in vitro
     4. Detailed tox study reports with full tabulations of data for each study primarily intended to support the safety of the proposed clinical investigation
     5. GLP Compliance Statement(s)

Table 1. (Continued)

Part 9   Previous Human Experience

Part 9   Previous Human Experience

Summary of known prior human experience with the investigational drug to include:

a. If previously investigated or marketed (anywhere):
    i. Detailed information about such experience relevant to safety of proposed investigation or rationale
    ii. If drug has been subject of controlled clinical trials detailed information on such trials relevant to an assessment of the drug's effectiveness for the proposed investigational use
    iii. Published material directly relevant to safety or effectiveness for the proposed investigational use—provide full copies.
    Published material less directly relevant—bibliography

b. For combination of drugs—Part 9a information for each drug.

c. Foreign marketing
    i. List of countries where marketed.
    ii. List of countries where drug has been withdrawn from marketing for reasons potentially related to safety or effectiveness.

*Adapted from 21 CFR 312.23

Ophthalmic drug clinical development generally follows the three phases, particularly if the drug is a new molecule and this is its first introduction into humans. If it is an old drug, such as an ocular dosage form of acetazolamide and the topical dose assuming 100% systemic bioavailability is much less than the oral dose exposure, then Phase 1 may be abbreviated and focus on the local toxicity profile with a concomitant measure of systemic exposure via blood and/or urine sampling.

In Phase 2 of clinical testing, the drug is usually first introduced into patients with the disease and a dose-response relationship is investigated. For oral drugs, the dose-response testing is a crucial parameter; however, it has not been a rigorous part of most topical ophthalmic drug development programs. The drug delivery researcher may find that these data are missing for his or her drug and needs to establish this relationship for optimization. An example of this occurred during the development of the Ocusert containing pilocarpine in which patients were given multiple microdoses of pilocarpine topically to establish the required release rate to provide the desired IOP-lowering response (7).

The final Phase 3 testing is essential to providing the substantial evidence from adequate and well-controlled studies required for proof of safety and effectiveness. It is particularly important that the endpoints used to measure the response of the delivery system be clinically relevant and that enough patients are included to detect a significant difference if one exists.

FDA has established standards for the conduct of clinical studies in order to ensure the quality and integrity of the data on which the safety and effectiveness decisions will be based and also, importantly, the protection of the rights and health of the participating subjects. These are commonly referred to as GCPs but are not embodied in one regulation. They are a combination of the Informed Consent regulation for clinical subjects (21 CFR 50), the Institutional Review Board (IRB) regulations (21 CFR 56), and the obligations of sponsors and investigators defined in the 1987 IND Rewrite regulations.

Table 2. Clinical Testing Phases

Phase 1: Initial introduction into man—closely monitored patients or normal volunteers. Primarily for side effects with increasing doses, ADME and clinical pharmacology and early readout on effectiveness. Used to design well-controlled, scientifically valid Phase 2 studies. Also used for structure-activity and mechanism of action studies as well as using drug as research tool to explore biology and disease processes. Usually involve less than 100 subjects.

Phase 2: Controlled studies for effectiveness in patients and determination of common short-term side effects and risks. Well-controlled and closely monitored studies in usually no more than several hundred patients. Used to screen out drugs with limited potential for safety and/or effectiveness. Data critical to design of Phase 3 studies particularly for dosage regimens and patient populations.

Phase 3: Expanded studies in patients both controlled and uncontrolled to gather data on safety and effectiveness needed to evaluate overall benefit-risk and provide basis for labeling. Usually involve several hundred to several thousand subjects.

Phase 4: Studies usually conducted after initial marketing. May be requested by FDA as condition of approval. May be used to examine specific patient subpopulations such as geriatric or pediatric or to increase exposure to further define benefit to risk ratio.

2. Preclinical Testing

The nonclinical or preclinical section addresses the biological data that support the pharmacological rationale for the intended use of the drug, the animal toxicology data to assess the safety risks for human exposure, and, if available, systemic and ocular pharmacokinetic data. These data may necessarily be limited at this point, particularly if the drug is a new molecule. If the delivery system is being developed with a known drug, then comparative tests will be useful to assess the risk. If the delivery system contains a new component, such

Table 3. Clinical Protocol Requirements

Objectives and purpose of study

Identification of each investigator and subinvestigator, research facilities and each IRB

Criteria for patient selection and exclusion and estimated number of patients

Study design including control group (if any) and methods to minimize bias on part of subjects, investigators and analysts

Method for determining doses to be used, the maximum dose and duration of patient exposure

Description of the observations and measurements to fulfill objectives of study

Description of clinical procedures, lab tests or other measures to monitor drug effects in subjects and to minimize risk as a polymer or surfactant to prolong ocular residence and/or enhance bioavailability, then additional safety testing may be required for the new component if the supplier has not already provided this information. In some cases, this component may have already been used in other drug applications or sometimes for food or cosmetic uses and have established a generally recognized as safe (GRAS) status. The toxicologist will have to assess the relevance of these data to the intended topical application.

FDA does not have specific requirements or guidelines to answer the often asked question—How much animal safety data do I need for an ophthalmic IND? In general, to begin clinical testing, FDA will require at least the same duration of testing in animals as proposed for human exposure. The requirements will vary with the particular drug and the novelty of the particular delivery system. The approach of one company in establishing the safety/toxicity profile of ophthalmic drugs and devices has recently been published (8).

FDA implemented GLP regulations in 1976 which established standards for the conduct and reporting of all animal safety-related studies to be used in support of an IND or NDA. This was a reaction to the discovery that some industrial and contract toxicology testing labs were conducting studies in a sloppy manner and in instances had falsified data that were submitted to FDA. FDA now routinely audits on a periodic basis all labs conducting such studies. Therefore, if animal safety data are generated in an academic institution and the results are to be used in support of an IND, the studies must meet GLP regulations and any deviations from these requirements must be explained. A certification of GLP compliance is required in the IND for each safety study (21 CFR 58).

3. Chemistry, Manufacturing, and Controls

The next major section of the IND describes the chemistry of the drug substance and the composition, manufacturing, packaging, quality control, and stability of the dosage forms to be used in the clinical trials. Inadequacies in this section can cause FDA to withhold the approval to conduct the proposed clinical trials, particularly if the deficiencies cause a concern related to safety.

a. Drug Substance

The drug substance must be characterized as to its structure and adequate analytical procedures be specified to analyze routinely the identity and purity of the drug. If the drug is in an official pharmacopeia, the monograph for the drug may be referenced; however, FDA is not bound by these requirements and may require additional tests and specifications. For example, the assay method for the drug should be stability indicating and some monographs may not meet this standard. Also, FDA will be interested in the major impurities and require specific tests and specifications for them which may not be part of a monograph.

The supplier of the drug substance is required to be identified and the methods of synthesis and controls used by the manufacturer. This will also be required for compendial drugs. Since the information on synthesis is usually considered proprietary, FDA has established a mechanism by which this confidential information can be supplied for their review directly from the manufacturer through a Drug Master File, or DMF (9). The manufacturer will send FDA a letter authorizing the IND sponsor to access this information in a specific DMF and the sponsor is required to include a copy of this letter of authorization in this section of the IND.

An authentic reference standard is required for each drug substance. If not available from USP, then it will have to be established independently, must be the highest purity available, and the method of synthesis and purification must be included.

b. Drug Product

The dosage form containing the active drug substance and its vehicle or delivery system must be described in detail:

Components—Listing of all active and inactive ingredients that are used in preparation of the finished product.

Inactive Components—The quality standard which is used and if other than compendial items, the actual tests and specifications.

Composition—The quantitative composition for the entire formula expressed in terms of percent, milligrams per milliliter, and a typical batch quantity.

Manufacturer—The name and address of each firm involved in the manufacture, packaging, labeling, and testing of the drug product.

Method of Manufacturing—The method of manufacturing, packaging, and labeling the product and the controls used in these processes.

Packaging Components—The packaging is identified and the components are described and specified. The USP specifies tests required for suitability of plastics in ophthalmic containers which are both physicochemical and biological (10). The tests should be conducted on the containers after they are cleaned and sterilized.

Stability—Sufficient stability data using stability-indicating methods should be submitted to assure a stable product for the duration of the clinical trials. GMPs require an expiration dating; however, FDA has proposed that this not be required for clinical supplies, since they are subject to strict control over their distribution.

Labeling—Copy of the labels to be applied to the containers of the clinical supplies. These are usually multipart labels so as to provide complete labeling information during shipment, which can be removed before given to the patient to mask the identity of the product from the patient and the physician. The label must bear the statement: "Caution: New Drug Limited by Federal Law to Investigational Use."

Placebo—Many studies require the drug to be compared to a placebo, which is usually the vehicle or delivery system itself. The same information described above for the active drug product is provided for the placebo dosage form.

Environmental Assessment—The environmental regulations provide for a categorical exclusion from preparing an environmental assessment for clinical trials if waste is controlled or any waste that may enter the environment would be in such a small amount so as to be considered nontoxic.* A justification for the categorical exclusion should be provided.

c. Sterilization

FDA regulation requires that all ophthalmic drug products be manufactured and packaged in a sterile manner. This can be accomplished basically in two ways; i.e., terminal sterilization or by aseptic combination of sterile components. Terminal sterilization is preferred, since it provides the greatest assurance of final product sterility. Often this is not feasible because of the heat lability of the ingredients or the packaging system.

---

*21 CFR 25.24(c)(4).

Terminal sterilization is usually done by radiation or steam under pressure. Many drug products are manufactured sterile by sterilizing the individual components, including the packaging materials, and then aseptically combining them in a sterile environment. FDA has provided guidelines for the proper validation of the aseptic process for sterile products (11).

Because of the much greater sterility assurance offered by a terminal sterilization process, FDA will require the applicant to justify the use of an aseptic process for sterilization (12). Data therefore should be generated during the development of the delivery system to determine the impact of a terminal sterilization process on the final packaged dosage form. This would usually involve chemical and physical analyses of the product for degradation products and any change in the toxicology profile.

d. Preservation

If the delivery system is a liquid in a multiple dose package, the requirement for addition of substance(s) to inhibit the growth of microorganisms during use needs to be considered. The regulation states that these substances must be added *or* the product packaged in such a manner that harmful contamination cannot reasonably occur during use (21 CFR 200.50). Therefore, the regulation does not absolutely require a preservative be used in all multidose packages. However, FDA has not given any published guidance as to their interpretation of what type of unpreserved multidose product would meet the requirements of this regulation.

The regulation specifically states a requirement for *liquid* products and provides no guidance for multidose semisolids such as aqueous gels. The drug delivery scientist should work closely with the microbiologist and packaging scientist to determine the best means to accomplish the safe administration of a sterile product irrespective of the possible loophole in current regulations.

New ophthalmic delivery systems in unit dose form offer the opportunity to improve the ability of the patient to comply with the prescribed dosage regimen and also obviate the need for the addition of a preservative agent.

e. GMPs for Clinical Supplies

Clinical supplies of the new ophthalmic drug delivery system should be manufactured in conformance with the GMP regulations. The pharmaceutical industry has recognized that the official GMP regulations are not always practical or suitable for clinical supplies. The quantities are usually small, and since this is a research and development process, changes will necessarily occur as experience is gained and the scale of manufacture increases. FDA has also recognized these facts and has issued guidelines which address the allowable differences in GMP compliance for clinical trial manufacture (13).

IV. REGULATORY REQUIREMENTS TO MARKET A NEW OPHTHALMIC DRUG DELIVERY SYSTEM FOR HUMAN USE

Once a manufacturer has obtained sufficient information from clinical trials in humans, safety testing in animals and chemistry and manufacturing experience to establish that the new drug is safe and effective for its intended use, he or she submits a New Drug Application (NDA) to obtain FDA approval to distribute it commercially within the United States and to export the product to other countries where it is approved.

A. New Drug Application (NDA)

The format and content requirements for the NDA is seen in Table 4. The first section is a comprehensive summary of the entire application. It is written in the style of a review article. A copy of this summary is provided to each reviewer of the application. The summary begins with a copy of the proposed labeling, i.e., package insert for the product which is annotated to the supporting information in the NDA. The applicant must be able to justify each statement in the proposed labeling.

There are six major technical sections comprising the data and information generated to support the approval.

1. Chemistry, Manufacturing, and Control for the drug substance and drug product
2. Microbiology—applicable only if an anti-infective drug
3. Human Pharmacokinetics—ADME data from human studies
4. Pharmacology—preclinical animal data for pharmacology, toxicology, and pharmaco-kinetics
5. Clinical—human data for safety and efficacy
6. Statistics—mathematical analyses of the human clinical data

FDA has issued guidelines for the format and content of each of these major technical sections (14).

7. A separate section ancillary to the chemistry review provides the documentation for the analytical methods validation package, the description of the drug substance, and drug product samples which the manufacturer is prepared to submit for laboratory evaluation and the product labeling, including the proposed package insert and the immediate container labels. The drug and product samples held by the manufacturer are submitted to one or more FDA district laboratories for analysis and validation of the regulatory analytical methods in the application. This allows FDA to verify the methods and examine the identity, purity, and strength of the drug and product in its own laboratories prior to approval so that FDA is prepared to check the product once marketed as part of the routine surveillance program or if a specific need arises. Under FDA's preapproval inspection program, a local FDA inspector may obtain the samples in person and inspect the documentation records.
8. A section is reserved for periodic updates of new safety information that may be obtained after the NDA was submitted, whereas under FDA review and just prior to final approval.
9. A major change in the NDA Rewrite of 1985 made it no longer required to submit a copy of each patient's Case Report Form (CRF). The information on the CRFs is the raw data from the clinical studies and is tabulated by entry into sophisticated computer databases for evaluation and statistical analysis. This reduced the size of NDA submissions substantially but still provided FDA with the basic data through submission of the patient by patient data tabulations. FDA may still request the original CRFs after submission. Original CRFs for discontinued patients with adverse events are still required routinely.

B. Computer-Assisted NDA (CANDA)

FDA now encourages applicants to submit the patient data tabulations in computer-readable formats such as relational databases and/or spreadsheets. These cannot be used to replace the official hard copy submission. No standard has yet been established by FDA for the clinical data in a CANDA. Each company should contact FDA before planning a CANDA submission. CANDAs have also been used for the toxicology and

Table 4.   NDA—Format and Content Outline*

1. INDEX TO ENTIRE APPLICATION

2. SUMMARY
   a. Labeling text annotated to both Summary & Technical Sections
   b. Pharmacological Class, Scientific Rationale, Intended Use(s) and Potential Clinical Benefits
   c. Foreign Marketing History—Applicant and others if known
       i. Countries in which marketed
      ii. Countries where withdrawn from market for safety or efficacy
     iii. Countries where marketing applications pending
   d. Summary of Chemistry, Manufacturing and Controls Section
   e. Summary of Nonclinical Pharmacology & Toxicology Section
   f. Summary of Human P-Kinetics & Bioavailability Section
   g. Summary of Microbiology Section
   h. Summary of Clinical Section including Statistical Analysis
   i. Concluding Discussion—Benefit/Risk consideration

3. CHEMISTRY, MANUFACTURING, AND CONTROLS SECTION
   a. DRUG SUBSTANCE
       i. Description of Chemical & Physical Characteristics
      ii. Stability
     iii. Source & Location of Manufacturer(s)
      iv. Synthesis, Purification and Controls
       v. Specifications & Analytical Methods
      vi. Reference Standard
   b. DRUG PRODUCT
       i. Components
      ii. Specs and Test Methods for Inactives
     iii. Composition
      iv. Name & Location of Each Manufacturer
       v. Manufacturing & Packaging Procedures & In-Process Controls
      vi. Acceptance Specifications for Each Batch
     vii. Analytical and Microbiological Test Methods
    viii. Packaging Container/Closure Systems
      ix. Stability Data & Protocols
       x. Proposed Expiry Dating & Storage Conditions
   c. Environmental Assessment of Manufacturing Process & Ultimate Use

4. SAMPLES, METHODS VALIDATION, LABELING
   a. Description & assay results of samples for FDA validation
   b. Methods Validation Package (Regulatory Specs & Methods)
   c. Container Labels & Package Insert Labeling

5. NONCLINICAL PHARMACOLOGY & TOXICOLOGY
   a. Pharmacology Studies
   b. Toxicology Studies
   c. Animal ADME Studies
   d. GLP Compliance Statements

Table 4. (Continued)

6. HUMAN PHARMACOKINETICS & BIOAVAILABILITY
   a. Waiver for topical or injectable product bioavailability studies
   b. For each human bio or pharmacokinetic study:
      i. Study report including analytical and statistical methods
      ii. IRB/Informed Consent Compliance Statements
   c. For specs or methods to assure bioavailability of drug or product:
      i. Rationale for establishing spec or method
      ii. Data and information supporting rationale
   d. Summary Discussion & Analysis of
      i. Pharmacokinetics & metabolism or active ingredient
      ii. Bioavailability and/or bioequivalence of drug product

7. MICROBIOLOGY (for Anti-Infectives Only)

8. CLINICAL DATA
   a. Clinical Pharmacology Studies
   b. Controlled Clinical Studies
   c. Uncontrolled Clinical Studies
   d. All other data and information relevant to evaluation of the safety and effectiveness of the drug product
   e. Integrated Summary of Effectiveness
   f. Integrated Summary of Safety
   g. Studies related to abuse potential or overdosages
   h. Integrated Summary of Benefits and Risks
   i. Compliance Statements (IRB & IC) for each clinical study
   j. Contract Research Organizations & Obligations Transferred
   k. List of studies where original subject records were audited or reviewed to verify accuracy of case reports

9. RESERVED FOR SAFETY UPDATE REPORTS
   a. Required AFTER NDA FILED at
      i. 4 months
      ii. Approvable letter and whenever FDA requests update
   b. New Safety Information from any source that may reasonably affect the labeling
   c. Case Report Forms for patients who died or were adverse event dropouts

10. STATISTICAL SECTION
    a. Copy of the following Clinical Data Sections
       i. Controlled Studies
       ii. Integrated Summary of Effectiveness
       iii. Integrated Summary of Safety
    b. Documentation and Supporting Statistical Analysis used to Evaluate each of the above Clinical Data Section

11. CASE REPORT TABULATIONS
    Data on each patient from
    a. Each adequate and well-controlled study (Phase 2 & 3)
    b. Each Phase 1 Clinical Pharmacology study
    c. Safety data from other clinical studies

Table 4. (Continued)

---

12. CASE REPORT FORMS
  a. Original application only for patients who:
     died during a clinical study or
     did not complete study due to adverse event whether or not thought to be drug related
        including patients on reference drug or placebo
  b. Additional CRFs may be requested after submission and must be submitted within 30
     days of FDA request

13. PATENT INFORMATION—Listing of all U.S. Patents which claim
  a. Drug
  b. Drug product composition
  c. Intended use

---

*Adapted from 21 CFR 314.50

biopharmaceutic data sections. An FDA committee is studying the feasibility of using CANDA for the chemistry sections as well. The NDA of the future will be submitted on one or more platters using Optical Disc Imaging technology integrated with digital computing technology.

C. Patent and Exclusivity

Prior to the passage of the Waxman-Hatch Act of 1984, FDA did not have to concern itself with information on patents. An NDA now must contain information on all unexpired patents for the drug substance, drug product composition, and methods of use. The applicant certifies the validity of the information provided and FDA upon approval publishes the information in the "Orange Book,"* so that subsequent generic applicants are put on notice as to the patents that may delay their entrance into the marketplace.

The new Act provides for periods of market exclusivity upon approval of most NDAs. The applicant submits a request for exclusivity, which is reviewed at the time the NDA is approved, and if it is granted, then FDA publishes the information in the "Orange Book" for notice to generic applicants. Basically an NDA can provide either a 5- or 3-year period of market exclusivity. Five years for the first approval of a new chemical entity and 3 years for all others when certain criteria, primarily the requirement for clinical studies essential to approval, are met. This period of market exclusivity is time in which generic equivalents cannot be legally marketed.

D. Patent Term Extension

Another feature of the Waxman-Hatch Act of benefit to the company obtaining an NDA approval is the possibility of extending the term of one unexpired patent. Within 60 days of the NDA approval, the patent holder may apply to the United States Patent and Trademark Office for extension of an eligible patent. The PTO and FDA then cooperate to determine if the patent is eligible and the amount of time to be extended. FDA verifies the two time

---

*Approved Drug Products with Therapeutic Equivalence Evaluations. Food and Drug Administration.

periods used to calculate the extension period; the times during the IND and NDA phases. The applicant chooses the patent to be extended subject to the rules for maximum times allowed (21 CFR 60).

E. Opportunities for New Ophthalmic Delivery Systems

The goal of developing an advanced drug delivery system is to provide an improved therapeutic regimen. This is often considered for existing or old drugs which have proved beneficial but have inherent limitations due to poor bioavailability or short duration. Another consideration is the protection of the product's franchise when it is due to go off patent and subject to generic competition. Development of a new dosage form with therapeutic advantages can help offset this market eventuality, and the same legislation that made the generic competition possible offers a further incentive to improve the drug by providing the possibility of a longer effective patent life and a head start of 3 to 5 years on generic competition even if there is no patent term remaining.

F. Expedited Availability of Certain New Drugs

The acquired immunodeficiency syndrome (AIDS) crisis has focused attention during the 1980s on the drug development and regulatory processes for making new therapies available for life-threatening and severely debilitating conditions, particularly where no approved therapy or suitable alternative therapies exist. FDA, under Commissioner Frank Young, instituted new procedures after a period of public comment to make promising new drug therapies available to treat patients as early in the drug development process as possible, whereas at the same time obtaining data on the drug's safety and effectiveness in clinical trials.

The treatment IND regulations finalized in 1987 (21 CFR 312.34) make it possible for patients to receive promising new drugs for certain serious and life-threatening conditions as early as Phase 2 or 3 while controlled clinical trials are still underway to make a final determination on the new drug's safety and effectiveness. In some cases, the manufacturer may charge for the investigational new drug product if necessary to undertake or continue the clinical trials. The sponsor of the new drug must apply to FDA for treatment use and provide available data supporting the drug's potential efficacy and safety. FDA may deny the request if the available scientific evidence, taken as a whole, is insufficient evidence supporting a reasonable conclusion that the drug may be effective for its intended use or would expose patients to unreasonable and significant additional risk of illness or injury. Also, clinical trials must be continuing to complete development and submission of an application to market the drug.

To expedite marketing approval, FDA has established the highest review priority for all AIDS products and approved the first AIDS therapy, azidothymidine (AZT), less than 4 months after NDA submission. This new initiative for expediting approval for drugs intended to treat life-threatening and severely debilitating illnesses places emphasis on increased consultation by the sponsor with FDA early in the developmental process prior to submitting an IND and after each phase of clinical testing with the goal that Phase 2 of testing be expanded to provide the data necessary for approval of the new drug. Agreement may be required to conduct additional postmarketing (Phase 4) studies to obtain additional information regarding risks, benefits, and optimal use (21 CFR 312.80).

REFERENCES

1. Nielsen, J. R. (1986). *Handbook of Federal Drug Law*, Philadelphia, Lea & Febiger.
2. *Pharmacy Law Digest*, (1991). page DC-4, J. L. Fink, et al. (eds.). Facts and Comparisons, Inc.
3. *Ibid.* p. DC-5 (1987).
4. *Federal Register*, (1987). 52(53):8798, March 19.
5. *Federal Register*, (1985). 50(36):7452, February 22.
6. *Federal Register*, (1982). 47(200):46139, October 15.
7. Lerman, S., and Reininger, B. (1971). *Can. J. Ophthalmol.*, 6:14.
8. Hackett, R. B. (1990). Nonclinical study requirements for ophthalmic drugs and devices in the United States, *Lens & Eye Toxic. Res.*, 7(3&4):181.
9. *Guideline for Drug Master Files*, September 1989, Center for Drug Evaluation and Research, FDA.
10. *United States Pharmacopeia XXII*, (1990). p. 1570.
11. *Guideline on Sterile Drug Products Produced by Aseptic Processing*, (1987). June, FDA.
12. *Federal Register*, (1991). 56(198):51354, October 11.
13. *Guideline on the Preparation of Investigational New Drug Products (Human & Animal)*, (1991). March, FDA.
14. Mathieu, M. (1990). *New Drug Development: A Regulatory Overview*. Parexel International Corporation, p. 121.

Index